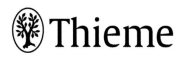

To our families and friends, who endure our quest to improve our medical and surgical skills on a daily basis, and to all our patients, who we hope will benefit from that quest.

Complications in Otolaryngology—Head and Neck Surgery

Edited by

Manuel Bernal-Sprekelsen, MD, PhD
Professor
Hospital Clinic
Department of Otorhinolaryngology
University of Barcelona
Barcelona, Spain

Ricardo L. Carrau, MD, FACS
Professor
Department of Otolaryngology–
Head and Neck Surgery
The Ohio State University Wexner Medical Center
Columbus, Ohio, USA

Stefan Dazert, MD
Professor and Chair
Department of Otorhinolaryngology,
Head and Neck Surgery
Ruhr University Bochum
Bochum, Germany

John L. Dornhoffer, MD, FACS
Professor and Sam McGill Chair in Otology Research
University of Arkansas for Medical Sciences
Little Rock, Arkansas, USA

Giorgio Peretti, MD
Professor
Department of Otorhinolaryngology–
Head and Neck Surgery
University of Brescia
Brescia, Italy

Marc A. Tewfik, MDCM, MSc, FRCSC
Assistant Professor
Department of Otolaryngology,
Head and Neck Surgery
Royal Victoria Hospital
Montreal, Quebec, Canada

Peter-John Wormald, MD
Professor
Department of Otorhinolaryngology,
Head and Neck Surgery
Queen Elizabeth Hospital
Woodville South, South Australia, Australia

With contributions by

Hassan Arshad, M. Demir Bajin, José-Luis Blanch, Gabriela P. B. Braga, Roberto Brusati, Miguel Caballero, Rodrigo Cadore Malfado, Giacomo Colletti, Francesca Del Bon, Leo F. S. Ditzel Filho, Richard Douglas, Albert Elmaraghy, Javier Gavilán, Michael B. Gluth, David S. Haynes, Jesús Herranz-González, Heinrich Iro, Arif Janjua, Amin B. Kassam, Karen M. Kost, Danielle de Lara, Andrea F. Lewis, Josep Llach, José Luis Llorente Pendas, Gabriele Materazzi, Paolo Miccoli, Amir Minovi, David A. Moffat, Philippe Monnier, Luc G. T. Morris, Salil B. Nair, Piero Nicolai, Matthew O. Old, Christopher L. Oliver, James P. O'Neill, Bradley A. Otto, Cesare Piazza, Daniel M. Prevedello, Alejandro Rivas, Ashok Rokade, Laura Samarà Piñol, Kishore Sandu, Levent Sennaroğlu, Jatin P. Shah, Ashok R. Shaha, Ralf Siegert, Ryan J. Soose, Carlos Suárez, Holger H. Sudhoff, Theodoros Teknos, Betty S. Tsai, Isabel Vilaseca, Stefan Volkenstein, Ian J. Witterick, Andrew Wood, Johannes Zenk.

361 illustrations

Thieme
Stuttgart · New York

Library of Congress Cataloging-in-Publication Data is available from the publisher.

Illustrator: Dr. Katja Dalkowski, Buckenhof, Germany

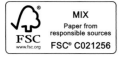

© 2013 Georg Thieme Verlag KG,
Rüdigerstrasse 14, 70469 Stuttgart, Germany
http://www.thieme.de
Thieme Medical Publishers, Inc., 333 Seventh Avenue,
New York, NY 10001, USA
http://www.thieme.com

Cover design: Thieme Publishing Group
Typesetting by Prepress Projects, Perth, UK
Printed in China by Everbest Co. Ltd

ISBN 978-3-13-160531-3

Also available as an e-book:
eISBN 978-3-13-173281-1

Important note: Medicine is an ever-changing science undergoing continual development. Research and clinical experience are continually expanding our knowledge, in particular our knowledge of proper treatment and drug therapy. Insofar as this book mentions any dosage or application, readers may rest assured that the authors, editors, and publishers have made every effort to ensure that such references are in accordance with **the state of knowledge at the time of production of the book.**

Nevertheless, this does not involve, imply, or express any guarantee or responsibility on the part of the publishers in respect to any dosage instructions and forms of applications stated in the book. **Every user is requested to examine carefully** the manufacturers' leaflets accompanying each drug and to check, if necessary in consultation with a physician or specialist, whether the dosage schedules mentioned therein or the contraindications stated by the manufacturers differ from the statements made in the present book. Such examination is particularly important with drugs that are either rarely used or have been newly released on the market. Every dosage schedule or every form of application used is entirely at the user's own risk and responsibility. The authors and publishers request every user to report to the publishers any discrepancies or inaccuracies noticed. If errors in this work are found after publication, errata will be posted at www.thieme.com on the product description page.

Editors

Senior Editor

Manuel Bernal-Sprekelsen, MD, PhD
Professor
Hospital Clinic
Department of Otorhinolaryngology
University of Barcelona
Barcelona, Spain

Section I Otology and Lateral Skull Base

John L. Dornhoffer, MD, FACS
Professor and Sam McGill Chair in Otology Research
University of Arkansas for Medical Sciences
Little Rock, Arkansas, USA

Stefan Dazert, MD
Professor and Chair
Department of Otorhinolaryngology, Head and Neck Surgery
Ruhr University Bochum
Bochum, Germany

Section II Rhinology and Anterior Skull Base

Peter-John Wormald, MD
Professor
Department of Otorhinolaryngology, Head and Neck Surgery
Queen Elizabeth Hospital
Woodville South, South Australia, Australia

Marc A. Tewfik, MDCM, MSc, FRCSC
Assistant Professor
Department of Otolaryngology, Head and Neck Surgery
Royal Victoria Hospital
Montreal, Quebec, Canada

Section III Complications of Head and Neck Surgery

Giorgio Peretti, MD
Professor
Department of Otorhinolaryngology–Head and Neck Surgery
University of Brescia
Brescia, Italy

Ricardo L. Carrau, MD, FACS
Professor
Department of Otolaryngology–Head and Neck Surgery
The Ohio State University Wexner Medical Center
Columbus, Ohio, USA

Contributors

Hassan Arshad, MD
Assistant Professor
Department of Head and Neck
Surgery/Plastic and Reconstructive
Surgery
Roswell Park Cancer Institute
Buffalo, New York, USA

M. Demir Bajin, MD
Assistant Professor
Department of Otolaryngology
Hacettepe University Faculty of
Medicine
Ankara, Turkey

Manuel Bernal-Sprekelsen, MD, PhD
Professor
Hospital Clinic
Department of Otorhinolaryngology
University of Barcelona
Barcelona, Spain

José-Luis Blanch, MD, PhD
Hospital Clinic
Section of Oncologic ENT Surgery
Barcelona, Spain

Gabriela P. B. Braga, MD
Assistant Professor
Otology Neurotology
Santa Casa de Misericórdia do Rio de
Janeiro
II Enfermaria de
Otorrinolaringologia
Rio de Janeiro, Brazil

Roberto Brusati, MD
Professor
Department of Maxillo-Facial
Surgery
University of Milan
San Paolo Hospital
Milan, Italy

Miguel Caballero, MD, PhD
Hospital Clinic
Department of Otorhinolaryngology
University of Barcelona
Barcelona, Spain

Rodrigo Cadore Malfado, MD
Research Fellow
Department of Neurosurgery
The Ohio State University Wexner
Medical Center
Columbus, Ohio, USA

Ricardo L. Carrau, MD, FACS
Professor
Department of Otolaryngology–
Head and Neck Surgery
The Ohio State University Wexner
Medical Center
Columbus, Ohio, USA

Giacomo Colletti, MD
Department of Maxillo-Facial
Surgery
University of Milan
San Paolo Hospital
Milan, Italy

Stefan Dazert, MD
Professor and Chair
Department of Otorhinolaryngology,
Head and Neck Surgery
Ruhr University Bochum
Bochum, Germany

Francesca Del Bon, MD
Department of
Otorhinolaryngology–Head and
Neck Surgery
University of Brescia
Brescia, Italy

Leo F. S. Ditzel Filho, MD
Clinical Fellow
Department of Neurosurgery
The Ohio State University Wexner
Medical Center
Columbus, Ohio, USA

John L. Dornhoffer, MD, FACS
Professor and Sam McGill Chair in
Otology Research
University of Arkansas for Medical
Sciences
Little Rock, Arkansas, USA

Richard Douglas, MD, FRACS, FRACP,
MRCP
Department of Surgery
University of Auckland
Auckland, New Zealand

Albert Elmaraghy, MD, FAAP
Department of Pediatric
Otolaryngology
Nationwide Children's Hospital
The Ohio State University Wexner
Medical Center
Columbus, Ohio, USA

Javier Gavilán, MD
Professor and Chairman
Department of Otolaryngology
La Paz University Hospital
Madrid, Spain

Michael B. Gluth, MD
Director
Comprehensive Listening Center
Division of Otolaryngology–
Head and Neck Surgery
University of Chicago
Chicago, Illinois, USA

David S. Haynes, MD, FACS
Professor of Otolaryngology,
Neurosurgery, and Hearing and
Speech Sciences
Neurotology Division/Fellowship
Program/Cochlear Implant Program
Director
Vanderbilt University Medical
Center
Nashville, Tennessee, USA

Jesús Herranz-González, MD, PhD
Complexo Hospitalario Universitario
A Coruña
Department of Otorhinolaryngology
University of Santiago de
Compostela
Santiago de Compostela, Spain

Heinrich Iro, MD, PhD
Professor and Medical Director
Hospital Clinic
Department of
Otorhinolaryngology–Head and
Neck Surgery
Friedrich-Alexander University
Hospital Erlangen-Nuremberg
Erlangen, Germany

Arif Janjua, MD, FRCSC
Endoscopic Sinus and Skull Base
Surgery
Vancouver General Hospital and
St. Paul's Hospital
Division of Otolaryngology–
Head and Neck Surgery
University of British Columbia
Vancouver, British Columbia, Canada

Amin B. Kassam, MD
Professor and Chair
Department of Neurosurgery
University of Ottawa
Ottawa, Ontario, Canada

Karen M. Kost, MD, FRCSC
Associate Professor
Department of Otolaryngology,
Head and Neck Surgery
Montreal General Hospital
Montreal, Quebec, Canada

Danielle de Lara, MD
Research Fellow
Department of Neurosurgery
The Ohio State University Wexner
Medical Center
Columbus, Ohio, USA

Andrea F. Lewis, MD
Assistant Professor
Department of Otolaryngology and
Communicative Sciences
University of Mississippi Medical
Center
Jackson, Mississippi, USA

Josep Llach, MD, PhD
Hospital Clinic
Endoscopic Unit IMDiM
University of Barcelona
Barcelona, Spain

José Luis Llorente Pendas
Department of Otorhinolaryngology
Hospital Universitario Central de
Asturias
University of Oviedo
Oviedo, Spain

Gabriele Materazzi, MD
Department of Surgery
University of Pisa
Pisa, Italy

Paolo Miccoli, MD
Department of Surgical Pathology
University of Pisa
Pisa, Italy

Amir Minovi, MD, PhD, MHA
Department of Otorhinolaryngology,
Head and Neck Surgery
Ruhr University Bochum
Bochum, Germany

David A. Moffat, BSc (Hons), MA
(Hon Cantab), MB BS, PhD, FRCS
Hunterian Professor of Surgery
University of Cambridge
Consultant in Neuro-Otology and
Skull Base Surgery
Addenbrooke's Cambridge
University Teaching Hospital
Cambridge, UK

Philippe Monnier, MD
Department of Otorhinolaryngology
–Head and Neck Surgery
Centre Hospitalier Universitaire
Vaudois – CHUV
Lausanne, Switzerland

Luc G. T. Morris, MD
Head and Neck Service
Department of Surgery
Memorial Sloan–Kettering Cancer
Center
New York, New York, USA

Salil B. Nair, MD, FRCS (ORL-HNS)
Consultant Rhinologist
Department of Otorhinolaryngology
Auckland City Hospitals
Auckland, New Zealand

Piero Nicolai, MD
Professor and Chairman
Department of
Otorhinolaryngology–Head and
Neck Surgery
University of Brescia
Brescia, Italy

Matthew O. Old, MD
Assistant Professor
Department of Otolaryngology–
Head and Neck Surgery
The Ohio State University Wexner
Medical Center
Columbus, Ohio, USA

Christopher L. Oliver, MD
Otolaryngology, Head and Neck
Surgery
Colorado Head and Neck Specialists
Centura Health
Denver, Colorado, USA

James P. O'Neill, MB, MRCSI, MD,
MBA, MMSc
Otolaryngology, Head and Neck
Surgery
The Royal College of Surgeons in
Ireland
Dublin, Ireland

Bradley A. Otto, MD
Assistant Professor
Department of Otolaryngology–
Head and Neck Surgery
The Ohio State University Wexner
Medical Center
Columbus, Ohio, USA

Giorgio Peretti, MD
Professor
Department of
Otorhinolaryngology–Head and
Neck Surgery
University of Brescia
Brescia, Italy

Cesare Piazza, MD
Spedali Civili of Brescia
Department of
Otorhinolaryngology–Head and
Neck Surgery
University of Brescia
Brescia, Italy

Daniel M. Prevedello, MD
Associate Professor
Department of Neurosurgery
The Ohio State University Wexner
Medical Center
Columbus, Ohio, USA

Alejandro Rivas, MD
Assistant Professor
Department of Otology and
Neurotology
Vanderbilt University Medical
Center
Nashville, Tennessee, USA

Ashok Rokade, MD, FRCS (ORL-HNS)
Rhinology Fellow
Royal Hampshire County Hospital
Winchester, UK

Laura Samarà Piñol, MD
Hospital Clinic
Department of Otorhinolaryngology
University of Barcelona
Barcelona, Spain

Kishore Sandu, MD
Head of Department
Otorhinolaryngology, Head and
Neck Surgery
Valais State Hospital – Centre
Hospitalier du Centre du Valais
Romand – CHCVR
Sion and
Centre Hospitalier Universitaire
Vaudois – CHUV
Lausanne, Switzerland

Levent Sennaroğlu, MD
Professor
Department of Otolaryngology
Hacettepe University Faculty of
Medicine
Ankara, Turkey

Jatin P. Shah, MD, PhD (Hon), FACS,
FRCS (Hon), FDSRCS (Hon), FRACS
(Hon)
Chief
Head and Neck Service
Department of Surgery
Memorial Sloan–Kettering Cancer
Center
New York, New York, USA

Ashok R. Shaha, MD, FACS
Professor of Surgery
Memorial Sloan–Kettering Cancer
Center
New York, New York, USA

Ralf Siegert, MD
Professor and Director
Department of Otorhinolaryngology,
Head and Neck Surgery
Prosper Hospital
Academic Teaching Hospital,
Ruhr University Bochum
Recklinghausen, Germany

Ryan J. Soose, MD
Director
Division of Sleep Surgery
Assistant Professor
Department of Otolaryngology
University of Pittsburgh School of
Medicine
Pittsburgh, Pennsylvania, USA

Carlos Suárez, MD, PhD
Department of Otorhinolaryngology
Hospital Universitario Central de
Asturias;
Instituto Universitario de Oncología
del Principado de Asturias
University of Oviedo
Oviedo, Spain

Holger H. Sudhoff, MD, PhD, FRCS,
FRCPath
Klinikum Bielefeld
Department of Otorhinolaryngology,
Head and Neck Surgery
Bielefeld, Germany

Theodoros Teknos, MD
Professor and Vice-Chairman
Division of Head and Neck Oncologic
Surgery
Department of Otolaryngology–
Head and Neck Surgery
The Ohio State University Wexner
Medical Center
Columbus, Ohio, USA

Marc A. Tewfik, MDCM, MSc, FRCSC
Assistant Professor
Department of Otolaryngology,
Head and Neck Surgery
Royal Victoria Hospital
Montreal, Quebec, Canada

Betty S. Tsai, MD
Assistant Professor
Department of Otorhinolaryngology
The University of Oklahoma Health
Sciences Center
Oklahoma City, Oklahoma, USA

Isabel Vilaseca, MD, PhD
Hospital Clinic
Department of Otorhinolaryngology
University of Barcelona
Barcelona, Spain

Stefan Volkenstein, MD
Department of Otorhinolaryngology,
Head and Neck Surgery
Ruhr University Bochum
Bochum, Germany

Ian J. Witterick, MD, MSc, FRCSC
Professor and Chair
Department of Otolaryngology–
Head and Neck Surgery
University of Toronto
Toronto, Ontario, Canada

Andrew Wood, BA, BM BCh
Department of Surgery
The University of Auckland
Auckland, New Zealand

Peter-John Wormald, MD
Professor
Department of Otorhinolaryngology,
Head and Neck Surgery
Queen Elizabeth Hospital
Woodville South, South Australia,
Australia

Johannes Zenk, MD, PhD
Professor and Deputy Medical
Director
Hospital Clinic
Department of
Otorhinolaryngology–Head and
Neck Surgery
Freidrich-Alexander University
Hospital Erlangen-Nuremberg
Erlangen, Germany

Foreword I

Having finished my residency training and military service, I did a fellowship with Dr. John Conley, the world's preeminent head and neck surgeon in 1967. I had very little training in head and neck surgery during my residency, and this year was meant to be a "remedial" year for me so that I could be well rounded in all aspects of our specialty and could become a member of an academic faculty.

Dr. Conley's practice was complex in many ways. It was a private practice populated by surgical oncologists from Memorial Sloan–Kettering Hospital, except for Dr. Conley, an otolaryngologist. Our outpatient office was quite a distance from St. Vincent's Hospital, which is where the surgery took place. Some of the complex cases that Dr. Conley saw were with far-advanced neglected cancers, many of which had already been treated with surgery and radiation. Those were the days prior to chemotherapy so we did not have to worry about that aspect. This was before the intensive care unit was invented and before nondelayed pedicle flaps had been introduced.

The surgeon assumes fundamental responsibility for all factors that might influence the success of his or her craft and so, in general, complications were accepted as part of head and neck surgery at that time. Most of the wound breakdowns and the fistulas we had to contend with, particularly in the patients who had been radiated, were blamed on the patient as having "poor protoplasm." I assisted on these cases and watched Dr. Conley and, later in the fellowship, I did the cases with Dr. Conley's assistance. I found myself spending more and more time in the hospital packing the wounds, taking care of the complications and making sure that the patients medical problems, as well as their surgical complications, were looked after.

I had the primary responsibility for the patients postoperative care. In an effort to improve the lot of these unfortunate patients and a bit in self defense motivated by the desire to see my family, I undertook an indepth study of complications.

I became quite analytical about these problems and I found this experience to be a provocative and educational process. I spent long hours analyzing each case to see how we could have done better and soon realized that, although the complications had been blamed on errors in technique in the operating room, the reality was that this was a multifactorial problem.

I soon came to realize that the prevention of complications begins the first time the patient is seen in the office. For instance, although it was easy to identify the patients who were malnourished, we never again gave much thought to nourishment being a big factor in healing. However, I soon realized its importance and we began to improve the patients nourishment prior to treatment. We knew that smoking was a biohazard in that it caused cancer, but we did not think so much about the effect on small vessels and the negative impact on healing.

After going through the analytical process, I organized many new ways of preventing complications, many of which admittedly had to do with surgical technique. After a few months our life was made easier by the introduction of the deltopectoral flap by Dr. Bakamjian, which allowed us the luxury of immediate reconstruction of these wounds whereas previously we had made oropharyngostomas to allow the neck to heal before closing the wound.

The realization that most complications are preventable is the concept that I carried throughout my entire 40-year surgical career. While it is not possible to go through such an extended period of time with no complications, I must say that we ended up with the bare minimum. I had the opportunity to train more than 150 residents and countless fellows in head and neck surgery in how to prevent complications rather than having to treat them.

I congratulate Professor Manuel Bernal-Sprekelsen and the remarkable group of experts that he has recruited into the writing and editing of this comprehensive book. I am impressed with their courage in undertaking the prodigious task of covering complications across the many subspecialty areas of our field. Although the main feature of this book will be diagnosis and management of complications, I am sure that there will be an emphasis on Benjamin Franklin's observation that "an ounce of prevention is worth a pound of cure."

I wish the editors and authors the best of success for this very important contribution to the literature in head and neck surgery.

Eugene N. Myers

Foreword II

It was with great interest that we received an invitation to review this book on complications in otorhinolaryngology—head and neck surgery, as the last complete opus in this field was published almost 50 years ago. Therefore *Complications in Otolaryngology—Head and Neck Surgery* fills an important gap in our discipline by examining complications in the area (excluding facial plastic and aesthetic surgery)

The comprehensive content covers procedures in the middle and inner ear and paranasal sinuses, endoscopic skull base surgery, airway management, laryngectomy, salivary gland and thyroid surgery, and much more. The book is a practical reference for the busy surgeon.

The special features of the book are as follows:

- It has been written by a team of leading worldwide authorities, who share tips, tricks, pearls, and clinical experience in every instructive chapter.
- The format makes it easily accessible and includes a definition of each complication and its sequelae, the incidence of occurrence, the point during surgery at which it is most likely to happen, tips for avoiding it, and techniques for managing it.

- The chapters include current scientific, evidence-based information throughout.
- It is generously illustrated, with more than 360 full-color intraoperative photographs, endoscopic images, and illustrations to help readers visualize surgical problems and solutions for every case, including revision surgery.

For the increasing number of ear, nose, and throat and neurosurgical teams that perform advanced endoscopic surgery of the anterior skull base beyond the paranasal sinuses, this book contains valuable information on complications. It is essential reading for all surgeons who need to prepare for and manage every contingency for the best possible outcomes in otorhinolaryngology and head and neck surgical procedures.

We believe that this is an international textbook that will certainly become a "must" in the library of every surgeon dealing with otorhinolaryngology—head and neck surgery.

Wolfgang Steiner
David Howard

Preface

Many years have passed since the publication of a book that comprehensively addresses the topic of surgical complications in otolaryngology and head and neck surgery.

Intraoperative and postoperative complications occur, even in the hands of skilled and experienced surgeons. Complications are not necessarily caused by the surgeon or the surgery, as sometimes they are a result of the underlying disease itself. A perilymphatic fistula on the lateral semicircular canal caused by cholesteatoma, erosion of the skull base by a benign tumor, or a carotid blowout caused by infiltration of the vessel by a metastatic cervical lymph node are just a few examples of complications that are not directly caused by surgery, and yet do pose risks and consequences for patients before, during, and after a surgical procedure.

Regardless of whether a complication was a direct result of the surgical procedure or caused by the disease itself, it has taken a great deal of candor and integrity to present these cases to both the medical and the lay audience, especially as some of the cases presented in this book are taken from our own experience. Furthermore, as an editor, I was especially pleased by the positive response from all my co-editors and contributors, who promptly accepted the invitation to write and illustrate their respective chapters in great detail.

Sequential learning and the acquisition of experience as a surgeon include complications, whether they are caused by our own actions or inactions or arise from other causes. Therefore, the aim of this "opus" is to, as much as possible, highlight the sources of perioperative risks in otolaryngology and head and neck surgery. In addition, we provide clinical "pearls" and suggestions for the beginner, and perhaps also for the experienced surgeon, on how to improve technical aspects of specific surgeries, and enhance their perioperative management, thus improving their safety.

Complications will continue to be part of our professional life. Patients and colleagues must take this fact into consideration. We as surgeons must also live with the consequences of complications, gain experience from them, and learn the proper lessons.

We hope that this book will provide the reader with practical suggestions on how to keep the number of complications to a minimum, and, when complications do occur, to implement prompt and proper treatment to avoid more severe consequences.

Manuel Bernal-Sprekelsen, Editor-in-Chief
Ricardo L. Carrau
Stefan Dazert
John L. Dornhoffer
Giorgio Peretti
Marc A. Tewfik
Peter-John Wormald

Table of Contents

Section II Rhinology and Anterior Skull Base

Section III Complications of Head and Neck Surgery

III A Surgery of the Oral Cavity and Oropharynx

III B Surgery of the Larynx, Trachea, Hypopharynx, and Esophagus

III C Surgery of the Major Salivary Glands

III D Surgery of the Thyroid and Parathyroid Glands

III E Surgery of the Neck

III F Reconstructive Surgery

Section I Otology and Lateral Skull Base

1 Outer Ear and External Auditory Canal

R. Siegert, S. Volkenstein, S. Dazert

Otoplasty and Surgery of the External Ear

R. Siegert

Introduction

Abnormalities of the external ear, especially protruding ears, are the most frequent malformations of the head and neck, affecting ~ 5% of the population. Therefore otoplasty is one of the most frequent procedures in facial plastic surgery and is often performed in children. It is estimated that 23,000 otoplasties are performed in Germany annually (i.e., 30 otoplasties in a population of 100,000 each year).[1] Furthermore, it is (almost) the only purely aesthetic procedure performed in children and is often asked for by parents when their children are at an age when they themselves are not concerned about their "abnormality". These are some of the unique features associated with otoplasty.

Otoplasty leads to one of the highest revision rates in facial plastic surgery, estimated to be greater than 20%.[1] There are no data to explain these unacceptably high complication rates, so we can only speculate that the operative challenge is tremendously underestimated. Although several of these complications (perichondritis, othematoma, keloid) may also occur under different circumstances, their treatment will be discussed with relation to otoplasty. More than 100 different techniques can be found in the literature for performing otoplasty, indicating that no single surgical technique has been found to correct all of the different types and degrees of protruding ears and other deformities.[2–4] Substantial experience in auricular surgery and adjustment to the patient's individual anatomy are the keystones for a predictable outcome with low complication rates. This is even more important when operating on young children who have no real psychologic stress from their abnormality. For the most frequent auricular procedure, the otoplasty for protruding ears, we distinguish between five operative techniques: the four standard methods and our own combined technique.

Overview of Techniques for the Correction of Protruding Ears

The Suture Technique

This technique was reported in 1960,[5] 1963[6] and 1967[7] by Mustardé. It should only be used in cases where ear cartilage has been found to be very thin and soft. We frequently find that this method results in an inexact transition between the concha and antihelix, somewhat soft and indistinct contours in the scapha and occasionally an overcompensation of the helix, which, from a frontal perspective, tends to sink back behind the antihelix, the so-called "hidden helix."

The Scoring Technique

This technique was described by Stenström in 1963[8] and a similar technique was reported in the same year by Ju et al,[9] Crikelair and Cosman[10] and Chongchet[11] using a postauricular approach and an incision in the scapha. The risk involved in using the Stenström technique is in the blind scoring of the anterior cartilage, which makes it impossible to maintain exact control over the folding of the antihelix. Excessive abrasion can lead to an uncontrolled weakening of the cartilage and bring about serious deformities or edges in the ear. This technique can also lead to serious complications, especially when accompanied by an excessive excision of postauricular skin.

The Scoring–Suture Technique

This technique was described in 1955 and 1963 by Converse and co-workers.[12,13] Here, too, incorrect scoring of cartilage can lead to edges and deformations. Moreover, excessive removal of postauricular skin can cause the ear to come too close to the mastoid and the auriculocephalic sulcus may become too small.

The Conchal Set-Back

This technique was described by Furnas in 1968[14] especially to correct hyperplasia of the conchal cavum. Using the postauricular incision, abundant connective tissue between the conchal cartilage and the mastoid planum is removed and the auricular cartilage is rotated toward the head (= conchal set-back). It is sutured to the periosteum of the mastoid planum and by doing so the projection of the auricle is adjusted.

Table 1.1 Synopsis for correcting protruding ears

Malformation	Characteristics	Technique
Antihelixhypoplasia	Very soft cartilage	Suture
	Average	Sutures and posterior scoring
	Strong	Sutures and anterior scoring
Cavumhyperplasia	High antihelix	Cavum rotation
Protruding lobule	Soft tissue tension or excess	Mattress suture Slight skin resection

The Combined Technique

Depending on the individual anatomy we suggest that these techniques be combined (**Table 1.1**). By doing so the particular structures that are abnormal are corrected, the forces to change the shape and position of the cartilage are distributed among various affected structures and harmony of the anatomical subunits of the auricle can be achieved. To optimize this combined technique, it is essential that a thorough analysis of all anatomical aspects and abnormalities is made preoperatively and that thorough planning is performed.

Complications

Apart from iatrogenic errors and complications there are several independent complications that can occur even after correct surgery. These include early events, which are defined as complications that occur within the first 14 days after the operation, and late complications after these first two postoperative weeks (**Table 1.2**).

Early Complications

Pain

Postoperative pain is normal to a certain extent because of the surgical trauma per se. As the auricle is more or less immobile, pain should be low, but the individual range of perceiving pain is broad. Intensive pain could be an important symptom for other arising problems like hematoma or infection.

Table 1.2 Overview of early and late complications

Early general complications	Late specific complications
Pain	Suture extrusion
Hematoma	Keloids
Infection	Stenosis of external ear canal
Pressure ulcer	"Bad" results

A complaint of pain always requires immediate clinical control. Regular postoperative findings of wound healing with moderate pain during the first and second postoperative days should be treated with "light" analgesic medication. In cases of severe pain, hematoma and infection need to be excluded. "Inappropriate" pain—and when the surgeon is in doubt—must lead to repeated clinical control of the wound. If indicated, early revision as described below can prevent serious sequelae.

Secondary Bleeding and Hematoma

- Slight secondary bleeding can be stopped by applying cold and a pressure bandage. If this is used it should only be applied for a short period of time to avoid the development of pressure ulcers.
- After performing anterior scoring techniques a hematoma can develop between the anterior skin and the cartilage. In these cases, mattress sutures tightened over small pieces of gauze can be used to reposition the elevated skin and re-establish the relief of the auricle.
- If pressure application is insufficient, open revision is indicated. The bleeding vessels are exposed and ligated or coagulated. If the bleeding is more or less diffuse, then hemostyptic biomaterials (e.g., Tabotamp [Ethicon Inc., Somerville, NJ, USA] or fibrin glue) might be applied into the wound.

> **Note**
> The best "treatment" of postoperative bleeding is its avoidance by meticulous intraoperative hemostasis. In addition, a small drain left in place for 1 day can help to avoid a hematoma.

Allergies

Before the operation, allergies to suture material or to topically applied ointments may be unknown. Although rare, allergic reactions can be avoided in most patients through taking careful note of the medical history. Removing the ointment and applying corticosteroids locally will alleviate an allergic reaction. Systemic administration of corticosteroids might be considered in severe reactions.

Infections

Otoplasty should be a sterile operation that does not generally require antibiotic prophylaxis. Nevertheless, short-term or one-shot perioperative antibiotic prophylaxis might reduce the risk of infection. Antimicrobial ointments (e.g., Betadine [providone–iodine], Mundipharma Laboratories Gmbh, Basel, Switzerland) and systemic antibiotics with high diffusion into cartilage (e.g., clindamycin) should be applied immediately and for a relatively long period because cartilage has hardly any cellular protective mechanisms.

Pressure Ulcers and Necrosis

The anterior auricular skin is one of the thinnest and most vulnerable of the whole body. In addition, it is located directly on cartilage, a tissue that has no blood supply of its own and therefore cannot "help" the skin to survive in a critical situation. Too much pressure from below due to a hematoma or from above due to the bandage can interrupt its flat, horizontally structured blood supply and lead to necrosis even after a few hours. Prophylaxis includes the avoidance and treatment of hematomas as discussed above and a meticulous bandage technique that avoids inadequate pressure on the auricular skin. We carefully cover the surface of the auricle with ointment and mold its contours with multiple pieces of gauze. To secure this we have developed a special foam dressing that is taped around the auricle to prevent it from being accidentally dislocated. It also has a special foam cap that fits exactly on to the taped foam and prevents pressure on the auricle from outside (Spiggle & Theis Medizintechnik Gmbh, Overath, Germany).

If necrosis has occurred it is often no longer a small, easy-to-treat issue. Up to a size of ~ 2 to 3 mm it might be closed directly; otherwise the necrotic tissue has to be removed and the defect of the auricle needs to be reconstructed according to the individual situation. We have described details of those reconstruction techniques in more detail elsewhere.[15-20]

Late Complications

Late complications are more common than early ones. They can "just happen" without being caused by any surgical mistake or they can be late sequelae of surgical deficiencies. This is influenced by the unique anatomy of the auricle with its very thin anterior skin, which can lead to prolonged periods of swelling over irregularities, sometimes for many months, and in the long-term can show up any deficiencies in reconstruction.

Suture Fistulae and Granulomas

There has been a long and still ongoing discussion as to whether sutures should be used, and if so, what type,

for the remodeling of the cartilage. If a technique that does not purely rely on scoring (i.e., a suture or combined technique, as we prefer) is used then one must understand the aim and mechanism of suturing. Sutures in the cartilage have to reshape and stabilize it. Cartilage is a bradytropic tissue—meaning that the speed of remodeling of its fibers is very slow. It takes many months for the turnover of its collagen before it is stable in its new shape on its own. This is much slower than the resorption of all kinds of nonpermanent sutures. If the sutures resorb while the corrected form is not stable, the cartilage will have a tendency to move back into its previous abnormality.

The only way to avoid a recurrence like this is to use permanent sutures. Otherwise a relapse—depending on the amount of tension in the cartilage—will occur. So if we use permanent sutures—and we suggest doing so in most cases of average or strong cartilage—they should be sufficiently covered by soft tissue. This can only be achieved when the sutures do not go all the way through the cartilage coming to lie directly under the very thin anterior skin, and posteriorly are covered sufficiently with the relatively thick skin that should not be sutured under tension. If sutures are exposed or lead to local irritation or infection they have to be removed. The wound should be cleaned carefully, granulation tissue also has to be removed and we apply some local antimicrobial treatment (e.g., framycetin).

Stenosis of External Ear Canal

The entrance to the external ear canal can become too narrow if the cavum rotation is performed in an anterior direction. To prevent this, it is much better to pull the auricle slightly posteriorly with the rotation suture. These sutures should not only pull the auricular cartilage toward the head, but also pull it slightly posteriorly. If the rotation has not been performed in this way, a stenosis of the entrance to the external ear canal might occur. This is caused by the cartilage of the conchal cavum, which might be pushed into the external ear canal. To widen it, cartilage and skin must be removed.

We prepare an H-flap with its central incision directly over the apex of the stenosis (**Fig. 1.1a**). Two U-flaps are then elevated to expose the cartilage (**Fig. 1.1b**). A crescent-shaped piece of cartilage is removed, and the skin flaps are appropriately trimmed and sutured back in place (**Fig. 1.1c**). This relatively small procedure is performed under local anesthesia in most patients.

Hypertrophic Scars and Keloids

Hypertrophic scars are thickened scars in the area of the previous wound. Keloids show a tendency to grow beyond the scar and develop a more or less unlimited growth. They can become huge and grow like a tumor, destroying

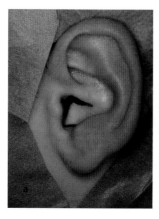 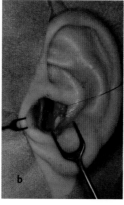 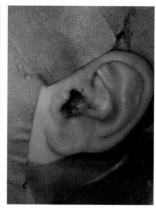

Fig. 1.1a–c Treatment of external ear canal stenosis.

a Marked H-flap with its central incision directly over the apex of the stenosis and two legs (not seen here) reaching medially into the external ear.

b U-flaps elevated.

c Skin flaps trimmed and sutured back in place after resection of a crescent-shaped piece of cartilage.

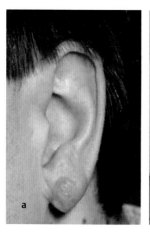 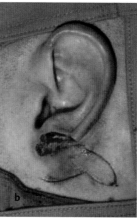 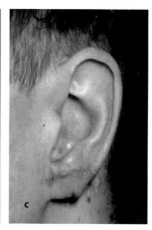

Fig. 1.2a–c Big recurrent keloid of the lobule (after partial resection at another institution) **(a)** before, and **(b)** after resection, and **(c)** after reconstruction with an anteriorly pedicled flap folded to itself (Gavello-flap).

the surrounding cartilage (**Fig. 1.2**). Sometimes they only start to develop years after surgery.

Many factors are thought to influence the development of keloids but none of these are the sole explanation.[21] Risk factors are individual disposition, race (more frequent in dark and Asian races), tension on the scar leading to increased activity of fibroblast with up to 12 times greater production of collagen in comparison to normal wounds and three times higher production of collagen in comparison to hypertrophic scar, localization of the wound (more frequent in ear, chest, and shoulders), and inflammation, which stimulates the liberation of growth factors. The latter causes can be influenced by the surgeon to a certain extent.

> **Note**
>
> Avoidance of tension along the wound closure is the most important advice. The position of the auricle should not rely on the skin sutures but on the remodeling of the cartilage. The resection of excess skin should be performed very conservatively, taking into account that, especially in young patients, folds will flatten over time.

Many different treatment options for keloids have been proposed, most of them with low evidence levels and no animal model has been established so far to study the development and treatment of keloids experimentally.[22]

Medical Treatment

Infiltrating mitomycin C, tamoxifen citrate, imidazola-quinolines, retinoic acid and other vitamin A derivatives, tacrolimus, phenylalkylamine calcium channel blockers, vascular endothelial growth factor, hepatocyte growth factor, basic fibroblast growth factor, transforming growth factor-β, methotrexate, mannose-6-phosphate, interleukin-10, antihistamines, prostaglandins, or Botox are all methods that lack long-term clinical control and follow-up.[23] Among the injectable agents, steroids are the only pharmaceuticals that are generally accepted in keloid treatment. We prefer Volon A (triamcinolone; 40 mg) injections into the scar region immediately after the surgical removal of the keloid and every 6 weeks afterward for 6 months. Nevertheless injections alone rarely remove a keloid completely, so that surgical removal is the treatment of choice. So-called minimal invasive therapies with the use of freezing techniques, laser therapy, or

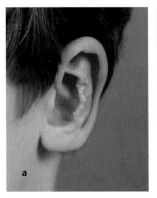 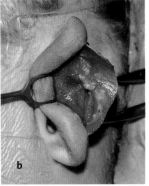 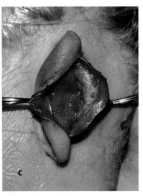 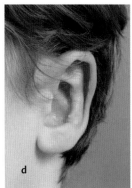

Fig. 1.3a–d Very insufficient result after otoplasty at another institution.

a Destruction of the antihelix.
b Open exposure.

c Meticulous reshaping of the cartilage, covering edges with free temporalis fascia and readjustment of the cartilage.
d Result after complex revision.

radiofrequency have not been proven to give predictable good long-term results.

Surgical Treatment

Although surgical resection of the keloid is considered to be the method of choice it is not clear how radical it should be. Intramarginal as well as radical excisions have been advocated with controlled clinical evidence. We tend to be not very radical in the first occurrence of a keloid but excise it more radically if the patient has a history of keloid formation or if it is a recurrent keloid. Even partial amputation of the auricle might be necessary in exceptional cases.

After the removal of the keloid it is of utmost importance to avoid any tension on the wound edges. Therefore we use a full thickness skin graft—most often harvested from the inguinal region—to cover the wound area. In addition, we use a thin layer of fibrin glue between the skin graft and the wound bed to avoid any accidental shear movements and press it on to the wound with a bolster of foam for 1 week. Alternatively, local flaps might be used for wound coverage, but again it is mandatory to avoid tension on the skin as far as possible. Steroids are injected at the end of the operation as described above.

- Postoperative radiation therapy[24] has been a matter of discussion for many years. If used, it is applied as a very superficial Roentgen-radiation with a total of 10 to 25 Gy. It has to start on the day of surgery or at least on the first postoperative day. Although no proven secondary malignancy has been reported linked to this kind of superficial low-dose radiation, we are reluctant to suggest it in primary keloids and young patients.

- Postoperatively, silicon foils and pressure bandages might be used, but both are difficult to fix on the postauricular scar even though devices with a spring or magnets have been described.

Poor Aesthetic Results

Although even experienced surgeons cannot guarantee a certain cosmetic result, many of these unsatisfying results are caused by improper techniques and could have been avoided. Treatment of poor aesthetic results can be very challenging. It ranges from reoperation for recurrences and minor corrections of the cartilage over open revisions, meticulous reshaping of the cartilage, covering minor edges with free temporalis fascia, and readjustment of the cartilage (**Fig. 1.3**) to complete auricular reconstructions (**Fig. 1.4**). Sufficient surgical experience in auricular reconstruction is mandatory to achieve good clinical results in these difficult and very individual challenges.

Surgery of the External Auditory Canal

S. Volkenstein

Surgery of the external auditory canal includes a wide variety of procedures for different indications and a heterogeneous group of patients. This includes malformations, atresia of the auricle or the external auditory canal (EAC), exostoses, posttraumatic, postinflammatory, and postoperative alterations such as blunting or stenosis, as well as benign and malignant tumors. Therefore, the appropriate type of anesthesia, preoperative examination

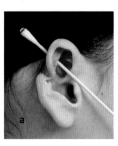 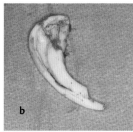 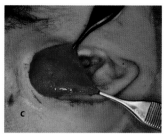 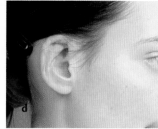

Fig. 1.4a–d Disastrous result after otoplasty at another institution with subtotal destruction of the cartilage and central perforation.

a Situation before reconstruction.
b Auricular framework carved out of autogenous rib cartilage.

c Auricular framework covered with pedicled superficial temporalis fascia.
d Result after complex reconstruction.

and preparation, imaging, and required tissue grafts have to be individually defined for each case to prevent unexpected developments and complications.

General Surgical Guidelines

Anesthesia

In adults, most surgeries of the EAC can be performed under local anesthesia. However, in our hands most surgical procedures of the ear are performed under general anesthesia. To reduce intraoperative bleeding, the use of local anesthesia (a ready-to-use mixture of 2% xylocaine with 1 : 200,000 epinephrine) is recommended in all cases. To allow the local anesthetic to work, the injection should take place at least 15 minutes before the skin incision.

Antibiotics

Surgery of the EAC may be associated with recurrent external otitis or chronic infection of the canal skin, so patients receive a single-shot antibiotic (i.e., cefuroxime or cotrimoxazol intravenously) as perioperative prophylaxis for wound infection.

Surgical Access

To achieve proper surgical access and allow for regular postoperative care, surgery of the EAC requires a wide entrance and lumen of the canal, no matter what kind of surgery is to be performed. The transmeatal route by an endaural incision is the most common surgical approach to remove EAC diseases.[25] This approach allows a small and atraumatic incision, usually with sufficient overview of the EAC. Potential difficulties include inadequate visibility or instrumental access to the medial portion of the EAC, especially in the anterior aspect. To provide a sufficient overview to the anterior tympanomeatal angle and to maximize conservation of the canal wall skin a postauricular approach is recommended in these cases.[26]

Hildmann and Sudhoff[27] described two effective ways to create a wide entrance to the external ear canal: creating a superiorly based skin flap in the cavum and folding it into a longitudinal incision of the ear canal or creating a pretragal pedicled flap, which is rotated into the endaural incision area. An additional gain in space may be achieved by removing bony edges from the posterior circumference (a prominent Henle spine or tympanosquamous fissure).

The partial removal of the EAC skin before widening the bony canal may be helpful to gain space for further preparation and usually does not cause any danger to the skin's viability. Widening the EAC should be performed until the entire tympanic membrane including the anulus is visible.

Resection and Grafting

Heat damage to the bone of the EAC during drill work must be avoided by sufficient irrigation. Areas of necrotic bone should be drilled down to healthy bone and then covered with split-thickness skin grafts. At the end of EAC surgery no bone should remain without any soft tissue cover. We usually recommend the use of split-thickness skin grafts harvested from the posterior side of the auricle with a No. 10 blade (Hildmann, personal communication).

To allow sufficient skin graft incorporation into the ear canal and to prevent early postoperative (re-)stenosis, careful coating with silicon foils and packing with gel foam of the EAC is suggested for ~ 3 to 4 weeks. After removing the packing it may be helpful to apply a corticosteroid/antibiotic ointment to EAC skin. This helps to reduce postoperative swelling and granulation tissue formation. In cases of persisting granulation tissue, local alcohol treatment of the EAC may be useful.[28] Return to water exposure should be avoided until at least 6 weeks after complete healing

Intraoperative Challenges

To prevent injuries of the tympanic membrane, the facial nerve, the jugular bulb, or the temporomandibular joint

(TMJ), a preoperative computed tomography scan may be helpful to investigate the extent of bony erosion or stenotic tissue.

The bony EAC may be widened with the bur until mastoid cells are shining through. When mastoid cells are opened, covering with cartilage chips or perichondrium is recommended.

The TMJ is located anteriorly and medially to the EAC, adjacent to the anterior wall. Herniation of the TMJ into the EAC may occur as a complication of otologic surgery.[29] After intraoperative opening of the joint with herniation of soft tissue into the EAC, cartilage, or more suitably a bone chip, (not soft tissue) should be placed using the underlay technique to cover the defect. Because of the high pressure that occurs when opening the mouth and chewing, the recurrence rate is relatively high. Larger defects are sometimes hard to control. Permanent herniation involving contact with the tympanic membrane and a disturbing loud sound when opening the mouth are possible outcomes. A firm packing of the EAC for at least 3 weeks should give the covered defect time to heal. A rare postoperative complication after entry into the TMJ is emphysema of the neck, as described in the literature.[30]

Postoperative Challenges

The entrance to the EAC may become stenotic after an endaural or retroauricular incision as the result of scar contraction. We recommend a sufficient meatoplasty during all procedures in chronic inflamed ears, as described above.

Postoperative complications often result from an incomplete tissue integration of the covering material, such as split skin or perichondrium, resulting in otorrhea, crusting, and odor.[31] After removal of the packing from the EAC there may still be a wet ear with uncovered bone and granulation tissue. Consequent cleaning and local treatment in the office and the use of a blow dryer by the patient to dry the ear several times a day for 5 minutes, as well as avoiding water exposure, are recommended. Postoperative stenosis or synechia of the EAC mostly require reoperation. Fibrous and scar tissue should be removed and split-thickness skin grafts should cover the epithelial defect. In selected cases a long-term stent may prevent postoperative canal stenosis.[32]

The integrity or precise reconstruction of the tympanomeatal angle needs special attention in middle ear surgery, and also during operations of the EAC. Manipulation and surgery in this area should be reduced to a minimum because of the risk of blunting. Blunting is considered to be the formation of scar or fibrous tissue in the tympanomeatal angle resulting in a blunt angle between the tympanic membrane and the anterior wall of the EAC. Blunting is a common problem after reconstruction of the tympanic membrane with the so-called overlay technique.[33] If reconstruction in the tympanomeatal angle is necessary, small split-thickness skin grafts should be precisely placed edge to edge at the site of the angle to avoid folding of the epithelium into the subepithelial layer resulting in a cholesteatoma.[34] However, if the problem of blunting cannot be solved by the techniques mentioned here, then an implantable hearing aid may be offered to the patient to overcome the air–bone gap.[35]

The development of a postoperative EAC cholesteatoma mostly occurs as an inclusion of epithelial cysts along the incision lines after ear surgery.[36] These cysts should be completely removed using a sickle knife to avoid further extension. The patients need to be followed until definite wound healing.

Complications in Disorders of the External Auditory Canal

Stenosis

Using morphology, stenosis of the EAC can be subdivided into bony or soft tissue stenosis, or using its origin, it can be divided into inherited, postoperative, postinflammatory, and posttraumatic stenosis.

Osteoma and Meatal Exostosis

Solitary osteoma of the EAC and multiple meatal exostosis (**Fig. 1.5**) are considered to be two different conditions. Neither of these findings usually involves the tympanic membrane. They can be removed by drilling or the use of a chisel. In experienced hands the use of the chisel is less traumatic to the canal skin, and allows the removal of exostoses in one piece. However, there is a certain

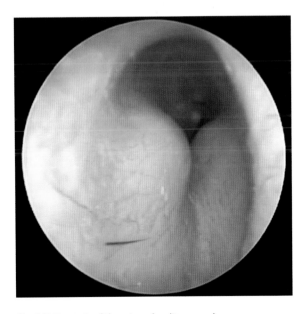

Fig. 1.5 Exostosis of the external auditory canal.

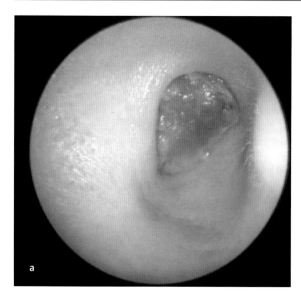

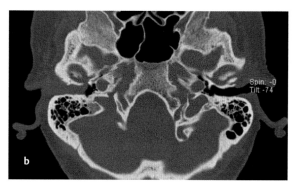

Fig. 1.6a,b Postinflammatory fibrosis of the external auditory canal.

a Otoscopic view.
b Computed tomography scan.

risk of damaging the facial nerve, the middle ear or even inner ear structures. The overlying meatal skin has to be removed carefully and may be replaced as a flap or a free graft at the end of surgery. Using a drill includes the risk of ripping off the skin flap when not removed temporarily. Using a large diamond bur is recommended for drilling the exostoses and widening the ear canal. At the end of the operation, the entire tympanic membrane including the circumference of the anulus should be visualized. In medial exostoses there is a risk of opening the middle ear or damaging the tympanic membrane. In these cases, a piece of temporal fascia, perichondrium or cartilage can be used to cover the lesion in an underlay technique. If noise trauma of the inner ear occurred by touching the short process of the malleus with the drill, the patient should receive intravenous corticosteroids according to guidelines for acute sensorineural hearing loss. Severe complications (inner ear trauma, facial nerve paralysis) are rare, minor complications (opening of the middle ear space, expositions of the capsule of the TMJ, prolonged healing) occur in up to 10% of patients.[37]

Postoperative complications of EAC surgery are the most important factors for a negative impact on the patient's health-related quality of life. Therefore, only patients with symptoms should have surgery.[38] External auditory exostoses recurred in 8 of 91 ears in a long-term follow-up, occurring up to 15 years after surgery.[39] Beside avoidance of cold water[40] and postoperative long-term packing of the ear canal, there are no known factors to sufficiently influence recurrence.

Acquired Stenosis or Atresia

Recurrent acute, subacute, or chronic infections of the EAC may result in thickened skin (at the beginning in the subepithelial layer) and sequential granulation tissue

formation that narrows or closes the EAC's lumen (postinflammatory stenosis, **Fig. 1.6**). The same conditions may develop posttraumatically where bony fragments can be enclosed.

Fibrotic tissue and bony fragments can be removed transcanal or by an endaural incision. All thickened skin has to be removed to prevent recurrence of the disease. Epithelial defects can be covered using split-thickness skin grafts from the back of the auricle. The main complication following surgery for acquired atresia of the EAC is recurrence, which occurs in almost 40% of patients.[41]

Aseptic Necrosis and Cholesteatoma of the External Auditory Canal

Aseptic necrosis (**Fig. 1.7**) and cholesteatoma of the EAC (**Fig. 1.8**) may be interpreted as different stages of the same pathologic entity. During this disease, epithelium grows into an aseptic necrosis of the bone followed by retention of debris and proliferative epithelium with a secondary cholesteatoma arising.[42,43] This underlying condition is caused by repeated microtrauma and diminished microcirculation.[44] In rare cases it is idiopathic, usually at the medial part/floor of the external ear canal. A location other than in the inferior portion of the EAC indicates a secondary form of the disease, for example, in the case of patients with atypically located carcinoma of the EAC after years of complete remission of Langerhans cell histiocytosis, which is considered a posttumor category and a specific late complication of this rare disease.[45] Cholesteatoma of the EAC with an intact tympanic membrane may occur spontaneously, following trauma or most often after ear surgery.[46,47]

Small cholesteatoma pearls or necrotic areas can be excised. The affected bone should be smoothed with a diamond bur and covered with split thickness skin grafts

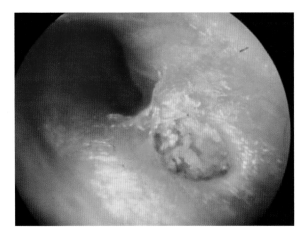

Fig. 1.7 Aseptic necrosis of the external auditory canal.

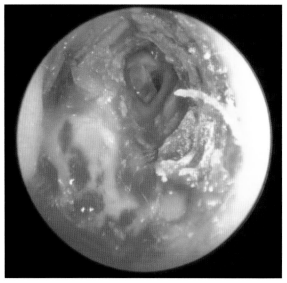

Fig. 1.9 Necrotizing otitis externa.

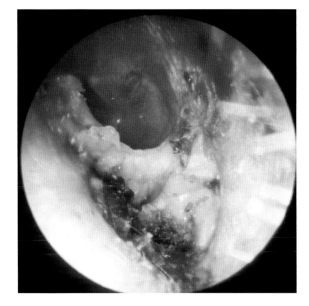

Fig. 1.8 Cholesteatoma of the external auditory canal.

or, in addition, with perichondrium or cartilage chips when mastoid cells are opened.

Malignant (Necrotizing) Otitis Externa

Malignant otitis externa is a rare infection involving the temporal bone and the skull in immunocompromised patients with potentially life-threatening complications of local bone erosion. The most frequent pathogen is *Pseudomonas aeruginosa.* Otorrhea, (nightly) pain, and granulation tissue in the EAC are the hallmarks of malignant otitis externa (**Fig. 1.9**).

Beside correction of the immunosuppression, a long-term systemic antibiotic therapy is mandatory. Surgical treatment should be reserved for limited cases when the disease is extensive or unresponsive to conservative treatment.[48] Bone sequestra and abscesses are treated surgically and mostly require extensive resection. Extensive surgery risks exposing healthy bone to the often persistent infection, which may lead to a further progression of the disease.[49] Cranial nerve involvement did not affect patient survival rate under an optimized medical treatment in a series of 23 patients, but all patients with lower cranial nerve palsy recovered normal function.[50]

Malignant Tumors

Malignant processes of the EAC are rare tumors, with bloody otorrhea as a hallmark symptom. Due to late diagnosis, surrounding structures are often already involved when diagnosed. Extended bone involvement significantly correlates with a worse prognosis than extended soft tissue involvement. Prognoses of patients with insufficient bone resection or no surgery are significantly poor.[51]

These tumors may require extensive surgical therapy (**Fig. 1.10**). In the case of an obliteration (e.g., with abdominal fat) of the external ear canal following (partial) petrosectomy, all squamous cell epithelium has to be removed to prevent creation of cholesteatoma. Surgical ablation may involve extended cutaneous structures and the auricle, the parotid gland, mandibula, etc. For reconstruction, multiple pedicled flaps, or in bigger defects, radial forearm free flaps may be used.[52] Postoperative radiotherapy is mandatory in almost all cases. Therefore, necessary reconstruction of the external ear is difficult. In the case of a postoperative prosthetic supply, the bone-anchor should be implanted before radiation, to allow the titanium screws to integrate into the bone.[53]

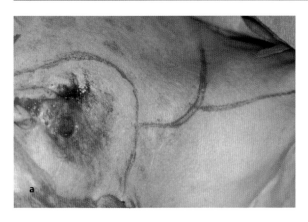

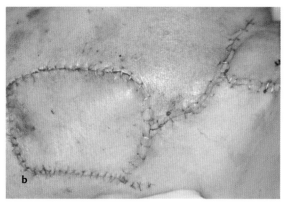

Fig. 1.10a,b Reconstruction of tissue defect after tumor surgery.

a Squamous cell carcinoma of the external auditory canal and intended surgical margins.

b Reconstruction with a radial forearm free flap.

References

1. Korczak D. Schönheitsoperationen: Daten, Probleme, Rechtsfragen. Bericht an die Bundesanstalt für Ernährung und Landwirtschaft, 2007
2. Weerda H, Siegert R. Complications of otoplasty and their treatment. [Article in German] Laryngorhinootologie 1994;73(7):394–399
3. Weerda H, Siegert R. Complications in otoplastic surgery and their treatment. Facial Plast Surg 1994;10(3):287–297
4. Weerda H, Siegert R. Die Ohrmuschelplastik und die Behandlung der Komplikationen. In: Bull AR, ed. Aesthetic Facial Surgery, 175–189, 1999
5. Mustardé JC. Effective formation of antihelix fold without incising the cartilage. In: Wallace J, ed. Transaction Int Soc Plast Surgeons, Baltimore: Williams, 1960
6. Mustardé JC. The correction of prominent ears using simple mattress sutures. Br J Plast Surg 1963;16:170–178
7. Mustardé JC. The treatment of prominent ears by buried mattress sutures: a ten-year survey. Plast Reconstr Surg 1967;39(4):382–386
8. Stenström SJ. A "Natural" Technique for Correction of Congenitally Prominent Ears. Plast Reconstr Surg 1963;32:509–518
9. Ju DMC, Li C, Crikelair GF. The Surgical Correction of Protruding Ears. Plast Reconstr Surg 1963;32:283–293
10. Crikelair GF, Cosman B. Another Solution for the Problem of the Prominent Ear. Ann Surg 1964;160:314–324
11. Chongchet V. A method of antihelix reconstruction. Br J Plast Surg 1963;16:268–272
12. Converse JM, Nigro A, Wilson FA, Johnson N. A technique for surgical correction of lop ears. Plast Reconstr Surg (1946) 1955;15(5):411–418
13. Converse JM, Wood-Smith D. Technical details in the surgical correction of the lop ear deformity. Plast Reconstr Surg 1963;31:118–128
14. Furnas DW. Correction of prominent ears by conchamastoid sutures. Plast Reconstr Surg 1968;42(3):189–193
15. Siegert R. On the surgical technique for auricle reconstruction. [Article in German] HNO 2006;54(10):737–741
16. Siegert R, Magritz R. Reconstruction of the external ear. [Article in German] Laryngorhinootologie 2007;86 (Suppl 1):S121–S140
17. Siegert R, ed. Auricular Reconstruction. Facial Plastic Surgery 25, 2009

18. Siegert R, Weerda H, Magritz, R. Basic techniques in autogenous microtia repair. Facial Plastic Surgery 2009;25(3):149–157
19. Siegert R, Magritz R. Special Reconstruction Techniques for Special Circumstances. Facial Plastic Surgery 2009; 25(3):204–211
20. Siegert R, Magritz R. Autologe Rekonstruktion schwerer Fehlbildungen und Defekte der Ohrmuschel. Journal für Ästhetische Chirurgie 2010;3:67–74
21. Crockett DJ. Regional keloid susceptibility. Br J Plast Surg 1964;17:245–253
22. Leventhal D, Furr M, Reiter D. Treatment of keloids and hypertrophic scars: a meta-analysis and review of the literature. Arch Facial Plast Surg 2006;8(6):362–368
23. Viera MH, Amini S, Valins W, Berman B: Innovative therapies in the treatment of keloids and hypertrophic scars. J Clin Aesthet Dermatol 2010;3(5):20–26
24. Fruth K, Gouveris H, Kuelkens C, Mann WJ. Radiofrequency tissue volume reduction for treatment of auricle keloids. Laryngoscope 2011;121(6):1233–1236
25. Rauch SD. Management of soft tissue and osseous stenosis of the ear canal and canalplasty. In: Nadol JB Jr, Schuhknecht HF, eds. Surgery of the Ear and Temporal Bone. New York: Raven Press; 1993:117–125
26. Perkins R. Canalplasty for exostoses of the external auditory canal. In: Brackmann DE, ed. Otologic Surgery. Philadelphia: WB Saunders Company; 1994: 28–35
27. Hildmann H, Sudhoff H. External Ear canal Surgery. In: Hildmann H, Sudhoff S, eds. Middle Ear Surgery. Heidelberg: Springer; 2006:67–72
28. Wollenberg B, Zenner HP. Erkrankungen von Trommelfell, Mittelohr und Mastoid. In: Zenner HP, ed. Praktische Therapie von HNO-Krankheiten. Stuttgart: Schattauer; 2008:95–101
29. Selesnick SH, Carew JF, DiBartolomeo JR. Herniation of the temporomandibular joint into the external auditory canal: a complication of otologic surgery. Am J Otol 1995;16(6):751–757
30. von Blumenthal H, Fisher EW, Adlam DM, Moffat DA. Surgical emphysema: a novel complication of aural exostosis surgery. J Laryngol Otol 1994;108(6):490–491
31. Graham MD, Larouere MJ. Miscellaneous External Auditory Canal problems. In: Brackmann DE, ed. Otologic Surgery. Philadelphia: WB Saunders Company; 1994:63–68
32. Moon IJ, Cho YS, Park J, Chung WH, Hong SH, Chang SO. Long-term stent use can prevent postoperative canal

stenosis in patients with congenital aural atresia. Otolaryngol Head Neck Surg 2012;146(4):614–620

33. Plester D, Pusalkar A. The anterior tympanomeatal angle: the aetiology, surgery and avoidance of blunting and annular cholesteatoma. Clin Otolaryngol Allied Sci 1981;6(5):323–328

34. Hildmann H, Sudhoff H. External ear canal surgery. In: Hildmann H, Sudhoff S, eds. Middle Ear Surgery. Heidelberg: Springer; 2006:30–37

35. Wagner F, Todt I, Wagner J, Ernst A. Indications and candidacy for active middle ear implants. Adv Otorhinolaryngol 2010;69:20–26

36. Venkatraman G, Mattox DE. External auditory canal wall cholesteatoma: a complication of ear surgery. Acta Otolaryngol 1997;117(2):293–297

37. Reber M, Mudry A. Results and extraordinary complications of surgery for exostoses of the external auditory canal. [Article in German] HNO 2000;48(2):125–128

38. Hempel JM, Forell S, Krause E, Müller J, Braun T. Surgery for outer ear canal exostoses and osteomata: focusing on patient benefit and health-related quality of life. Otol Neurotol 2012;33(1):83–86

39. House JW, Wilkinson EP. External auditory exostoses: evaluation and treatment. Otolaryngol Head Neck Surg 2008;138(5):672–678

40. King JF, Kinney AC, Iacobellis SF II, et al. Laterality of exostosis in surfers due to evaporative cooling effect. Otol Neurotol 2010;31(2):345–351

41. Magliulo G. Acquired atresia of the external auditory canal: recurrence and long-term results. Ann Otol Rhinol Laryngol 2009;118(5):345–349

42. Meyer M. Über Entstehung, knochenzerstörende Ausbreitung und theoretische Einordnung des sekundären Cholesteatoms und über den Einfluss auf die Pneumatisation des Warzenfortsatzes. Arch Ohr-Nas-Kehlk-Heilk. 1934;139:127–149

43. Jahnke K, Lieberum B. Surgery of cholesteatoma of the ear canal. [Article in German] Laryngorhinootologie 1995;74(1):46–49

44. Farrior J. Cholesteatoma of the external ear canal. Am J Otol 1990;11(2):113–116

45. Dubach P, Häusler R. External auditory canal cholesteatoma: reassessment of and amendments to its categorization, pathogenesis, and treatment in 34 patients. Otol Neurotol 2008;29(7):941–948

46. Holt JJ. Ear canal cholesteatoma. Laryngoscope 1992;102(6):608–613

47. Brookes GB. Post-traumatic cholesteatoma. Clin Otolaryngol Allied Sci 1983;8(1):31–38

48. Carfrae MJ, Kesser BW. Malignant otitis externa. Otolaryngol Clin North Am 2008;41(3):537–549, viii–ix

49. Amorosa L, Modugno GC, Pirodda A. Malignant external otitis: review and personal experience. Acta Otolaryngol Suppl 1996;521:3–16

50. Mani N, Sudhoff H, Rajagopal S, Moffat D, Axon PR. Cranial nerve involvement in malignant external otitis: implications for clinical outcome. Laryngoscope 2007;117(5):907–910

51. Ito M, Hatano M, Yoshizaki T. Prognostic factors for squamous cell carcinoma of the temporal bone: extensive bone involvement or extensive soft tissue involvement? Acta Otolaryngol 2009;129(11):1313–1319

52. Rosenthal EL, King T, McGrew BM, Carroll W, Magnuson JS, Wax MK. Evolution of a paradigm for free tissue transfer reconstruction of lateral temporal bone defects. Head Neck 2008;30(5):589–594

53. Volkenstein S, Dazert S, Jahnke K, Schneider M, Neumann A. Prosthetic supply of tissue defects in head and neck surgery. [Article in German] Laryngorhinootologie 2007;86(12):854–860

2 Tympanic Membrane Reconstruction: Difficult Situations and Complications

L. Sennaroğlu, M. D. Bajin

Anatomy

The tympanic membrane is a semi-transparent membranous structure that constitutes a wide part of the lateral wall of the tympanic cavity at the end of the bony external ear. The membrane is placed obliquely (45°), at a sharp angle to the inferior wall of the external auditory canal (EAC), and its lateral surface is directed downward and forward. The adult tympanic membrane extends ~ 8 to 9 mm horizontally and 9 to 10 mm vertically. The larger area of the membrane is tense (pars tensa), but superiorly there is a soft portion (pars flaccida, Shrapnell membrane). The annulus fibrosus of the tympanic membrane anchors it into the tympanic sulcus. The anulus fibrosus does not fully encircle the tympanic membrane; the ends of the fibrous ring meet in the area of the processus brevis. The extension in front is called the stria anterior and the one at the back the stria posterior, and these ligaments carry the malleus–incus complex, forming malleolar folds by encircling the striae. The lateral process of the malleus together with the posterior and anterior malleolar folds separate the pars flaccida from the pars tensa. The Shrapnell membrane serves as the lateral wall of the Prussak space.[1,2]

> **Note**
> To facilitate the definition and localization of the lesions, the tympanic membrane is divided into four quadrants with horizontal and vertical imaginary lines going through the umbo.

Etiology and Classification of Tympanic Membrane Perforations

Tympanic membrane perforations result mainly from infectious and traumatic etiologies. Among the infectious etiologies are acute otitis media, chronic otitis media, and tuberculous otitis media. Penetrating trauma, non-explosive and explosive blast injuries and iatrogenic causes are among the traumatic etiologic factors.

It is possible to classify the perforations according to their localizations and the area where they affect the tympanic membrane. The tympanic membrane is divided by a vertical line through the umbo, so that perforations can be classified as anterior and posterior. In addition, perforations can be categorized clinically as central when located within the limits of the anulus fibrosus, and marginal where the anulus is destroyed. Finally, the terms "total" or "subtotal" can also be used based on the perforation area that affects the tympanic membrane.[3]

Aim of Surgery

Although tympanic membrane reconstruction is generally considered to be an "easy" operation, it is one of the most difficult otologic surgeries to perform successfully. This is because there are two goals of the operation that must be accomplished for it to be regarded as a successful surgery. First, the perforation must be repaired successfully; and second, hearing is expected to be improved while the ear's function and other structures are preserved. Failure to reach these goals may cause patient dissatisfaction.[4]

Surgical Approaches for Tympanic Membrane Reconstruction

Three different surgical approaches are being used for membrane reconstruction. These are the endaural, postauricular, and endomeatal approaches. Each approach has its advantages and disadvantages. In the endaural approach there is less bleeding and trauma compared with the postauricular approach,[5] and a natural meatoplasty is obtained by leaving the inferior part of the incision unsutured. In the postauricular approach, it is easier to expose the anterior remnant of the tympanic membrane in subtotal perforations. This also applies to cases where the anterior wall is prominent. The endomeatal approach is preferred in perforations, especially those located in the posterior part of the tympanic membrane, and it provides a cosmetic advantage because there is no visible incision. As there is less tissue trauma, it is possible to maintain natural tissue integration.

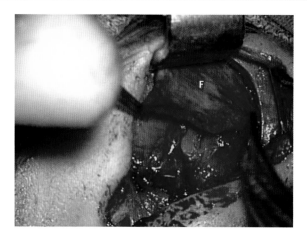

Fig. 2.1 Harvesting the temporalis muscle fascia graft in the endaural approach.
F: fascia

Graft Materials

Fascia temporalis is the most frequently used grafting material in tympanoplasty, with a rate of success reaching 95%[6,7] (**Fig. 2.1**). However, this rate decreases in some patients. Lower success rates occur in chronic tubal dysfunction, adhesive process, tympanosclerosis, and recurrent perforations. In such cases, cartilage grafts are more commonly preferred.[8,9] The primary reasons for preferring the cartilage graft are mechanical stability and resistance to high negative pressure changes in the middle ear.[10] Subtotal perforations are also cases where fascia grafting has lower success rates; failure in these patients generally stems from graft dislocation from the anterior wall. The primary reasons for failure are:

- Decrease in the medial support of the graft by absorbable gelatin sponges placed in the anterior mesotympanum that is displaced toward the eustachian tube over time.
- Decreased visibility of the area in cases with a prominent anterior canal wall.
- After the graft is placed anteriorly, it may be dislocated while the surgeon is conducting manipulation in the posterior part of the graft.

There are certain techniques that can be applied to prevent the graft from moving away from the anterior edge of the tympanic membrane. One technique involves placing the graft under the anterior external ear canal skin and anulus fibrosus. However, this is a difficult technique, and there is a risk of blunting in the anterior part of the EAC. Pulling the edges of the graft through a small incision of the tympanic membrane at the site of the anulus is another method that can be applied. A further option is to apply overlay tympanoplasty. Although there is a greater chance of success in overlay tympanoplasty, it has

some known complications, such as the longer recovery period, anterior blunting, graft lateralization, and epithelial pearl formation.[11] Many studies suggest that the overlay technique has more disadvantages and that it is prone to more complications.[12]

In recent years there has been an increased tendency to use cartilage grafts in tympanoplasty. The most significant reason for this is their strength and the high graft success rate. There are various techniques for cartilage tympanoplasty, but the most frequently used are the "palisade" and "island" techniques.[9] In our clinic we use an anterior cartilage reinforced tympanoplasty technique for total and anterior perforations, and an island technique for revision cases. Cartilage is used from the tragus or conchal part of the auricular cartilage. In the anterior cartilage reinforced tympanoplasty technique, after the placement of absorbable gelatin sponges in the middle ear up to the drum level, the cartilage graft is placed under the remnant of the tympanic membrane in front. The fascia graft is then placed, using an underlay technique, between the drum remnant and the cartilage. Posteriorly, the fascia lies over the bony EAC. The purpose of this technique is to minimize detachment of the fascia graft anteriorly. The placement of cartilage in the anterior hypotympanum supports the fascia graft medially. In the event that the fascia graft moves away from the anulus, epithelialization may continue over the cartilage (**Figs. 2.2 and 2.3**). In addition, it is possible to observe the middle ear in the postoperative period, as regards cholesteatoma or effusion, because cartilage is only present on the medial part of the anterior part of the newly formed membrane.

Intraoperative Complications

Bleeding

Bleeding may occur during surgery and in the postoperative period. Maintaining a blood-free surgical field is important if one is to perform a correct and successful graft placement.

A meticulous preparation technique is very important to obtain a bloodless field. Bleeding may initially come from the incision, and preoperative injection of the incision line with 2% lidocaine and 1:100,000 epinephrine helps to reduce bleeding. It is important, particularly during the graft harvesting, to dissect the correct surgical plane between the fascia and the muscle; injury of the muscle tissue under the temporalis fascia leads to troublesome bleeding. Another location of bleeding may be the anterior superior part of the bony EAC, where the posterior tympanic artery may be damaged during elevation of the skin flaps.[2] Hypertension may also cause generalized bleeding from many locations. Introduction of new hypotensive agents such as remifentanil (Ultiva;

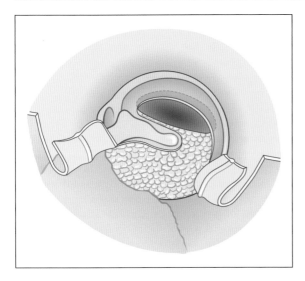

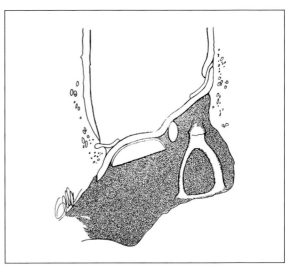

Fig. 2.2 Diagram of anterior reinforced cartilage myringoplasty. (Adapted from an image supplied with courtesy of S. Saraç, MD).

Fig. 2.3 Coronal view of anterior reinforced cartilage myringoplasty. (Image courtesy of S. Saraç, MD.)

GlaxoSmithKline, Philadelphia, PA, USA) has greatly improved surgical vision and manipulation during microsurgery by reducing bleeding. If the middle ear has had a recent infection, this may also cause bleeding from the granulation tissues. All these bleeding points should be cauterized or controlled with epinephrine-soaked gelatin sponges before proceeding, otherwise the surgeon may be faced with difficulty during graft placement.

When working on or in close proximity to the facial nerve, arterial bleeding may also occur. This should be controlled with gelatin sponges. It should also warn the surgeon of the proximity of the nerve.

Preoperative high-resolution computed tomography of the temporal bone is routinely obtained at Hacettepe University before tympanoplasty). In addition, to evaluate the middle ear or mastoid pathology, axial and coronal imaging shows if there is a high jugular bulb or an aberrant internal carotid artery.[13] Although these entities are rare, they can lead to devastating consequences if the surgeon fails to recognize them. Accidental injury to a highly placed or uncovered jugular bulb can be treated by applying oxidized cellulose (Surgicel; Ethicon Company, Somerville, NJ, USA)). Ideally, the pieces of oxidized cellulose (Surgicel) should be larger than the defect, and they should cover the jugular bulb without being pushed into the lumen, to avoid pulmonary embolism.[14]

Damage to the Tympanomeatal Flap

Preservation of the ear canal flaps is very important for rapid and uncomplicated healing in the postoperative period; they may support graft epithelialization and avoid scar and stenosis formation in the EAC.[15] They have to be handled with care and should be intact at the end

of the operation. Usually it is necessary to elevate the skin from the tympanosquamous suture anterosuperiorly, up to the 6 o'clock position (right ear) inferiorly before using the bur. If the meatal skin cannot be removed sufficiently from the drilling area, the flap may also be removed and retransplanted at the end of the surgery. Enlargement of the bony canal by drilling is a routine part of the myringoplasty to obtain a better exposure of the middle ear and improve postoperative care. During this process the flaps may be damaged by the bur. It is good practice to protect the flaps with suction while the bur is being used; if the ear canal skin is properly elevated and protected, the risk of damage by the bur is very low.

Due to the enlargement of the bony EAC, the original canal skin is generally not enough to completely cover the bony surface at the end of the operation. Additional fascia can be used to cover the bone, which is placed under the skin, to improve regular wound healing and avoid unwanted scar formation in the EAC.

Enlargement of the Bony Ear Canal

Enlarging the bony ear canal is a routine part of the myringoplasty procedure in our department. The aim is to improve the surgical exposure (**Fig. 2.4**). First the lateral part of the bony canal is widened, and this is continued medially, removing the tympanosquamous suture and all the overhanging bone to obtain a full visualization of the anulus from the 6 o'clock position to the 2 o'clock position (right ear). A cutting bur should be used at the beginning. If preoperative high-resolution computed tomography of the temporal bone demonstrates a small temporal bone where the distance between the EAC and the dura is relatively small, then manipulation of the bur

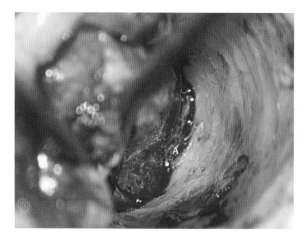

Fig. 2.4 Enlarged ear canal up to the level of the anulus. A: anulus.

may cause dural damage at this stage. It is mandatory to use fresh cutting burs at all times. It is not infrequent to expose the dura and even use it as the landmark (the dura is the surgeon's friend), but dural laceration should be avoided by using fresh cutting burs and avoiding unnecessary pressure.

Damaging the Temporomandibular Joint

It is very important to visualize the anterior part of the tympanic membrane perforation before placing the graft. De-epithelialization of the anterior part of the perforation may even decrease the exposure. To properly place the graft underneath the drum remnant, usually the bony bulge of the anterior canal wall should be removed with a bur. After a circumferential and two radial incisions, the anterior canal skin is elevated and retracted medially. It is important to avoid damaging the skin, which can be protected by preparing a round piece of suture cover (6 to 7 mm in diameter). It is preferable to use diamond burs at this stage. Care must be taken to avoid entering the temporomandibular joint. Tilting the patient toward the front enables the surgeon to recognize the fibrotic capsule of the temporomandibular joint before it is damaged.[16]

Elevating the Tympanic Anulus and Entering the Middle Ear

To lift the tympanic membrane the anulus should be elevated from the bony sulcus using instruments such as a 45° pick or the Plester knife, taking care not to leave any part of the skin attached to the bone to avoid iatrogenic cholesteatoma. The middle ear mucosa is identified as a transparent blueish membranous structure. This is penetrated with a 45° pick with its tip pointing toward the middle ear to avoid damage of the tympanic membrane. A House elevator can then be used for further elevation of the tympanic membrane. The risk of iatrogenic cholesteatoma is more likely in cases of marginal perforations and severe retraction pockets, where the skin is both thinner and posteriorly more retracted, making it more difficult to identify and preserve.[17]

Injury to the Chorda Tympani Nerve

Surgeons should do their best to avoid damage to the chorda tympani nerve (CTN). The CTN can be damaged during the elevation of the anulus and while entering the middle ear. Preservation of the CTN is very important to avoid future taste disturbance. After identification, it is freed from the posterior ear canal wall and mucosal attachments with a 45° pick and then dissected using a House elevator. In some cases the tympanic membrane or part of the cholesteatoma is completely attached to the CTN. In these situations the nerve may have to be sacrificed.

The possibility of taste disturbances and mouth dryness due to chorda tympani nerve injury must be included as part of the informed consent before myringoplasty.[18] It is also stated that stretching causes more symptoms than transecting the nerve.[19,20] The goal of the otologist should be protecting the nerves as far as possible. Complete recovery has been reported in 76% of patients.

Sensorineural Hearing Loss

Sensorineural hearing loss is a rare complication after tympanic membrane reconstruction. However, this situation may be a devastating complication for the patient; it must therefore be included in every informed consent before surgery. This is particularly important in a patient undergoing the operation for the only hearing ear. In case of total hearing loss in this situation, the necessity of cochlear implantation should also be mentioned preoperatively.

This complication is most commonly associated with abnormal manipulation of the ossicular chain.[21,22] It is a common practice to check the mobility of the ossicles in tympanoplasty. To see the complete ossicular chain, a limited atticotomy is necessary to observe the footplate mobility. During the atticotomy the surgeon must be cautious not to touch the ossicular chain with the high-speed drill. This transmits high vibrational energy to the inner ear and may cause inadvertent sensorineural hearing loss.[23] In our practice, initially the lateral part of the ear canal is enlarged by drilling with a cutting bur until the ear canal attains a conical shape where the anulus is fully visible from the 6 o'clock to 2 o'clock positions (right ear). This not only increases visibility of the middle ear structures and helps in maneuvering the graft, but also allows better exposure during atticotomy (**Fig. 2.5**). Then the attic should be opened carefully from inside, going backward until the long process of the incus and stapes footplate

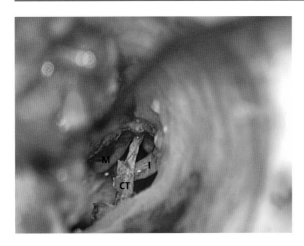

Fig. 2.5 Limited atticotomy for ossicular exposure. M: malleus; I: incus; CT: chorda tympani nerve.

is visible. Usually more exposure is not necessary unless there is a cholesteatoma. Gentle palpation on the malleus and observation of the movement of the stapes, and particularly the footplate, is necessary for checking the movement of the ossicular chain. Excessive manipulation should be avoided as it may cause sensorineural hearing loss. However, if there is tympanosclerosis around the ossicles they should be removed to mobilize the chain. Sometimes the tympanosclerotic plaques are very adherent to the stapes, and manipulation of the ossicles may cause sensorineural hearing loss.[24] In addition, the stapes may be accidentally dislocated during these maneuvers. A meticulous preparation technique is required during this part of the surgery. Removal of the tympanosclerotic plaques from the stapes should be performed as the last step of the surgery before graft placement.

Inner ear integrity may be checked using the Weber test on the following day. If there is vertigo and nystagmus, it is recommended to check bone conduction on the first postoperative day. If there is a drop in the bone conduction levels, the patient should be hospitalized and treated in the same way as for acute sensorineural hearing loss, with steroids and intravenous dextran.

Facial Nerve Injury

Facial nerve injury is unlikely during tympanic membrane reconstruction. Facial nerve palsy can occur without direct injury to the nerve, especially in the case of a dehiscent Fallopian canal and overuse of local anesthetics.[25] The surgeon must be careful to use the correct amount of local anesthetics in the correct location.

There may be situations where the nerve can be damaged during tympanoplasty as well. The facial nerve may be dehiscent in 8.6% of cases in the tympanic portion.[26] If the angled instruments are used in the medial part of the incus, facial nerve injury may occur. Sometimes

tympanosclerotic plaques form layers on top of the tympanic segment of the facial nerve, which may inhibit the movements of the ossicular chain. They should therefore be removed during tympanoplasty to obtain the mobility of the stapes. During the removal of these layers it may be difficult to distinguish the facial nerve. This is another situation where the nerve can be damaged. These layers should be elevated gently with appropriate picks and a House elevator. It is important to find the facial canal at the normal anatomical position, and then proceed proximally or distally and remove the plaques that cause stapes fixation.

Thermal damage of the facial nerve is another important point. Continuous irrigation during drilling is mandatory to avoid this complication.

If the patient has facial palsy in the immediate postoperative period and the surgeon is confident with the surgery, it is best to wait for a few hours until the effect of local anesthesia diminishes and the facial functions return to normal. In the case of doubtful surgical experience, it may be better to revise the surgery with an experienced surgeon as soon as possible.

De-epithelialization of the Perforation Edge

The underlay grafting technique requires the complete de-epithelialization of the medial part of the tympanic membrane edge. The surgeon should learn to perform a de-epithelialization without enlarging the perforation. This is particularly important in patients with near total perforations. To do this properly the surgeon needs an angled sharp hook and should make an incision between the lateral and medial surfaces of the tympanic membrane remnant, then remove the medial part of the remnant preserving the outer layer (**Fig. 2.6**). Insufficient

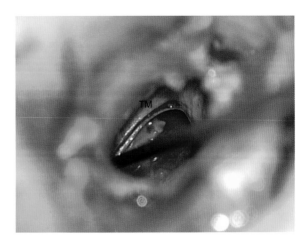

Fig. 2.6 De-epithelialization of the medial part of the tympanic membrane remnant without enlarging the perforation. TM: tympanic membrane.

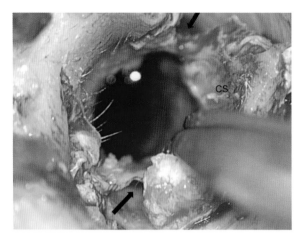

Fig. 2.7 Canal skin incisions for increasing exposure. CS: canal skin, black arrows indicate incision lines.

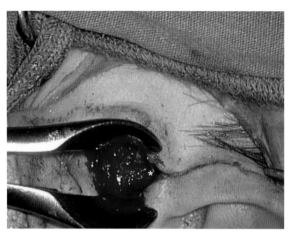

Fig. 2.9 Natural meatoplasty in the endaural approach. Note that the inferior part of the incision is unsutured (white asterisk)

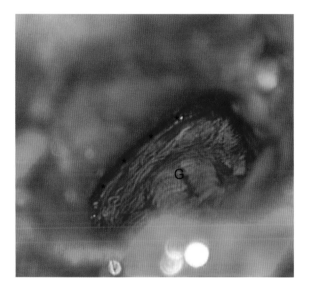

Fig. 2.8 Underlay grafting technique with temporalis fascia graft under the tympanic membrane remnant. G: graft, black asterisks: anterior tympanic membrane remnant.

de-epithelialization may bend epithelial remnants under the tympanic membrane, resulting in epithelial cysts. In our surgical approach we do not use the swing door technique where the canal skin is completely incised from the most lateral part to the anulus; it has been observed that skin edges on the medial side tend to fold inward in this method. We prefer to raise the skin in the lateral two-thirds of the ear canal while the medial one-third is preserved intact (**Fig. 2.7**). This avoids inward rotation of the skin edges and the formation of cholesteatoma pearls over the graft during wound healing. It also supports the epithelialization of the graft.

Graft Placement

After thorough de-epithelialization, the middle ear is filled with absorbable gelatin sponges up to the level of the drum remnant. It is important to place a few larger pieces around the orifice of the eustachian tube to avoid postoperative graft medialization when the patient starts swallowing. If the gelatin sponges are insufficient there will be a dehiscence between the drum remnant and the graft, resulting in persisting perforation. It is important to place the graft completely under the drum remnant (**Fig. 2.8**). Posteriorly, part of the graft is placed over the bony ear canal for support. Anteriorly the only support is given by the gelatin sponges. If some epithelial tissues are left around the drum remnant, they may turn medially and produce cholesteatoma in the long term.

Repositioning the Flaps

Proper repositioning of the skin flaps is very important to avoid postoperative stenosis of the ear canal. The subcutaneous part of the skin of the ear canal may be thinned to aid in rotation of the flaps. The ear canal is filled with pieces of loose gelatin sponges to keep the flaps in position.

Meatoplasty

Enlargement of the EAC supports the surgical approach to the middle ear and also improves wound healing and postoperative care. This can be regarded as a mild meatoplasty. In the endaural approach a natural meatoplasty is easily obtained by leaving the inferior part of the incision unsutured (**Fig. 2.9**). Meatoplasty is also advisable in the postauricular approach if the ear canal is slightly enlarged.

Postoperative Complications

Wound Infection

Wound infection and perichondritis are rare complications, and they present themselves as pain, hyperemia, and swelling around the incision and auricle. Ninety percent of otologic wounds are colonized at the time of surgery, and therefore chronic ear surgery is accepted as clean-contaminated or contaminated. As in any type of surgery, the main principle is to minimize the colony counts so that host defense mechanisms can overcome the potential infection. To maintain a low colony count many otologists use prophylactic antibiotics. However, a study by Jackson points out that prophylactic antibiotics are harmless, but useless.[27] Perichondritis after the end-aural approach close to incision has been reported, but it is rare and can be treated with antibiotics. Drainage may be necessary in the case of abscess formation.

Bleeding

Postoperative wound hematoma or bleeding from the incision may occur as a result of increased blood pressure or insufficient hemostasis during surgery. Hematoma will prolong the healing period.[28] The treatment is immediate removal of the clot, clamping the bleeding artery or vein, and compression with a mastoid dressing. If the patient is a child, these interventions should be made in the operating room with sedation or under general anesthesia.

Iatrogenic Cholesteatoma

The lateral surface grafting technique also demands a complete de-epithelialization of the lateral surface of the drum remnant. Care should be directed especially to the anteroinferior part of the canal 1 mm lateral to the anulus, where the skin attachment is tight. If there is a concern about the thoroughness of the de-epithelialization, a portion of the remnant can be removed. In case of incomplete removal of all the epithelium, cholesteatoma cysts may develop.[29] Removing the epithelial cysts and the keratin debris can be done in an office setting.

Tympanic Membrane Retraction

In case of eustachian tube dysfunction, postoperative graft retraction or persistent effusion and conductive hearing loss can be seen. This is sometimes hard to identify, especially in cartilage tympanoplasty. Some surgeons place a ventilation tube, as an additional procedure during myringoplasty. If the contralateral drum is retracted, or in cases such as Down syndrome and craniofacial anomalies where there is pervading eustachian tube dysfunction, it is sensible to do both tympanic membrane reconstruction and ventilation tube placement at the same time. To avoid retraction, the temporalis fascia graft and the perichondrium of the cartilage graft should be positioned over the posterior bony canal.

Facial Nerve Paralysis

In the postoperative period a temporary facial nerve palsy caused by local anesthetics can be seen. This will recover completely after a couple of hours.[23] There are also some reported cases of delayed facial paralysis after middle ear surgery. The clinical presentation is ipsilateral facial nerve palsy that appears more than 72 hours after an uneventful middle ear procedure, without symptoms of any infection. These cases are attributed to viral activation and varicella zoster is the suspected organism.[30,31] They should be treated like Bell's palsy. The prognosis is very good.

Lateralization of the Tympanic Membrane

This is mainly due to an inability to place the graft under the manubrium mallei. It usually occurs after 6 months following the surgery and causes conducting hearing reduction. During ear examination the manubrium mallei is not visualized within the tympanic membrane, which appears more lateral than its usual location. The treatment is reoperation and placing the graft under the manubrium mallei.

Blunting in the Anterior Sulcus

Complete removal of ear canal skin is part of the overlay technique. Blunting in the anterior sulcus occurs if the anulus is separated from the bony sulcus in the anterior part of the membrane. Excessive fibrosis in this area causes blunting. This complication usually results in a conductive hearing loss. Since successful reoperation is difficult, implantable hearing aids are considered to be an option.

References

1. Gulya AJ. Gulya and Schuknecht's Anatomy of the Temporal Bone and its Surgical Implications. New York: Informa Healthcare USA; 2007
2. Gulya AJ. Developmental anatomy of the temporal bone and skull base. In: Gulya AJ, Minor LB, Poe DS, eds. Glasscock-Shambaugh Surgery of the Ear. Shelton: PMPH-USA; 2010
3. Sheehy JL. Tympanoplasty. J R Soc Med 1981;74(6):467–468
4. Wullstein H. Theory and practice of tympanoplasty. Laryngoscope 1956;66(8):1076–1093
5. Tos M. Approaches, myringoplasty, ossiculoplasty and tympanoplasty. In: Manual of Middle Ear Surgery. Stuttgart: Georg Thieme Verlag; 1993:88–127
6. Perkins R, Bui HT. Tympanic membrane reconstruction using formaldehyde-formed autogenous temporalis

fascia: twenty years' experience. Otolaryngol Head Neck Surg 1996;114(3):366–379

7. Gierek T, Slaska-Kaspera A, Majzel K, Klimczak-Golab L. Results of myringoplasty and type I tympanoplasty with the use of fascia, cartilage and perichondrium grafts. [Article in Polish] Otolaryngol Pol 2004;58(3):529–533

8. Yung M. Cartilage tympanoplasty: literature review. J Laryngol Otol 2008;122(7):663–672

9. Dornhoffer J. Cartilage tympanoplasty: indications, techniques, and outcomes in a 1,000-patient series. Laryngoscope 2003;113(11):1844–1856

10. Zahnert T, Hüttenbrink KB, Mürbe D, Bornitz M. Experimental investigations of the use of cartilage in tympanic membrane reconstruction. Am J Otol 2000;21(3):322–328

11. Glasscock ME III. Tympanic membrane grafting with fascia: overlay vs. undersurface technique. Laryngoscope 1973;83(5):754–770

12. Singh M, Rai A, Bandyopadhyay S, Gupta SC. Comparative study of the underlay and overlay techniques of myringoplasty in large and subtotal perforations of the tympanic membrane. J Laryngol Otol 2003;117(6):444–448

13. Sauvaget E, Paris J, Kici S, et al. Aberrant internal carotid artery in the temporal bone: imaging findings and management. Arch Otolaryngol Head Neck Surg 2006;132(1):86–91

14. Huang BR, Wang CH, Young YH. Dehiscent high jugular bulb: a pitfall in middle ear surgery. Otol Neurotol 2006;27(7):923–927

15. Aggarwal R, Saeed SR, Green KJ. Myringoplasty. J Laryngol Otol 2006;120(6):429–432

16. Nunn DR, Strasnick B. Temporomandibular joint prolapse after tympanoplasty. Otolaryngol Head Neck Surg 1997;117(6):S169–S171

17. Hough JV. Revision tympanoplasty including anterior perforations and lateralization of grafts. Otolaryngol Clin North Am 2006;39(4):661–675, v

18. Gopalan P, Kumar M, Gupta D, Phillipps JJ. A study of chorda tympani nerve injury and related symptoms following middle-ear surgery. J Laryngol Otol 2005;119(3):189–192

19. Nin T, Sakagami M, Sone-Okunaka M, Muto T, Mishiro Y, Fukazawa K. Taste function after section of chorda tympani nerve in middle ear surgery. Auris Nasus Larynx 2006;33(1):13–17

20. Michael P, Raut V. Chorda tympani injury: operative findings and postoperative symptoms. Otolaryngol Head Neck Surg 2007;136(6):978–981

21. Ballantyne J. Iatrogenic deafness. J Laryngol Otol 1970; 84(10):967–1000

22. Weber PC. Iatrogenic complications from chronic ear surgery. Otolaryngol Clin North Am 2005;38(4):711–722

23. Dawes PJ. Early complications of surgery for chronic otitis media. J Laryngol Otol 1999;113(9):803–810

24. Ho KY, Tsai SM, Chai CY, Wang HM. Clinical analysis of intratympanic tympanosclerosis: etiology, ossicular chain findings, and hearing results of surgery. Acta Otolaryngol 2010;130(3):370–374

25. Green JD Jr, Shelton C, Brackmann DE. Iatrogenic facial nerve injury during otologic surgery. Laryngoscope 1994;104(8 Pt 1):922–926

26. Kim CW, Rho YS, Ahn HY, Oh SJ. Facial canal dehiscence in the initial operation for chronic otitis media without cholesteatoma. Auris Nasus Larynx 2008;35(3):353–356

27. Jackson CG. Antimicrobial prophylaxis in ear surgery. Laryngoscope 1988;98(10):1116–1123

28. Schwager K. Acute complications during middle ear surgery: part 1: Problems during tympanoplasty—what to do? [Article in German] HNO 2007;55(4):307–315, quiz 316–317

29. Pulec JL, Deguine C. Iatrogenic cholesteatoma. Ear Nose Throat J 2004;83(7):445

30. Gyo K, Honda N. Delayed facial palsy after middle-ear surgery due to reactivation of varicella-zoster virus. J Laryngol Otol 1999;113(10):914–915

31. De Stefano A, Neri G, Kulamarva G. Delayed facial nerve paralysis post middle ear surgery: herpes simplex virus activation. B-ENT 2009;5(1):47–50

3 Management and Prevention of Complications in Stapes Surgery and Ossicular Chain Reconstruction

S. Dazert, A. Minovi

Introduction

Surgery for ossicular chain reconstruction and stapes surgery begins with the proper approach. In general, we recommend the endaural approach for stapes surgery. Some other centers (especially in the United States) prefer the transcanal approach. In ossicular chain reconstruction surgery the most appropriate approach depends on the pathology. For cholesteatoma surgery or operations that include the mastoid area, the postauricular approach is recommended because this allows comfortable control of the mastoid, the skull base, or the internal auditory canal.[1] In cases of tympanic membrane perforations close to the anterior anulus, the postauricular approach allows better visualization of the operation site.

In general, the otologic surgeon should consider that surgery of the middle ear is "landmark" surgery. Important anatomical structures, such as Henle spine, the round window niche, the oval niche, and the facial nerve, need to be identified and inspected. One of the most consistent anatomic landmarks is the round window niche, which serves as the first anatomical orientation in revision surgeries.

In our department, the majority of middle ear surgeries are performed under general anesthetic. However, the standard application of local anesthesia ~ 15 to 20 minutes before surgery is mandatory to reduce intraoperative bleeding. Many other centers prefer local anesthesia for the entire surgery. Usually 3 to 4 mL local anesthesia containing a mixture of 2% xylocaine with 1:200,000 epinephrine is injected postauricularly and into all four quadrants of the external auditory canal. This should be done before disinfection to allow the local anesthesia time to take effect.[2] In addition, it is particularly important to inject the anterior part of the external auditory canal when performing stapes surgery.

If unexpected intraoperative diffuse bleeding should occur, irrigation with physiologic solutions is recommended. For continuous bleeding, application of 0.5 mL of pure epinephrine solution (1:1,000) for several minutes is recommended. Especially in stapes surgery, an almost bloodless operative field is mandatory for a successful outcome. However, epinephrine should only be applied before the footplate is opened.

> **Tips for Middle Ear Surgery**
> - Preoperative planning of the appropriate approach is mandatory to facilitate surgery and prevent complications.
> - Proper positioning of the patient's head (supine, open angle) allows comfortable surgical dissection.
> - Visualization of important anatomical landmarks is essential for safe surgery
> - A standardized and proper local anesthesia technique is mandatory.
> - Intraoperative application of undiluted epinephrine 1:1,000 allows profound reduction of bleeding.

Stapes Surgery

Stapes surgery requires precise surgical skills that come with experience. It is better to refer the patient to a specialist than to perform only the occasional stapes surgery. **Table 3.1** summarizes the management of complications in stapes surgery.

Intraoperative Challenges and Complications

Approach

Minimizing complications in stapes surgery starts with the correct approach. In Europe most surgeons prefer the endaural incision over the transcanal approach.[3,4] We usually perform the endaural incision using a middle-sized speculum, a No. 10 blade for the intercartilaginous incision, and a No. 15 blade for lifting the meatal skin flap. The tympanomeatal flap should not be too short because a short flap length may not allow sufficient coverage of the curetted lateral attic wall, particularly if extensive drilling of the scutum in a far posteriorly located footplate is required. In these cases we perform an underlay tympanoplasty using a small piece of fascia.[5]

Table 3.1 Complications and their management in stapes surgery

Complication	Management
Tympanic membrane perforation	Underlay tympanoplasty with fascia
Chorda tympani lesion	Transect nerve rather than extensively stretch
Persistent stapedial artery	Try displacement, if not possible, then coagulate
Floating footplate	Drill and carefully remove footplate
Gusher	Insertion of prosthesis if possible
Fracture of the lenticular process	More proximal fixation of the prosthesis
Overhanging facial nerve with complete occlusion of the footplate	Insertion of the prosthesis into a drilled promontory window
Narrowed oval niche	Lowering of the bony pyramid with a fine drill
Obliterative otosclerosis	Stapedotomy with Skeeter drill
Mild postoperative vertigo	Corticosteroids, daily examination
Severe vertigo with profound sensorineural hearing loss	Corticosteroids, immediate revision

Tympanic Membrane Perforation

Tympanic membrane perforation in stapes surgery may occur during the elevation of the anulus. This can happen when an inexperienced surgeon slides over the anulus rather than elevating it from its bony sulcus. However, a tympanic membrane perforation is not considered to be a major complication. If it occurs, an underlay myringoplasty using temporalis fascia or tragal perichondrium is recommended, and these grafts can be harvested using the same approach. However, it is important to harvest the graft before continuing with the stapes surgery and opening the footplate.

Chorda Tympani Lesion

There are several steps during stapes surgery when the chorda tympani nerve may be injured. First, it can be damaged during the elevation of the anulus in the region where the nerve enters its bony canal. Second, the nerve may be injured during the curettage of the scutum. For a complete mobilization of the nerve it is also important to discontinue its attachment to the manubrium.[6] The nerve should be preserved whenever possible; however, if maximum mobilization of the nerve does not allow sufficient exposure of the oval window, the nerve should be transected rather than extensively stretched.[7] Several studies have shown that chorda tympani lesions do not lead to permanent taste disturbances in the majority of patients.[8]

Luxation of Incus

A luxation of the incus can occur during the removal of the lateral attic wall using a curette. The luxation can be into an anterior direction when the curette unintentionally slips toward the lenticular process or into a posterior direction when the curette slips toward the short process of the incus.[5] To avoid this complication, we recommend the following technique for removal of the scutum.[4] In a right ear the surgeon should use the left hand and rotate the curette counterclockwise (**Fig. 3.1**). In a left ear the surgeon should use the right hand and rotate the curette in a clockwise direction (**Fig. 3.2**). The curettage of the scutum should be continued until the insertion of the stapedius tendon into the pyramidal process can be seen. If the bone of this area is very thick, we prefer using the diamond drill to reduce the scutum (**Fig. 3.3**).

Fracture of Lenticular Process

Fracture of the lenticular process may occur during the separation of the incudostapedial joint, fixation of the prosthesis, or removal of the scutum. It is usually possible to fix the prosthesis in more proximal regions of the lenticular process. If this is not possible a malleovestibulopexy may be needed.

Persistent Stapedial Artery

A persistent stapedial artery running through the stapes crura may obscure the view to the oval window (**Fig. 3.4**). This has been reported to occur in 1 of 1,000 ear surgeries.[9] Schuknecht[10] recommends removing the stapes suprastructure and placing the artery anteriorly, which allows a safe insertion of the prosthesis. If this maneuver does not allow adequate exposure to the oval window, then discontinuation of the surgery is recommended by some authors.[3] As recommended by others, we perform coagulation of the artery if the oval window is obscured.[4,11]

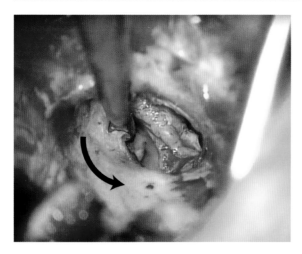

Fig. 3.1 Scutum curettage with the left hand in a right ear in counterclockwise direction.

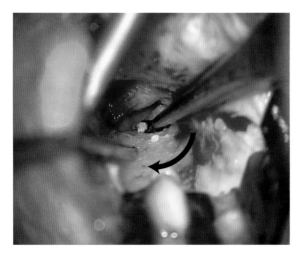

Fig. 3.2 Scutum curettage with the right hand in a left ear in clockwise direction.

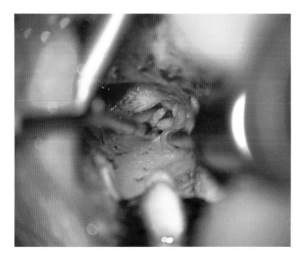

Fig. 3.3 Left ear: Scutum resection with the diamond bur.

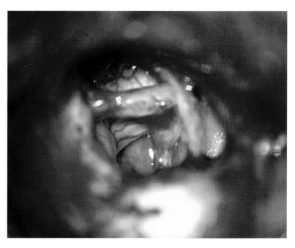

Fig. 3.4 Right ear: Persistent stapedial artery running through the tympanic cavity.

Narrowed Oval Niche

A thick bony promontory wall may cause a profoundly narrowed oval niche. In these cases, the bony area can be removed using a fine diamond bur at low rotation speed after the stapes suprastructure is removed. It is important to perform this technique before the footplate is opened.[12] Sometimes an abnormal low-running or dehiscent facial nerve can partially or completely occlude the view to the oval window. In most cases of a partially occluded oval window, insertion of the prosthesis is still possible (**Fig. 3.5**). If the oval window is completely blocked, some authors recommend termination of the surgery.[13] In our department, a windowing of the promontory is performed.[3] Häusler[3] reported on 39 patients with stapedectomies and abnormal positioning of the facial nerve, and in 82% of these patients a postoperative conductive hearing loss of less than 20 dB was achieved. There was no case of facial palsy or deafness after surgery.

Obliterative Otosclerosis

In cases of an obliterative footplate with broad thickening of the footplate, a fine diamond bur (e.g., Skeeter drill) is used for perforation of the footplate to achieve a small opening to the vestibule (**Fig. 3.6**). The incidence of obliterative otosclerosis ranges between 1 and 16%.[5]

Floating Footplate

A free-floating footplate is a serious intraoperative event during stapes surgery. It describes a completely mobile footplate, which may occur during the perforation of the footplate, especially when the footplate has a "biscuit-type" thickening of the middle part. If a floating footplate occurs, we recommend drilling a small perforation on the promontory side of the vestibule using a fine diamond bur (0.6 mm) and carefully lifting and removing the footplate

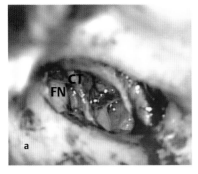
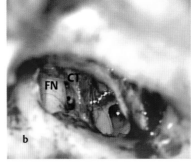
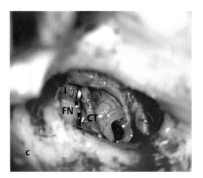

Fig. 3.5a–c Right ear. FN: facial nerve; CT: chorda tympani; I: incus.

a Footplate partially covered by overhanging facial nerve.

b Stapedotomy in the posterior region of the footplate.

c Insertion of prosthesis.

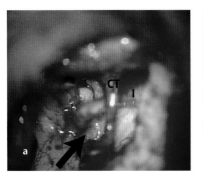
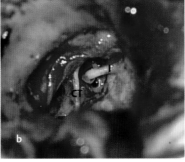
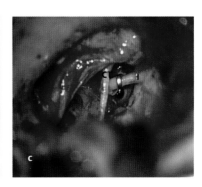

Fig. 3.6a–c Left ear. CT: chorda tympani; I: incus.

a Obliterative otosclerosis with thick footplate.

b Condition after stapedotomy with the Skeeter drill.

c Insertion of prosthesis.

using a small hook.[14] If all or part of the footplate is displaced into the vestibule, it is best to leave it there. If such is the case, we recommend covering the footplate with connective tissue and discontinuing the stapes surgery. If parts of the footplate are fractured, a small hook is inserted into the posterior portion of the footplate and the fractured piece is carefully pulled out.

Gusher

Another intraoperative condition is the "gusher" phenomenon, which describes an intense and massive flow of perilymph/cerebrospinal fluid after perforation of the footplate. A patent cochlear aqueduct is believed to cause this phenomenon, and it is more often seen in patients with inner ear anomalies.[11] There are more reports of a gusher on the left side than on the right.[15] In cases of a heavy gusher, the surgery should be discontinued and a "waterproof" closure of the oval window should be made using fat or connective tissue. The "oozer" is a milder gusher and can often be controlled by the quick insertion of the prosthesis and sealing with connective tissue. In cases of a more extensive discharge of cerebrospinal

fluid, a lumbar drain can help to reduce the pressure of the cerebrospinal fluid.[16]

Prosthesis

The distance between the lenticular process and the footplate varies between 3.9 and 5 mm. In most cases, we use a 4.5-mm prosthesis. A prosthesis that is too long may come into contact with the utricle or saccule, which can cause profound vertigo and tinnitus. The tip of the prosthesis should not penetrate more than 0.5 mm into the vestibule.

Immediate Postoperative Complications

Vertigo

Immediate postoperative vertigo can be caused by a loss of perilymph, mechanically induced irritation of the inner ear, or a serous labyrinthitis.[3] Symptoms usually subside after a few days. If inner ear damage is suspected, an application of high-dose corticosteroids (250 to 1,000 mg intravenous prednisone once daily on three consecutive days) is recommended.[17] Loosening of the packing of the ear canal may also improve the symptoms.

Vertigo combined with fluctuating hearing can be a characteristic sign of a perilymphatic fistula. If a fistula is suspected, immediate revision and closure of the oval window by connective tissue should be performed. Progressing sensorineural hearing loss and persistent vertigo despite conservative therapy (high-dose corticosteroids and antibiotics) also necessitate an immediate surgical revision.[18] For early detection of these complications, it is necessary to perform continuous examination of the patient using the glasses of Frenzel and a tuning fork. In cases of immediate revision with removal of the prosthesis, revision surgery for hearing improvement can be performed after 6 months.

Inflammation

To prevent inflammation of the auricular canal and tympanic membrane the patient has to be advised not to wear hearing aids for at least 1 week before surgery. In cases of an infection with herpes simplex or other infection of the upper airway, stapes surgery should be postponed.[19]

Hearing Loss

Hearing loss is considered to be the most serious complication after stapes surgery. Most authors estimate the risk at 1%, but there is wide variation in the incidence of this complication in different studies.[3] In most cases the reason for postoperative deafness is unclear.[20] Some surgical methods that pose an increased risk for the inner ear and subsequent hearing loss have been abandoned (e.g., coverage of the oval niche with Gelfoam, which was accompanied by an increased risk of inner ear fistulas[21]). If an inner ear complication is suspected, then high-dose therapy with corticosteroids as well as antibiotics should be initiated.[17] In addition, before surgery, patients should be informed about the alternative treatment of hearing aid fitting.

Reparative Granuloma

Another postoperative complication, which usually occurs within 7 to 15 days after surgery, is a reparative granuloma. A major symptom is progressive inner ear hearing loss after immediate postoperative hearing improvement. Otoscopic examination will show an erythematous and thickened tympanic membrane.[15] If there is suspicion of this complication, immediate revision surgery is recommended.

Long-term Postoperative Complications

Vertigo that persists for months after surgery is usually a sign of a prosthesis extending too far into the vestibule. In such cases, the revision and replacement of the prosthesis against a shorter piston is necessary.

Impairment of hearing with increase of the air–bone gap can happen several years following stapes surgery.[18] An indication for revision surgery is a persistent or new conductive hearing loss of 20 dB or more.[22] The most common finding in revision stapes surgery is incus erosion with displacement of the prosthesis. In most of these cases a more proximal fixation of the prosthesis at the long process of the incus is successful. If this is not possible, a malleovestibulopexy will be necessary. The risk of damage to the inner ear after revision surgery is estimated at ~ 2.2%.[3]

Ossicular Chain Reconstruction

Ossicular chain reconstruction may be necessary for several indications, such as trauma, tympanosclerosis, or cholesteatoma. Potential complications during surgery are usually dependent on the extent of surgery and the disease of origin. The critical point in the proper management of ossicular chain reconstruction is to choose the right technique in the right case. In general, we recommend that beginners of ear surgery perform one learned technique (grafting with fascia or cartilage, use of prosthesis, etc.) in at least 100 to 200 cases before starting to develop new or modified methods. Our focus here is to highlight the main complications and barriers in ossicular chain reconstruction and how to deal with these problems. **Table 3.2** summarizes the main principles.

Intraoperative Challenges and Complications

Bleeding

Bleeding is a general problem and is more probable in cases of severe infection or during surgery involving vascularized processes (e.g., paragangliomas). Prevention of bleeding starts with the proper positioning of the patient on the operating table (head up, feet down). Bleeding during the opening procedure needs to be immediately controlled to prevent continuous bleeding from blocking the surgeon's view. Diffuse bleeding from the middle ear mucosa may be controlled by the application of epinephrine (1:1,000). Epinephrine may be administered either as a direct fluid injection or as a Gelfoam application. During this time any necessary grafts, such as cartilage,

Table 3.2 Complications and their management in ossicular chain reconstruction

Intraoperative complications	Management
Diffuse bleeding	Epinephrine solution 1:1,000 for few minutes
Jugular bulb laceration	Immediate forced packing of the hypotympanum with Surgicel
Facial nerve injury	Superficial: coverage with cartilage Transection: immediate interposition with greater auricular nerve
Footplate fracture	Immediate coverage with tissue 1,000 mg prednisolone Intravenous antibiotics
Postoperative complications	Management
Vertigo, inner ear hearing loss	Corticosteroids, antibiotics; if no response then revision
Facial nerve palsy	Wait and scan If no resolution within 6 hours then think about revision Refer to special center
Intraoperative challenges	Management
Medially rotated malleus	Transection of tensor tympani tendon
Incus erosion	Short: bridging with cement Long: incus interposition Cholesteatoma: titanium prosthesis
Medially rotated stapes	Insertion of total ossicular replacement prosthesis between the stapes crura directly on the footplate
Instable prosthesis on the footplate	Cartilage or cartilage shoe

can be harvested. In severe cases of bleeding, packing of the tympanic cavity with hemostyptics such as Surgicel (Ethicon Company, Somerville, NJ, USA) is an option. Finally, interventional obliteration of the bleeding vessel by the neuroradiologist may be considered.

Massive intraoperative bleeding while working in the hypotympanon is usually a result of laceration of a dehiscent high jugular bulb. The incidence of a high jugular bulb is reported to be between 0.5 and 25%.[23–25] A high jugular bulb may be suspected after noticing a blue transparency behind the tympanic membrane. Paracentesis and injuries during middle ear preparation may result in severe bleeding. Usually immediate compression with Surgicel for several minutes stops the bleeding, and the surgery can be continued. The dehiscent area of the high jugular bulb should be covered with cartilage. If this management fails and the bleeding persists, the tympanic membrane can be reconstructed and a pressure packing put in the external auditory canal.[26]

Malleus

The distance between the handle of the malleus and the stapes or promontory varies widely. In chronic and adhesive otitis media, the umbo area of the malleus may be closely positioned to the promontory or even adherent to it. Tympanic membrane reconstruction may be difficult or impossible when the ossicular chain is intact. To elevate the handle of the malleus from the promontory, the tensor tympani tendon can be cut. Disconnection of the ossicular chain should only be considered if no other solution is suitable. When an incus interposition is planned, the height of the shaped incus has to be adapted to the distance between the malleus handle and stapes. In most cholesteatoma cases, when there is need of ossicle separation, we recommend resecting the head of the malleus. By transecting the tensor tympani tendon, it is possible to rotate the malleus handle upward. This maneuver allows restoration of the normal distance between the malleus handle and promontory in most cases. The handle of the malleus should be preserved whenever possible because it plays an important role in the audiometric success of the ossiculoplasty.[27]

A fixation of the malleoincudal joint in chronic otitis media may be the reason for relevant conductive hearing loss. Different options for remobilization should be considered. According to Tos[28] obstructing plaque can be removed at the site of the joint over an atticoantrotomy after partially resecting the attic wall with a curette. This method allows the preservation of an intact chain but does carry risk for refixation. Alternatively, removal of the incus and shaping with the drill, followed by interposition of the autograft between the head of the stapes and the handle of the malleus may be considered. An alloplastic prosthesis (e.g., titanium partial ossicular replacement prosthesis [PORP]) can also be interpositioned. In this case the plate of the PORP needs to be covered with a flat piece of cartilage to prevent protrusion.[29]

Incus

One of the main pathologic findings in the ossicles that demands a proper reconstruction is discontinuity of the incudostapedial joint. This condition is usually the result of an erosion of the lenticular process. It may occur in chronic middle ear infections, such as tympanic membrane retraction, or in an adhesive process with a spontaneous type III situation (contact of tympanic membrane with incus). In most cases, a fibrous connection between the incus and stapes is still present and does not allow proper sound conduction.

Several ossiculoplasty techniques are described in the literature based on the extent of erosion. For short defects, some authors recommend using a small piece of cortical bone to bridge the interruption and report good results.[30,31] Others recommend using cement for the reconstruction, which is called incudostapedial rebridging ossiculoplasty. Several authors report good results applying this technique, with an air–bone gap closure of less than 20 dB in the majority of cases.[30,32] The incudostapedial gap can also be bridged using a prosthesis, based on the technique described by Plester.[33] In our department, an incus interposition is the favorable surgical technique in chronic otitis media. PORP autograft incus interposition (see above) can be performed in several ways.[11,14,28,29] We recommend fixing the removed incus in a blood vessel clamp and reducing the long process to the level of the incus body. The short process is then drilled back to the necessary length to bridge the distance between the stapes and malleus. In addition, a small groove to accommodate the stapes head is drilled into the short process.[29]

In cholesteatoma surgery, we prefer using a titanium prosthesis instead of the incus. Only in special cholesteatoma cases, like small congenital cholesteatomas when there is no sign of ossicle erosion, do we recommend an incus interposition.

Fixation of the incus usually occurs in the malleoincudal joint and is treated as mentioned above. A fixation at the incudostapedial joint is rare.[34] A bony connection between both ossicles may be seen in cases of small middle ear malformations (conglomerate ossicles).[35] If the stapes footplate is also fixed, stapes surgery or malleovestibulopexy may be an option. Total ossicular replacement prosthesis (TORP) autograft incus interposition between the stapes footplate and malleus is not recommended because of the risk of a bony fixation of the graft with the surrounding structures (e.g., canal of facial nerve) over time.

Stapes

The structures of the stapes can be involved in several pathologies of the middle ear, including trauma, tympanosclerosis, otosclerosis, and malformation. The stapes footplate may also be used to couple the transducer (e.g., Floating Mass Transducer, Vibrant Soundbridge) of an implantable hearing aid. A serious complication of middle ear surgery is fracture of the footplate, with subsequent perilymph fistula and possible inner ear damage or complete deafness. Especially in cholesteatoma surgery with stapes involvement, dissection work on the footplate can mobilize or fracture the footplate. If this happens, the footplate should be immediately covered with connective tissue and 1,000 mg prednisolone and antibiotics should be intravenously administered. Hearing restoration surgery should then be performed 1 year later in a second-look operation.

Conductive hearing loss may be a result of tympanosclerotic stapes fixation. Tympanosclerotic plaques need to be removed to allow the ossicles to vibrate. Stapes mobilization usually only results in a short-term hearing improvement because of the high risk of refixation.[36] Therefore, in most cases a stapedotomy with the insertion of a stapes prosthesis is recommended. Because of the bacterial involvement of the sclerotic plaques,[37] there is a higher risk of deafness in tympanosclerosis than in otosclerosis if the inner ear is opened. Therefore, it is very important not to mobilize the stapes.

Our strategy depends on the following clinical findings. If the patient is deaf in the contralateral ear, a stapedoplasty is contraindicated and hearing aids are recommended. If the patient has normal hearing in the contralateral ear, then a staged stapedoplasty can be discussed.[36] Surgical manipulation at the site of the stapes footplate should only be considered when the tympanic membrane is intact. In all other cases, a second-look procedure for hearing improvement should be performed. If stapes surgery seems too risky for inner ear or vestibular injury, the adaptation of an implantable hearing aid may be promising. There is some evidence that the coupling of the Floating Mass Transducer to the round window even works effectively when the footplate is fixed.[38]

Another important challenging intraoperative finding is the condition of the stapes. According to Tos[39] several defects of the stapedial arch may be found. In his series, the incidence of stapes erosion varied between 3% in chronic otitis media up to 10% in cholesteatomas.[28,40] One important variation is the missing stapes head, which makes the insertion of a PORP difficult. In this situation, and also when there are erosions or missing parts of the anterior or posterior arch, we do not recommend using PORPs. Instead, and when there is a highly medially rotated stapes, it is better to use a TORP, which is placed directly between the stapes arches on the footplate (**Fig. 3.7**).

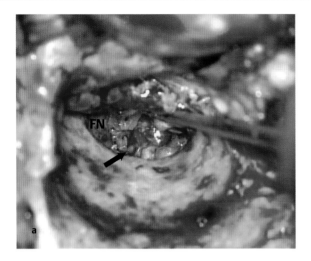

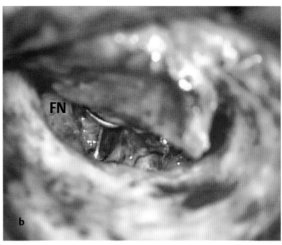

Fig. 3.7a,b Right ear. FN: facial nerve.

a Medially rotated stapes (black arrow) after incus interposition.

b Insertion of a total ossicular replacement prosthesis between the stapes crura on the footplate.

It was mentioned earlier that a TORP incus interposition on the stapes footplate is not recommended because of potential osseus fixation.[41] Also, PORP interpositions on the head of the stapes may develop a tightly fixed connection over time, leading to difficult separation of the ossicles during revision surgery. Usually ossifications can best be opened with gentle movements of the sickle knife tip or the needle. Because of these complications, some authors recommend the insertion of alloplastic prostheses in all reconstruction procedures of the ossicular chain. However, although titanium prostheses are reported to have high middle ear biocompatibility, without osseus fixation,[42] a fixed bony connection between the foot of a titanium TORP and the stapes footplate has been reported.[43] During revision surgery, the prosthesis was removed along with the adherent footplate. Tight fixations between alloplastic materials and bony parts of the middle ear have to be considered as potential complications, and these may be loosened with the sickle knife or with the laser (beware the facial nerve!).

In severely infected ears, the stapes may be completely integrated into granulation tissue, and gentle probing with a microinstrument can give evidence of stapes integrity and mobility. If the stapes is integrated into granulation tissue, it should be left alone. Our experience is that if the surgeon succeeds in creating a well-aerated middle ear, the granulations will usually heal and disappear.

Insertion of the Prosthesis

The chosen prosthesis must fit easily and stably into the designated space of the ossicular chain. Too high a pressure on the head of the stapes or the footplate may cause vertigo. Too much force to the tympanic membrane may result in protrusion.

The lengths of PORPs and TORPs in ossicular chain reconstruction depend on the experience of the surgeon. As described by others, in most cases we use a 2.0-mm PORP and a 4.0-mm TORP.[44] However, if there is a flat or high tympanic cavity, other prostheses may be needed. Less experienced ear surgeons who feel uncertain in estimating the length of the prosthesis should not hesitate to test the length with commercially available silicone dummies (TORP and PORP) (**Fig. 3.8**).

Proper positioning and adaptation of the TORP at the site of the stapes footplate is mandatory for successful sound transduction to the inner ear. In most cases the foot of the prosthesis can be placed without additional stabilization. If the prosthesis tends to slip off the footplate, there are different options to prevent dislocation. In some selected cases we prefer using the cartilage shoe (**Fig. 3.9**). A cartilage shoe can be punched out of a piece

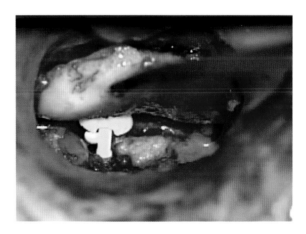

Fig. 3.8 Measuring the height of a total ossicular replacement prosthesis using a silicone dummy.

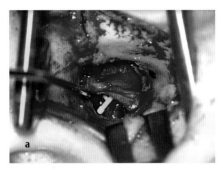 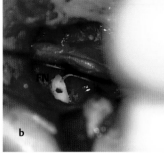 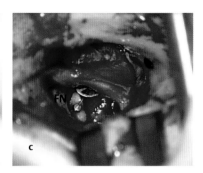

Fig. 3.9a–c Using a cartilage shoe. FN: facial nerve.

a Measuring the height of a total ossicular replacement prosthesis (TORP) using a silicone dummy.

b Cartilage shoe on the footplate.

c Condition after securing a TORP on the footplate with the cartilage shoe.

of cartilage using a commercially available instrument (Atos Medical Company, Hörby, Sweden). The cartilage shoe is similar to the medium shape and size of the footplate, and a central hole to accommodate the foot of the prosthesis is created at the same time.[45] Another option is the use of the so-called Ω-connector (Kurz Company, Dusslingen, Germany), which is placed on the footplate. This is a titanium device with a coupling system that allows connection to the foot of the TORP.[46] When using the Ω-connector, the prosthesis should be 0.5 mm shorter than without the device.

Facial Nerve

The facial nerve is the most delicate structure of the temporal bone, and every otologic surgeon has to know its exact course from the internal auditory canal through the tympanic cavity and the mastoid to the stylomastoid foramen. To study the route of the nerve and prevent iatrogenic damage, repeated drilling of cadaver temporal bone are strongly recommended. Most frequently, the site of the dehiscence is in the tympanic cavity (**Fig. 3.10**). A facial nerve dehiscence is more often seen in cholesteatoma than in chronic otitis media. It is also more often reported in adults and in revision surgeries.[47,48]

The facial nerve can be found without any bony covering at different parts of the temporal bone. This may occur spontaneously or after exposure to temporal bone diseases, such as cholesteatoma, or after trauma. In cases of an uncovered facial nerve inside the tympanic cavity next to the oval niche, care has to be taken during the placement of the prosthesis. Alloplastic materials should not come into contact with the perineurium, and no pressure should be applied to the nerve tissue. Connective tissue may be placed between the prosthesis and the nerve to prevent nerve injury. If there is any danger of nerve compression or if the nerve covers the stapes footplate, the adaptation of an implantable hearing aid (e.g., Vibrant Soundbridge) to the round window should be considered instead of ossicular chain reconstruction.

In situations where the footplate is not suitable for ossicular chain reconstruction, fenestration surgery may be considered, where the prosthesis can be adapted to the inner ear via the promontory or the lateral semicircular canal. However, since the successful introduction of implantable hearing devices, fenestration surgery has become relatively uncommon.

Monitoring of the facial nerve during temporal bone surgery does not replace anatomical knowledge but may be helpful in difficult ear cases, such as extended cholesteatomas, paragangliomas, malformations, or revision surgery. It is recommended that the surgeon does not rely primarily on facial nerve monitoring but, instead, uses monitoring to reconfirm identification of the facial nerve according to anatomical findings and surgical knowledge. To reduce iatrogenic damage to the facial nerve, we recommend electrophysiologic monitoring of the nerve in cholesteatoma revision surgeries. In this situation the risk of facial nerve damage is higher because of the modified anatomy. In anatomically challenging situations caused

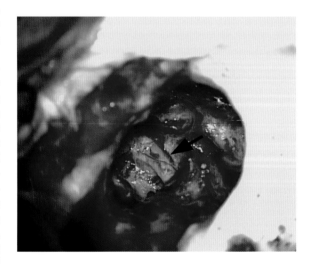

Fig. 3.10 Partly uncovered facial nerve (tympanic part) in revision surgery.

by several surgeries or anomalies, a high-resolution computed tomography scan can give good information on the course of the facial nerve.

With modern navigation software, navigated surgery of the temporal bone and the lateral skull base is also an option. Particularly in cases of temporal bone tumors, vestibular schwannomas, paragangliomas, malformations, or difficult cases of revision surgery, computer navigation may be considered. If necessary, matched imaging of magnetic resonance images and computed tomography scans is possible.

If intraoperative iatrogenic damage to the facial nerve does occur, the treatment depends on the extent of the injury. If only the epineural sheath is injured, the nerve is covered with cartilage. If there is a complete transection of the nerve, a nerve interponation from the greater auricular nerve is performed.[49]

Chorda Tympani

Damage of the chorda tympani may result in severe discomfort for the patient, along with ipsilateral malsensation of the lateral tongue and an inconvenient metallic taste. These symptoms usually disappear after several months.[50] However, the chorda tympani should be preserved whenever possible. If the chorda tympani hinders the approach to middle ear structures, transection should be preferred over distension.[7] Our experiences show that the chorda tympani is more vulnerable in cases of otosclerosis than in chronic infectious ear diseases such as cholesteatoma.

Immediate Postoperative Complications

Vertigo and Inner Ear Damage

Vertigo after tympanoplasty may have different causes, such as direct damage to the vestibular system or the inner ear or a dislocated or oversized prosthesis. Treatment has to be individually adapted to the patient findings. Dizziness may be tolerated as long as the tuning fork lateralizes to the operated ear. Loosening or partial removal of the packing from the external auditory canal may reduce the symptom. Also, high doses of corticosteroids can protect the inner ear from further damage.

If vertigo does not improve or even deteriorates under the mentioned therapy or the tuning fork lateralizes to the contralateral ear, revision surgery should be considered. Usually any alloplastic prosthesis will be removed, and a second-look operation will be scheduled after several months.

The treatment for sensorineural hearing loss following ear surgery is the same as the therapy for vertigo. High doses of corticosteroids are administered, and if the

tuning fork lateralizes to the nonoperated ear, revision surgery with removal of the prosthesis is necessary.[49]

Facial Nerve Palsy

Facial nerve palsy after middle ear surgery is a severe problem and needs to be further evaluated. First, the effect of local anesthesia to the nerve needs to be considered. If this is the case, nerve function should be normal after several hours. The surgeon needs to decide whether direct nerve damage during the operation may be the origin. In such cases, the palsy is present during the immediate postoperative period, and immediate surgery with decompression or readaptation of the facial nerve may be advisable. If facial nerve damage progressively develops during the postoperative period, nerve swelling inside the Fallopian canal has to be considered. In such cases, if nerve decongestion with high doses of corticosteroids fails, then reoperation with nerve decompression will be necessary. It is then advisable to refer the patient to an experienced otologic surgeon or to a special department with profound expertise in ear surgery.[49]

Long-term Postoperative Complications

In chronic otitis media, postoperative protrusion of alloplastic prostheses may occur for several reasons. Rejection of alloplastic materials may be one cause. However, since the advent of titanium prostheses, which provide high middle ear biocompatibility, rejection is less of an issue.[42]

In cases of progressive middle ear diseases, protrusion of the prosthesis may occur because of continuous retraction of the tympanic membrane caused by negative pressure inside the tympanic cavity. To prevent protrusion, the plate of the prosthesis facing the tympanic membrane should be covered by a flat piece of cartilage.[29,41] In addition, all attempts to improve middle ear aeration may help to prevent this complication. In poorly aerated ears a mastoidectomy or tubal dilatation[51] may be considered. If protrusion of the prosthesis[52,53] re-occurs, middle ear implantable hearing systems may be an option.

References

1. Sudhoff H, Hildmann H. Cholesteatoma surgery. In: Sudhoff H, Hildmann H, eds. Middle Ear Surgery. Heidelberg: Springer; 2006:67–72
2. Helms J. Local anesthesia of the Ear. In: Jahrsdoerfer RA, Helms J, eds. Ear Head and Neck Surgery. Stuttgart: Thieme; 1996
3. Häusler R. Advances in stapes surgery. In: Jahnke K, ed. Middle Ear Surgery. Recent Advances and Future Directions. Stuttgart: Thieme; 2004:95–140
4. Sudhoff H, Hildmann H. Stapes surgery. In: Sudhoff H, Hildmann H, eds. Middle Ear Surgery. Heidelberg: Springer; 2006:112–119

5. Tos M. Surgical solutions for conductive hearing loss. Manual of Middle Ear Surgery, Vol. 4. Stuttgart: Thieme; 2000

6. Perkins R. Prevention of complications in stapes surgery. In: Wiet RJ, ed. Ear and Temporal Bone Surgery Minimizing Risks and Complications. New York: Thieme; 2006:81–89

7. Michael P, Raut V. Chorda tympani injury: operative findings and postoperative symptoms. Otolaryngol Head Neck Surg 2007;136(6):978–981

8. Miuchi S, Sakagami M, Tsuzuki K, Noguchi K, Mishiro Y, Katsura H. Taste disturbance after stapes surgery—clinical and experimental study. Acta Otolaryngol Suppl 2009;(562):71–78

9. Marion M, Hinojosa R, Khan AA. Persistence of the stapedial artery: a histopathologic study. Otolaryngol Head Neck Surg 1985;93(3):298–312

10. Schuknecht HF. Otosclerosis surgery. In: Nadol JB, Schuknecht HF. eds. Surgery of the Ear and Temporal Bone. New York: Raven Press; 1993

11. Sanna M, Sunose H, Mancini F, Russo A, Taibah A. Middle Ear and Mastoid Microsurgery. Stuttgart: Thieme; 2003

12. Naumann HH, Wilmes E. Operations for stapes ankylosis. In: Jahrsdoerfer RA, Helms J. eds. Head and Neck Surgery Vol II Ear. New York: Thieme; 1996:229–261

13. Welling DB, Glasscock ME III, Gantz BJ. Avulsion of the anomalous facial nerve at stapedectomy. Laryngoscope 1992;102(7):729–733

14. Fisch U. Tympanoplasty, Mastoidectomy, and Stapes Surgery. Stuttgart: Thieme; 2008

15. Roland PS, Meyerhoff WL. Otosclerosis. In: Bailey BJ, ed. Head and Neck Surgery—Otolaryngology. Philadelphia: Lippincott Williams & Wilkins; 2001

16. Schwager K. Acute complications during middle ear surgery: part 2: Accidents in classical stapes surgery and their solutions. [Article in German] HNO 2007;55(5):411–416, quiz 417–418

17. Dornhoffer JL, Milewski C. Management of the open labyrinth. Otolaryngol Head Neck Surg 1995;112(3):410–414

18. Dazert S, Hildmann H. Stapes revision surgery. In: Hildmann H, Sudhoff H. eds. Middle Ear Surgery. Heidelberg: Springer; 2006:131–133

19. Minovi A, Probst G, Dazert S. Current concepts in the surgical management of otosclerosis. [Article in German] HNO 2009;57(3):273–286

20. Mann WJ, Amedee RG, Fuerst G, Tabb HG. Hearing loss as a complication of stapes surgery. Otolaryngol Head Neck Surg 1996;115(4):324–328

21. Sheehy JL, Perkins JH. Stapedectomy: gelfoam compared with tissue grafts. Laryngoscope 1976;86(3):436–444

22. Jahnke K, Solzbacher D, Dost P. Revision stapes surgery. Adv Otorhinolaryngol 2007;65:314–319

23. Huang BR, Wang CH, Young YH. Dehiscent high jugular bulb: a pitfall in middle ear surgery. Otol Neurotol 2006;27(7):923–927

24. Overton SB, Ritter FN. A high placed jugular bulb in the middle ear: a clinical and temporal bone study. Laryngoscope 1973;83(12):1986–1991

25. Savic D, Djeric D. Surgical anatomy of the hypotympanum. J Laryngol Otol 1987;101(5):419–425

26. Moore PJ. The high jugular bulb in ear surgery: three case reports and a review of the literature. J Laryngol Otol 1994;108(9):772–775

27. Bared A, Angeli SI. Malleus handle: determinant of success in ossiculoplasty. Am J Otolaryngol 2010;31(4):235–240

28. Tos M. Manual of Middle Ear Surgery. Vol. 1: Approaches, Myringoplasty, Ossiculoplasty, Tympanoplasty. Stuttgart: Thieme; 1993

29. Sudhoff H, Hildmann H. Ossicular Chain Reconstruction. In: Sudhoff H, Hildmann H. eds. Middle Ear Surgery. Heidelberg: Springer; 2006:49–54

30. Celik H, Aslan Felek S, Islam A, Demirci M, Samim E, Oztuna D. The impact of fixated glass ionomer cement and springy cortical bone incudostapedial joint reconstruction on hearing results. Acta Otolaryngol 2009;129(12):1368–1373

31. Solomons NB, Robinson JM. Bone pâté repair of the eroded incus. J Laryngol Otol 1989;103(1):41–42

32. Baglam T, Karatas E, Durucu C, et al. Incudostapedial rebridging ossiculoplasty with bone cement. Otolaryngol Head Neck Surg 2009;141(2):243–246

33. Maassen MM, Zenner HP. Tympanoplasty type II with ionomeric cement and titanium-gold-angle prostheses. Am J Otol 1998;19(6):693–699

34. Suzuki M, Kanebayashi H, Kawano A, et al. Involvement of the incudostapedial joint anomaly in conductive deafness. Acta Otolaryngol 2008;128(5):515–519

35. Teunissen EB, Cremers WR. Classification of congenital middle ear anomalies. Report on 144 ears. Ann Otol Rhinol Laryngol 1993;102(8 Pt 1):606–612

36. Gurr A, Hildmann H, Stark T, Dazert S. Treatment of tympanosclerosis. [Article in German] HNO 2008;56(6):651–657, quiz 658

37. Asiri S, Hasham A, al Anazy F, Zakzouk S, Banjar A. Tympanosclerosis: review of literature and incidence among patients with middle-ear infection. J Laryngol Otol 1999;113(12):1076–1080

38. Colletti V, Soli SD, Carner M, Colletti L. Treatment of mixed hearing losses via implantation of a vibratory transducer on the round window. Int J Audiol 2006;45(10):600–608

39. Tos M. Tympanoplasty in partial defects of the stapedial arch. J Laryngol Otol 1975;89(3):249–257

40. Tos M. Pathology of the ossicular chain in various chronic middle ear diseases. J Laryngol Otol 1979;93(8):769–780

41. Zahnert T. Hearing disorder. Surgical management. [Article in German] Laryngorhinootologie 2005;84(Suppl 1):S37–S50

42. Schwager K. Titanium as an ossicular replacement material: results after 336 days of implantation in the rabbit. Am J Otol 1998;19(5):569–573

43. Sudhoff H, Lindner N, Gronemeyer J, Dazert S, Hildmann H. Study of osteointegration of a titanium prosthesis to the stapes: observations on an accidentally extracted stapes. Otol Neurotol 2005;26(4):583–586

44. Dornhoffer JL. Cartilage tympanoplasty. Otolaryngol Clin North Am 2006;39(6):1161–1176

45. Beutner D, Luers JC, Huttenbrink KB. Cartilage 'shoe': a new technique for stabilisation of titanium total ossicular replacement prosthesis at centre of stapes footplate. J Laryngol Otol 2008;122(7):682–686

46. Schmid G, Steinhardt U, Heckmann W. The omega connector—a module for jointed coupling of titanium total prostheses in the middle ear. [Article in German] Laryngorhinootologie 2009;88(12):782–788

47. Kim CW, Rho YS, Ahn HY, Oh SJ. Facial canal dehiscence in the initial operation for chronic otitis media without cholesteatoma. Auris Nasus Larynx 2008;35(3):353–356

48. Magliulo G, Colicchio MG, Ciniglio M. Facial nerve dehiscence and cholesteatoma. Ann Otol Rhinol Laryngol 2011;120(4):261–267

49. Schwager K. Acute complications during middle ear surgery: part 1: Problems during tympanoplasty–what to do? [Article in German] HNO 2007;55(4):307–315; quiz 316–317

50. Guinand N, Just T, Stow NW, Van HC, Landis BN. Cutting the chorda tympani: not just a matter of taste. J Laryngol Otol 2010;124(9):999–1002

51. Ockermann T, Reineke U, Upile T, Ebmeyer J, Sudhoff HH. Balloon dilatation eustachian tuboplasty: a clinical study. Laryngoscope 2010;120(7):1411–1416

52. Iñiguez-Cuadra R, Alobid I, Borés-Domenech A, Menéndez-Colino LM, Caballero-Borrego M, Bernal-Sprekelsen M. Type III tympanoplasty with titanium total ossicular replacement prosthesis: anatomic and functional results. Otol Neurotol 2010;31(3):409–414

53. Sheehy JL. TORPs and PORPs: causes of failure—a report on 446 operations. Otolaryngol Head Neck Surg 1984;92(5):583–587

4 Complications of Mastoidectomy

M. B. Gluth, J. L. Dornhoffer

Mastoidectomy is one of the fundamental surgical techniques in otologic surgery. Not only is it commonly indicated, but it also acts as a building block for numerous other temporal bone surgical procedures. Accordingly, an understanding of the principles related to the prevention and management of mastoidectomy complications is a worthy topic of discussion and learning for otolaryngologists at all levels of expertise. To this end, an overview of the most common mastoidectomy-related complications is reviewed in this chapter.

Preoperative Considerations

Otologic surgeons must recognize and minimize poor operating conditions that could increase the risk of mastoidectomy complications. Many of these factors are outlined in **Fig. 4.1**. It is the surgeon's responsibility as a patient advocate to assume control of and take responsibility for the quality of the operating environment. Furthermore, when conditions are poor but surgery is nonetheless indicated, novice temporal bone surgeons should

---

- Malfunctioning operating room equipment
- Defective surgical instruments
- Disruptive noise or commotion
- Operating room staff and anesthesia colleagues unfamiliar with otologic surgery
- Excessively bloody surgical field
  - Insufficiently hypotensive anesthesia
  - Poor preoperative local vasoconstrictor medication infiltration
  - Coagulopathy
  - Severe acute tympanomastoid inflammation
- Distorted tissue planes
  - Trauma
  - Previous surgery
  - Tumor
  - Infection
- Unfavorable patient anatomy
  - Large body habitus
  - Poor neck flexibility
  - Prominent shoulder and/or chest

Fig. 4.1 Factors that may contribute to poor otologic surgical conditions.

---

be under direct constant supervision or should assume an observational role.

When the risk of complications is deemed to be higher than normal, as with congenital anomalies, cholesteatoma, trauma, or revision surgery, the authors recommend acquisition and close scrutiny of preoperative high-resolution computed tomography (HRCT) imaging. Controversy exists regarding the need for acquisition of imaging before every mastoidectomy procedure,[1] and there is no clear published evidence that such imaging prevents surgical complications; however, it is our assertion that HRCT is a valuable tool for anticipating the extent of disease, the type and scale of surgery required, and the anatomical subtleties unique to each patient.[2–5] All of this has value in preoperative patient counseling.

Intraoperative Complications

Facial Nerve Injury

Outlook and Prevention

There is arguably no more feared complication in mastoid surgery than unintentional injury to the facial nerve. Not only are there significant negative medical consequences to such an injury (e.g., corneal exposure, paralytic ectropion, oral incompetence), but the psychosocial effects of facial disfigurement are profound, including negative self-image, depression, and social rejection. It is therefore imperative for surgeons to go to great lengths to avoid this complication.

The incidence of iatrogenic facial nerve injury is variable and depends on the skill and experience of the surgeon. Reported rates of injury are around 1 case in 1,000 with experienced surgeons, but may be higher with inexperienced surgeons at a teaching facility.[6–8] For revision surgery, the risk of injury is probably increased. The most common site of injury during mastoidectomy has been reported to be the second genu at the junction of the tympanic and mastoid segments. Unlike the tympanic segment, which is often noted to be partially dehiscent in small areas, the second genu is usually covered by bone, except in rare cases of very extensive erosive cholesteatoma. Hence, most of these injuries can be traced to mistakes in drilling of the overlying bone.

Drill-related injuries to the facial nerve are usually related to a failure to properly identify the nerve in a controlled and systematic manner or failure to assure sufficient irrigation to prevent thermal injury. This phenomenon can be witnessed in the setting of training in the temporal bone laboratory, where novice surgeons often recklessly drill small, deep, and narrow mastoidectomy cavities with the aim of rapid and direct entry into the antrum. In a sclerotic mastoid, this faulty technique may result in drilling in a trajectory that is more inferior than intended, resulting in potential fenestration of the lateral semicircular canal and injury to the adjacent facial nerve. In contrast, proper safe technique requires wide methodical saucerization of the mastoid cavity that progresses with stepwise identification of one known anatomical landmark after another.

The authors' preferred sequence in mastoid drilling is as follows (see **Fig. 4.2**). First, the boundaries of the Macewen triangle are vaguely delineated. Then, broad strokes are used with a large bur around the temporal line (only a rough guide) until the tegmen is clearly identified at its lateral then inferior aspects. The sigmoid sinus is then widely demarcated in a similar manner. Next, with broad drill strokes, triangular dissection is executed that allows wide passage through the central tract of air cells and Koerner septum before progressing to controlled entry into the antrum. To be executed properly, one of the corners of the triangular dissection field must be located far enough anteriorly to lie deep to the zygomatic root. The lateral semicircular canal and the lateral process of the incus are then identified with careful widening of the antral opening. Next, drilling of the sinodural angle posteriorly and delineation of the digastric ridge inferiorly are undertaken.

The final sequence proceeds with copious irrigation and a medium-sized coarse diamond bur. This involves identification of the facial nerve by thinning the bone of the external auditory canal with slow controlled strokes

1. Broadly delineate tegmen
2. Skeletonize sigmoid sinus
3. Perform wide triangular dissection through central air cell tract and Koerner septum using tegmen and zygomatic root as guide marks to locate antrum
4. Widen antrum; identify lateral semicircular canal and incus
5. Thoroughly define sinodural angle and digastric ridge
6. Thin external auditory canal and identify facial nerve
7. Drill tip, perilabyrinthine, infralabyrinthine, retrolabyrinthine, and retrosigmoid air cells as needed
8. Open epitympanum with drilling of zygomatic root up to anterior attic wall

Fig. 4.2 Recommended sequence for mastoidectomy.

that span from just inferior to the lateral semicircular canal toward the mastoid tip and digastric ridge. The latter acts as a rough depth gauge of where one should expect to encounter the inferior aspect of the facial nerve. As is the case with skeletonization of the tegmen and sigmoid, exposure of the nerve over a broad front is desired. In most cases, it is preferable to preserve a thin layer of bone over the nerve once it is properly identified. In doing so, focal punctate bleeding vessels may be encountered in a vascular area supplied by the stylomastoid artery, commonly known as "sentinel bleeders." If hemostasis is required, gentle application of bone wax or other topical hemostatic agents are used in lieu of cauterization.

As a policy, it is beneficial to identify (but not expose) the facial nerve in every mastoidectomy procedure. Not only does this facilitate completeness of the operation, but it also leaves no room for doubt in the mind of the surgeon as to the status of the nerve at the completion of surgery. As one saying goes, "make the facial nerve your friend." Once identified, subsequent advanced techniques, such as removal of the mastoid tip or posterior tympanotomy, can be safely and confidently executed under direct visualization of a valuable landmark.

There is some debate as to the role of facial nerve monitoring as an adjuvant in mastoid surgery.[9,10] This pertains not only to the general question of use or nonuse, but also to whether it is indicated routinely or only in complicated and revision cases. There is no definitive evidence that facial nerve monitoring lowers the incidence of iatrogenic facial nerve injury in mastoidectomy. Nevertheless, the authors recommend routine monitoring in centers where otologic surgical training is undertaken and otherwise in cases that portend an increased risk of injury (e.g., congenital anomaly, cholesteatoma, trauma). The facial nerve monitor provides the additional advantage of affording nerve stimulation for identification when this is in question, such as in the case of extensive mastoid granulation tissue.

Management

Clinical trials in this area are generally not feasible, so acute management of iatrogenic facial nerve injury is based on both anecdotal guidelines and a general knowledge of principles applicable to motor nerve injury.[11] **Fig. 4.3** outlines a general scheme of management based on the timing of recognition and the severity of the injury, versions of which have been frequently cited over decades in otologic surgical teaching. In addition, it is common practice for most surgeons to treat these injuries with courses of high-dose intravenous corticosteroids that may be extended well into the postoperative recovery period with an oral dosing taper.

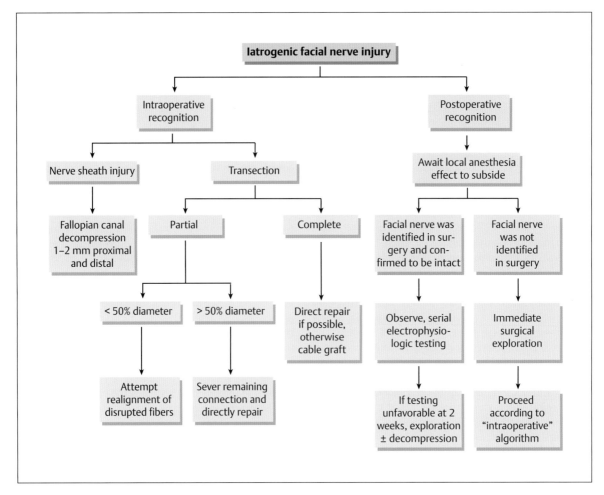

Fig. 4.3 Management scheme for iatrogenic facial nerve injury.

Sigmoid Sinus Injury

Outlook and Prevention

The sigmoid sinus is a major landmark in mastoid surgery; for this reason, the need to manage sigmoid sinus bleeding will arise on at least a few occasions throughout the career of most otologic surgeons. For those unfamiliar with this situation, it can be a very dramatic and fear-invoking experience as the surgical field may be rapidly and completely flooded with blood. Fortunately, the vast majority of these injuries can be easily controlled with simple measures if they are properly anticipated and calmly handled.[12] Sigmoid sinus bleeding is low-flow venous output.

Most sigmoid sinus injuries are the result of drill-related trauma. In some cases the sigmoid may be located in a position only a few millimeters under the cortical bone of the mastoid, placing it at risk of trauma even from a few initial shallow drilling strokes with a cutting bur. Additionally, in a sclerotic mastoid, the sigmoid sinus is

at risk by virtue of being displaced far further anteriorly than usual. Both of these conditions can be recognized on preoperative HRCT images. When drilling is undertaken in an intentional manner to completely remove overlying bone, the sigmoid is fairly resilient to direct contact with a large diamond bur; however, interface with a cutting bur or a small caliber diamond bur places the sigmoid at risk for tear or puncture, respectively.

Management

Small points of sigmoid bleeding, especially those encountered at the junction between the sigmoid and smaller feeding veins, can usually be controlled with focal bipolar cauterization. Use of monopolar cautery is not recommended because it may further open and widen the bleeding point.

For brisker bleeding (**Fig. 4.4**), a large piece of Gelfoam (Baxter International, Deerfield, IL, USA) that is much larger than the injured area, to prevent embolization, or a piece of autologous muscle is applied at the bleeding

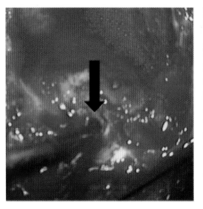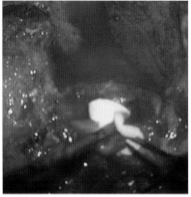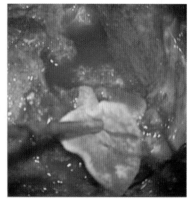

Fig. 4.4 Management of sigmoid sinus bleeding.

a Sigmoid bleeding is initially managed with suction and pressure.

b As soon as possible, a piece of Gelfoam (Baxter International, Deerfield, IL, USA), significantly larger than the bleeding defect, is is positioned to prevent embolization.

c Gelfoam is held in place with a cotton sponge and pressure is applied with a suction cannula for approximately 1 minute. Pressure is then withdrawn, but the cotton sponge is left in place for an additional 5 minutes, after which it can usually be gently removed leaving the underlying Gelfoam in place.

source. The Gelfoam or muscle is then held in place under pressure by a suction tip with a cotton sponge acting as an interface. Generally, pressure with the suction tip is required for no longer than a minute, after which the suction may be withdrawn, leaving the cotton sponge and Gelfoam in situ. Work can be resumed at another site, with final removal of the cotton sponge occurring roughly 10 minutes thereafter. The vast majority of sigmoid sinus injuries can be successfully controlled in this manner.

Very rarely, a large sigmoid tear occurs that will require a more complex repair. If the lumen of the sigmoid is widely exposed, it can be occluded with dense packing of a single piece of muscle into the lumen that is fixed in place with sutures to prevent migration. Alternatively, vascular balloon catheters may be inserted and inflated proximal and distal to the injury site to allow primary suture repair (4.0 nonabsorbable monofilament, tapered needle) of the sinus wall. This nonocclusive primary repair technique may be particularly required if there is concern about the status of contralateral venous outflow.

In the case of a very large sigmoid sinus injury, especially when the lumen and inner walls of the sinus can be seen, an alert for the possibility of an air embolus should be raised and communicated to the anesthesiologist. To minimize this risk, Trendelenburg's position is instituted immediately and the surgical field is temporarily flooded with physiologic solution while direct pressure is maintained on the bleeding site and preparations for definitive repair are finalized.

Management principles for the jugular bulb are the same as these described for the sigmoid sinus.

Labyrinthine Injury

Outlook and Prevention

Similar to the discovery of a transected facial nerve, the unexpected discovery of "snake eyes," indicating inadvertent violation of a semicircular canal, is a sight that all otologists hope to avoid.

Although labyrinthine fistulas are regularly managed in the setting of erosive cholesteatoma, experienced surgeons who are adept at recognizing the hallmark characteristics of dense ivory-colored labyrinthine bone should rarely encounter iatrogenic fistulas.[7,13,14]

The lateral semicircular canal is at greatest risk because of its exposed location relative to the antrum. Injuries to the lateral semicircular canal in this location can be attributed to many of the same errors in technique that have been discussed in relation to facial nerve injuries, especially narrow-field drilling toward the antrum in a sclerotic mastoid. In fact, the horrific scenario of concurrent iatrogenic lateral semicircular canal fenestration and injury to the second genu of the facial nerve has been reported. The posterior and superior semicircular canals are also at risk of violation with drilling of the infralabyrinthine and supralabyrinthine air cell tracts, respectively.

Management

Although the presence of an iatrogenic labyrinthine fistula generates a significant risk of sensorineural hearing loss and severe vertigo, these do not occur with absolute certainty. In fact, there are numerous reports of iatrogenic labyrinthine fistulas wherein hearing and/or partial vestibular function has been preserved. Perhaps this is not surprising given what we know about similar results for surgery that involves intended and controlled fenestration or occlusion of the labyrinth.

The keys to optimal management of this complication seem to be early recognition and avoidance of further trauma to the membranous labyrinth. As such, if a labyrinthine fistula is recognized, drilling should immediately cease and suction to the area should be strictly avoided. A prompt seal of the fistula can then be achieved by plugging the exposed semicircular canal with bone wax and/or fascia. An extended course of antibiotic therapy with an appropriate medication that passes through the blood–brain barrier is prescribed to prevent bacterial labyrinthitis and meningitis, especially in the case of an infected surgical field. As with a facial nerve injury, high-dose systemic corticosteroids may also be of benefit.

Acoustic Trauma

Even though the presence of a temporary shift in bone conduction thresholds has been described immediately after routine mastoid surgery, drilling-related acoustic trauma is not felt to be a significant cause of permanent sensorineural hearing loss in uncomplicated cases.[15] The one notable exception to this rule is the situation where prominent drilling on the incus or other ossicles has occurred.[16,17] Such cases can be associated with a large degree of high-frequency sensorineural hearing loss, generally at 4000 Hz and above.

Incudal drill trauma most often occurs during haphazard drilling within the aditus ad antrum. This situation is recognized by the presence of an unnaturally flattened aspect on the lateral surface of the incus, suggestive of drill bit contact. This complication can be avoided by early identification of the short process of the incus when drilling in this region. Pooled irrigation fluid within the antrum causes bending of light at the air–fluid interface and the ability to view the incus "around the corner," where it can be gently palpated with a blunt hook. Widening of the aditus ad antrum is best undertaken on the posterolateral margin, with drilling and curettage only of bone that is completely visible; as such, inside-out removal of bone that involves blind introduction of instruments into the aditus ad antrum is not acceptable.

In cases where manipulation of the ossicular chain is felt to be likely for whatever reason, or when removal of ossicles is planned preoperatively, such as with canal-wall down surgery, the incudostapedial joint is ideally disarticulated before drilling.

Dura Mater Exposure and Injury

Outlook and Prevention

Mastoid surgery requires the ability to engage and safely manipulate the dura of the middle and posterior cranial fossae. Defects in the bone-covering dura may be idiopathic, secondary to tympanomastoid disease, or iatrogenic. Although most of these defects are of no clinical consequence, some can result in delayed herniation of meninges or brain into the tympanomastoid compartment, resulting in leakage of cerebrospinal fluid (CSF), conductive hearing loss, pulsatile tinnitus, or increased susceptibility to meningitis. Hence, intraoperative decision-making is required during mastoidectomy to determine when exposed dura is limited and inconsequential or large and complicating.

Trauma to the dura resulting from drilling during mastoid surgery may result in a tear, with exposed brain and CSF leakage. In many ways, the dura is similar to the sigmoid sinus in that it too is reasonably resilient to contact with a large diamond bur; whereas cutting burs and small burs of all kinds are more likely to result in penetration. In elderly patients, the dura may be particularly prone to tearing.

Fear of dural injury on the part of surgeons may lead them to avoid definitive identification during mastoidectomy. This is a mistake. As with identification of the facial nerve, clear visualization of the anatomical boundaries of the dura, especially the middle cranial fossa, is critical to performing thorough and safe mastoid surgery.

The most common error in surgical judgment that may result in drill-related exposure or injury of the dura involves failure to anticipate and estimate the natural curvature of the floor of the middle cranial fossa. In practice, this means that the surgeon must keep in mind that the height limit of the tegmen in its superior–inferior aspect will gradually dip inferiorly into the mastoid cavity as one progresses in drilling from the lateral aspect to the medial aspect through the central mastoid air cell tract toward the antrum. Hence, aggressive drilling with a cutting bur in a direct medial trajectory from the site of middle fossa dura identification at its lateral aspect can be dangerous. Once the dura is identified and skeletonized laterally, the authors advocate removal of all adjacent air cells with a large extra-coarse diamond bur using broad drill strokes. At times, bleeding dural vessels are encountered that can easily be managed with bipolar cautery.

Management

It has traditionally been suggested in otologic teaching that dural defects that are 1 cm² or greater in size should be routinely repaired to prevent delayed complications; however, these recommendations are anecdotal. A variety of materials and techniques are available to deal with excessively exposed dura, including fascia, bone pâté, cartilage, muscle, bone wax, and varieties of commercially available cranioplastic bone replacement products.[18,19] Local soft tissue flaps consisting of combinations of fascia, muscle, and pericranium may also be used.

In routine instances where there is no herniation of cranial vault contents or CSF leakage, the authors' preferred technique involves simple application of bone pâté acquired from cortical bone (do not harvest from infected mastoid air cells) as a replacement for absent bone. This is generally covered by a simple overlay with fascia or other soft tissue in the tympanomastoid compartment.

When a small herniation or CSF leakage is present, more elaborate layered techniques are generally required that involve blind retrograde elevation of adjacent dura off the cranial floor circumferentially through the defect via the mastoid. Repair material (preferably something relatively rigid, like cartilage) is then passed through the defect, where it lies sandwiched under the elevated dura and residual cranial floor bone, thereby closing the defect. Layers of other materials, and possibly fibrin glue if CSF leakage is still present, are then added in an overlay fashion for further reinforcement.

In the case of dural tear and CSF leakage, effort should be made to close the dura primarily with interrupted sutures (5.0 nonabsorbable monofilament, tapered needle) as much as possible. For large defects, it may be necessary to sew in a dural patch graft comprising fascia or commercially available dura replacement materials to attain watertight closure. Suture techniques such as these in a confined space can be technically challenging.

When there is concern about the quality of dural closure because of ongoing CSF leakage despite attempted repair or when the cranial floor defect is extremely large, a small middle fossa craniotomy is performed to provide improved surgical exposure of the affected area and to afford more definitive repair of dura and bone defects. Once the dura is elevated off the middle cranial fossa floor, repair of the bone defect with a sufficiently large piece of in-set autologous muscle, with or without an accompanying piece of cartilage or cortical bone graft, will repair the problem in most cases. Commercially available neurosurgical cranioplastic bone cements comprised primarily of hydroxylapatite may also be useful.

In the postoperative period, patients are treated with stool softeners and directed to avoid activities associated with excessive straining or Valsalva-associated events for several weeks. A sufficient course of treatment with antibiotics that cross the blood–brain barrier are especially warranted when CSF leakage is encountered in a grossly infected surgical field or when nonautologous materials have been used for repair. If underlying high CSF pressure is suspected, a lumbar drain may be helpful postoperatively.

Miscellaneous Intraoperative Complications

With more advanced mastoidectomy techniques, a few other complications are possible. When drilling of the facial recess is required, trauma to the chorda tympani nerve is a possibility that can result in postoperative taste disturbance. As a general rule, if the chorda tympani

appears significantly traumatized, the resultant symptoms are probably less bothersome in the long term if it is intentionally transected completely.[20]

If drilling of the infralabyrinthine or peritubal air cells is required, carotid injury is possible; however, risk to the carotid artery should be extraordinarily low in routine mastoid surgery. Carotid injuries generally require significant penetrating trauma with sharp instrumentation or a cutting drill bur. Only the smallest pinpoint carotid bleeding can be controlled with secure packing consisting of topical hemostatic agents. For larger injuries, primary repair (5.0 non-absorbable monofilament, tapered needle) is ideal when technically feasible. Otherwise, carotid injuries must be dealt with using endovascular methods by an interventional radiologist. Injuries associated with the need for extended temporary or permanent carotid occlusion may result in stroke.

Postoperative Complications

Unfavorably Displaced Pinna

Some degree of alteration of the conchal–mastoid angle is commonplace following mastoidectomy. Most often this is not particularly noticeable because it is usually limited and it is surprisingly uncommon to view the pinnae at the same time from a symmetric frontal viewpoint. Moreover, partial hair coverage will often mask such alterations. However, when excessive, pinna displacement can be a genuine cosmetic issue, especially for patients with short hair. This may be a particular risk in cases that involve a widely saucerized mastoidectomy defect.

Preventative measures are particularly helpful in dealing with this problem. Although it is not a perfect analogy, the pinna and postauricular incision site can be considered similar to the lower eyelid. Whereas a subciliary incision poses a risk of cicatricial ectropion, an incision deep within the postauricular sulcus bears a similar risk because of scarring of the skin and underlying postauricular musculature. Ideally, a reasonably wide margin (at least 1 cm) of undisturbed postauricular skin and soft tissue is maintained to avoid pinna displacement through scar contracture.[21] Although there is a temptation to attempt to hide the postauricular incision deep within the sulcus, a more posteriorly placed incision (even as far as the hairline) will only rarely have any notable cosmetic implications.

On occasion, the postauricular soft tissues overlying a mastoidectomy defect will scar inward. Such cases can be easily addressed surgically by reopening the incision and releasing the scar tissue that is binding the pinna. In some cases it may also be helpful to then rotate a thin soft tissue flap, such as temporoparietal fascia, to act as a barrier between the mastoidectomy defect and the overlying skin envelope to prevent repeat contracture.

In cases that do not involve an infected surgical field,

postoperative inward scarring may also be dealt with by reconstructing the lateral aspect of the mastoidectomy defect with titanium mesh or commercially available cranioplastic bone replacement products.[22] This may be particularly useful for large mastoidectomy defects associated with lateral skull base surgical procedures.

Infection

Infection following mastoidectomy can be divided into two broad categories although there can be some degree of overlap. The first category involves infection of the postauricular soft tissues, similar to a surgical wound infection encountered at almost any site of the body. The risk factors for such an infection are well known to most surgeons and include wound dehiscence, hematoma, defective sterile technique, unsatisfactory postoperative local wound care, and poor patient primary healing factors (i.e., malnutrition, diabetes, tobacco use). *Staphylococcus aureus* is often implicated in this category of infection. Treatment of surgical infections of this nature requires culture-directed antibiotic therapy, surgical drainage of an abscess or hematoma, and local wound care consisting of packing and debridement while the infection clears and healing occurs.

The second type of infection encountered following mastoidectomy may be considered a continuation of, or failure to eradicate, a primary tympanomastoid infectious condition that generally would have acted, at least in part, as an indication for mastoidectomy in the first place.[23] Some of these cases can be attributed to atypical or antimicrobial-resistant strains of infectious pathogens. Treatment of such infections should be directed by acquiring swab and tissue specimens for broad laboratory testing, including appropriate stain and culture techniques to detect fungus and mycobacteria. Formal medical consultation with infectious disease specialists may also be helpful, especially when medical conditions, such as immunodeficiency or poorly controlled blood sugar, are felt to be contributing factors. Biopsy specimens are also helpful for histopathology to rule out the presence of a compounding neoplastic, granulomatous, or atypical inflammatory process.

Unfortunately, rare cases do exist where persistent postoperative infection may be related to inadequate surgical management of affected soft tissues, bone, and/or air cells.[24] When infection is the overriding indication for mastoidectomy, it is important to completely remove all involved air cells as far as is possible. Commonly neglected areas include the tegmen, retrolabyrinthine, tip, retrofacial, anterior supralabyrinthine (including the anterior epitympanic sinus/supratubal recess), and sinal (between the sigmoid and tegmen) air cells. Significant extension of infection into the petrous apex can also be encountered, but rarely.

In the case of severe otomastoiditis with bony erosion noted on preoperative imaging, incomplete removal of devitalized bone may preclude the resolution of infection by leaving devascularized necrotic foci that harbor chronic infection. This is particularly an issue in an immunocompromised host, where risk for the development of osteomyelitis of the skull base is possible. Such cases require long-term intravenous antibiotic therapy and occasionally serial surgical debridement of the temporal bone.

The Unstable Open Mastoid Cavity

Defining an unstable open mastoid cavity may be a subjective endeavor that can vary from patient to patient and is impacted not only by the specific anatomical parameters of the cavity itself, but also by the personality and lifestyle of the patient. For example, one patient may be perfectly content to adhere to strict water precautions and routine follow-up every few months for cleaning, whereas another may be displeased by any day-to-day inconveniences and required office visits more frequent than once per year. Of course, many unstable mastoid cavities are self-evident, such as the case of chronic otorrhea that does not respond to local care and medical therapy.

Office management of a discharging mastoid cavity is common practice for most otologic surgeons, the hallmark of which involves meticulous and complete suction debridement of all retained debris and infected elements. Drying and acidifying agents are often used to combat the accumulation of granulation tissue and fungal overgrowth. Ethanol and boric or acetic acid preparations are popular for this purpose although patient tolerance due to pain can be a problem in some instances.

Ototopical antibiotics are helpful to treat infection with culture-directed therapy used in refractory cases; however, fungal overgrowth (which is often already a compounding issue) can occur, especially with the use of steroid-containing agents. In an effort to promote a dry environment, serial topical application of petroleum-based antimicrobial ointment, in lieu of aqueous drops, may be advantageous. Treatment of granulation tissue with focal application of silver nitrate is also popular; however, provision for the location of the facial nerve and other vital structures must be made.

The causes of an unstable cavity may be related to its anatomical characteristics, physiologic factors, and host behavior.[25–27] These are outlined in **Figure 4.5**. Anatomical characteristics may play the greatest role in determining the long-term stability of a cavity, and these are the same factors that are most dependent upon the quality of surgical technique. When unfavorable anatomy is noted in an unstable cavity, potential for surgical correction should be recognized and offered as a management option to the unsatisfied patient.[28] The anatomical factors most commonly cited as problematic include a high facial ridge, an

- Anatomical characteristics
  - Excessive volume
  - Gravity-dependent sump effect
  - High facial ridge
  - Inadequate saucerization/ridge irregularity
  - Excessively "hourglassed" at meatus
- Physiologic factors
  - Lack of barrier separation of mucosalized middle ear and epithelialized cavity
  - Neotympanic membrane atelectasis
  - Recurrent cholesteatoma
  - Incompletely eradicated diseased air cells
  - Antimicrobial resistant pathogens
  - Immunodeficiency
  - Poor blood supply
  - Excessive moisture
  - Insufficient acidity
- Host behavioral factors
  - Neglect of follow-up care
  - Poor hygiene
  - Hearing aid usage
  - Active outdoor lifestyle

Fig. 4.5 Factors that may contribute to mastoid cavity instability.

inadequately large meatoplasty, and a voluminous open mastoid tip.

Failure to lower the facial ridge has a few negative consequences. First, a large step-off between the native external auditory canal and the mastoid cavity creates a partial partition that discourages self-cleaning and epithelial migration. Furthermore, a gravity-dependent reservoir is created within the posterior and inferior aspects of the cavity. This causes a "sump" effect by promoting the accumulation of debris and moisture in these areas. Accordingly, complete lowering of the facial ridge over the entire mastoid segment of the facial nerve should be a routine step in open-cavity mastoid surgery.

A meatoplasty is deemed insufficient if it does not functionally meet the demands of the underlying mastoid cavity. The minimum size criteria will differ depending on the size and dimensions of the mastoid cavity, to the point that only minimal enlargement may be required in a very small or partially obliterated cavity. For examination and cleaning purposes, the meatoplasty must afford access to every anatomical subunit. Furthermore, an "hourglass" effect, wherein a large cavity is expected to self-clean via a relatively small meatus, should be avoided when possible. As a general rule, the external auditory meatus should extend until it is favorably oriented with the posterior boundary of the cavity, creating a tapered conical orientation rather than an hourglass. This almost always requires resection of a wedge of conchal cartilage. Conversely, an excessively large meatoplasty should be avoided for reasons of poor cosmesis and difficulties related to hearing aid fitting.

Amputation of the mastoid tip at the digastric ridge affords several advantages. First, a large open tip will contribute to the aforementioned sump effect and will greatly increase the overall cavity volume. However, a fact lost on many ear surgeons is that removal of the mastoid tip also greatly reduces cavity volume by lowering the lateral cavity depth and inviting inward collapse of adjacent soft tissues. By doing so, the boundaries of the open cavity may then be shifted to the anterior edge of the sigmoid sinus, which in most instances is only ~ 2 cm from the anterior wall of the native external auditory canal, even in a well-pneumatized mastoid. The superior–inferior dimension is also decreased as measured from the tegmen, as the new inferior limit (bend of the sigmoid toward the jugular bulb) is usually ~ 1 cm superior to the lower margin of the mastoid tip. If the surgeon wishes to pursue these favorable effects, the tip must be completely amputated (even in a sclerotic mastoid) as inward fracture is not sufficient.

A properly saucerized open mastoid cavity is one that is most likely to auto-obliterate. This situation is akin to placing a wet piece of canvas over a hole dug into the ground. By rounding and widening the outer edges of the hole like a saucer, inward collapse and reduction of volume by medial draping of the overlying wet canvas is attained without altering the ultimate depth of the hole. Accordingly, broad skeletonization of the tegmen, mastoid cavity, and tympanic bone are desirable when shaping an open mastoid cavity.

To achieve a small-volume cavity, the favorably shaped mastoid cavity will usually only require limited obliteration or, in many cases, no obliteration at all. Numerous mastoid obliteration techniques have been described using autologous materials, such as bone pâté, cartilage chips, and vascularized soft-tissue flaps.[29-34] In the authors' opinion, obliteration techniques are generally effective and safe in properly selected instances where residual cholesteatoma is not of concern. Obliteration is a helpful adjuvant in the reduction of open mastoid cavity volume; however, it must be stressed that obliteration techniques should not be used as a replacement for the other surgical principles outlined in this section.

Vertigo

Vertigo following mastoidectomy can have several causes. First, similar to sensorineural hearing loss, the mechanical effects of surgery itself may result in peripheral vestibular end-organ damage. This is usually manifested by vertigo and nystagmus that present during the immediate postoperative period. This usually lasts for a few days, followed by a variable period of instability that persists until compensation occurs. Such damage is most likely to occur in the setting of cholesteatoma that requires intraoperative management of a labyrinthine fistula. Other similar, but rare, causes of postoperative vertigo are infectious and inflammatory labyrinthitis. In contrast to mechanical vestibular injuries, these usually present in the slightly delayed acute postoperative setting. In the setting of an open mastoid cavity, patients may complain of ongoing caloric-effect vertigo that occurs with wind or water exposure.[35] This is especially common when a large meatoplasty is present.

Treatment of postoperative vertigo consists of judicious use of vestibular suppressant and antiemetic medications. Similar to the situation of vestibular neuritis, a course of systemic corticosteroid therapy may also be of benefit. In cases where concern for inner ear pathogen contamination is present, antimicrobial therapy that crosses the blood–brain barrier is indicated. After the acute vertiginous stage has subsided, it is critical to discontinue vestibular suppressants and to encourage ambulation as soon as possible so as not to delay compensation. For patients with prolonged or excessive instability, early vestibular rehabilitation is advantageous. Obliteration techniques have been shown to reduce caloric-effect vertigo in an open mastoid cavity.[36]

Mastoid–Cutaneous or Mastoid–Canal Fistula

An unwanted open epithelialized communication between the mastoid cavity and the postauricular skin or between the mastoid cavity and the external auditory canal constitutes a mastoid–cutaneous or mastoid–canal fistula, respectively. Development of a mastoid–cutaneous fistula may be the result of an interplay between several complicating factors during the postoperative healing phase. These factors may include dehiscence of the postauricular incision, wound infection, or an excessively thin soft tissue envelope overlying the mastoidectomy cavity.[37] In contrast, a mastoid–canal fistula is generally attributed to a flaw in technique during intact-canal wall mastoid surgery, specifically in assuring that the lateral external auditory canal skin is properly reset and sealed completely within the bony external auditory canal during surgical closure. A mastoid–canal fistula is generally encountered at the bone–cartilaginous junction.

Both of these conditions usually present with unwanted discharge of pus or mucous, incomplete healing, and granulation tissue from the postauricular area or external auditory canal. Treatment of both types of mastoid fistula is surgical, and the basic underlying principles are similar. The fistula tract and granulation tissue must be completely excised and the resultant defect is closed in a meticulous layered fashion. Often this will require introduction and interposition of a soft tissue barrier between the mastoidectomy cavity and the involved structure. The postauricular region generally requires a pedicled soft tissue flap whereas the canal can generally be managed with a fascia or cartilage graft.

Cerebrospinal Fluid Leak and Meningoencephalocele

Leakage of CSF is suspected in the postoperative period if the patient is experiencing persistent unilateral watery rhinorrhea or otorrhea. This can also be manifested by excessive watery saturation of mastoid dressing materials, a positive "halo sign" (differential circumferential separation of blood from clear fluid when applied to paper), headache, or meningitis. Definitive diagnosis is made by acquisition of a specimen for laboratory analysis for the presence of β-transferrin. After a fluid sample is obtained (0.5 mL or greater is usually required), it should be refrigerated for transit to, and testing in, the laboratory.

Small CSF leaks will often seal spontaneously if underlying CSF pressures are normal. Therefore, a period of initial observation and conservative management is usually acceptable in most cases encountered following mastoidectomy that was not a component of a major lateral skull-base surgical procedure. Generally these patients are placed on bedrest, with elevation of the head of the bed, and are given stool softeners as well as antibiotics if a contaminated mastoidectomy field was involved. Antibiotic coverage is controversial if the surgical field was not contaminated as this may simply select for antibiotic-resistant pathogens.[38] If these measures are unsuccessful, placement of a lumbar drain is indicated.

When CSF leakage persists despite conservative measures, when mastoidectomy was a component of a major lateral skull-base procedure, or when a meningoencephalocele is noted to be present, surgical management is indicated. The general principles of dural and tegmen repair have been covered in the preoperative section of this chapter. In addition, it should be noted that difficult cases of CSF leakage may require more aggressive measures, such as eustachian tube plugging and blind sac closure of the external auditory canal with comprehensive removal of all epithelial contents from the tympanomastoid compartment. These procedures are often performed in combination with mastoid obliteration using a rotational temporalis muscle flap or free fat graft, although the latter should never be performed in a grossly infected surgical field.

In the case of meningoencephalocele, amputation of the devitalized herniated brain and dura must be undertaken via bipolar cautery.[39] Definitive repair of the dura and skull base is then undertaken as previously described, with provision for antiseizure prophylaxis. A middle fossa craniotomy is usually required to properly repair CSF leakage accompanying meningoencephalocele.[40]

Conclusions

With thoughtful planning and adherence to sound surgical techniques, avoidance of mastoidectomy complications can be achieved. Yet, for the busy otologic surgeon who regularly engages in difficult and revision cases, dealing with complications is inevitable. Therefore, a working knowledge of the management schemes outlined in this chapter can be applied to deal with these complications as they occur to minimize associated morbidity.

References

1. Banerjee A, Flood LM, Yates P, Clifford K. Computed tomography in suppurative ear disease: does it influence management? J Laryngol Otol 2003;117(6):454–458
2. Blevins NH, Carter BL. Routine preoperative imaging in chronic ear surgery. Am J Otol 1998;19(4):527–535, discussion 535–538
3. Chee NW, Tan TY. The value of pre-operative high resolution CT scans in cholesteatoma surgery. Singapore Med J 2001;42(4):155–159
4. Jackler RK, Dillon WP, Schindler RA. Computed tomography in suppurative ear disease: a correlation of surgical and radiographic findings. Laryngoscope 1984;94(6):746–752
5. Alzoubi, FQ, Odat HA, Al-Balas HA, Saeed SR. The role of preoperative CT scan in patients with chronic otitis media. Eur Arch Otorhinolaryngol 2009;266(6):807–809
6. Green JD Jr, Shelton C, Brackmann DE. Iatrogenic facial nerve injury during otologic surgery. Laryngoscope 1994; 104(8 Pt 1):922–926
7. Harkness P, Brown P, Fowler S, Grant H, Ryan R, Topham J. Mastoidectomy audit: results of the Royal College of surgeons of England comparative audit of ENT surgery. Clin Otolaryngol Allied Sci 1995;20(1):89–94
8. Nilssen EL, Wormald PJ. Facial nerve palsy in mastoid surgery. J Laryngol Otol 1997;111(2):113–116
9. Greenberg JS, Manolidis S, Stewart MG, Kahn JB. Facial nerve monitoring in chronic ear surgery: US practice patterns. Otolaryngol Head Neck Surg 2002;126(2):108–114
10. Prass RL. Iatrogenic facial nerve injury: the role of facial nerve monitoring. Otolaryngol Clin North Am 1996;29(2):265–275
11. Green JD Jr, Shelton C, Brackmann DE. Surgical management of iatrogenic facial nerve injuries. Otolaryngol Head Neck Surg 1994;111(5):606–61
12. Graham MD. The jugular bulb: its anatomic and clinical considerations in contemporary otology. Laryngoscope 1977;87(1):105–125
13. Jahrsdoerfer RA, Johns ME, Cantrell RW. Labyrinthine trauma during ear surgery. Laryngoscope 1978;88(10): 1589–1595
14. Wormald PJ, Nilssen EL. Do the complications of mastoid surgery differ from those of the disease? Clin Otolaryngol Allied Sci 1997;22(4):355–357
15. Urquhart AC, McIntosh WA, Bodenstein NP. Drill-generated sensorineural hearing loss following mastoid surgery. Laryngoscope 1992;102(6):689–692
16. Gjuric M, Schneider W, Buhr W, Wolf SR, Wigand ME. Experimental sensorineural hearing loss following drill-induced ossicular chain injury. Acta Otolaryngol 1997;117(4):497–500
17. Jiang D, Bibas A, Santuli C, Donnelly N, Jeronimidis G, O'Connor AF. Equivalent noise level generated by drilling onto the ossicular chain as measured by laser Doppler vibrometry: a temporal bone study. Laryngoscope 2007;117(6):1040–1045
18. Wootten CT, Kaylie DM, Warren FM, Jackson CG. Management of brain herniation and cerebrospinal fluid leak in revision chronic ear surgery. Laryngoscope 2005;115(7):1256–1261
19. Pelosi S, Bederson JB, Smouha EE. Cerebrospinal fluid leaks of temporal bone origin: selection of surgical approach. Skull Base 2010;20(4):253–259
20. Michael P, Raut V. Chorda tympani injury: operative findings and postoperative symptoms. Otolaryngol Head Neck Surg 2007;136(6):978–981
21. Shekhar C, Bhavana K. Aesthetics in ear surgery: a comparative study of different post auricular incisions and their cosmetic relevance. Indian J Otolaryngol Head Neck Surg 2007;59:187–190
22. Jung TT, Park SK. Reconstruction of mastoidectomy defect with titanium mesh. Acta Otolaryngol 2004; 124(4):440–442
23. Pillsbury HC III, Carrasco VN. Revision mastoidectomy. Arch Otolaryngol Head Neck Surg 1990;116(9):1019–1022
24. Nadol JB Jr. Causes of failure of mastoidectomy for chronic otitis media. Laryngoscope 1985;95(4):410–413
25. Wormald PJ, Nilssen EL. The facial ridge and the discharging mastoid cavity. Laryngoscope 1998;108(1 Pt 1):92–96
26. Bhatia S, Karmarkar S, DeDonato G, et al. Canal wall down mastoidectomy: causes of failure, pitfalls and their management. J Laryngol Otol 1995;109(7):583–589
27. Phelan E, Harney M, Burns H. Intraoperative findings in revision canal wall down mastoidectomy. Ir Med J 2008;101(1):14
28. Dornhoffer JL. Surgical modification of the difficult mastoid cavity. Otolaryngol Head Neck Surg 1999;120(3):361–367
29. Leatherman BD, Dornhoffer JL. Bioactive glass ceramic particles as an alternative for mastoid obliteration: results in an animal model. Otol Neurotol 2002;23(5):657–660; discussion 660
30. Leatherman BD, Dornhoffer JL. The use of demineralized bone matrix for mastoid cavity obliteration. Otol Neurotol 2004;25(1):22–5; discussion 25–26
31. Mahendran S, Yung MW. Mastoid obliteration with hydroxyapatite cement: the Ipswich experience. Otol Neurotol 2004;25(1):19–21
32. Ramsey MJ, Merchant SN, McKenna MJ. Postauricular periosteal–pericranial flap for mastoid obliteration and canal wall down tympanomastoidectomy. Otol Neurotol 2004;25(6):873–878
33. Roberson JB Jr, Mason TP, Stidham KR. Mastoid obliteration: autogenous cranial bone pAte reconstruction. Otol Neurotol 2003;24(2):132–140
34. Singh V, Atlas M. Obliteration of the persistently discharging mastoid cavity using the middle temporal artery flap. Otolaryngol Head Neck Surg 2007;137(3):433–438
35. Kos MI, Castrillon R, Montandon P, Guyot JP. Anatomic and functional long-term results of canal wall-down mastoidectomy. Ann Otol Rhinol Laryngol 2004;113(11):872–876
36. Beutner D, Helmstaedter V, Stumpf R, et al. Impact of partial mastoid obliteration on caloric vestibular function in canal wall down mastoidectomy. Otol Neurotol 2010;31(9):1399–1403
37. Choo JC, Shaw CL, Chong YCS. Postauricular cutaneous mastoid fistula. J Laryngol Otol 2004;118(11):893–894
38. Brodie HA. Prophylactic antibiotics for posttraumatic cerebrospinal fluid fistulae. A meta-analysis. Arch Otolaryngol Head Neck Surg 1997;123(7):749–752
39. Mosnier I, Fiky LE, Shahidi A, Sterkers O. Brain herniation and chronic otitis media: diagnosis and surgical management. Clin Otolaryngol Allied Sci 2000;25(5):385–391
40. Sanna M, Fois P, Russo A, Falcioni M. Management of meningoencephalic herniation of the temporal bone: Personal experience and literature review. Laryngoscope 2009;119(8):1579–1585

5 Complications in Cochlear Implants and Implantable Hearing Devices

B. S. Tsai, G. P. B. Braga, A. Rivas, D. S. Haynes

Introduction

In recent decades, technologic advances, such as cochlear implants and osseointegrated implants, commonly referred to as bone-anchored hearing aids (BAHA), have increased the access to sound for hearing-impaired patients who previously had limited options with hearing aids. As indications for these surgical devices grow, they have increasingly played more significant roles in the management of both children and adults with hearing impairment. Although the safety of the devices has improved as the surgical techniques are refined, they are not without their complications. Understanding the potential complications will not only allow clinicians to provide better informed consent, but also help in preventing such complications and developing a good treatment plan should the need arise.

Complications in Cochlear Implants

Cochlear implants are the first human-made device to replace a sensory organ. In patients whose hearing end-organ, the cochlea, no longer provides useful input, the cochlear implant bypasses the sensory cells to directly provide electrical stimulation of the auditory nerve. Among its many indications, it is most commonly used for the treatment of bilaterally profound sensorineural hearing loss. It has also been shown to benefit patients with auditory neuropathy spectrum disorder. The surgical procedure comprises a cortical mastoidectomy with facial recess drill out followed by a cochleostomy. Additionally, for some implants, a bony well to seat the implant under the temporalis muscle needs to be drilled out. During any part of the surgery, injury to the adjacent anatomical structures can lead to unwanted complications. Also, the implant itself can be the source of complications. Because complications of a mastoidectomy are already discussed in Chapter 4, this chapter will primarily focus on complications specific to the facial recess and cochleostomy drill outs as well as device complications.

Nerve Injury Secondary to Cochlear Implantation

After completing the mastoidectomy, the facial recess is widely opened to expose the round window niche. Anatomical variations in the relative location of the facial and chorda tympani nerves can place them at risk for injury.

Facial Nerve Injury

The course of the facial nerve from the brainstem to the facial musculature can be divided into three segments: intracranial, intratemporal, and extratemporal or peripheral.[1] The intracranial portion of the facial nerve extends from the brainstem to the porus acusticus of the internal auditory canal. The intratemporal portion begins at the porous acousticus at the medial internal auditory canal, travels a tortuous course within the temporal bone and exits via the stylomastoid foramen. This segment is further subdivided into meatal, labyrinthine, tympanic, and mastoid segments. The meatal portion is located between the porus acusticus and the fundus and the labyrinthine segment travels from the fundus to the geniculate ganglion before the nerve turns at an acute angle to form the tympanic segment in the middle ear. It then makes a second genu and becomes the mastoid segment and travels toward the stylomastoid foramen. The petrous temporal bone protects the meatal and labyrinthine segments of the intratemporal facial nerve. From the mastoid segment, the chorda tympani, a branch of the facial nerve, travels anterolaterally to join the lingual nerve to provide taste sensation. The extratemporal or peripheral portion of the facial nerve begins at the stylomastoid foramen, from which it enters the parotid and branches to innervate the facial musculature.

During routine otologic surgery, the tympanic and mastoid segments are at increased risk for injury. However, in cochlear implantation, the mastoid segment with the second genu and chorda tympani nerve are of interest because they serve as the boundaries of the facial recess for the posterior tympanotomy. To visualize the cochlea adequately, a wide enough opening must be created. The proximity of the two nerves to the recess opening may result in injury to one or both nerves.

Variations in facial nerve anatomy can further increase the likelihood of inadvertent injury especially when the facial nerve is not easily visualized while entering into the facial recess. The most common variation is an anteromedial facial nerve distal to the oval window that runs inferior or over the location of the round window.[2] Traumatic injuries to the facial nerve typically present as neural edema, especially if the facial palsy presents within the early postoperative days.[3] Potential sources of injury include thermal injury by the bur and direct trauma. For that reason, copious irrigation is used when drilling around the facial nerve. Preoperative radiologic evaluation with a noncontrast computed tomography scan of the temporal bone will alert the surgeon to potential course deviations of the facial nerve to minimize inadvertent injury. Although commonly used during otologic surgery, intraoperative facial nerve monitoring has not been shown to decrease the incidence of facial palsy.

Other causes of facial paresis after cochlear implantation surgery include herpes virus reactivation, acute nerve compromise, and postoperative wound infection. Reactivation of herpes simplex virus type I secondary to surgical trauma, although rare, is a well-documented cause resulting in facial palsy after otologic surgery, especially when there is direct manipulation of the nerve root.[4] Reactivation then results in inflammation, demyelination and palsy. Vrabec previously showed that increased manipulation of the sensory branches of the facial nerve resulted in an increased incidence of delayed facial palsy, and other studies have demonstrated that the raising of the tympanomeatal flap disrupts cutaneous branches of the facial nerve that could precipitate viral reactivation.[5,6] As a result, several studies have suggested that injury to the chorda tympani nerve could serve as a likely trigger for reactivation.[3,7] Confirmation that viral reactivation is the cause of the facial paresis can be obtained by sampling nerve tissue or endoneural fluid; however, these methods are not without risks. Because delayed facial palsy carries a favorable prognosis, surgical exploration or decompression with biopsy is not indicated.[3] Acute nerve compromise can result from vasospasm triggered by local blood breakdown products, ischemia of the nerve, or venous outflow obstruction, resulting in neural edema.[3,4] Despite these theories, the mechanism of delayed facial lesion remains elusive, and no etiologic factors have been found.[3,6]

Facial palsy after cochlear implantation tends to present in a delayed fashion. In a retrospective study of 705 patients who were implanted between 1980 and 2002, the incidence was 0.71% with all nerve injuries presenting in a delayed fashion. When the patient presents with this type of paresis, the treatment is medical with the prompt initiation of a high-dose corticosteroid taper, with or without antiviral medication.[3] Additionally, if the weakness is severe, resulting in incomplete eye closure, lubrication with artificial tears and ointment is extremely important. The addition of a moisture chamber at night can also help to protect against corneal drying and subsequent ulceration. If the eye becomes painful or erythematous, a consultation with an ophthalmologist early in the course may be required.

Chorda Tympani Injury

The chorda tympani nerve carries preganglionic secretomotor fibers that innervate the submandibular and sublingual glands and taste fibers from the anterior two-thirds of the tongue. They are carried with the lingual nerve through the infratemporal fossa and enter the tympanic cavity through the petrotympanic fissure and iter chordae anterius, also known as the Canal of Hugier. It crosses the tympanic cavity along the posterior superior middle ear space, medial to the neck of the malleus, and then exits the tympanic cavity via the iter chordae posterius as it proceeds inferiorly to join the vertical portion of the facial nerve within the mastoid bone.

By virtue of its location, during the cochlear implant surgery, more specifically, during the drilling of the facial recess, this nerve is at increased risk of injury, resulting in dysgeusia, a change in sensation of taste. These alterations in taste are often described as a metallic, bitter or salty taste in the mouth. Patients occasionally complain of tongue numbness. Lloyd et al[8] compared the outcomes of patients who underwent cochlear implantation with preservation of the chorda tympani nerve, with the outcomes of patients whose nerves were sectioned. They showed that about half of the patients with an intact nerve presented with alterations in taste and 42% of these patients had subsequent resolution of their symptoms. However, in patients whose nerve was sectioned, although 86% had taste disturbances, 67% had resolution of their symptoms. These results were found to be similar to other studies that described postoperative dysgeusia in otologic surgery.

Infectious Complications of Cochlear Implantation

Infections after cochlear implantation are relatively rare with an incidence between 1.7 and 3.3%, but can present with management challenges.[9-11] The most dreaded complication is meningitis and has been widely discussed in the literature as well as local media. However, wound complications are far more common. With increasing numbers of children receiving cochlear implantation, the incidence of otitis media after cochlear implantation has risen and prompt treatment is necessary to prevent more severe sequelae.

Meningitis

Meningitis is a serious infection that can present after cochlear implantation with the majority presenting within the first year of implantation.[12] Many papers have been published about the risk of meningitis after cochlear implants, but the precise cause is still under debate. It has been suggested that the incidence of meningitis in profoundly deaf patients is higher than in the general population.[13] That same study showed that the incidence of postimplant meningitis due to *Streptococcus pneumoniae* was 138.2 cases per 100,000 person-years, at least 30 times greater than that of the general population in 2000.[13] Risk factors include an age less than 5 years, impaired immune status, presence of intracranial foreign bodies such as a ventricular shunt, and a history of meningitis. Additionally, a history of otitis media as well as inner ear malformations may place patients at increased risk.[14] In many cases, meningitis, especially when it occurs 30 days postimplantation, is often preceded by an episode of acute otitis media.[15] Previously, an additional consideration that predisposed cochlear implant patients to meningitis was the use of positions that created further trauma to the osseous spiral lamina and modiolus. This allowed pneumococcal meningitis to spread via an otogenic route.[16] As a result such implants have been withdrawn from the market.

Various theories have been proposed regarding the pathophysiology of meningitis after cochlear implantation. The two most common theories are via otogenic or hematogenous spread. Otogenic spread can be from direct invasion of the bacteria from the middle ear to the meninges through a tegmen defect or via the inner ear in patients with cochlear implants. The latter is the more commonly accepted view.[12] By creating a cochleostomy and inserting an implant, the barriers separating the middle ear from the inner ear are compromised, potentially allowing bacteria easier access into the inner ear, especially when the cochleostomy seal is inadequate. Alternatively, bacteria can enter the inner ear through the round window membrane. Bacterial toxins, antibiotics and other substances have been shown to pass through the round window membrane.[17] Once in the inner ear, bacteria access the meninges and the cerebrospinal fluid (CSF) through the labyrinth, infiltration of the cochlear turns, along the electrode into the bony channels of Schuknecht, or through perineural or perivascular routes into the internal auditory canal.[15] Additionally, the presence of cochlear malformation is often associated with an enlarged cochlear aqueduct, providing a more open channel between the cochlea and central nervous system.[18–20] Evidence also exists for the hematogenous spread of bacteria as the cause of meningitis with a subsequent retrograde spread of infection toward the inner and middle ears.[21–23] Infection in patients with bacteremia may seed in compromised tissues within the inner ear, such as areas of tissue necrosis related to the electrodes or positioner, with subsequent spread to the meninges and CSF.[24] The likelihood of meningitis may be related to the duration and severity of the bacteremia, as these variables determine the concentration of bacteria reaching the subarachnoid space.[25]

Although not necessarily causative, the presence of an electrode within the inner ear has been shown to be associated with an increased risk of meningitis, especially within the first 2 months after implantation.[24] The presence of the implant has been shown to reduce the threshold level of bacteria required to induce meningitis.[1] It has been postulated that the presence of the electrode may reduce local inner ear immunity, making it more susceptible to inoculation with subsequent spread to the central nervous system. Alternatively, the presence of the implant could reduce the global central nervous system immunity, breaking down the blood–brain barrier and allowing for hematogenous spread from the systemic circulation.[1] Traumatic insertions of the cochlear implant have been shown to be a risk factor for pneumococcal meningitis, especially in those patients whose implants had a positioner before 2002. Reefhuis et al[11] demonstrated in a study of 4,264 children that although only 19% of these children had implants with a positioner, a wedge that rests in the cochlea next to the electrodes, 71% of these children developed meningitis.[24] Despite achieving a better electrode position for stimulation of the cochlear nerve, the positioner may result in increased trauma to the inner ear with subsequent necrosis and absorption of the modiolus and osseous spiral lamina resulting in higher susceptibility to infection.[2] Even though the risk of meningitis is elevated in these patients beyond 24 months of implantation, removal of these implants or their positioners is not recommended.[24]

Preventive Measures

The most common pathogens responsible for meningitis in cochlear implant recipients are *Streptococcus pneumoniae* (most frequent) and, *Haemophilus influenzae*, including type b and nontypeable species. Because this is a preventable infection that could result in undesirable consequences, the U.S. Food and Drug Administration (FDA) and many other government organizations around the world have recommended universal immunization for all implant recipients in an effort to reduce the incidence of meningitis. Because all children in the United States are required to have the Hib (*H. influenza* type b conjugate) vaccine in infancy and early childhood, the only additional vaccination recommended by the Center for Disease Control and Prevention is against *S. pneumoniae*. The most commonly used vaccines are the heptavalent pneumococcal conjugate vaccine (PCV7; Prevnar, Wyeth-Lederle Vaccines, Madison, NJ, USA) and the 23-valent pneumococcal polysaccharide vaccine (PPV23; pneumovax 23, Merck & Co. Inc., Whitehouse Station, NJ, USA; and Pnu-Immune 23; Lederle Laboratories, Madison, NJ, USA).[12,26] It is expected that all children considered for cochlear implantation will be up-to-date for all their vaccinations. The immunization guidelines for cochlear implant candidates and recipients are summarized as follows:

- Children under the age of 24 months are expected to have completed the pneumococcal conjugate vaccine (Prevnar) series. If their last dose was given before 12 months of age, an additional Prevnar dose should be given between 12 and 15 months of age. When they turn 24 months old, they should be given the PPV23 vaccine.
- Children older than 24 months old should have completed the Prevnar series already. If they have not, they should be immunized according to a high-risk schedule. All patients should receive the PPV23 vaccine, with at least 2 months after the last Prevnar dose.[27]
- Children between 24 and 59 months who have not yet been immunized should receive two doses of the Prevnar vaccine spaced at least 2 months apart, followed by one dose of the PPV23 vaccine 2 months later.[27]
- Persons older than 5 years old, should receive a single dose of PPV23.[23,28]
- Patients planning to receive a cochlear implant should have their pneumococcal vaccination up-to-date.[27]

It is recommended that the patient complete all vaccinations at least 2 weeks before implantation. Some would even argue that the patients should be immunized a month before surgery, because a study in 2005 of 120 cochlear implant patients between the ages of 5 and 27 years, who received the PPV23 vaccine, demonstrated that serum antibody levels to vaccine-specific serotypes increased significantly within 4 weeks after vaccination.[29]

Because cochlear trauma is thought to increase the risk of developing meningitis, some have advocated the use of soft surgical techniques whenever possible.[2] The advance off-stylet technique minimizes force on the lateral wall of the cochlea to reduce structural damage to the inner ear.[30] Cochleostomy placements that are more inferior and anterior to the round window have also been shown to decrease displacement of electrodes from the scala tympani.[31,32]

Wound Infection

Wound infections after cochlear implantation can potentially have severe consequences, especially if it requires the removal of the device. Often, after removal of the implant, it cannot be immediately replaced. During this time, there is the possibility that the scala tympani can become scarred making future reimplantation more difficult or even, if possible, resulting in poorer performance. For that reason, the electrode array is often severed at the cochleostomy and left in place until the time of reimplantation.

Infectious complications range from 1.7% to 8.2%, although typically lower for severe complications.[14,25,33] Clinically they present as tenderness over the receiver site, progressing with edema, erythema, and eventually sometimes to an abscess. Because all efforts should be made to minimize the chance of implant removal, conservative medical treatment with broad-spectrum intravenous antibiotics is often initiated. If cultures can be obtained without compromising implant integrity, the antibiotics can be tailored accordingly. Appropriate intraoperative wound debridement with culture-guided antibiotics can often salvage the implant.

In treating infectious complications of cochlear implants, one must consider the presence of bacterial biofilms. These are composed of bacterial communities that produce a polymeric matrix of exopolysaccharides with the ability to attach and persist on the surface of biomaterials. The presence of a biofilm requires a minimum of 6 weeks of antibiotic treatment to eradicate the offending organisms. However, the persistence of the biofilm may require removal of the device, leaving only the electrode within the cochlea.[25] Antonelli et al[34] demonstrated that *Staphylococcus aureus* has been the most common pathogen identified in such infections, suggesting a non-otologic source. Sterile technique with intraoperative antibiotic irrigation may minimize the seeding of bacteria at the time of implantation.

Middle Ear and Mastoid Disease

Middle ear and mastoid disease are common not only in children but also in adults. As cochlear implantation becomes increasingly popular in young children and infants with profound sensorineural hearing loss, prompt treatment of middle ear or mastoid infections over the course of the lifetime of patients with cochlear implants becomes increasingly important. As the incidence of acute otitis media is 60 to 80% within the first 6 years of life, even though there are no studies that demonstrate a higher incidence of acute otitis media in children with cochlear implants, its management remains a challenge in these patients.[35] Previously, cochlear implantation was contraindicated in patients with otitis media because of the increased risk of tympanic membrane perforation, recurrent cholesteatoma, meningitis and electrode extrusion.[28] However, recent studies have shown that cochlear implantation is safe in these patients. One prospective study even demonstrated that the incidence of acute otitis media decreased postimplantation after adequate control of the disease preimplantation.[28] The literature emphasizes the importance of controlling acute otitis media before implantation to minimize bacterial contamination of the device and meningitis.

Patients with a dry perforation can undergo cochlear implantation after a successful tympanoplasty. Some argue that the tympanoplasty should precede the cochlear implantation by at least 3 months to ensure adequate healing as a persistent perforation at the time of implantation may increase postoperative complications from an exposed electrode. In the setting of a dry perforation, some have advocated a one-stage closure and implantation. Others have advocated procedures such as meatal closure or radical mastoidectomy to perform the cochlear implant in a single-stage surgery. However, after a meatal closure, otoscopic surveillance is impossible, and therefore, early diagnosis and prompt treatment of middle ear diseases is limited, thereby increasing the risk of meningitis.[28]

Patients with cholesteatoma have an elevated risk of intracranial complications, such as meningitis, and other complications such as device extrusion.[36] Therefore, complete eradication of the disease should be obtained before implantation. Intact canal wall mastoidectomy and radical mastoidectomy are both options to remove the disease depending on the extent and likelihood of recurrence. It is recommended that the implant be placed at least 3 to 6 months after eradication of the disease.[28] As revision surgery is performed 6 to 12 months after the first surgery, the same waiting period should apply toward cochlear implantation surgery.[28]

Device-Related Complications of Cochlear Implantation

Device Failure

Device failure is one of the major complications in cochlear implantation, given the potential need to explant and reimplant the device. Cohen in 2004, in his review, found that the most common reason for cochlear reimplantation is device failure, occurring most frequently in children, as a result of head trauma.[37,38] Other device failures can occur immediately, as the result of factory defects or damage during surgical manipulation. They can be divided into hard and soft failures. Hard device failures account for 42 to 83% of revision surgeries whereas soft failures account for 15 to 41.7% of the surgeries.[39–42]

A cochlear implant with a hard failure is defined as one that is out of compliance with the manufacturer's specifications with in vivo integrity testing revealing abnormal implant performance.[41] A soft failure, on the other hand, is a diagnosis of exclusion, typically manifesting as deteriorations in implant performance or poor patient progression with the implant. In vivo integrity testing is typically unable to demonstrate any detectable defect in soft failures.[43] Certain steps should be taken when a device failure is suspected. The audiologist should interrogate the device, adjust program settings and exchange the external component as needed. A medical evaluation including an otologic examination and imaging of the implant to assess its placement is performed.

Suspected device failure (soft failure), can be the result of an inability of the internal receiver to maintain a lock with the external speech processor, a complete loss of connectivity between the receiver and the electrode array or a gradual disconnection, or a short circuiting of the electrodes. The patient may also develop some symptoms such as pain, vertigo, headache, aberrant sounds, increased loudness, facial nerve stimulation, intermittent cochlear implant function or programming difficulties. Despite being classified as a soft failure, 38 to 86% of devices removed have subsequently been found to have a detectable defect during bench testing.[39,41] This emphasizes the importance of close follow-up on a patient's performance postoperatively to promptly diagnose these soft failures. When dealing with symptoms related to device failures, revisional cochlear implant surgery should be considered.

Device Extrusion

Device failure, wound and flap-related problems, electrode extrusion, device upgrade and cholesteatoma formation, are the most common causes for device extrusion and have already been addressed in this chapter.

Facial Nerve Stimulation

Because of the close proximity of the facial nerve to the cochlear nerve, the most common nonauditory stimulation related to cochlear implant surgery is inadvertent facial nerve stimulation by the cochlear implant electrodes in 1 to 14% of cases.[15,36,44,45] Various etiologies have been suggested: the close proximity of the labyrinthine segment of the facial nerve to the basal turn of the cochlea, especially in inner ear malformations; a change in the electrical conduction of bone, more common in otosclerosis; the proximity of the electrodes to the modiolus; and the design of the cochlear implant electrode.

Electrical current passing through the electrode to reach the spiral ganglion cells stimulates the nearby facial nerve resulting in symptoms that can vary from simple perception to facial spasm.[46] This is believed to be a result of the proximity of the labyrinthine portion of the facial nerve to the basal turn of the cochlea.[47] Additionally, the change in bone matrix properties in abnormal bone remodeling can change the conductive pathway of the electrical current through the cochlear bone. Facial nerve stimulation is mostly seen in patients with cochlear bony dysplasias such as cochlear otosclerosis, cochlear labyrinthitis ossificans, or those with new bone formation in the cochlea.[46] It has been suggested that the use of a modiolar hugging electrode array, which tends to direct the current toward the spiral ganglion as opposed to the outer rim of the cochlea, can decrease facial nerve stimulation.[48] Despite the concerns regarding electrode positioning, Ahn et al in 2009,[46] found that in normal cochleas, the prevalence of facial nerve stimulation remains unchanged regardless of type of electrode used. Different options can be presented to cochlear implant recipients who experience facial nerve stimulation. The most conservative strategy consists of reprogramming the device, reduction of the stimulation levels, and selective deactivation of electrodes. Although these measures can reduce the discomfort caused by facial nerve stimulation, increasing channel deactivation with reduction of stimulus levels will limit the benefit that patients receive from cochlear implants. Reimplantation can also be considered, whether it be on the same or the contralateral side. The use of a perimodiolar electrode array may help to decrease the likelihood of facial nerve stimulation.[46]

Magnet-related Complications

A potential device after cochlear implantation is the migration or displacement of the magnet from its central location within the receiver-stimulator pocket.[49–54] This is more common in the newer implants whose magnets are surrounded by silastic and removable in an outpatient surgery setting if necessary. Whereas these new implants provide the patients with the possibility of performing magnetic resonance imaging after the magnet is removed, they have an increased risk of magnet displacement compared with older ceramic implants in which the magnet was completely encased. This can result in the need for reimplantation of the magnet.

The most frequent cause of magnet displacement is head trauma in children, who tend to suffer more minor head injuries than adults. Not only do they have a smaller skull with a bigger curvature of the skull, they have thinner skin compared with adults, which results in less protection against trauma and nearby magnets, such as those in toys. Once the magnet is displaced, the skin flap overlying it is at increased risk of breaking down and the magnetic coil may not lock on to the receiver properly.

Usually an outpatient surgery to reposition the magnet will be required. Until then, patients are advised not to wear their device to minimize skin flap injury. To repair this, a separate incision posterior to the receiver is made and the skin flap is elevated over the fibrous capsule overlying the receiver. The magnet is identified and is then repositioned in the correct orientation.[49] To reduce the incidence of magnet displacement, manufacturers have modified the magnet well, reducing its diameter from 6 to 5.3 mm.[42]

External magnet retention difficulty is another rare complication after cochlear implantation. When the external coil does not attach to the receiver properly, initial stimulation and programming of the device can be difficult even though this complication is not always reported in the literature. Magnet fixation problems can be intermittent, fluctuating or present as a noisy signal from the device; a drop in auditory performance differentiates magnet retention difficulty from a soft failure.[55] The most common cause of magnet retention difficulty is the presence of a thick skin flap. When the thickness

is greater than 7 mm the appropriate coupling and signal transmission to the receiver-stimulator can become difficult.[55]

Within the first year of cochlear implantation, the flap thins naturally from the compression between the external and internal magnets.[56] When there is concern regarding the thickness of the flap, a percutaneous puncture or the use of an ultrasound can be used to determine the thickness.[55] Conservative treatment consists of increasing the magnet strength of the headpiece, hair shaving at the magnet site, or the use of a headband to secure the headpiece. However, these techniques are not always successful and can lead to irritation or erythema of the skin flap.[57] Alternatively, surgical revision of the skin flap may be considered with other risks such as increased flap breakdown, ulceration, necrosis, and potential magnet exposure.[14,50,58]

Other Complications and Challenges of Cochlear Implantation

When cochlear implants first gained popularity, inner ear malformations were a contraindication to surgery.[59] In 1983, Mangabeira-Albernaz[60] reported the first successful implantation in a patient with Mondini dysplasia, a cochlear malformation. Challenges to cochlear implantation that present in patients with ear malformations include difficult access to the cochlea, an aberrant facial nerve, perilymph or CSF fistula resulting in a gusher, abnormal cochlear nerve, and unwanted facial nerve stimulation.[61] In all children suspected of middle ear malformations, proper radiographic studies including a computed tomography temporal bone scan and magnetic resonance image of the internal auditory canals must be obtained to evaluate the patency and development of the cochlea, location of the facial nerve, and presence of the cochlear nerve as this can affect candidacy for cochlear implantation.

Aberrant Facial Nerve

The presence of an inner ear abnormality should alert the physician to the possibility of an aberrant facial nerve. In certain malformations such as the common cavity and cochlear hypoplasia, the vertical segment of the nerve can be dislocated anteromedially toward the promontory, overlying the round and oval windows.[59,62] Patients with cochlear hypoplasia often have accompanying semicircular canal abnormalities, which have been associated with an aberrant course through the second genu and mastoid segment.[59] Although in most cases the nerve is displaced anteriorly, it has also been described as more lateral and posterior to its usual course in the setting of a hypoplastic lateral semicircular canal.[59] Even though most surgeons already use intraoperative facial nerve monitoring during cochlear implantation, it is crucial for patients with inner ear abnormalities, especially where there is an aberrant or dehiscent nerve.

Approach to the Cochlea in a Malformed Ear

Whereas in most patients, the standard transmastoid–facial recess approach can be used to access the cochlea, the presence of complex malformations may require modification of the approach. In a study by McElveen, of 71 patients who had inner ear abnormalities, six patients required the use of alternative approaches including a transcanal approach and a transmastoid labyrinthotomy approach.

Cerebrospinal Fluid Leak and Gusher

Cerebrospinal fluid leak during cochlear implantation can be a result of a dural breach or arise from an abnormal communication between the cochlea and the CSF compartment, resulting in a "gusher." The former is considered a technical error and can be easily avoided with proper drilling techniques and identification of landmarks, the latter is related to the patient's anatomy and understanding the risk factors may help the surgeon to identify and manage the leak in a timely fashion. Abnormal development of the otic capsule and trauma are commonly encountered in the presence of a CSF leak. Common malformations of the inner ear include common cavity deformity, cochlear hypoplasia, an unusually patent cochlear aqueduct and enlarged vestibular aqueduct syndrome.[59,63] Of these, the most frequently encountered associated with a gusher during the creation of the cochleostomy is the common cavity deformity.[64] However, there are instances in which a CSF gusher may present in ears with a normal cochlea. Although the overall incidence of a cochleostomy gusher is 6.7% in a large case series of 298 children, multiple studies have demonstrated a 50% leak rate in those with abnormal cochleovestibular anatomy.[63,65–67] Nevertheless, in a study by Wootten et al,[64] normal cochlear anatomy was encountered in half of the patients with gushers, showing that although malformations of the inner ear may be predictive of a CSF gusher, the presence of a normal cochlea cannot exclude the risk of one.

In most cases, CSF leak can be managed conservatively. An algorithm proposed by Wootten et al.[64] is given in **Fig. 5.1**. Upon encountering the gusher, the electrode should be placed followed by immediate packing of the cochleostomy and middle ear with temporalis fascia and muscle, with or without fibrin glue, for "tight" packing. The patient can be placed in reverse Trendelenburg position to decrease the CSF flow. Other measures to stop the flow of CSF include hyperventilation to decrease $PaCO_2$ to 27 to 29 mmHg, administration of mannitol, and keeping the head of the bed elevated in addition to compression dressings. A watertight closure is performed. Occasionally a lumbar drain may be required if the leak persists after packing the middle ear space. Leaks that cannot be controlled with a lumbar drain may require obliteration of the middle ear with fat and oversewing of the ear canal.[64]

Vestibular Dysfunction

Because of the close relationship between the cochlea and vestibular labyrinth, transient vertigo has been described in less than 10 to 74% of patients after cochlear implantation.[68–70] Various reasons for vertigo after cochlear implantation have been suggested. In some patients, cross stimulation of the vestibular system by the cochlear implant electrode has been reported.[71–73] A coactivation of the inferior vestibular nerve or the saccular macula by electrical stimulation has been suggested given the presence of increased vestibular evoked myogenic potentials in some patients after cochlear implant activation.[74] On the other hand, the majority of patients have decreased vestibular evoked myogenic potential responses after cochlear implantation, which is thought to be from insertion trauma by the electrode, impairing the integrity of the vestibular receptors in the saccule.[75] Other studies have also shown significant postoperative vestibular loss after implantation, between 30 and 60%.[76,77]

Risk factors associated with increased postoperative vestibular symptoms include: preimplantation vestibular symptoms, especially in patients with Meniere disease, older age at time of implantation (> 59 years old), age at onset of hearing loss (> 26 years old), abnormal dynamic posturography preimplantation.[69] Whereas the preoperative caloric testing results were not predictive of those who would suffer vertigo postoperatively, those who were symptomatic had a greater degree of unilateral weakness.[78] However, there have been reports of improvement in computerized dynamic posturography after cochlear implantation.[58]

Patients with persistent vestibular symptoms, lasting more than 1 week after cochlear implant surgery could benefit from vestibular rehabilitation. Patients have benefited from exercises that stimulate the vestibular–ocular reflex with faster compensation and recovery times after unilateral vestibular loss.[78]

Complications of Osseointegrated Implants

The osseointegrated implant, more commonly referred to as the bone-anchored hearing aid (BAHA) is a percutaneous implant introduced in 1977 that was originally designed for patients with unilateral conductive hearing loss, either congenital or acquired, who cannot wear a hearing aid.[79–81] Since then, the indications for the BAHA have expanded to include bilateral conductive or mixed

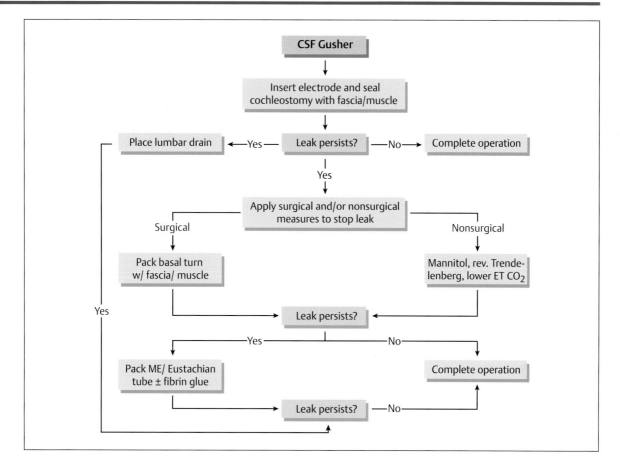

Fig. 5.1 Management of intraoperative cochleostomy gusher. (From Wootten et al, 2006.[64] Reprinted with permission from John Wiley and Sons.)

hearing loss as well as unilateral sensorineural deafness. Although the surgical technique has evolved over the years, wound and flap complications continue to be the most frequent problems. Multiple institutions have published their complication rates over the years ranging from as low as 8% to as high as 89%.[82-94] Despite these complications, the BAHA has been shown to improve hearing outcomes and quality of life.[88,95-99] Most BAHA complications can be classified under two main categories: bony and soft tissue.[19] Other, rarer complications such as paresthesia, dural perforation, osteonecrosis, subdural hematoma and meningitis have also been described.[99]

Bony Complications of Osseointegrated Implants

Bone-anchored hearing aids rely on an osseointegrated titanium implant to attach the device to the skull. Chronic inflammation and infection can develop at the site of the implant interface with the skull and may result in bone overgrowth or extrusion of the implant. The most common bony complication of BAHA surgery is failure of osseointegration with fixture loss. It has been reported

in the literature to be between 5.3 and 40% especially in children under 5 years old.[85,96] In some cases, this presents as a loose abutment–fixture complex that falls out. In others, a fibrous attachment keeps the fixture in place but the complex spins freely, resulting in patients experiencing little or no sound or complaining of sound distortion.[100]

Risk factors affecting osseointegration include a thin calvarium, poor surgical technique, trauma, and new bone growth.[94] Of these, the most common problem encountered in the insertion of fixtures is inadequate calvarial thickness resulting in failure to osseointegrate.[94] This is often seen in younger children and in those with abnormal craniofacial syndromes. For that reason, the FDA guidelines recommend a lower limit of 5 years for implantation because most children at this age have calvarial thickness that can hold a 3-mm fixture.[100] Fixtures less than 3 mm in length have been shown to have a higher failure rate.[101-103] When thin bone is encountered, the surgeon has the option of closing the wound and returning 6 to 12 months later when the temporal bone is thicker, or performing a two-stage procedure in which the bone is augmented around a 3-mm fixture in which

1 mm of the fixture is exposed above the skull. The space is packed with bone chips and dust and secured with a synthetic material.[100,104,105] Alternatively, a fixture that is slightly longer than the thickness of the skull may be placed (i.e., 3-mm fixture for bone that is 2.5 mm thick) with a longer waiting period for osseointegration before loading the implant.[94,103,106]

Poor surgical technique resulting in a loosely fitted fixture can also increase the likelihood of failure to osseointegrate. According to the study of 51 children by Zeitoun et al, they were incompletely inserted into bone 4.7% of the time. However, some of these fixtures were able to osseointegrate after leaving the fixture unloaded for a longer waiting period. Because of the higher failure rate in younger children, some authors recommend placing sleeper fixtures at the same time as the primary surgery.

Trauma, although rare (1 to 2.8%), was seen more often in older children as a cause for fixture loss.[82,94] New bone formation has also been described in the literature, typically in children between the ages of 5 and 11 where there is rapid bony growth of their temporal and parietal bones.[102,106] This bone can be carefully removed to salvage the fixture without requiring reimplantation.[107] Alternatively, longer fixtures have been placed to minimize the need for reimplantation in the presence of bony or even skin overgrowth.

Soft Tissue Complications of Osseointegrated Implants

Soft tissue complications especially around the abutment are common in BAHA implants. They may range from 2.4% to 44%, with variable severity.[96,108,109] Skin overgrowth (granulation tissue, hypertrophic skin, local dermatitis and cellulitis), loosening of the abutment, and infectious complications resulting in implant extrusion were the soft tissue complications found most often. The treatment varies with the skin reaction ranging from conservative treatment with antibiotic ointments to revision surgery. The Holger classification system (**Table 5.1**) has commonly been used to describe skin reactions. Typically, for grade 1 reactions, local antibiotic ointment is recommended. Grade 2 reactions may require reapplication of the healing cap and wrapping the area with antibiotic gauze for a period of time. Often, grade 3 and 4 reactions require revision surgery.[100]

Studies have shown that skin reactions may be related to surgical technique. Early BAHA implantation with the two-stage technique tended to produce later onset of skin reactions, often years after implantation, whereas single-stage technique BAHA implantation has been associated with a higher incidence of skin reactions within the first year of surgery but becoming less common as the surgery date becomes more remote.[110] Other studies have shown differences in skin complication rates between the use of a dermatome, postauricular skin graft, and various skin flap methods. Tamarit Conejeros et al[111] showed in a study of 27 patients that use of the dermatome produced a higher rate of skin reactions (74%) compared with those patients who had a U-shaped skin flap (34%). Van Rompaey et al,[81] in a retrospective study of 138 patients between 1998 and 2008, also found a high incidence of skin complications associated with the dermatome such that the authors have since used a linear incision technique to decrease their complication rate.[88,98,111,112]

Skin overgrowth can also be a problem with the BAHA. Conservative management with topical steroids has been shown to be helpful in early stages.[100] For more severe skin reactions, local steroid injections can be considered in addition to the application of steroid creams. However, they should not be used when there is suspected or known delay in wound healing. Furthermore, the skin surrounding the abutment may be removed as an office procedure. If conservative measures fail, the patient may need revision of the skin flap, which requires removal of all soft tissue down to the level of the periosteum. Alternatively, the abutment may be replaced with a longer one, especially in cases of chronic skin overgrowth.

Conclusions

Implantable devices have allowed hearing impaired patients to function in society in ways that hearing aids are unable to. However, the procedures to implant these devices are not without risks or complications. As surgeons continue to understand the complications, new methods of minimizing and treating them will continue

Table 5.1 The Holger classification system for grading soft tissue reactions[112]

Grade	Skin reaction	Incidence[105,110,112]
0	Reaction-free skin around abutment	90–95%
1	Redness with slight swelling around abutment	3–5%
2	Redness, moistness, and moderate swelling	1–4%
3	Redness, moistness, and moderate swelling with tissue granulation around abutment	0.5–1.5%
4	Overt signs of infection resulting in removal of implant	< 0.5%

to evolve. It is imperative that before surgery patients understand the risks because some may have devastating consequences.

References

1. Wei BP, Shepherd RK, Robins-Browne RM, Clark GM, O'Leary SJ. Threshold shift: effects of cochlear implantation on the risk of pneumococcal meningitis. Otolaryngol Head Neck Surg 2007;136(4):589–596

2. Wei BP, Shepherd RK, Robins-Browne RM, Clark GM, O'Leary SJ. Pneumococcal meningitis post-cochlear implantation: preventative measures. Otolaryngol Head Neck Surg 2010; 143(5, Suppl 3)S9–S14

3. Fayad JN, Wanna GB, Micheletto JN, Parisier SC. Facial nerve paralysis following cochlear implant surgery. Laryngoscope 2003;113(8):1344–1346

4. Lalwani AK, Butt FY, Jackler RK, Pitts LH, Yingling CD. Delayed onset facial nerve dysfunction following acoustic neuroma surgery. Am J Otol 1995;16(6):758–764

5. Shea JJ Jr, Ge X. Delayed facial palsy after stapedectomy. Otol Neurotol 2001;22(4):465–470

6. Vrabec JT. Delayed facial palsy after tympanomastoid surgery. Am J Otol 1999;20(1):26–30

7. Joseph ST, Vishwakarma R, Ramani MK, Aurora R. Cochlear implant and delayed facial palsy. Cochlear Implants Int 2009;10(4):229–236

8. Lloyd S, Meerton L, Di Cuffa R, Lavy J, Graham J. Taste change following cochlear implantation. Cochlear Implants Int 2007;8(4):203–210

9. Hoffman RA, Cohen NL. Complications of cochlear implant surgery. Ann Otol Rhinol Laryngol Suppl 1995;166:420–422

10. Yu KC, Hegarty JL, Gantz BJ, Lalwani AK. Conservative management of infections in cochlear implant recipients. Otolaryngol Head Neck Surg 2001;125(1):66–70

11. Telian SA, El-Kashlan HK, Arts HA. Minimizing wound complications in cochlear implant surgery. Am J Otol 1999;20(3):331–334

12. Wei BP, Shepherd RK, Robins-Browne RM, Clark GM, O'Leary SJ. Pneumococcal meningitis post-cochlear implantation: potential routes of infection and pathophysiology. Otolaryngol Head Neck Surg 2010; 143(5, Suppl 3) S15–S23

13. Reefhuis J, Honein MA, Whitney CG, et al. Risk of bacterial meningitis in children with cochlear implants. N Engl J Med 2003;349(5):435–445

14. Bhatia K, Gibbin KP, Nikolopoulos TP, O'Donoghue GM. Surgical complications and their management in a series of 300 consecutive pediatric cochlear implantations. Otol Neurotol 2004;25(5):730–739

15. Niparko JK, Oviatt DL, Coker NJ, Sutton L, Waltzman SB, Cohen NL. Facial nerve stimulation with cochlear implantation. VA Cooperative Study Group on Cochlear Implantation. Otolaryngol Head Neck Surg 1991;104(6):826–830

16. Wei BP, Shepherd RK, Robins-Browne RM, Clark GM, O'Leary SJ. Effects of inner ear trauma on the risk of pneumococcal meningitis. Arch Otolaryngol Head Neck Surg 2007;133(3):250–259

17. Goycoolea MV. Clinical aspects of round window membrane permeability under normal and pathological conditions. Acta Otolaryngol 2001;121(4):437–447

18. Phelps PD, King A, Michaels L. Cochlear dysplasia and meningitis. Am J Otol 1994;15(4):551–557

19. Ohlms LA, Edwards MS, Mason EO, Igarashi M, Alford BR, Smith RJ. Recurrent meningitis and Mondini dysplasia. Arch Otolaryngol Head Neck Surg 1990;116(5):608–612

20. Bluestone CD. Prevention of meningitis: cochlear implants and inner ear abnormalities. Arch Otolaryngol Head Neck Surg 2003;129(3):279–281

21. Igarashi M, Saito R, Alford BR, Filippone MV, Smith JA. Temporal bone findings in pneumococcal meningitis. Arch Otolaryngol 1974;99(2):79–83

22. Igarashi M, Schuknecht HF. Pneumococcal otitis media, meningitis, and labyrinthitis. Arch Otolaryngol 1962;76: 126–130

23. Merchant SN, Gopen Q. A human temporal bone study of acute bacterial meningogenic labyrinthitis. Am J Otol 1996;17(3):375–385

24. Rubin LG, Papsin B; Committee on Infectious Diseases and Section on Otolaryngology-Head and Neck Surgery. Cochlear implants in children: surgical site infections and prevention and treatment of acute otitis media and meningitis. Pediatrics 2010;126(2):381–391

25. Rivas A, Wanna GB, Haynes DS. Revision cochlear implantation in children. Otolaryngol Clin North Am 2012;45(1):205–219

26. Hausdorff WP, Bryant J, Paradiso PR, Siber GR. Which pneumococcal serogroups cause the most invasive disease: implications for conjugate vaccine formulation and use, part I. Clin Infect Dis 2000;30(1):100–121

27. Centers for Disease Control and Prevention (CDC). Advisory Committee on Immunization Practices. Pneumococcal vaccination for cochlear implant candidates and recipients: updated recommendations of the Advisory Committee on Immunization Practices. MMWR Morb Mortal Wkly Rep 2003;52(31):739–740

28. Hellingman CA, Dunnebier EA. Cochlear implantation in patients with acute or chronic middle ear infectious disease: a review of the literature. Eur Arch Otorhinolaryngol 2009;266(2):171–176

29. Hey C, Rose MA, Kujumdshiev S, Gstoettner W, Schubert R, Zielen S. Does the 23-valent pneumococcal vaccine protect cochlear implant recipients? Laryngoscope 2005; 115(9):1586–1590

30. Roland JT Jr. A model for cochlear implant electrode insertion and force evaluation: results with a new electrode design and insertion technique. Laryngoscope 2005;115(8):1325–1339

31. Briggs RJ, Tykocinski M, Stidham K, Roberson JB. Cochleostomy site: implications for electrode placement and hearing preservation. Acta Otolaryngol 2005;125(8):870–876

32. Skinner MW, Holden TA, Whiting BR, et al. In vivo estimates of the position of advanced bionics electrode arrays in the human cochlea. Ann Otol Rhinol Laryngol Suppl 2007;197:2–24

33. Hopfenspirger MT, Levine SC, Rimell FL. Infectious complications in pediatric cochlear implants. Laryngoscope 2007;117(10):1825–1829

34. Antonelli PJ, Lee JC, Burne RA. Bacterial biofilms may contribute to persistent cochlear implant infection. Otol Neurotol 2004;25(6):953–957

35. Lin YS. Management of otitis media-related diseases in children with a cochlear implant. Acta Otolaryngol 2009;129(3):254–260

36. Kelsall DC, Shallop JK, Brammeier TG, Prenger EC. Facial nerve stimulation after Nucleus 22-channel cochlear implantation. Am J Otol 1997;18(3):336–341

37. Achiques MT, Morant A, Muñoz N, et al. [Cochlear implant complications and failures]. Acta Otorrinolaringol Esp 2010;61(6):412–417

38. Cohen NL. Cochlear implant candidacy and surgical considerations. Audiol Neurootol 2004;9(4):197–202

39. Rivas A, Marlowe AL, Chinnici JE, Niparko JK, Francis HW. Revision cochlear implantation surgery in adults: indications and results. Otol Neurotol 2008;29(5):639–648

40. Venail F, Sicard M, Piron JP, et al. Reliability and complications of 500 consecutive cochlear implantations. Arch Otolaryngol Head Neck Surg 2008;134(12):1276–1281

41. Brown KD, Connell SS, Balkany TJ, Eshraghi AE, Telischi FF, Angeli SA. Incidence and indications for revision cochlear implant surgery in adults and children. Laryngoscope 2009;119(1):152–157

42. Cullen RD, Fayad JN, Luxford WM, Buchman CA. Revision cochlear implant surgery in children. Otol Neurotol 2008;29(2):214–220

43. Balkany TJ, Hodges AV, Buchman CA, et al. Cochlear implant soft failures consensus development conference statement. Otol Neurotol 2005;26(4):815–818

44. Rayner MG, King T, Djalilian HR, Smith S, Levine SC. Resolution of facial stimulation in otosclerotic cochlear implants. Otolaryngol Head Neck Surg 2003;129(5):475–480

45. Cohen NL, Hoffman RA, Stroschein M. Medical or surgical complications related to the Nucleus multichannel cochlear implant. Ann Otol Rhinol Laryngol Suppl 1988;135:8–13

46. Ahn JH, Oh SH, Chung JW, Lee KS. Facial nerve stimulation after cochlear implantation according to types of Nucleus 24-channel electrode arrays. Acta Otolaryngol 2009;129(6):588–591

47. Gulya AJ, Minor LB, Poe DS, eds. Glasscock-Shambaugh's Surgery of the Ear. 6th ed. Shelton: PMPH-USA; 2010

48. Polak M, Ulubil SA, Hodges AV, Balkany TJ. Revision cochlear implantation for facial nerve stimulation in otosclerosis. Arch Otolaryngol Head Neck Surg 2006;132(4):398–404

49. Nichani JR, Broomfield SJ, Saeed SR. Displacement of the magnet of a cochlear implant receiver stimulator package following minor head trauma. Cochlear Implants Int 2004;5(3):105–111

50. Migirov L, Taitelbaum-Swead R, Hildesheimer M, Kronenberg J. Revision surgeries in cochlear implant patients: a review of 45 cases. Eur Arch Otorhinolaryngol 2007;264(1):3–7

51. Yun JM, Colburn MW, Antonelli PJ. Cochlear implant magnet displacement with minor head trauma. Otolaryngol Head Neck Surg 2005;133(2):275–277

52. Stokroos RJ, van Dijk P. Migration of cochlear implant magnets after head trauma in an adult and a child. Ear Nose Throat J 2007;86(10):612–613

53. Wilkinson EP, Dogru S, Meyer TA, Gantz BJ. Case report: cochlear implant magnet migration. Laryngoscope 2004;114(11):2009–2011

54. Deneuve S, Loundon N, Leboulanger N, Rouillon I, Garabedian EN. Cochlear implant magnet displacement during magnetic resonance imaging. Otol Neurotol 2008; 29(6):789–790

55. Posner D, Scott A, Polite C, Lustig LR. External magnet displacement in cochlear implants: causes and management. Otol Neurotol 2010;31(1):88–93

56. Raine CH, Lee CA, Strachan DR, Totten CT, Khan S. Skin flap thickness in cochlear implant patients – a prospective study. Cochlear Implants Int 2007;8(3):148–157

57. Cohen NL, Hoffman RA. Surgical complications of multichannel cochlear implants in North America. Adv Otorhinolaryngol 1993;48:70–74

58. Buchman CA, Higgins CA, Cullen R, Pillsbury HC. Revision cochlear implant surgery in adult patients with suspected device malfunction. Otol Neurotol 2004;25(4):504–510, discussion 510

59. Sennaroglu L. Cochlear implantation in inner ear malformations—a review article. Cochlear Implants Int 2010;11(1):4–41

60. Mangabeira-Albernaz PL. The Mondini dysplasia—from early diagnosis to cochlear implant. Acta Otolaryngol 1983;95(5-6):627–631

61. Graham JM, Phelps PD, Michaels L. Congenital malformations of the ear and cochlear implantation in children: review and temporal bone report of common cavity. J Laryngol Otol Suppl 2000;25:1–14

62. Romo LV, Curtin HD. Anomalous facial nerve canal with cochlear malformations. AJNR Am J Neuroradiol 2001;22(5):838–844

63. Fahy CP, Carney AS, Nikolopoulos TP, Ludman CN, Gibbin KP. Cochlear implantation in children with large vestibular aqueduct syndrome and a review of the syndrome. Int J Pediatr Otorhinolaryngol 2001;59(3):207–215

64. Wootten CT, Backous DD, Haynes DS. Management of cerebrospinal fluid leakage from cochleostomy during cochlear implant surgery. Laryngoscope 2006;116(11):2055–2059

65. Papsin BC. Cochlear implantation in children with anomalous cochleovestibular anatomy. Laryngoscope 2005; 115(1 Pt 2, Suppl 106)1–26

66. Luntz M, Balkany T, Hodges AV, Telischi FF. Cochlear implants in children with congenital inner ear malformations. Arch Otolaryngol Head Neck Surg 1997;123(9):974–977

67. Weber BP, Dillo W, Dietrich B, Maneke I, Bertram B, Lenarz T. Pediatric cochlear implantation in cochlear malformations. Am J Otol 1998;19(6):747–753

68. Dutt SN, Ray J, Hadjihannas E, Cooper H, Donaldson I, Proops DW. Medical and surgical complications of the second 100 adult cochlear implant patients in Birmingham. J Laryngol Otol 2005;119(10):759–764

69. Fina M, Skinner M, Goebel JA, Piccirillo JF, Neely JG, Black O. Vestibular dysfunction after cochlear implantation. Otol Neurotol 2003;24(2):234–242, discussion 242

70. Steenerson RL, Cronin GW, Gary LB. Vertigo after cochlear implantation. Otol Neurotol 2001;22(6):842–843

71. Bilger RC, Black FO. Auditory prostheses in perspective. Ann Otol Rhinol Laryngol Suppl 1977; 86(3 Pt 2, Suppl 38)3–10

72. Black FO. Effects of the auditory prosthesis on postural stability. Ann Otol Rhinol Laryngol Suppl 1977; 86(3 Pt 2, Suppl 38)141–164

73. Black FO, Lilly DJ, Peterka RJ, Fowler LP, Simmons FB. Vestibulo-ocular and vestibulospinal function before and after cochlear implant surgery. Ann Otol Rhinol Laryngol Suppl 1987;96(1 Pt 2):106–108

74. Jin Y, Nakamura M, Shinjo Y, Kaga K. Vestibular-evoked myogenic potentials in cochlear implant children. Acta Otolaryngol 2006;126(2):164–169

75. Jin Y, Shinjo Y, Akamatsu Y, et al. Vestibular evoked myogenic potentials evoked by multichannel cochlear implant – influence of C levels. Acta Otolaryngol 2008; 128(3):284–290

76. Huygen PL, Hinderink JB, van den Broek P, et al. The risk of vestibular function loss after intracochlear implantation. Acta Otolaryngol Suppl 1995;520(Pt 2):270–272

77. Limb CJ, Francis HF, Lustig LR, Niparko JK, Jammal H. Benign positional vertigo after cochlear implantation. Otolaryngol Head Neck Surg 2005;132(5):741–745

78. Enticott JC, Tari S, Koh SM, Dowell RC, O'Leary SJ. Cochlear implant and vestibular function. Otol Neurotol 2006;27(6):824–830

79. Macnamara M, Phillips D, Proops DW. The bone anchored hearing aid (BAHA) in chronic suppurative otitis media (CSOM). J Laryngol Otol Suppl 1996;21:38–40

80. Browning GG, Gatehouse S. Estimation of the benefit of bone-anchored hearing aids. Ann Otol Rhinol Laryngol 1994;103(11):872–878

81. Van Rompaey V, Claes G, Verstraeten N, et al. Skin reactions following BAHA surgery using the skin flap dermatome technique. Eur Arch Otorhinolaryngol 2011; 268(3):373–376

82. Hobson JC, Roper AJ, Andrew R, Rothera MP, Hill P, Green KM. Complications of bone-anchored hearing aid implantation. J Laryngol Otol 2010;124(2):132–136

83. Kraai T, Brown C, Neeff M, Fisher K. Complications of bone-anchored hearing aids in pediatric patients. Int J Pediatr Otorhinolaryngol 2011;75(6):749–753

84. House JW, Kutz JW Jr. Bone-anchored hearing aids: incidence and management of postoperative complications. Otol Neurotol 2007;28(2):213–217

85. Davids T, Gordon KA, Clutton D, Papsin BC. Bone-anchored hearing aids in infants and children younger than 5 years. Arch Otolaryngol Head Neck Surg 2007;133(1):51–55

86. Gillett D, Fairley JW, Chandrashaker TS, Bean A, Gonzalez J. Bone-anchored hearing aids: results of the first eight years of a programme in a district general hospital, assessed by the Glasgow benefit inventory. J Laryngol Otol 2006;120(7):537–542

87. Kohan D, Morris LG, Romo T III. Single-stage BAHA implantation in adults and children: is it safe? Otolaryngol Head Neck Surg 2008;138(5):662–666

88. Lloyd S, Almeyda J, Sirimanna KS, Albert DM, Bailey CM. Updated surgical experience with bone-anchored hearing aids in children. J Laryngol Otol 2007;121(9):826–831

89. Lustig LR, Arts HA, Brackmann DE, et al. Hearing rehabilitation using the BAHA bone-anchored hearing aid: results in 40 patients. Otol Neurotol 2001;22(3):328–334

90. McDermott AL, Williams J, Kuo M, Reid A, Proops D. The Birmingham pediatric bone-anchored hearing aid program: a 15-year experience. Otol Neurotol 2009;30(2):178–183

91. Shirazi MA, Marzo SJ, Leonetti JP. Perioperative complications with the bone-anchored hearing aid. Otolaryngol Head Neck Surg 2006;134(2):236–239

92. Wazen JJ, Young DL, Farrugia MC, et al. Successes and complications of the Baha system. Otol Neurotol 2008;29(8):1115–1119

93. Yellon RF. Bone anchored hearing aid in children—prevention of complications. Int J Pediatr Otorhinolaryngol 2007;71(5):823–826

94. Zeitoun H, De R, Thompson SD, Proops DW. Osseointegrated implants in the management of childhood ear abnormalities: with particular emphasis on complications. J Laryngol Otol 2002;116(2):87–91

95. Mylanus EA, van der Pouw KC, Snik AF, Cremers CW. Intraindividual comparison of the bone-anchored hearing aid and air-conduction hearing aids. Arch Otolaryngol Head Neck Surg 1998;124(3):271–276

96. McDermott AL, Sheehan P. Bone anchored hearing aids in children. Curr Opin Otolaryngol Head Neck Surg 2009;17(6):488–493

97. McDermott AL, Williams J, Kuo M, Reid A, Proops D. Quality of life in children fitted with a bone-anchored hearing aid. Otol Neurotol 2009;30(3):344–349

98. Tietze L, Papsin B. Utilization of bone-anchored hearing aids in children. Int J Pediatr Otorhinolaryngol 2001;58(1):75–80

99. Weber PC. Medical and surgical considerations for implantable hearing prosthetic devices. Am J Audiol 2002;11(2):134–138

100. Battista RA, Littlefield PD. Revision BAHA Surgery. Otolaryngol Clin North Am 2006;39(4):801–813, viii viii

101. Tjellström A, Granström G. One-stage procedure to establish osseointegration: a zero to five years follow-up report. J Laryngol Otol 1995;109(7):593–598

102. Granström G, Bergström K, Odersjö M, Tjellström A. Osseointegrated implants in children: experience from our first 100 patients. Otolaryngol Head Neck Surg 2001;125(1):85–92

103. Papsin BC, Sirimanna TK, Albert DM, Bailey CM. Surgical experience with bone-anchored hearing aids in children. Laryngoscope 1997;107(6):801–806

104. Proops DW. The Birmingham bone anchored hearing aid programme: surgical methods and complications. J Laryngol Otol Suppl 1996;21:7–12

105. Reyes RA, Tjellström A, Granström G. Evaluation of implant losses and skin reactions around extraoral bone-anchored implants: a 0- to 8-year follow-up. Otolaryngol Head Neck Surg 2000;122(2):272–276

106. Jacobsson M, Albrektsson T, Tjellström A. Tissue-integrated implants in children. Int J Pediatr Otorhinolaryngol 1992;24(3):235–243

107. Sunkaraneni VS, Gray RF. Bony overgrowth onto fixture component of a bone-anchored hearing aid. J Laryngol Otol 2004;118(8):643–644

108. McDermott AL, Barraclough J, Reid AP. Unusual complication following trauma to a bone-anchored hearing aid: case report and literature review. J Laryngol Otol 2009;123(3):348–350

109. Mani N, Rothera M, Sheehan P. Two-stage BAHA with one general anaesthetic in children. Clin Otolaryngol 2009;34(3):269–270

110. Badran K, Arya AK, Bunstone D, Mackinnon N. Long-term complications of bone-anchored hearing aids: a 14-year experience. J Laryngol Otol 2009;123(2):170–176

111. Tamarit Conejeros JM, Dalmau Galofre J, Murcia Puchades V, Pons Rocher F, Fernández Martínez S, Estrems Navas P. Comparison of skin complications between dermatome and U-graft technique in BAHA surgery. [Article in Spanish] Acta Otorrinolaringol Esp 2009;60(6):422–427

112. de Wolf MJ, Hol MK, Huygen PL, Mylanus EA, Cremers CW. Nijmegen results with application of a bone-anchored hearing aid in children: simplified surgical technique. Ann Otol Rhinol Laryngol 2008;117(11):805–814

6 Complications in Surgery of the Lateral Skull Base

H. H. Sudhoff, D. A. Moffat

Introduction

The lateral skull base has a complex anatomy and contains the pyramidal temporal bone with its sensory end organs and neurovascular structures as well as important adjacent intracranial and extracranial structures. Surgery to this anatomical region inevitably, therefore, carries a risk of complications, the outcome of which may significantly affect quality of life and may be devastating for the patient.

The combination of a prolonged and complex neuroanesthesia and extended tumor resection by a multidisciplinary team including otologists, neurosurgeons, head and neck, vascular and plastic surgeons, as well as the necessity for a complex reconstruction exponentially increases the risk of potential complications.[1] Patients considered for skull base surgery, therefore, generally exhibit a unique set of factors predisposing them to complications of which their anatomical site and their histopathologic heterogeneity are of paramount importance.

Skull base lesions are frequently beyond a single surgeon's area of expertise.

A multidisciplinary team approach, therefore, is essential to plan a resection involving major vascular, central nervous system, cranial nerve, and pharyngeal components of tumor management. The patient's age, general health and in particular their cardiovascular and pulmonary status necessitates careful consideration because the surgery is major and protracted. Fluid balance with volume replacement as necessary is critical in both perioperative and postoperative care. The risk of neurologic deficit and in particular aspiration either perioperatively or intraoperatively must be considered and managed appropriately. The ability and willingness to cope with skull base tumor management is also influenced by the patient's psychosocial status. Previous therapy may also affect the surgical resection and reconstruction plan. The majority of patients have failed previous therapy and the consequences of surgery following radiation therapy significantly increases the potential for complications. The concept of the "learning curve" in the early years of consultant appointment is no longer acceptable and yet, for most complex operations, learning is a career-long process. Subspecialization offers part of the solution to this problem by concentrating expertise, but there remains the question of how to introduce new team members without adversely affecting patient outcome.[2] "Dove-tailing" with an inexperienced surgeon working alongside a senior surgeon for several years as well as proleptic surgical appointments can be very successful in minimizing the effects of the surgical learning curve.

This chapter outlines the differential diagnosis and therapeutic options of patients with complications from lateral skull base surgery. The management of complications of the lateral skull base is a highly complex part of this surgery, which is generally performed by otolaryngologists and neurosurgeons as part of a multidisciplinary team. The subspecialty encompasses the preoperative evaluation, discussion of the most suitable approach and the postoperative management. Evaluation of patients with diseases affecting the lateral skull base can be complex both from an investigative viewpoint and in terms of surgical management. A wide variety of pathologic conditions may occur in lateral skull base surgery. Numerous surgical approaches and procedures have been described for dealing with them. There are many very important neurovascular structures in this anatomical region and surgery will inevitably result in complications. There is not necessarily one single right solution to the management of any particular problem in lateral skull base surgery. Multiple factors have to be considered in dealing with complications resulting from surgery. We need to audit our own results and outcomes and compare them with published data. Only then will patients be able to give informed consent to our surgical intervention.

The diagnosis and management of minor and major complications during lateral skull base surgery and in the postoperative period are highlighted and discussed.

Preoperative Counseling

Careful and detailed discussion and counseling preoperatively is important to provide the patient and family members with sufficient information to make a balanced judgment on optimal management and to give informed consent to the surgical procedure. This understanding may subsequently help them to cope with the sequelae and complications should they occur.

The patient's expectations of the treatment must be realistic and the risk of complications must be defined and quantified. Alternative treatment options like watch, wait and rescan strategies and radiation therapies such as stereotactic radiotherapy either by single-dose gamma-knife radiosurgery, cyberknife or by multiple-fraction linear accelerator should be discussed with an oncologist in a multidisciplinary team setting.

Associated Sequelae and Complications of Skull Base Surgery

The fine distinction between a sequela and a complication must be discussed with the patient and family preoperatively. There are many consequences of surgery that are unavoidable and are inevitable sequelae of the procedure and not a complication of it.[1] These, however, may be viewed as complications retrospectively by the patient or the family if they are not adequately informed and consented. Patient satisfaction with the care received is increased if there is an ongoing preoperative and postoperative discussion between the surgical team and the patient and relatives explaining the reason for the clinical course and its likely final surgical outcome. Some expected sequelae of lateral skull base surgery may be incisional hair loss, altered facial sensation, possible change in facial contour, temporary facial or permanent segmental or complete facial paralysis, eustachian tube dysfunction, conductive or sensorineural hearing loss, vertigo, tinnitus, variable trismus and malocclusion, atrophy of temporal fossa, diplopia, hoarseness and swallowing difficulty.[1]

Imaging

In view of the anatomical localization of most tumors involving the skull base, the preoperative physical examination must be complemented by detailed high-resolution contrast-enhanced computed tomography with bone window sequences and gadolinium-enhanced magnetic resonance imaging.[3] Patients with tumors involving the petrous carotid artery should undergo preoperative angiography with cross-flow studies. This involves test balloon occlusion of the ipsilateral carotid system. First, a standard angiogram is completed and then the test balloon occlusion is performed with a soft balloon catheter. The occlusion is performed in the internal carotid artery with the patient awake. Subsequently with the assistance of an anesthetist to monitor the vital signs the blood pressure is pharmacologically lowered until the patient develops neurologic symptoms and signs.

Approximately 10% of patients tested fail to tolerate the balloon occlusion test. There is potential for clotting proximal to the balloon and subsequent embolization distal to the deflated balloon at the conclusion of the balloon occlusion test. Arterial spasm and hypoperfusion, particularly in the medial cerebral distribution, may occur. In elderly or previously irradiated patients, inflation of the balloon in a manner that produces an elongation of the balloon within the artery can fracture the intima or even rupture the arterial wall.

Positioning of the Patient on the Operating Table

Surgery of the lateral skull base can be performed with the patient in a lateral supine position or in a sitting position depending on the surgical team's preference.[4] Some neurosurgeons advocate the "park bench" position.

Lateral Supine Position

The lateral supine position is suitable for the majority of lateral skull base procedures and has been used predominantly in vestibular schwannoma surgery, where in many centres it has become the position of choice. This position is also preferable in patients with an open foramen ovale.

The patient is placed in a supine position with a cushion supporting and elevating the ipsilateral shoulder. The head may be placed in a three-point headring with a "mayo clamp" and the head is rotated through 45 degrees to the opposite side (this may vary depending on the size and anatomical localization of the tumor). The head is then clamped in the optimal position under the direction of the surgeon. It is imperative to protect the patient from falling off the table with two wide straps, one around the thorax and the other over the superior iliac crests because it might be necessary to tilt the table during surgery.[4]

The risk of skin or nerve pressure injury during long surgical procedures can be avoided by meticulous positioning of the patient and the careful use of gel cushions and pneumatic mattresses as well as using cotton wool pads between the patient's arms and the armrests.

Sitting Position ("Beach Chair Position")

Complex cerebellopontine angle (CPA) tumor procedures can be performed with the patient in a sitting position if the suboccipital or retrosigmoidal approach is used.[4,5] This approach offers perfect conditions for microsurgical manipulation because all fluids drain out of the operative field. The surgeon has both hands free for surgical maneuvers because the necessity for suction of cerebrospinal fluid is significantly reduced. The sitting position, however, embraces the risk of air embolism. This can be reduced significantly by placing a special cushion under the patient's legs to lift the legs to the level of the heart and the teeth to the same level as the frontal region. If the venous sinus is opened during surgery the assistant should irrigate the operative field copiously resulting in aspiration of fluid through the defect and not air. If air is detected by transesophageal echocardiography, it can be aspirated by the anesthetist using a central-line catheter. If a definite sinus laceration cannot be detected, speedy compression of the jugular vein by the anesthetist may

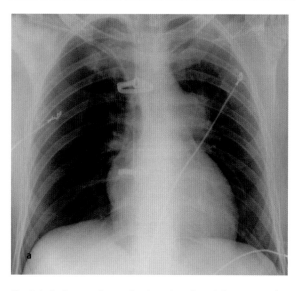
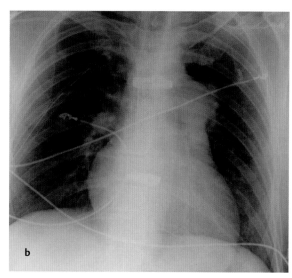

Fig. 6.1a,b Pneumothorax after insertion of a subclavian central venous catheter.

a Postoperative chest X-ray showing a right pneumothorax caused by insertion of a subclavian central venous catheter.

b Drainage in place with reduction of the pneumothorax 3 days after transtemporal surgery for a left-sided acoustic neuroma.

be helpful and the head should be immediately lowered below heart level and the legs raised. It is also necessary to cover the surgical field with soaked cottonoid patties or strips of lintine. The risk of air embolism is the reason why the sitting position is rarely used in the United States, the United Kingdom or the Netherlands. Neurosurgeons in these countries prefer the lateral position.

Potential Anesthetic Complications

General anesthesia requires careful and meticulous preparation. All available monitoring techniques should be used, including arterial lines, central venous pressure monitoring, pulse oximetry, electroencephalography, temperature probe, and urinary catheterization with output measurement and frequent blood gas measurement, intraoperative hematologic evaluation including clotting studies if there is a risk of diffuse intravascular coagulopathy. If necessary a brain pressure probe can be used.

The complications of neuroanesthesia include those due to the anesthetic agents themselves, such as hypotension and hypoxia, unsatisfactory control of the $PaCO_2$ and subsequent brain swelling.

Pneumothorax is a potentially dangerous condition that may arise unexpectedly during anesthesia or after insertion of a subclavian central venous catheter (**Fig. 6.1**). The diagnosis is one of exclusion, as initial changes in vital signs (cardiorespiratory decompensation and difficulties with ventilation) may be nonspecific. The other causes of such changes are more common than

pneumothorax. Additionally, local signs may be difficult to elicit, especially without full access to the chest. The diagnosis may be made by chest aspiration in suspected cases and correct insertion of a chest drain is essential for the further safe conduct of anesthesia and surgery.[6]

A fluid volume overload needs to be avoided in lateral skull base surgery. The use of intraoperative mannitol to reduce intracranial pressure must be carefully monitored. Abnormalities of fluid and electrolyte balance may adversely affect organ function and surgical outcome. Perioperative fluid therapy has a direct bearing on outcome, and prescriptions should be tailored to the needs of the patient. The goal of fluid therapy in the elective surgical setting is to maintain an effective circulatory volume while avoiding interstitial fluid overload whenever possible.[7]

Medical complications that occur after skull base procedures may be pulmonary, including atelectasis, aspiration pneumonia and respiratory failure, or cardiovascular, such as myocardial infarction and hypertension. Air emboli are more likely to occur in the sitting position. A degree of postsurgical pneumocephalus occurs in all patients with craniotomies,[8] and is usually resorbed within 2 or 3 days.

Several factors can increase a patient's risk of deep vein thrombosis, including advanced age (the highest risk factor) and prolonged surgery, which is likely in lateral skull base procedures. Deep vein thrombosis is the formation of a thrombus in a deep vein, most commonly in the legs. Besides acquired risk factors such as old age, obesity and smoking, there are other factors like high fibrinogen levels and inherited risk factors, e.g., antithrombin deficiency and Protein C deficiency/Protein S deficiency. An

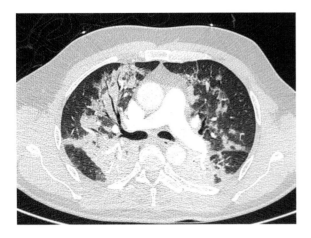

Fig. 6.2 Computed tomography of the lung after translabyrinthine surgery on the left ear for a 2.2-mm acoustic neuroma. The patient failed to have sufficient respiration and required intubation. The 54-year-old male patient developed, intraoperatively, a deep vein thrombosis with a mild pulmonary embolism and developed atypical pneumonia.

abnormal D-dimer level at the end of treatment might signal the need for continued treatment among patients with a first unprovoked proximal deep vein thrombosis. Pulmonary embolism is a blockage of the main artery of the lung or one of its branches by a substance that has travelled from elsewhere in the body through the bloodstream (**Fig. 6.2**).

Renal complications comprise urinary tract infection and renal failure. Hematologic problems like bleeding diathesis, transfusion reaction or transfusion-transmitted disease may occur.

Intraoperative Surgical Complications

Morbidity

The majority of intraoperative complications are instantly visible and treatable.

Hemorrhage may occur during skeletonization of the the sigmoid sinus or on lowering the jugular bulb.[9] The bleeding can be controlled by placing a square of Surgicel (Ethicon Inc., Somerville, NJ, USA) over the defect and then simple pressure with a neurosurgical lintine under a Yassergil retractor, compression of a bone wax oval on to the defect if there is a rim of bone to retain it, suturing a roll of Surgicel over the defect, or suturing a piece of muscle over the defect in the sinus. If the damage to the venous structures is significant then, very rarely, ligation may become necessary. This carries with it the risk of developing benign intracranial hypertension, particularly if it is the dominant sinus.

Cranial Nerve Deficits

Cranial nerve deficits can have a significant negative impact on the patient's quality of life.[10] Patients with lower cranial nerve palsies may be dependent on nasogastric feeding or percutaneous gastrostomy tubes and tracheotomies.

Facial Nerve Injury

Comprehensive evaluation and documentation of injury is required to determine the most suitable timing and method of surgical intervention.[11] The majority of nerve injuries are limited and direct repair or simple nerve grafting are the indicated treatment modalities.

The management of facial nerve injuries requires a multidisciplinary surgical team with several available methods of reconstruction.[12] Facial nerve palsy in patients with House–Brackmann (HB) Grades IV to VI and in some patients with HB III results in very significant deterioration in the patient's quality of life. Hypromellose or "false tears" for the eye during the day and Lacrilube at night will help to prevent exposure keratitis and corneal ulcers. A temporary or permanent lateral or medial tarsorrhaphy or blepharoplasty may be necessary. Gold or platinum weights in the upper eyelid will allow the eyelid to close under the force of gravity and it may be necessary to enlist the help of a plastic surgery colleague with microvascular expertise to consider a variety of delayed static or dynamic surgical procedures for permanent facial weakness.

Trigeminal Nerve Damage

Injury to the fifth cranial nerve may rarely occur in the excision of large vestibular schwannomas. This can result in anesthesia in the distribution of the injured nerve. Rarely a trigeminal trophic syndrome may be caused by trigeminal nerve damage (**Figs. 6.3 and 6.4**).[13]

Cerebellar and Brainstem Injury

Cerebellar and brainstem injuries are the major and most feared complications of lateral skull base surgery. Cerebellar compression injury is more likely with the retrosigmoid than the translabyrinthine approach because in the latter, access is obtained by bony removal rather than by cerebellar retraction. Cerebellar contusion can be induced by direct compression of neural tissues with retractors, the use of the ultrasonic cavitron surgical aspirator, by intrinsic hemorrhage and edema, or by extrinsic pressure from blood clotting in the CPA.[14]

Hemorrhage

Hemorrhage into the posterior fossa or subdural or extradural hemorrhage in the immediate or late postoperative

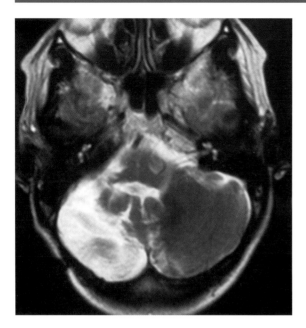

Fig. 6.3 T2-weighted magnetic resonance image showing severe gliosis in the cerebellum 20 years after suboccipital acoustic neuroma removal in a 72-year-old Caucasian female patient. The previous neurosurgeon had also injured the trigeminal nerve during the acoustic neuroma removal (see **Fig. 6.4**).

period can result in brainstem compression and rapid death or severe neurologic deficits (**Fig. 6.5**). The prevention of secondary bleeding relies on strict hemostasis, and it is essential to coagulate both ends of any minor surface vessels during tumor resection. Bipolar coagulation enables meticulous hemostasis.

Injury to Arteries

Vascular complications after lateral skull base surgery are potentially devastating and should be identified as early as possible. Expeditious postoperative extubation allows a systematic neurologic assessment. The facility for immediate postoperative computed tomography scanning should be available. Rapid return to theater to evacuate intracranial blood clot and to secure hemostasis may be necessary.

Vasospasm

Vasospasm after resection of skull base tumors is a rare complication that often produces serious ischemic sequelae,[15] which may complicate the patient's postoperative course. The cause of vasospasms appears to be multifactorial and the surgical approach may contribute to the pathogenesis of vasospasm.

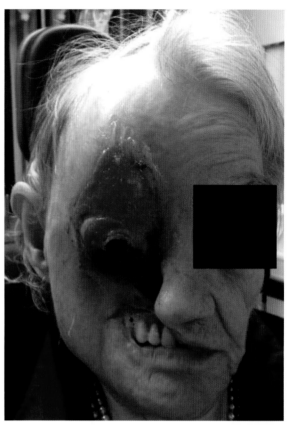

Fig. 6.4 A trigeminal trophic syndrome occurs in this patient (see **Fig. 6.3**) weeks after initial surgery. The patient was treated with an exenteration of the eye. The defect was covered with a free radial forearm flap.

The Anterior Inferior Cerebellar Artery

The anterior inferior cerebellar artery (AICA) is the most significant vascular structure within the CPA and is closely related to cranial nerves VI to VIII. Commonly arising as a single trunk from the basilar artery, it may also arise as two separate branches. In rare cases, it originates as a branch of the posterior inferior cerebellar artery. As the AICA travels from anterior to posterior, it first follows the ventral surface of the brainstem, but within the CPA it may take a long loop laterally to the porus acusticus (**Fig. 6.6**). In 15 to 20% of patients, the AICA actually passes into the lumen of the internal auditory canal before turning back on itself toward the posterior surface of the brainstem. The AICA can be divided into the premeatal, meatal, and postmeatal segments. Injury to the AICA results in brainstem and cerebellar infarction of variable degrees, depending on its size and the area of its terminal artery (**Fig. 6.6**).[16] Hemorrhage from the AICA bears a high risk of brainstem and cerebellar compression and infarction.

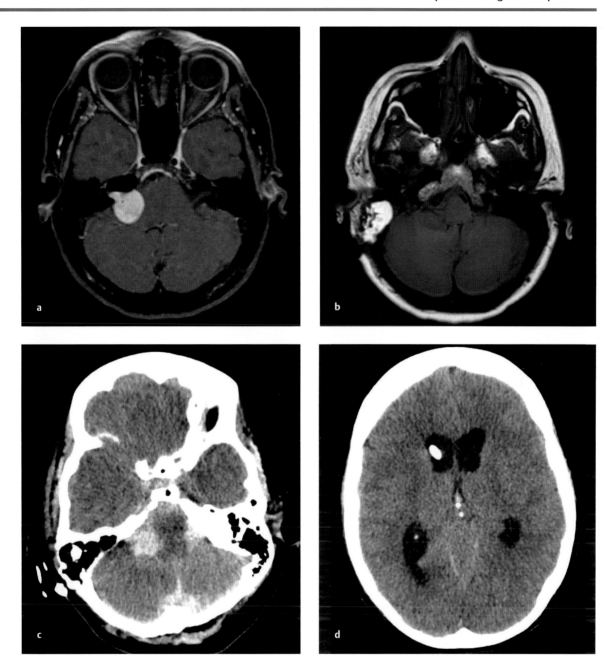

Fig. 6.5a–d Brainstem compression after hemorrhage.

a Gadolinium-enhanced magnetic resonance imaging showing a right-sided intrameatal and extrameatal acoustic neuroma with brainstem compression.

c The 54-year-old female patient became unconscious and was intubated for 4 days due to postoperative hemorrhage.

b T2-weighted postsurgical magnetic resonance image with fat obliteration of the mastoid cavity.

d A ventricular drain was placed initially after intubation to release and monitor an increased intracranial pressure.

Veins

Two venous structures have to be observed during surgical procedures involving the lateral skull base. The veins are more variable in position and number. The petrosal vein (of Dandy) carries returning venous blood from the cerebellum and lateral brainstem to the superior or inferior petrosal sinus. It is generally encountered in the area of the trigeminal nerve anterior to the porus acusticus. The petrosal vein often carries enough venous blood for its obstruction to lead to venous infarction and cerebellar edema. Its integrity should be preserved at all times

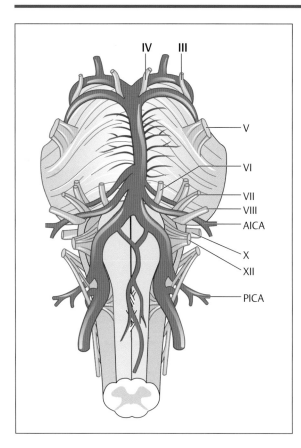

Fig. 6.6 Illustration revealing the anterior view of the brainstem, midbrain, pons, medulla oblongata with the cranial nerves (left) and arteries (right).

unless this is not possible. Additional venous blood reaches the superior petrosal sinus through a series of bridging veins that cross the CPA. Although every attempt should be made to preserve these veins, their sacrifice is generally inconsequential.

The vein of Labbé carries returning venous blood from the inferior and lateral surfaces of the temporal lobe to the superior petrosal sinus, tentorial venous lakes, or the transverse sinus. Its configuration and anatomy are variable. However, obstruction, obliteration, or occlusion of the superior petrosal sinus may, in some cases, result in occlusion of the vein of Labbé. Sudden occlusion of the vein of Labbé carries a high risk of venous infarction of the temporal lobe and rapid life-threatening cerebral edema.

Postoperative Complications

Other Forms of Postoperative Intracranial Bleeding

Bleeding and brain swelling may develop after CPA tumor surgery. If this occurs a subsequent operation may be necessary to reopen the wound to arrest bleeding and

allow the brain to expand.[1] This complication can result in paralysis or death. The possibility of interventricular or interparenchymal bleeding caused by intraoperative or postoperative diathesis is a potential danger.

Hydrocephalus

Patients occasionally require a ventriculoperitoneal shunt for hydrocephalus within a few weeks of the operation (**Figs. 6.7 and 6.8**). Initially a lumbar drain is used to significantly reduce intracranial pressure. If the problem is persistent a ventriculoperitoneal shunt is inserted.[12]

Central Nervous System

Vascular damage may result in stroke or death. Intracranial or parenchymal bleeding may worsen cerebral edema and result in a mass/volume intracranial effect. Pneumocephalus, seizure, meningitis and cerebritis are further serious complications (**Figs. 6.9 and 6.10**).

Mortality

There has been a continuous lowering of mortality and morbidity rates in the 20th century, thanks to increasing microsurgical experience and newer technologies in neuroanesthesia, surgical instrumentation, endoscopy, and neuronavigation. Vestibular schwannomas are located adjacent to vital brainstem neural pathways that control breathing, blood pressure and heart function. As the tumor enlarges it may become firmly adherent to and compress the brainstem and often becomes intertwined with the blood vessels supplying these areas of the brain. Careful tumor dissection, with the help of an operating microscope, usually allows avoidance of these complications.[17] Charpiot et al[18] reported mortality of 0.8% during the first year of translabyrinthine acoustic neuroma removal. If the blood supply to vital brain centers is compromised, serious complications may result: loss of muscle control, paralysis, even death (**Figs. 6.11 and 6.12**). This is now a very rare occurrence in vestibular schwannoma surgery.

Completeness of Resection

In most patients a vestibular schwannoma originates from the vestibular nerve and only compresses the cochlear nerve.[19] More than 95% of acoustic neuromas arise from vestibular fascicles.[20] Samii and Matthies[20] in their series of 1,000 acoustic neuromas have observed that only 1.1% of the CPA tumors arise from the cochlear nerve. Therefore, although tumor cells are commonly seen between the fascicles of the cochlear nerve, an attempt to seek complete tumor removal by excision of the cochlear nerve may not be advised by some authors. The importance of complete tumor removal and the effect it has on recurrence is well known. In 1989, Hardy et al[3] reported

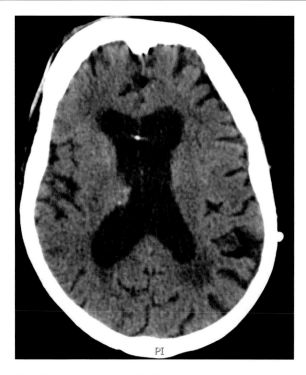

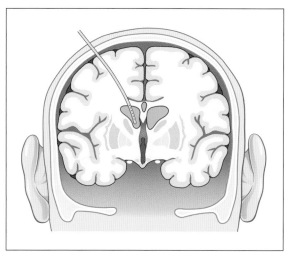

Fig. 6.8 The treatment of a hydrocephalus is surgical, generally using various types of cerebral shunts. It involves the placement of a ventricular catheter into the cerebral ventricles as shown.

Fig. 6.7 Hydrocephalus is defined by an abnormal accumulation of cerebrospinal fluid (CSF) in the ventricles. The computed tomography scan was taken 3 months after surgery for acoustic neuroma for new headaches.

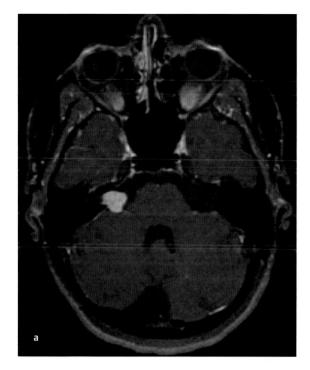

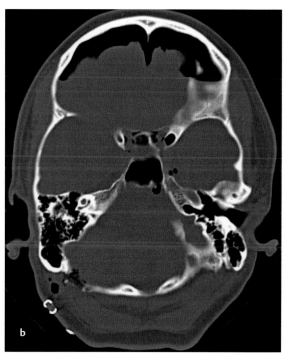

Fig. 6.9a,b Pneumocephalus after removal of an acoustic neuroma.

a The gadolinium-enhanced magnetic resonance image reveals a right-sided intrameatal and extrameatal acoustic neuroma. The hearing threshold was normal. Hearing dropped by 25–30 dB after suboccipital acoustic neuroma removal on the operated side.

b Computed tomography scan showing a postsurgical pneumocephalus 1 day after surgery that was uneventfully resorbed 3 days later.

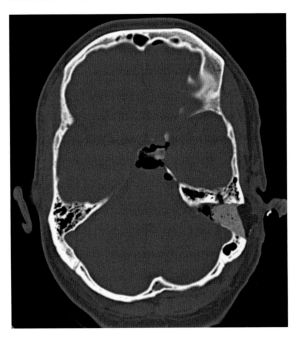

Fig. 6.10 Mild postsurgical pneumocephalus after translabyrinthine acoustic neuroma removal in a 54-year-old patient. The bony defect was covered with autologous bone dust.

only three perioperative deaths among 100 translabyrinthine acoustic neuroma excisions, which was reasonable in those days, and the postoperative morbidity was low.

Subsequently these authors report a current mortality of 0.3% (Moffat, personal communication).

Complete tumor excision was achieved in 97% of patients and no recurrences were seen during follow-up of 1 to 7 years. In that series, because of the surgical approach used, hearing preservation was of no concern.[3]

Cerebrospinal Fluid Leakage

Early or delayed cerebrospinal fluid (CSF) leakage from the wound, CSF rhinorrhea, or CSF otorrhea can occur even if all precautions have been taken to avoid it. It is extremely important to obtain a watertight closure. The pathway of CSF leakage is most commonly through mastoid air cells that were opened during the craniotomy into the middle ear and then down the eustachian tube to present as CSF rhinorrhea. Closure of mastoid air cells with bone wax is essential. The eustachian tube can be occluded with small pieces of fascia lata and the middle ear and attic can be filled with fat globules, having divided the tensor tympani tendon to obtain access to the anterior malleolar recess anterior to the COG (attic bony plate). A patch of fascia lata is then glued to the bony external canal wall to cover the aditus and is then wrapped over the Fallopian canal and curled over the medial aspect of the promontory. Although a current CSF leak rate of 4% has been achieved using this technique, a vicryl hernia net (similar to those used in abdominal surgery) and autologous fibrin glue using the Vivostat system (Vivostat

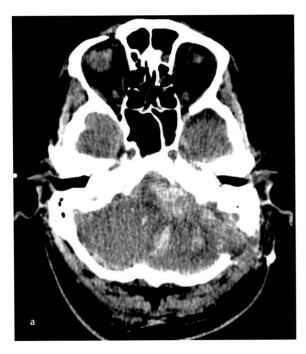

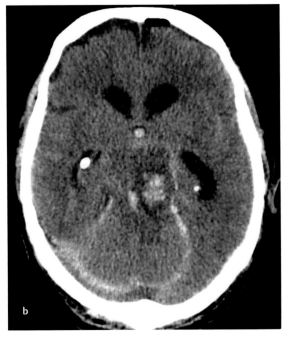

Fig. 6.11a,b Fatal intracranial bleeding complications.

a Fatal bleeding and brain swelling in the posterior cranial fossa 2 days after left-sided suboccipital acoustic tumor removal in a 65-year-old patient.

b A fourth intraventricular clot causing additional pressure to the hemorrhage and edema of the posterior cranial fossa.

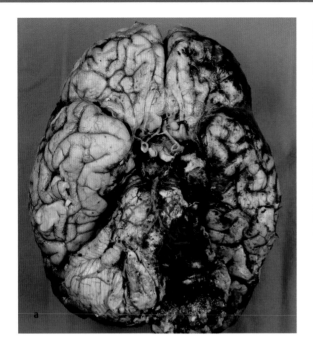

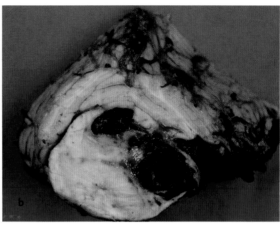

Fig. 6.12a,b Fatal massive intracranial hemorrhage.

a Brain dissection of the 65-year-old patient, with fatal massive intracranial hemorrhage (see **Fig. 6.11**), during autopsy.

b Detailed microphotograph of the brainstem and cerebellum showing massive hemorrhage of the left cerebellopontine angle after acoustic neuroma surgery.

A/S, Alleroed, Denmark) are currently being investigated in an attempt to reduce the incidence of CSF leakage even further. Postoperative CSF leakage following lateral skull base surgery can be managed with lumbar subarachnoid drain insertion for 4 days in most patients. This management is, however, more likely to be successful after translabyrinthine surgery than after retrosigmoid surgery. Failure to control the leak with lumbar drainage or recurrent CSF leakage make revision surgery necessary[21] in 1% of patients. A transient increase in CSF pressure and decrease in craniospinal compliance is known to be provoked by surgery.[22]

Postoperative Infection

Infection rarely occurs in patients following lateral skull base surgery. When it does occur it can lead to meningitis, an infection of the fluid and meninges surrounding the brain. Following confirmation of the infection by examination, analysis and culture of the CSF, treatment with high doses of antibiotics is indicated. Complications from antibiotic treatment are rare. Aseptic meningitis may also occur and may be a result of the irritant effect of bone dust in CSF of the CPA and usually responds to steroid treatment.

Postoperative Headache

Headache following vestibular schwannoma excision is common in the early postoperative period. In some rare cases, headache may be prolonged. Postoperative headache is significantly more common in the retrosigmoid approach, where it may manifest as occipital neuralgia, or it may be due to dural stretching at the craniotomy site.

Occipital neuralgia can be confirmed by injection of local anesthetic into the nerve as it exits the occipital foramen. This will abolish the pain transiently and is used diagnostically. Drugs used for neuropathic pain, such as amitriptyline, carbamazepine or gabapentin, can be effective in some patients; however, phenol injection of the nerve may be necessary. Screwing a titanium mesh sheet to the bony defect of the craniotomy may abolish headache related to stretching of the dura on raising intracranial pressure.

Revision Lateral Skull Base Surgery

Postoperative cranial deficits and complications are more common after revision skull base surgery compared with primary surgery. Complete resection without recurrence can be achieved in revision skull base surgery.[5] Modern reconstruction techniques can reduce major postoperative complications and morbidity from cranial nerve deficits. Complete microsurgical removal of acoustic neuromas after failed stereotactic radiotherapy is challenging. The functional outcome generally tends to be worse than in untreated patients. Surgery after previous partial tumor removal and stereotactic surgery are most challenging and related to poorer outcomes.[5,16]

Conclusions

Careful selection of patients from a multidisciplinary team meeting, meticulous surgical and anesthetic management, and intensive postoperative care are essential in helping to prevent the complications of lateral skull base surgery.

References

1. Wiet RJ, Teixido M, Liang JG. Complications in acoustic neuroma surgery. Otolaryngol Clin North Am 1992;25(2):389–412

2. Sharp MC, MacFarlane R, Hardy DG, Jones SE, Baguley DM, Moffat DA. Team working to improve outcome in vestibular schwannoma surgery. Br J Neurosurg 2005;19(2):122–127

3. Hardy DG, Macfarlane R, Baguley D, Moffat DA. Surgery for acoustic neurinoma. An analysis of 100 translabyrinthine operations. J Neurosurg 1989;71(6):799–804

4. Hildmann H, Sudhoff H. Middle Ear Surgery. Berlin, Heidelberg, New York: Springer-Verlag, 2006

5. Gerganov VM, Giordano M, Samii A, Samii M. Surgical treatment of patients with vestibular schwannomas after failed previous radiosurgery. J Neurosurg 2012;116(4):713–720

6. Bacon AK, Paix AD, Williamson JA, Webb RK, Chapman MJ. Crisis management during anaesthesia: pneumothorax. Qual Saf Health Care 2005;14(3):e18

7. Lobo DN, Macafee DA, Allison SP. How perioperative fluid balance influences postoperative outcomes. Best Pract Res Clin Anaesthesiol 2006;20(3):439–455

8. Hernández-Palazón J, Martínez-Lage JF, de la Rosa-Carrillo VN, Tortosa JA, López F, Poza M. Anesthetic technique and development of pneumocephalus after posterior fossa surgery in the sitting position. Neurocirugia (Astur) 2003;14(3):216–221

9. Moffat DA, Quaranta N, Chang P. Management of the high jugular bulb in translabyrinthine surgery. Laryngoscope 2003;113(3):580–582

10. Lloyd SK, Kasbekar AV, Baguley DM, Moffat DA. Audiovestibular factors influencing quality of life in patients with conservatively managed sporadic vestibular schwannoma. Otol Neurotol 2010;31(6):968–976

11. Prasai A, Jones SE, Cross J, Moffat DA. A facial nerve schwannoma masquerading as a vestibular schwannoma. Ear Nose Throat J 2008;87(9):E4–E6

12. Hardy DG, Macfarlane R, Baguley DM, Moffat DA. Facial nerve recovery following acoustic neuroma surgery. Br J Neurosurg 1989;3(6):675–680

13. Litschel R, Winkler H, Dazert S, Sudhoff H. Herpes zoster-associated trigeminal trophic syndrome: a case report and review. Eur Arch Otorhinolaryngol 2003;260(2):86–90

14. Roche PH, Ribeiro T, Fournier HD, Thomassin JM. Vestibular schwannomas: complications of microsurgery. Prog Neurol Surg 2008;21:214–221

15. Aoki N, Origitano TC, al-Mefty O. Vasospasm after resection of skull base tumors. Acta Neurochir (Wien) 1995;132(1–3):53–58

16. Kania R, Lot G, Herman P, Tran Ba Huy P. Vascular complications after acoustic neurinoma surgery. [Article in French] Ann Otolaryngol Chir Cervicofac 2003;120(2):94–102

17. Shiobara R, Ohira T, Inoue Y, Kanzaki J, Kawase T. Extended middle cranial fossa approach for vestibular schwannoma: technical note and surgical results of 896 operations. Prog Neurol Surg 2008;21:65–72

18. Charpiot A, Tringali S, Zaouche S, Ferber-Viart C, Dubreuil C. Perioperative complications after translabyrinthine removal of large or giant vestibular schwannoma: outcomes for 123 patients. Acta Otolaryngol 2010;130(11):1249–1255

19. Horrax G, Poppen JL. The end results of complete versus intracapsular removal of acoustic tumors. Ann Surg 1949;130(3):567–575

20. Samii M, Matthies C. Management of 1000 vestibular schwannomas (acoustic neuromas): the facial nerve—preservation and restitution of function. Neurosurgery 1997;40(4):684–694

21. Allen KP, Isaacson B, Purcell P, Kutz JW Jr, Roland PS. Lumbar subarachnoid drainage in cerebrospinal fluid leaks after lateral skull base surgery. Otol Neurotol 2011;32(9):1522–1524

22. Laing RJ, Smielewski P, Czosnyka M, Quaranta N, Moffat DA. A study of perioperative lumbar cerebrospinal fluid pressure in patients undergoing acoustic neuroma surgery. Skull Base Surg 2000;10(4):179–185

Section II Rhinology and Anterior Skull Base

7 Complications Following Surgery of the Septum and Turbinates

R. Douglas, A. Wood

Septoplasty and inferior turbinate reduction are very commonly performed procedures,[1] usually for the surgical treatment of nasal obstruction. Although major complications are rare, minor complications are not infrequent. This chapter will outline these complications, their management, and strategies to reduce the risk of them occurring.

When treating a patient with nasal obstruction secondary to deviation of the septum, it is common practice to perform a procedure to reduce the size of the inferior turbinates, which serves to increase the cross-sectional area at the region of the nasal valve and to improve airflow. When the inferior turbinates are large but the nasal septum is in the midline, inferior turbinate surgery may be performed alone. In this chapter, these two procedures will be discussed separately.

Septoplasty

Indications

Some degree of nasal septal deviation is extremely common.[2] Septoplasty is most commonly performed for those deviations that are severe enough to cause obstruction of nasal airflow.[3] If there is significant associated deviation of the external nose, a septorhinoplasty is usually performed.[4]

The role played by deviation of the nasal septum in causing nasal symptoms is not easily measured objectively because there is poor correlation between physical measurements of nasal airflow and a patient's subjective appreciation of the severity of obstruction.[5] Nonetheless, most patients with septal deviation sufficiently severe to warrant septoplasty report an improvement in both nasal symptoms and quality of life after the procedure.[6,7]

Many cases of septal deviation are congenital, and may be related to birth trauma.[8] Any retrospective study would be expected to be subject to significant recall bias but a proportion of septal deviations are acquired, being clearly related, by patients, to external trauma.[9]

Any part of the septum may be deviated from the midline. The three most common patterns of septal deviation seen in rhinology practice are a convex deviation away from the sagittal plane, which is usually maximal in the region of the osseochondral junction, septal spurs, which are usually formed by the vomer, and very caudal cartilaginous deflections.[10] The nature of the deviation (and there are often several in combination) alters the surgical approach and consequently the potential for complications to occur. The septum is most commonly approached endonasally via hemitransfixion or Killian incisions. Visualization can be facilitated by a speculum and headlight, or a nasal endoscope.

> **Note**
> The efficacy and complication rate using either of these approaches would appear to be equivalent in the few comparative studies that have been reported to date.[11,12] Severe caudal deflections, and deflections that involve the nasal tip are generally best approached externally.[13]

Preoperative Planning

Septal deviation and rhinitis are both very common, and when a patient presents with nasal obstruction it is not easy to assess the relative contributions of these two factors toward the patient's symptoms. When coexistent rhinitis is suspected, a trial of medical therapy (including at least several weeks treatment with a topical nasal corticosteroid spray) is indicated. Many patients will have sufficient relief from medical therapy alone so that septoplasty is no longer required.[14]

If chronic rhinosinusitis is suspected on clinical grounds, a computed tomography scan of the sinuses is indicated. It is not uncommon for patients with chronic rhinosinusitis to have a septoplasty and inferior turbinate reduction procedure performed without adequate investigation to exclude chronic rhinosinusitis, only to return postoperatively with inadequate relief of symptoms due to persisting sinusitis.

The majority of cases of septoplasty are performed under general anesthesia. The general health status of the patient needs to be assessed preoperatively because it may impact on the safety of general anesthesia. Although nasal obstruction may have a significant impact on quality of life, septal surgery indications are nearly always relative, and septoplasty should be undertaken circumspectly in patients with significant cardiovascular risk factors. Anticoagulant or antiplatelet medication and possibly nonsteroidal anti-inflammatories should be stopped an appropriate numbers of days before surgery.[15] If the risk of stopping anticoagulant and antiplatelet medication outweighs the perceived benefit of the surgery we would advocate postponing surgery until the medication is no longer required.

> **Note**
>
> Systemic conditions that may affect the septum also need to be considered preoperatively. Cocaine abuse, cigarette smoking, and inflammatory conditions such as Wegener granulomatosis may impact on the presentation and postoperative course of patients requiring a septoplasty.[16–18]

Anesthesia

The risk of general anesthesia can be avoided by performing a septoplasty under local anesthesia. There is evidence to suggest that the use of local anesthesia reduces overall operating time.[19] However, it is our experience that the procedure is better tolerated under general anesthetic than under local anesthetic.

Optimizing operating conditions improves visualization and so reduces the possibility of intraoperative complications occurring. Preparing the nasal mucosa by the application of topical vasoconstrictors such as epinephrine, oxymetazoline, or cocaine reduces intraoperative bleeding. Injecting the septal mucosa with a combination of topical anesthetic and epinephrine reduces mucosal blood flow further, and injection into the subperichondral plane may facilitate dissection of the mucosal flaps. There is however a lack of consensus on the most appropriate regimen for topical preparation of the nose before surgery.[20,21]

> **Note**
>
> General anesthetic conditions affect intraoperative blood flow. Placing the patient in a reverse Trendelenburg position facilitates venous return, and induction of relative hypotension and bradycardia reduces bleeding further.[22]

Obstacles and Complications

Hemorrhage

Because septoplasty is largely performed within avascular planes, there is usually little associated blood loss. Most of the bleeding that occurs comes from the initial mucosal incision or from fractured or incised bone edges. Accordingly, persistent epistaxis after septoplasty alone is uncommon and rarely severe.[23] However, small volumes of blood can collect in the potential space between the mucosal flaps to form a septal hematoma. This can cause nasal obstruction, but a far more serious complication occurs if the hematoma becomes infected.[24] The septal abscess can break down the septal cartilage, and a saddle defect can result.[25]

The risk of a septal hematoma forming may be reduced by placing a posterior incision in one of the intact flaps (assuming no mucosal tears occur during the raising of

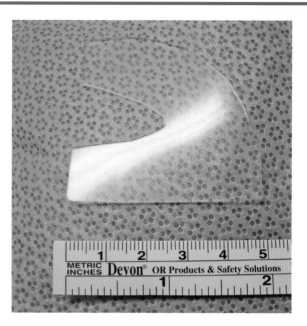

Fig. 7.1 A Silastic splint that has been cut to sit parallel to the nasal septum after endoscopic sinus surgery and septoplasty. The superior limb lies in the middle meatus and the inferior limb lies under the horizontal ground lamella against the posterior part of the septum.

the flaps). Preventing or limiting the collection of blood in the space between the two flaps can be achieved by placing septal quilting sutures.[26] Bilateral packing can achieve the same result, but packing universally causes obstruction until its removal. In some patients this can cause systemic effects, the most significant of which is compromising of oxygen saturation in the early postoperative period.[27] There is some evidence that thin Silastic sheets (Dow Corning, Midland, MI, USA) placed against the nasal septum may improve postoperative healing (**Fig. 7.1**)[28] but routine packing of the nose for hemostasis following septal surgery appears to be unnecessary.[29]

Saddle Deformity

A saddle deformity presents both cosmetic and functional problems and arises because of destabilization of the septal cartilage (**Fig. 7.2**).[30] The mid-third of the nasal dorsum is depressed and widened. In more severe cases the lack of support causes the nasal tip to become over-rotated and there is columellar retraction. It can result from the inadvertent division of the attachment of the quadrangular cartilage from the perpendicular plate of the ethmoid bone at its superior end. At least 1 cm of superior attachment of the cartilage to the perpendicular plate needs to be left intact to prevent this cosmetically displeasing deformity from developing. It is safer to start the incision made at the osseochondral junction at its superior extent, ensuring at least a 1-cm margin of safety above the tip of the Freer elevator, and then continue it inferiorly toward the maxillary crest (**Fig. 7.3**).

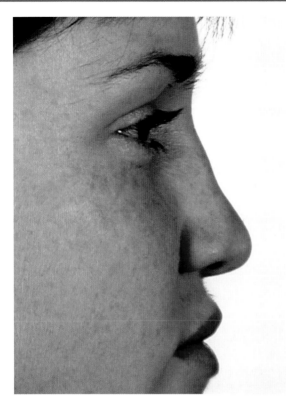

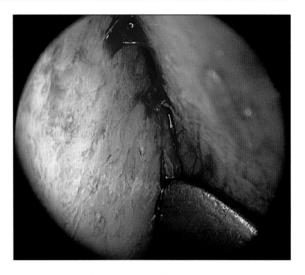

Fig. 7.3 Dividing the osseochondral junction with a Freer's elevator. At least the superior 1 cm of this junction must be preserved to prevent the possibility of a saddle deformity occurring. The incision is best made from its superior extent toward the maxillary crest.

Fig. 7.2 Saddle deformity in a patient who has previously undergone a septoplasty. Excessive dissection of the quadrilateral cartilage has led to a depression of the mid-third of the nasal dorsum.

Another way in which the bony support can be disrupted is by fracturing the anterior end of the perpendicular plate of the ethmoid from its attachment to the nasal bones. This usually occurs as a consequence of twisting the superior part of the perpendicular plate. It is possible to control the site of fracture of the ethmoid plate by making a cut with turbinectomy scissors from the superior extent of the osseochondral incision, in a direction parallel to the nasal bones. This bony incision reduces the possibility of twisting the superior attachment of the ethmoid plate from the nasal bones and so reduces the risk of both saddle deformity and cerebrospinal fluid (CSF) leak[30] (**Fig. 7.4**).

Should a saddle deformity occur, the defect can be concealed using techniques such as the placement of camouflage cartilage grafts over the depression. This procedure requires an external rhinoplasty approach and is usually performed some time after the septoplasty.[31]

Cerebrospinal Fluid Leak

This is a very rare but significant complication of septoplasty.[32] It results from either the instruments used to elevate the periosteal flap being driven inadvertently through the cribriform plate or alternatively the cribriform plate being cracked by the use of excessive twisting

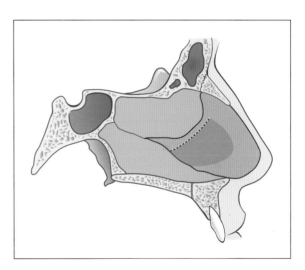

Fig. 7.4 A diagram illustrating the anatomy of the septum. The interrupted line shows the site of incision through the septal cartilage just anterior to the osseochondral junction. The key area is immediately above the superior extent of this incision. This is where the septal cartilage, perpendicular plate of the ethmoid and nasal bones intersect. Disruption of this area can lead to a saddle deformity. The crosshatched area of the septal cartilage can usually be removed safely. A 10- to 15-mm L-shaped strut of septal cartilage must be kept intact to prevent saddle deformity or ptosis of the nasal tip.

force while removing the perpendicular plate of the ethmoid. Patients with low cribriform plates are more at risk of this complication.[33] It is noted however that if required, the septal cartilage can be safely removed anterior to the middle turbinate without threatening the skull base.[34]

A CSF leak may be recognized intraoperatively by the flow of clear fluid from the region of the cribriform plate, or postoperatively by the persistence of clear rhinorrhea that is positive for the presence of β_2-transferrin protein.[35] If a CSF leak is suspected, then a thin-slice computed tomography scan is required to delineate the extent of the disruption of the cribriform plate. Intraoperative identification of the site of the leak may be facilitated by the intrathecal administration of a small quantity of fluorescein via a lumbar puncture performed immediately preoperatively. The majority of traumatic leaks are amenable to endoscopic multilayer closure.[36]

Perforation

Septal perforation is the most common of the significant complications that follow septoplasty. Although septal perforation may occur as a late and consequently unrecorded complication, reported prevalence rates after septoplasty range from 1 to 6.7%.[30] The severity of the symptoms caused by a septal perforation are a function of both its size and site. Paradoxically, small perforations are often more problematic than larger ones because the velocity and turbulence of airflow through smaller perforations is greater (**Fig. 7.5**). Small perforations can produce a whistling sound that can be particularly disturbing at night. Anterior and inferior perforations tend to be more symptomatic than posterior or superior perforations. This is because there is physiologic turbulence in the posterior nose but anteriorly the abnormal turbulent air flow caused by a perforation desiccates nasal mucosa, leading to crusting, local infection, mucosal granulation and bleeding.[37]

Septal perforation occurs when the mucosal blood flow to adjacent sides of the septal mucosa is disrupted. This may result from local tears in the mucosa of both septal flaps. This situation is best managed by avoidance and an intraoperative injury to the mucosa on one side of the septum should prompt a particularly cautious and conservative approach to the remaining dissection. It is common practice to elevate the mucosal flap on the concave side of the septal deviation to improve the chance of raising this flap intact.[4] Septal tears are very easily created around sharp vomerine spurs (**Figs. 7.6 and 7.7**). Fortunately, should a perforation occur it is likely to be sufficiently posterior that symptoms are unlikely to result.

> **Note**
>
> The risk of septal perforation is increased if the plane of dissection is superficial to the deepest layer, the perichondrium. The perichondrium is the strongest component of the septal flap, and its disruption increases the possibility of the flap breaking down.[38]

When overlapping small mucosal tears occur during the performance of a septoplasty, the mucosal edges can be opposed by the careful placement of quilting sutures (**Fig. 7.8**). The use of septal splints may support the septal mucosa and encourage healing of the mucosal tears (see **Fig. 7.1**). Although not specifically reported in most published studies of the etiology of septal perforation,[39] intuitively it seems likely that technical factors reducing local blood flow to the septal mucosa, such as excessive quilting or tension on sutures anchoring a septal splint, may predispose to perforation and should be avoided. Only sufficient tension need be placed on quilting sutures

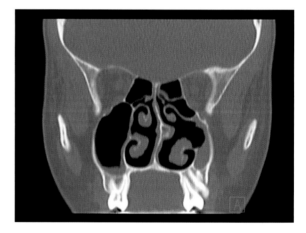

Fig. 7.6 A computed tomographic scan showing a septal spur. The right uncinate and posterior fontanelle are very atelectatic on this scan.

Fig. 7.5 A septal perforation. This perforation is small and anterior and caused troublesome crusting and whistling.

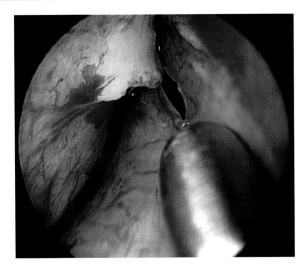

Fig. 7.7 It is very difficult not to split the septal mucosa when elevating it off septal spurs. These tears usually heal well unless there is an opposing tear in the contralateral mucosal flap.

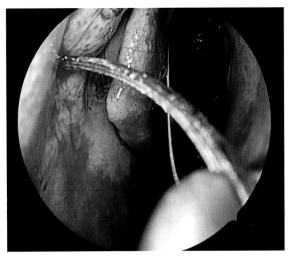

Fig. 7.8 A septal quilting suture being placed. This suture has already been passed through the middle turbinates to medialize them as the ethmoid sinuses have been dissected. Endoscopy permits careful placement of the quilting suture so that accidental tears can be accurately closed.

to eliminate the potential volume between the mucosal flaps.[30]

Nasopalatine Nerve

The nasopalatine nerve is a branch of the sphenopalatine nerve that runs from the anterior face of the sphenoid and along the septum to the incisive foramen. As it passes over the maxillary crest, it is vulnerable to injury if the crest is resected aggressively. Injury to the nerve results in numbness of the upper lip and upper incisors. Fortunately, persisting symptoms are unusual, with gradual resolution over weeks or months being the usual postoperative course should this complication occur, most likely because of overlap with the innervation from the anterior palatine nerves in this region.[40] This complication can be largely avoided by not resecting the anterior part of the maxillary crest. The nerve is particularly endangered by the use of osteotomes to divide the maxillary crest flush from the horizontal plates of the hard palate or by the use of electrocautery in this region.[41]

Infection

Infective complications usually become apparent within a few days of the procedure. Minor crusting and erythema at the site of the septal incision is not uncommon. This often settles without further treatment, but if symptomatic or progressive, it requires a course of appropriate antibiotics. Most postseptoplasty infections are caused by *Staphylococcus aureus*, with a much smaller proportion being caused by *Haemophilus influenzae* and other pathogens. There is a surprising paucity of objective microbiologic data on postoperative infections in this setting.[24]

In general, however, the incidence of infective complications following septoplasty is low and there is a consensus that prophylactic antibiotics are not indicated in routine cases.[42] A recent randomized controlled trial of a single dose of prophylactic cefuroxime before septoplasty did conclude that there may be some benefit to its use in prolonged surgery or if there were significant crusting or purulence preoperatively.[43]

Septal abscess is a much less common but much more severe complication. It occurs when a septal hematoma becomes infected. An abscess presents in very much the same manner as a hematoma, with nasal obstruction, local discomfort and septal swelling. An abscess may be distinguished on clinical grounds by greater tenderness and erythema, and by aspiration of pus from the septum.

Septal abscesses need to be drained acutely. This usually requires a general anesthetic, opening of the mucosal incision, drainage of the pus and remnants of the hematoma, and copious lavage.[30] We would advocate placing a small drain into the space between the mucosal flaps and packing the nasal passages bilaterally to prevent the abscess reforming.

> **Note**
>
> Nasal packing can rarely lead to toxic shock syndrome resulting from the release of exotoxins by *Staphylococcus aureus* colonizing the packing. The exotoxins have superantigen activity and can cause severe and widespread systemic effects.[44] The risk of toxic shock syndrome has been used as an argument against the use of nasal packing after septoplasties. If packing is used it is generally advised to prescribe an antibiotic while the packing is in place.

Persisting Obstruction

Although the majority of patients who have had a septoplasty performed report relief of nasal obstruction, some do not. There are several potential causes for failure of the procedure. A common cause of an unsatisfactory result is failure to recognize and treat coexistent rhinitis and sinusitis. It is our practice to obtain a computed tomography sinus scan in all patients listed for septoplasty, and to perform routinely a turbinate reduction procedure at the same time as the septoplasty is performed.

Another easily missed cause of nasal obstruction is collapse of the lateral nasal wall in the region of the external valve.[4] In cases of lateral wall collapse it is our usual practice to perform a septoplasty and inferior turbinate reduction procedure first and see if nasal function is improved satisfactorily. If it is not, then a procedure to address the lateral nasal wall is performed at a later date. If the cause of lateral wall collapse is from malformed (usually malrotated) lower lateral cartilages, then the crural J-flap procedure can be performed, in which a J-shaped slice of mucosa and cartilage is removed from the anteroinferior aspect of the lower lateral cartilage, and the incised edges approximated with sutures to increase lateral wall tension[45] (**Fig. 7.9**). If however the lateral wall collapse is to the result of soft tissue thinning and flaccidity then a batten procedure is performed to stiffen the lateral nasal wall.[46]

Another common cause of failure of septoplasty is incomplete reversal of the deviation. The septal cartilage is a structure in which both surfaces are under tension. When the tension is imbalanced, a deviation results. Overcoming the tension producing the deviation is not always easily achieved. It is a not an infrequent experience during septoplasty surgery to achieve intraoperative straightening of the cartilage, only to find that the septum has resumed its preoperative shape by the first follow-up appointment. Failure to reverse a septal deviation also occurs when caudal or dorsal septal deformities are not properly identified and addressed.[47]

Several techniques have been developed to overcome this difficulty. Scoring of the cartilage on the concave side of the deviation can sometimes be helpful. Mustardé sutures have been used with success.[48] Excising a sliver of cartilage over the length of the maxillary crest

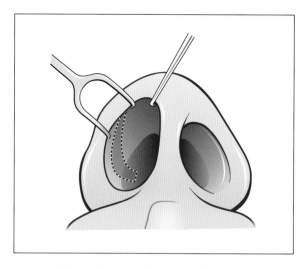

Fig. 7.9 A diagram illustrating the incisions from a crural J-flap procedure (after O'Halloran, 2003[45]). The first incision is made immediately caudal to the lower lateral cartilage. A J-shaped strip of mucosa and cartilage is then excised. The suturing of the wound increases tension in the lateral nasal wall in the region of the external valve.

and anterior nasal spine allows the septum to swing into a more midline position. A reliable method to overcome persisting deviations that fail to respond to less aggressive techniques is to excise as much of the deviated cartilage and ethmoid plate as possible (essentially performing a submucosal resection). Nasal packing for a few days postoperatively may also reduce the tendency of deviations to resume their preoperative position.

Very caudal deflections and very marked deviations are difficult to correct via an endonasal approach. Performing an external septoplasty and straightening the septum on the table before reinserting and reattaching it to the surrounding bone and soft tissue, is generally regarded as the most reliable technique to correct such deformities.[9]

Although there are clearly cases where an external approach is advantageous it must be remembered that this brings with it extra risks. The patient is committed to an external scar and the extra dissection most likely incurs a longer anesthetic and greater risk of infection. There is also an increased risk of late columellar retraction caused by scar contraction.[30]

Inferior Turbinate Reduction Procedures

Procedures to reduce the size of the inferior turbinates are indicated in two circumstances. The first of these are when the inferior turbinates are increased in size by inflammatory conditions such as allergic rhinitis. The second is in conjunction with a septoplasty when normal inferior turbinates are reduced to further increase the cross-sectional area of the nasal passages.[49] Patients with a septal deviation often have a degree of inferior turbinate enlargement, with particular compensatory enlargement on the side of the septal concavity.[50] Determining the relative contribution of these two factors to a patient's symptoms is not easy, and so it is common for both procedures to be performed simultaneously.

The complications that result from inferior turbinate reduction procedures are dependent on the surgical techniques used. A myriad of different techniques have been described, and each has its own profile of strengths and weaknesses. The techniques include cautery applied to the mucosa or submucosa, resection of submucosal tissue, elevation of mucosal flaps and resection of the inferior conchal bone and partial or complete amputation of the inferior turbinate. An excellent randomized trial comparing several different techniques has been performed.[51] After long-term follow-up the authors concluded that the best techniques to achieve lasting nasal patency are those that include resection of much of the inferior conchal bone. Techniques that reduce the soft tissues only tend to be more frequently associated with relapse, particularly after a year's follow-up.

Complications after Inferior Turbinate Reduction

Bleeding

Inferior turbinates are highly vascular. Most of their blood supply comes from the inferior conchal artery, which courses from posterior to anterior just medial to the horizontal part of the inferior conchal bone.[52]

Intraoperative bleeding can be reduced by the same techniques that reduce bleeding during the performance of septoplasty: the topical application of vasoconstrictors, the submucosal injection of epinephrine, the reverse Trendelenburg position and hypotensive general anesthesia. Intraoperative bleeding can be controlled by the application of bipolar or monopolar cautery. If the technique used involves the incision of mucosa then dressings such as Surgicel (Ethicon Inc., Somerville, NJ, USA) or Nasopore (Polyganics, Groningen, the Netherlands) can be applied to the mucosal edges to both control hemorrhage and keep the mucosal flaps in place.

Postoperative hemorrhage can be primary or secondary. Minor primary hemorrhage is common after techniques involving mucosal incisions. Hemostasis that appeared adequate during conditions of anesthesia may be found wanting if the blood pressure becomes elevated after emergence from anesthesia. Sitting the patient up and controlling the blood pressure usually settles primary hemorrhage. Occasionally packing is required.

Reactive hemorrhage usually occurs about a week postoperatively. It is caused by the displacement of fibrin clots. If the bleeding is brisk, packing or cautery may sometimes be required.

Crusting and Scarring

Mucosal crusting is a significant problem in the postoperative period if mucosal cautery techniques are used. It is not uncommon for crusting to persist for three or more weeks after the procedure is performed. Nasal lavage may help to control this problem, but the frequency of its occurrence and persistence provide a strong argument against using techniques that disrupt a large surface of the turbinate mucosa.

Injury of the turbinate mucosa also increases the possibility of postoperative adhesions forming between the medial aspect of the inferior turbinate and the nasal septum.[51] The risk of adhesions developing may be reduced by placing packing or splints within the nasal cavity. Early and regular debridement is also likely to control crusting and reduce the risk of adhesion formation.

Inadequate Relief of Symptoms

Inferior turbinate reductions can provide an inadequate nasal airway in the early postoperative period because of too small a reduction of turbinate size. Partial inferior turbinectomies are easy to perform, but may not always relieve obstruction adequately if the posterior part of the turbinate is bulky and left in situ. For this reason, we usually perform a turbinoplasty or total turbinectomy.

Some techniques of inferior turbinate reduction may successfully control symptoms for a period of many months before a slow recurrence of symptoms. This seems to be particularly the case for techniques in which cautery alone is applied to the mucosa or submucosa. Excising the inferior conchal bone would appear to be the best approach to ensure long-lasting benefit from the procedure (**Fig. 7.10**).[51]

Inferior turbinate reduction procedures are usually effective at reducing obstructive symptoms. It has been reported that turbinate reduction produces some long-lasting improvement in symptoms of allergic rhinitis such as sneezing, itch and rhinorrhea.[53] It is our experience however that this is less marked than the improvements in nasal obstruction and so we typically warn patients that treatment with topical corticosteroid sprays or antihistamines may still be required after the procedure.

It has been reported that excessive resection of the inferior turbinates can lead to the development of "empty nose syndrome." Although successful attempts have been made to treat this disorder[54] it is best avoided and a balance needs to be struck between improvement of the nasal airway and excessive resection of the turbinates.[55] Unfortunately it is a poorly understood disorder and the optimum extent of turbinate reduction has not yet been clearly defined.

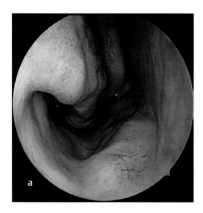 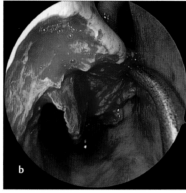 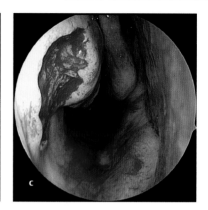

Fig. 7.10a–c Excision of the inferior conchal bone.

a Right inferior turbinate before a turbinoplasty is performed. Topical vasoconstrictor has been applied so the turbinate mucosa does not appear swollen.

b A medial septal flap has been elevated exposing the vertical part of the inferior conchal bone.

c The conchal bone is reduced and the shortened flap is replaced.

Summary

Septoplasty and inferior turbinate reduction are commonly performed procedures that result in significant improvements in nasal symptoms and quality of life. In the majority of situations they are completed with minimal morbidity. There is, however, a wide range of potential complications related to pitfalls occurring at all stages of the procedures and these are summarized in **Table 7.1**.

Table 7.1 Summary of major potential pitfalls and ways to avoid them

Stage in the surgical encounter	Potential pitfalls	Avoiding problems
Preoperative assessment	Failure to relieve symptoms due to neglect of either dorsal septal deflection or external valve collapse	Appreciate the role for external septoplasty and procedures for nasal valve collapse
Consent	Postoperative dissatisfaction due to incomplete discussion of potential complications	Full discussion of complications outlined above
Anesthesia	Poor intraoperative visualization	Intraoperative hypotension, bradycardia and reverse Trendelenburg position
Topical preparation of the nose	Intraoperative bleeding, early postoperative pain and bleeding	Use local anesthesia and vasoconstrictor(s)
Elevation of septal flaps	Septal perforation due to injury of mucoperichondral flaps	Ensure the correct tissue plane is entered before elevation and care is taken elevating over septal spurs
Resection of septal cartilage and/or bone	Cerebrospinal fluid leak, saddle deformity, septal perforation or nasopalatine nerve injury due to excessive resection	Familiarity with septal anatomy and unsafe regions for resection
Closure of septum	Septal hematoma and/or abscess due to failure to eliminate dead space	Ensure that a small septal incision is made in a posterior flap and that the septum is quilted without tension
Inferior turbinate reduction	Long-term failure of symptom control owing to preservation of inferior conchal bone	Use a technique that includes reduction of conchal bone volume

References

1. Cullen KA, Hall MJ, Golosinskiy A. Ambulatory surgery in the United States, 2006. Natl Health Stat Report 2009;(11):1–25
2. Pérez-Piñas, Sabaté J, Carmona A, Catalina-Herrera CJ, Jiménez-Castellanos J. Anatomical variations in the human paranasal sinus region studied by CT. J Anat 2000;197(Pt 2):221–227
3. Cottle MH, Loring RM. Surgery of the nasal septum; new operative procedures and indications. Ann Otol Rhinol Laryngol 1948;57(3):705–713
4. Dobratz EJ, Park SS. Septoplasty pearls. Otolaryngol Clin North Am 2009;42(3):527–537
5. André RF, Vuyk HD, Ahmed A, Graamans K, Nolst Trenité GJ. Correlation between subjective and objective evaluation of the nasal airway. A systematic review of the highest level of evidence. Clin Otolaryngol 2009;34(6):518–525
6. Gandomi B, Bayat A, Kazemei T. Outcomes of septoplasty in young adults: the Nasal Obstruction Septoplasty Effectiveness study. Am J Otolaryngol 2010;31(3):189–192
7. Schwentner I, Dejakum K, Schmutzhard J, Deibl M, Sprinzl GM. Does nasal septal surgery improve quality of life? Acta Otolaryngol 2006;126(7):752–757
8. Gray LP. Prevention and treatment of septal deformity in infancy and childhood. Rhinology 1977;15(4):183–191
9. Gubisch W. Extracorporeal septoplasty for the markedly deviated septum. Arch Facial Plast Surg 2005;7(4):218–226
10. Lee M, Inman J, Callahan S, Ducic Y. Fracture patterns of the nasal septum. Otolaryngol Head Neck Surg 2010;143(6):784–788
11. Chung BJ, Batra PS, Citardi MJ, Lanza DC. Endoscopic septoplasty: revisitation of the technique, indications, and outcomes. Am J Rhinol 2007;21(3):307–311
12. Paradis J, Rotenberg BW. Open versus endoscopic septoplasty: a single-blinded, randomized, controlled trial. J Otolaryngol Head Neck Surg 2011;40(Suppl 1):S28–S33
13. Chaaban M, Shah AR. Open septoplasty: indications and treatment. Otolaryngol Clin North Am 2009;42(3):513–519
14. Benninger M, Farrar JR, Blaiss M, et al. Evaluating approved medications to treat allergic rhinitis in the United States: an evidence-based review of efficacy for nasal symptoms by class. Ann Allergy Asthma Immunol 2010;104(1):13–29
15. Georgalas C, Obholzer R, Martinez-Devesa P, Sandhu G. Day-case septoplasty and unexpected re-admissions at a dedicated day-case unit: a 4-year audit. Ann R Coll Surg Engl 2006;88(2):202–206
16. Congdon D, Sherris DA, Specks U, McDonald T. Long-term follow-up of repair of external nasal deformities in patients with Wegener's granulomatosis. Laryngoscope 2002;112(4):731–737
17. Fuchs HA, Tanner SB. Granulomatous disorders of the nose and paranasal sinuses. Curr Opin Otolaryngol Head Neck Surg 2009;17(1):23–27
18. Slavin SA, Goldwyn RM. The cocaine user: the potential problem patient for rhinoplasty. Plast Reconstr Surg 1990;86(3):436–442
19. Fedok FG, Ferraro RE, Kingsley CP, Fornadley JA. Operative times, postanesthesia recovery times, and complications during sinonasal surgery using general anesthesia and local anesthesia with sedation. Otolaryngol Head Neck Surg 2000;122(4):560–566
20. Demiraran Y, Ozturk O, Guclu E, Iskender A, Ergin MH, Tokmak A. Vasoconstriction and analgesic efficacy of locally infiltrated levobupivacaine for nasal surgery. Anesth Analg 2008;106(3):1008–1011.
21. Higgins TS, Hwang PH, Kingdom TT, Orlandi RR, Stammberger H, Han JK. Systematic review of topical vasoconstrictors in endoscopic sinus surgery. Laryngoscope 2011; 121(2):422–432
22. Wormald PJ, van Renen G, Perks J, Jones JA, Langton-Hewer CD. The effect of the total intravenous anesthesia compared with inhalational anesthesia on the surgical field during endoscopic sinus surgery. Am J Rhinol 2005;19(5):514–520
23. Bajaj Y, Kanatas AN, Carr S, Sethi N, Kelly G. Is nasal packing really required after septoplasty? Int J Clin Pract 2009;63(5):757–759
24. Mäkitie A, Aaltonen LM, Hytönen M, Malmberg H. Postoperative infection following nasal septoplasty. Acta Otolaryngol Suppl 2000;543:165–166
25. Beekhuis GJ. Saddle nose deformity: etiology, prevention, and treatment; augmentation rhinoplasty with polyamide. Laryngoscope 1974;84(1):2–42
26. Hari C, Marnane C, Wormald PJ. Quilting sutures for nasal septum. J Laryngol Otol 2008;122(5):522–523
27. Zayyan E, Bajin MD, Aytemir K, Yılmaz T. The effects on cardiac functions and arterial blood gases of totally occluding nasal packs and nasal packs with airway. Laryngoscope 2010;120(11):2325–2330
28. Jung YG, Hong JW, Eun YG, Kim MG. Objective usefulness of thin silastic septal splints after septal surgery. Am J Rhinol Allergy 2011;25(3):182–185
29. Suzuki C, Nakagawa T, Yao W, Sakamoto T, Ito J. The need for intranasal packing in endoscopic endonasal surgery. Acta Otolaryngol Suppl 2010; (563):39–42
30. Bloom JD, Kaplan SE, Bleier BS, Goldstein SA. Septoplasty complications: avoidance and management. Otolaryngol Clin North Am 2009;42(3):463–481
31. Pribitkin EA, Ezzat WH. Classification and treatment of the saddle nose deformity. Otolaryngol Clin North Am 2009;42(3):437–461
32. Onerci TM, Ayhan K, Oğretmenoğlu O. Two consecutive cases of cerebrospinal fluid rhinorrhea after septoplasty operation. Am J Otolaryngol 2004;25(5):354–356
33. Keros P. Ober die praktische Bedeutung der Niveau-Unterschiede der Lamina cribrosa des Ethmoids. Laryngol Rhinol Otol (Stuttg) 1962;41:808–813
34. Wormald PJ. Salvage frontal sinus surgery: the endoscopic modified Lothrop procedure. Laryngoscope 2003; 113(2):276–283
35. Fransen P, Sindic CJ, Thauvoy C, Laterre C, Stroobandt G. Highly sensitive detection of beta-2 transferrin in rhinorrhea and otorrhea as a marker for cerebrospinal fluid (C.S.F.) leakage. Acta Neurochir (Wien) 1991;109(3–4):98–101
36. Liu P, Wu S, Li Z, Wang B. Surgical strategy for cerebrospinal fluid rhinorrhea repair. Neurosurgery 2010;66(6 Suppl Operative):281–285; discussion 285–286
37. Grützenmacher S, Mlynski R, Lang C, Scholz S, Saadi R, Mlynski G. The nasal airflow in noses with septal perforation: a model study. ORL J Otorhinolaryngol Relat Spec 2005;67(3):142–147
38. Kim DW, Egan KK, O'Grady K, Toriumi DM. Biomechanical strength of human nasal septal lining: comparison of the constituent layers. Laryngoscope 2005;115(8):1451–1453
39. Døsen LK, Haye R. Nasal septal perforation 1981–2005: changes in etiology, gender and size. BMC Ear Nose Throat Disord 2007;7:1
40. Langford RJ. The contribution of the nasopalatine nerve to sensation of the hard palate. Br J Oral Maxillofac Surg 1989;27(5):379–386
41. Chandra RK, Rohman GT, Walsh WE. Anterior palate sensory impairment after septal surgery. Am J Rhinol 2008;22(1):86–88
42. Georgiou I, Farber N, Mendes D, Winkler E. The role of antibiotics in rhinoplasty and septoplasty: a literature review. Rhinology 2008;46(4):267–270

43. Lilja M, Mäkitie AA, Anttila VJ, Kuusela P, Pietola M, Hytönen M. Cefuroxime as a prophylactic preoperative antibiotic in septoplasty. A double blind randomized placebo controlled study. Rhinology 2011;49(1):58–63

44. Nahass RG, Gocke DJ. Toxic shock syndrome associated with use of a nasal tampon. Am J Med 1988;84(3 Pt 2):629–631

45. O'Halloran LR. The lateral crural J-flap repair of nasal valve collapse. Otolaryngol Head Neck Surg 2003;128(5):640–649

46. Yarlagadda BB, Dolan RW. Nasal valve dysfunction: diagnosis and treatment. Curr Opin Otolaryngol Head Neck Surg 2011;19(1):25–29

47. André RF, Vuyk HD. Reconstruction of dorsal and/or caudal nasal septum deformities with septal battens or by septal replacement: an overview and comparison of techniques. Laryngoscope 2006;116(9):1668–1673

48. Byrd HS, Salomon J, Flood J. Correction of the crooked nose. Plast Reconstr Surg 1998;102(6):2148–2157

49. Devseren NO, Ecevit MC, Erdag TK, Ceryan K. A randomized clinical study: outcome of submucous resection of compensatory inferior turbinate during septoplasty. Rhinology 2011;49(1):53–57

50. Jun BC, Kim SW, Kim SW, Cho JH, Park YJ, Yoon HR. Is turbinate surgery necessary when performing a septoplasty? Eur Arch Otorhinolaryngol 2009;266(7):975–980

51. Passàli D, Passàli FM, Damiani V, Passàli GC, Bellussi L. Treatment of inferior turbinate hypertrophy: a randomized clinical trial. Ann Otol Rhinol Laryngol 2003;112(8):683–688

52. Padgham N, Vaughan-Jones R. Cadaver studies of the anatomy of arterial supply to the inferior turbinates. J R Soc Med 1991;84(12):728–730

53. Mori S, Fujieda S, Yamada T, Kimura Y, Takahashi N, Saito H. Long-term effect of submucous turbinectomy in patients with perennial allergic rhinitis. Laryngoscope 2002;112(5):865–869

54. Jang YJ, Kim JH, Song HY. Empty nose syndrome: radiologic findings and treatment outcomes of endonasal microplasty using cartilage implants. Laryngoscope 2011;121(6):1308–1312

55. Chhabra N, Houser SM. The diagnosis and management of empty nose syndrome. Otolaryngol Clin North Am 2009;42(2):311–330, ix

8 Complications Following Surgery of the Nasolacrimal System

S. B. Nair, A. Rokade, M. Bernal-Sprekelsen

Introduction

Surgery of the nasolacrimal system can be performed via an external or endoscopic approach. This chapter will focus on the complications associated with endoscopic dacryocystorhinostomy (DCR) surgery, although some of the complications mentioned are common to both techniques.

The lacrimal drainage system allows tears to drain from the lacrimal lake to the inferior meatus. Malfunction of the system results in overflow tearing or epiphora. Many procedures have been described to treat epiphora resulting from nasolacrimal duct pathology. These include the application of lasers, using cold steel, and using specially designed drills.[1,2] None of these are perfect and all are associated with potential complications. Over the last decade, a better understanding of the endonasal anatomy of the lacrimal gland and improvements in surgical technique and equipment have resulted in better endonasal DCR success rates.[3] Nevertheless complications

can occur that are both specific to nasolacrimal surgery and generally related to endoscopic sinus surgery. A thorough knowledge of the relevant anatomy is important to minimize the risk of complications and this will be covered in the following section.

Anatomy

The nasolacrimal system is simple in design but rather more complex in its function. The tear film flows medially to drain through inferior and superior puncta located in the nasal portion of each eyelid. The puncta open up into the superior and inferior canaliculi, which travel vertically for ~ 2 mm before turning sharply medially, paralleling the eyelid margin and diving posteriorly for ~ 8 mm toward the lacrimal sac.[4] In 90% of patients, these two canaliculi join to form the common canaliculus before entering the lacrimal sac at the junction of the middle and upper third (**Fig. 8.1**).

The lacrimal fossa is at the junction of the frontal process of the maxilla anteriorly and the lacrimal bone posteriorly. The lacrimal sac sits in the lacrimal fossa with a small portion of it, ~ 5 mm, sitting above the medial canthal tendon and 10 mm below the tendon. It opens inferiorly into the nasolacrimal duct. The duct resides in a bony canal within the maxilla and terminates in the inferior meatus as the valve of Hasner. Endonasally, the nasolacrimal system corresponds to the maxillary line, which is a curvilinear eminence, of variable prominence, extending from the axilla of the middle turbinate superiorly to the root of the inferior turbinate inferiorly.[5]

The lacrimal sac and duct are intimately related to the structures on the lateral nasal wall. The nasolacrimal duct lies between 1 and 8 mm anterior to the attachment of the uncinate process. The natural maxillary ostium is a similarly close posterior relationship to the duct. Pneumatization of the agger nasi cell can extend anteriorly to the region of the frontal process and lacrimal bone. This makes the sac and duct more vulnerable.[5] In children, these distances are smaller and one must be aware of the proximity of the anterior skull to the fundus of the sac.

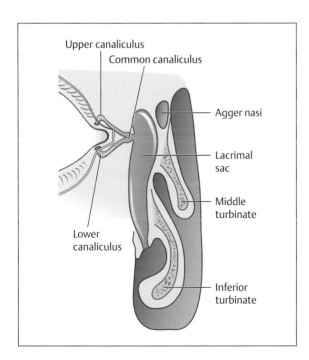

Fig. 8.1 Anatomy of the nasolacrimal duct system.

Complications Defined by Each Surgical Step

Preoperative Planning

Sinonasal Pathology

If patients have concomitant sinonasal pathology it is best practice to use maximum medical therapy before surgery. The use of antibiotics and in selected cases oral and or topical corticosteroids aims to reduce the load of inflammatory mediators.

Comorbidities

The majority of the patients undergoing endoscopic DCR are elderly and likely to have systemic comorbidities that may increase surgical bleeding. Conditions such as hypertension and peripheral vascular disease should be optimally managed perioperatively as maintaining controlled hypotension during surgery could pose a significant anesthetic challenge. Patients with mitral valve stenosis can have increased bleeding as the result of a rise in venous pressure. Total intravenous anesthesia has been shown to provide an excellent surgical field with ideal hypotensive bradycardia conditions for endoscopic sinonasal surgery.[6]

If patients have any coagulopathies as a result of liver disease, renal disease, chronic alcohol abuse, malnutrition, or inherent bleeding diathesis, appropriate control of coagulation profile should be achieved preoperatively with the help of medical colleagues.

Medications

Certain common medications like aspirin and similar drugs belonging to the family of nonsteroidal anti-inflammatory drugs (NSAIDs) can inhibit platelet function by inhibiting the formation of thromboxane A2. These drugs produce a systemic bleeding tendency and consequently prolong the bleeding time. Aspirin exerts these effects by irreversibly blocking the cyclooxygenases (COX-1 to a greater extent than COX-2) and, therefore, its actions persist for the circulating lifetime of the platelet. NSAIDs inhibit cyclooxygenase reversibly so the duration of their action depends on specific drug dose, serum level, and half-life. The clinical risks of bleeding with aspirin or nonaspirin NSAIDs are enhanced by the concomitant use of alcohol or anticoagulants and by associated conditions, including advanced age, liver disease, and other coexisting coagulopathies.[7]

Some authors have reported that the incidence of postoperative bleeding is higher in patients taking NSAIDs. Of patients who had bled, 40% had been taking NSAIDs compared with 16% of patients who had not bled.[8] It is advisable to stop aspirin at least 1 week before surgery and NSAIDs 2 to 3 days before surgery. Certain herbal remedies and nutritional supplement treatments such as ginkgo biloba, can also affect platelet function. Ginkgo has been linked with bleeding events and postoperative hemorrhage in general surgery.[9] Increased risk is associated with the following agents: feverfew (*Tanacetum parthenium*), used to treat headache; garlic (*Allium sativum*), used as an antimicrobial and diuretic; ginger (*Zingiber officinale*), an antiemetic; and ginseng (*Panax* spp.), used to treat anxiety and gastric upset.[10] We advise our patients to stop any such treatments at least 1 week before surgery.

Nasal Preparation

As with most endoscopic procedures it is important to achieve the best surgical field possible. Topical and local application of vasoconstrictors is important for maintaining the optimum surgical field. We have found that the use of neurosurgical patties soaked in a mixture of 2 mL 4% cocaine, 1 mL 1:1,000 epinephrine, and 7 mL saline very useful, provided there is no contraindication to the use of cocaine. However, where there are concerns regarding potential cardiac side effects this can be substituted for 1% oxymetazoline. The potential complications of topical agents have been well described.[11] The use of a combination of local anesthetic and vasoconstrictor infiltrate in the region of the lacrimal sac just anterior to the axilla of the middle turbinate provides excellent vasoconstriction. A commonly used agent is a mixture of 2% lignocaine and 1:80,000 epinephrine. It is important to allow sufficient time for topical and local vasoconstrictors to work.

Raising the Mucosal Flaps— Intraoperative Strategies

The positioning of the patient during surgery is important. Maintaining the reverse Trendelenburg position with 30 to 40° head up lowers the arterial pressure and prevents venous congestion, thereby reducing bleeding. Controlled hypotension throughout the surgery with ideal mean arterial blood pressure below 60 to 75 mmHg and the ideal heart rate to be less than 60 beats/min, is helpful in reducing bleeding.[12] Total intravenous anesthesia is better than inhaled anesthetic agents in achieving this because it causes less vasodilatation.[6]

Diligent handling of nasal endoscopes and surgical instruments is vital to avoid unnecessary collateral mucosal trauma, which can result in troublesome bleeding. One should have a low threshold of performing a septoplasty if the intranasal access is compromised by septal deviations or spurs. An "access" submucosal resection can be performed endoscopically without the need for a formal septoplasty. The septal mucoperichondral flaps elevated during the procedure should be well approximated by placing absorbable quilting sutures. Septoplasty can increase the risk of postoperative hemorrhage. A septoplasty as an access procedure may be necessary in nearly half of all patients undergoing an endoscopic DCR.[1,2]

Minor oozing from mucosal incisions can be dealt with by using topical vasoconstrictors on neurosurgical patties or bipolar diathermy. The use of an endoscope irrigation system is helpful because it reduces the need for repeatedly removing the endoscope for cleaning. It is not unusual to have some increase in bleeding when the patient comes out of general anesthesia. This is the result of an increase in venous pressure that can occur during extubation, particularly if the patient coughs. This usually settles with the patient being nursed in a 30°, head up position. Temporary neurosurgical patties soaked in a vasoconstrictor solution can be placed in the nasal cavity to control minor bleeding, and then be removed in the recovery room. For more than minor bleeding, a nasal pack or tampon can be placed for 12 to 24 hours. Rarely is a nasal pack required for longer than 24 hours. If this is the case the use of prophylactic antibiotic cover is recommended.

Creating a Rhinostomy

It is important to create a good rhinostomy that fully exposes the intranasal portion of the lacrimal sac. There are several methods that can be used alone or in combination to achieve this. Rongeurs, lasers, and drills are all associated with potential complications. The most likely complication arising during this part of the operation would be an orbital breach with fat exposure and bleeding. Damage to the skull base with a resultant cerebrospinal fluid leak has only been reported in association with a correction of nasal septal deviation where the septum was said to have been inserted unusually on the cribriform plate instead of the crista galli.[13]

Orbital Fat Exposure and Periorbital Emphysema

The most common intraoperative complication of endoscopic DCR appears to be inadvertent exposure of periorbital fat. The overall incidence of this appears to be 1.25%,[14] but some series have reported rates as high as 10.5%.[15] As long as this is recognized early and further entry into the orbit is not made, it is not a major complication and should not pose a significant problem. However, one must be cautious when using high-speed drills and suction to avoid pulling more fat into the operative field and so risk damage to the underlying muscle and vascular structures.

This complication can occur if the surgeon strays away from anatomical landmarks. Orbital fat exposure is more likely if the dissection proceeds posterior to the uncinate process; as long as the surgeon stays anterior to the insertion of the uncinate process, orbital entry is unlikely.

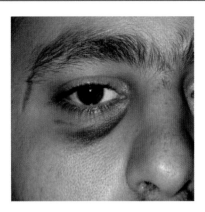

Fig. 8.2 Cheek ecchymosis.

When the agger nasi cell is absent or poorly pneumatized, penetration behind the hard frontal process of the maxilla puts the surgeon at risk of entering the orbit.

The chances of orbital entry increase when ancillary endoscopic sinus surgical procedures are performed simultaneously. This is particularly the case if a traditional uncinectomy is performed. It is not uncommon to have no ethmoid cells separating the uncinate process from the lamina papyracea. An incision as small as 2 mm through the uncinate process can penetrate the lamina and so breach the orbit. A retrograde uncinectomy is favored to reduce the likelihood of orbital entry.

If the lamina papyracea is breached this may result in a minor ecchymosis, which usually settles down in 3 to 5 days (**Fig. 8.2**). Orbital fat herniation occurs if there is a breach in the orbital periosteum. If a breach of the lamina is suspected, one can ballot the ipsilateral closed eye, which results in abrupt movement of the fat. The orbital fat should be left alone and not manipulated further. Ideally, one should refrain from trying to push the fat back into the orbit, pulling it out, or cauterizing it. This may make matters worse rather than improving the situation. Unless the fat herniation is extensive, abandoning surgery is unnecessary. One can use either a moist neurosurgical pattie or a piece of Silastic film (Dow Corning, Midland, MI, USA) placed over the fat to protect the area while continuing with the rest of the procedure. Again, as mentioned above, powered instruments should be used cautiously in this instance.

Postoperatively patients should not blow their nose for up to 10 days. Keeping the mouth open during unavoidable sneezing during this period can help to avoid periorbital emphysema. It is important to monitor ocular vital signs such as pupillary reflexes and vision. Simple palpation of the globe at the end of the procedure will give the surgeon some indication of the orbital pressure. This is important should the situation deteriorate and orbital bleeding occur. In this situation, lateral canthotomy should be considered and the opinion of an ophthalmologist should be sought. The patient should be given postoperative prophylactic antibiotics to avoid the risk of developing periorbital cellulitis.

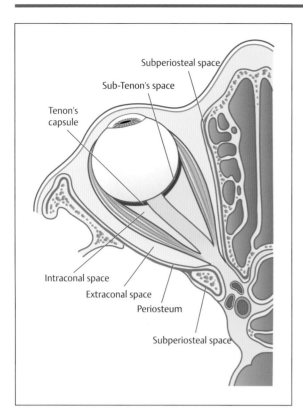

Fig. 8.3 Orbital compartments. The four rectus muscles and their fibrous septa divide the contents of the orbit in to two compartments: an extraconal (peribulbar) and intraconal (retrobulbar) space.

Major Orbital Complications

Serious orbital complications leading to visual loss following endoscopic DCR surgery have not been reported in the literature. Diplopia secondary to transient medial rectus palsy has been described. This is thought to occur as a result of local anesthetic infiltration.[16] Intervention is not warranted because the effects of local anesthesia wear off without any permanent sequelae. There is a case report of inadvertent damage to the medial rectus during surgery resulting in diplopia that resolved within a few weeks.[17]

Hemorrhage is a rare complication of regional ophthalmic anesthesia. Such bleeding can range from minor, with only spot ecchymosis of the eyelid, to severe, with retrobulbar hemorrhage (intraconal) and raised intraocular pressure.[18] Peribulbar (extraconal) hemorrhage (**Fig. 8.3**) is rare in endonasal DCR although cases have been reported.[16] It would appear that this can occur as a result of inadvertent infiltration of local anesthetic around the orbit. This can be managed conservatively with the application of an intraocular pressure reducer such as a Honan balloon. If this is not available one could use a mercury bag. This treatment has been described for retrobulbar hemorrhage in cataract surgery. It involves the

placement of the pressure reducer or mercury bag over the closed affected eye.[19] After 5 to 10 minutes the eye can be reassessed. If there is a satisfactory reduction in intraocular pressure, digital pressure and further application of the mercury bag or intraocular pressure reducer can be continued intermittently for up to 20 minutes. Significant retrobulbar (intraconal) hemorrhage, has not been reported in endoscopic DCR surgery.

The likelihood of major orbital complications is increased if an ancillary procedure such as endoscopic sinus surgery is performed. However, the surgeon should, as always, be aware of the potential complications and take steps to minimize these. The management of these complications is described in detail in other sections of this book.

Bleeding

Primary Hemorrhage

During endoscopic DCR surgery some mucosal bleeding is expected but troublesome intraoperative bleeding is unusual. Boezaart and van der Merwe Grading is a useful system for grading bleeding during endoscopic sinus surgery (**Table 8.1**).[20]

- Minor bleeding, which does not obscure the surgical site (approximately < 10 mL) and requires only infrequent suction, occurs in more than 50% of cases.[17,21] This is easily managed with topical vasoconstrictors, surgical patties and if necessary bipolar diathermy. This level of bleeding rarely requires nasal packing.
- Moderate bleeding, which requires repeated suctioning and can obscure the surgical field, is managed in a similar fashion. Anesthetic measures to improve heart rate and keep this below 60 beats/min have been shown to significantly improve the surgical bleeding grade.[12]
- Major bleeding (Grade 4 and 5) impairing surgery is not very common in endoscopic DCR on its own. It is more common if ancillary procedures such as septal surgery and endoscopic sinus surgery are undertaken. It is reported in around 5 to 11% of cases.[21]
- Epistaxis requiring perioperative nasal packing is reported in around 5% of patients.[17]

Bleeding may increase the postoperative stay in the hospital. Very rarely, surgery might have to be abandoned due to excessive bleeding despite local measures and systemic drugs used to induce hypotensive bradycardia. Some patients might need nasal packing or further surgical intervention to control bleeding. The use of topical antifibrinolytic drugs may be useful in reducing bleeding. Drugs such as tranexamic acid can be used systemically but are most effective topically in this situation.[22]

Major arterial bleeding is not reported with endoscopic DCR alone. There have been reports of significant

Table 8.1 Grading system for bleeding during endoscopic sinus surgery

Grades	Surgical field
Grade 1	Cadaveric conditions with minimal suction required
Grade 2	Minimal bleeding with infrequent suction required
Grade 3	Brisk bleeding with frequent suction required
Grade 4	Bleeding covers surgical field after removal of suction before surgical instruments can perform maneuver
Grade 5	Uncontrolled bleeding. Bleeding out of nostril on removal of suction

bleeding, which can occur if the anterior ethmoid artery is damaged during concurrent sinus surgery. This can be controlled endoscopically using special endoscopic bipolar diathermy forceps.[15]

Bleeding can be minimized by careful preoperative planning and by optimizing perioperative conditions (discussed earlier).

Reactionary Hemorrhage

This can occur in the first 12 hours following surgery, as a result of bleeding from minor blood vessels, which had gone into spasm during surgery. These blood vessels may open up as a result of relaxation or fibrinolysis of the occluding clot. This should ideally be managed by selective cautery of the offending vessels under direct vision. If this is not feasible then a nasal pack and/or balloon may be required to control the bleeding.

Secondary Hemorrhage

Secondary hemorrhage is unusual following endoscopic DCR surgery. It may occur 2 to 8 days after surgery. It might occur as a result of the dissolution of a blood clot at the surgical site or as a result of postoperative infection. The secondary hemorrhage rate is reported to be around 3.8 to 11%.[8,23]

Following a thorough endoscopic examination any clots and crusts can be debrided following the application of local anesthetic spray. If there is evidence of an infection it may be necessary to use oral or intravenous antibiotic. Troublesome bleeding will require a nasal tampon or targeted bipolar diathermy.

Exposing the Sac

Using anatomical landmarks one can easily remove much of the ascending process of the maxilla with either a 45° or 90° Kerrison or a forward-biting Hajek–Koeffler punch. However, exposing the fundus of the sac will often require the use of a drill. Without adequate irrigation, the drill may burn the bone itself. If the drill used is not specifically designed for endonasal surgery one can burn the nostril. Removing the thick bone with a hammer and chisel requires angling the chisel toward the orbit and needs good previous training of the helping hand.

When using cold fiber lighting to illuminate the sac to identify its location, one must be aware that transillumination highlights the thin bone, which is usually at its posterior part toward the lacrimal bone, in close proximity to the orbit.

Opening the Sac

Once the sac is exposed, including the fundus superiorly, it can be opened. Usually the mucosa of the agger nasi is exposed while removing the bone in the region of the axilla of the middle turbinate. It can be difficult to distinguish the sac wall from the agger nasi cell mucosa or the skin. A lacrimal probe or light pipe should be passed through the inferior canaliculus, which should enter without any resistance into the lacrimal sac. The light pipe or lacrimal probe helps to illuminate or tent the sac mucosa, allowing easier identification (avoiding potential complications of light fiber intubation—see section above).

The probe can be visualized endonasally by the tenting of the sac mucosa medially. When the tip of the probe is seen clearly through a single layer of mucosa, it is safe to incise the sac using the probe as a marker. Incising the sac too far posteriorly can result in orbital fat exposure. Rarely is this troublesome and surgery can usually be completed without much hindrance. Managing orbital fat prolapse has been dealt with in the previous section.

Intubating the Canalicular System

Either during probing before opening the sac, or following intubation, it is possible to create a false passage. This is more likely if there is canalicular stenosis. It is therefore important to visualize the common canaliculus opening during stenting to ensure that both probes emerge from the same opening. This highlights the importance of adequate bone removal over the fundus of the sac, which allows inspection of this area.

Following DCR surgery, depending on the pathology, silicone tubing can be used to "stent" the canalicular and nasolacrimal system. Being relatively inert this is usually well tolerated. However, complications can occur. Tubes that are secured too tightly in the nose can cheesewire through the canaliculi (**Figs. 8.4 and 8.5**). This would affect the lacrimal pump system. To avoid this complication, it is important to pull a loop of tubing at the punctal portion, to allow enough slack, before securing the intranasal portion of the tube. This can easily be checked by

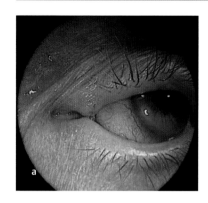

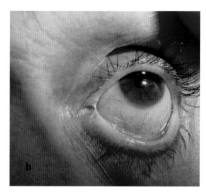

Fig. 8.4a,b Complications of silicone tubing.

a Tubes too tight.

b Canalicular scarring.

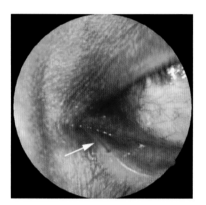

Fig. 8.5 Cheesewiring of the inferior canaliculus (white arrow).

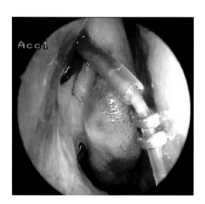

Fig. 8.6 Silastic collar.

anesthetic topical medication. It is not uncommon to see granulations on the anterior edge of the lacrimal sac–nasal mucosa junction in patients who have undergone silastic tube stenting. This is usually easily treated with removal of the stent and granuloma and cautery with silver nitrate of the granulation base.

Immediate Postoperative Issues

Periorbital Emphysema

Air can be forced into the soft tissues around the eye if the lamina papyracea is breached at the time of surgery and the patient has blown their nose or sneezed, which leads to a sharp increase in intranasal pressure. The incidence of this occurrence is around 2%.[14,15] It would be prudent for the surgeon to inform the anesthetist of any breach of lamina papyracea noticed during the surgery. This should prompt the anesthetist to be cautious when providing ventilation via a facemask after extubation. It is suggested that one should avoid a fixed valve on the ventilation circuit, which could lead to a build up of intranasal pressure.

Surgical emphysema usually resorbs within 3 to 5 days. Some authors recommend the use of prophylactic antibiotics to minimize the risk of developing periorbital cellulitis.[24]

Facial Subcutaneous Emphysema and Ecchymosis

Subcutaneous emphysema and ecchymosis can occur over the premaxillary area. This can occur as a result of injury to the subcutaneous tissue and skin while removing the frontal process of maxilla by use of either rongeurs or drills. In the experience of one of the senior authors, the incidence of subcutaneous emphysema and that of minor cheek ecchymosis (**Fig. 8.6**) is ~ 9% and up to 44%, respectively.[15]

Using an inferiorly based mucoperichondral flap from the agger nasi down to the inferior turbinate, which at

retraction of the eyelids, which should allow a portion of tubing to sit comfortably between the upper and lower canaliculi.

If there is too much slack with the tubes, subluxation can occur. The knot can then migrate through the rhinostomy into the lacrimal sac. This can result in a corneal abrasion or pyogenic granuloma at the puncta. Using a silastic collar around the tubes as a spacer does help to reduce migration (**Fig. 8.6**). The subluxed tubes either need to be pulled back intranasally and secured, or if no longer required, can be removed. Pyogenic granulomas should be excised and cauterized. Corneal abrasions are treated in conjunction with the ophthalmologist using a combination of antibiotic, corticosteroid and, if required,

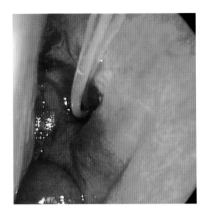

Fig. 8.7 Inferiorly based mucosal flap. The flap is outlined with the head of the middle turbinate (MT) being inferomedial.

the end of the procedure covers the lateral wall again as described by Massegur et al,[25] significantly reduces the incidence of ecchymosis (**Fig. 8.7**).

If a drill is used, one can minimize trauma to the sac and collateral tissue by using a diamond bur. Both, facial emphysema and hematoma are usually self limiting and usually absorbed within 2 to 4 days. The use of postoperative prophylactic antibiotics, to avoid cellulitis, is recommended.[15]

Infection, Crusting, and Adhesions

The nose is not a sterile site and any surgical intervention in the nose can result in a postoperative infection. In the case of nasolacrimal surgery, the mucosal incision on the lateral nasal wall and trauma from drilling or the use of rongeurs can predispose to infection. The use of a single dose of antibiotics given at the start of surgery is recommended. When the lacrimal sac is potentially infected, as in the presence of a chronic dacryocystitis or the maxillary sinus is inadvertently entered during surgery, the use of prophylactic postoperative antibiotics is appropriate.

Fibrin exudation and adhesion formation following endoscopic endonasal DCR surgery is not uncommon. As with all endoscopic sinonasal surgery, attention to detail is important and minimizing collateral damage is crucial in preventing adhesion formation. The incidence of adhesions in endoscopic sinus surgery is between 4 and 6%,[24] and is likely to be similar in DCR surgery. Similarly,

control of hemostasis prevents excessive clot formation and subsequent adhesions[26] (**Fig. 8.8a**). The presence of adhesions can affect sinonasal function and studies have suggested that it is likely to significantly affect the outcome of a DCR procedure.[27] Fibrous adhesion bands within the marsupialized sac can potentially cause a lacrimal sump syndrome. Mitomycin C has been used, with limited success, to reduce adhesion formation.[28]

If necessary, adhesions that are limiting nasal function can usually be easily divided, in the clinic, using through-cutting forceps. Adhesions or scarring at the rhinostomy site can be detected on direct endoscopy while syringing the nasolacrimal system (**Fig. 8.8b**). If affecting the transit of tears, these adhesions will need to be divided. Occasionally one might need to reintubate the nasolacrimal system using silicone tubes for a period of 4 to 8 weeks.

Crusting is common following any sinonasal surgery, and nasolacrimal surgery is no exception. This is a consequence of surgery rather than a complication. However, significant crusting can be associated with infection and may occur as a result of inadequate douching. Many studies have highlighted the positive effects of postoperative nasal douching. This helps to reduce crusting and adhesion formation in the early postoperative period.[29]

Special Circumstances

Complications of Conjunctivodacryocystorhinostomy

In the presence of canalicular stenosis, when other treatment modalities have failed, a conjunctivodacryocystorhinostomy can provide symptomatic relief. The procedure involves the insertion of a Lester Jones pyrex glass bypass tube, which creates a lacrimal drainage route from the conjunctiva into the nose, bypassing the canaliculi and sac. However, tube extrusion, obstruction, migration, infection and granuloma formation are not uncommon. Correct placement of the Lester Jones tube with respect to intranasal anatomy is important. The intranasal portion should not be in contact with the middle turbinate

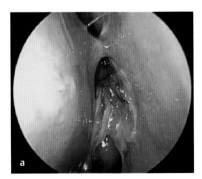
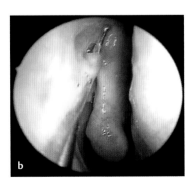

Fig. 8.8a,b Adhesions and crusting.

a Adhesion between septum and lateral wall. Crusting around rhinostomy and silastic tubing.

b Adhesion band across rhinostomy. A ball probe is inserted under the band after the fluorescein dye test.

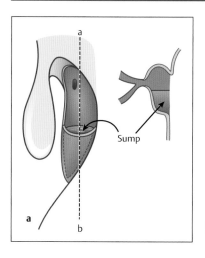

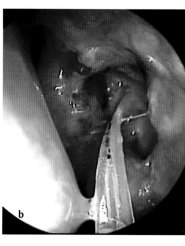

Fig. 8.9a,b Lacrimal sump syndrome.

a Schematic coronal view (left) and cross-sectional view (right).

b Showing a pouch in the inferior aspect of the sac.

or nasal septum. Choosing the correct tube length prevents migration or granulation formation. Angling the tube posteroinferiorly allows dependent tear drainage. The caruncle is easily removed by grasping it with a pair of forceps and cutting it flush with a pair of tenotomy scissors. This prevents the redundant conjunctiva from obstructing the medial canthal portion of the tube.[30]

Laser-assisted DCR Surgery

Lasers are excellent in achieving hemostasis and can ablate bone and soft tissue depending on the lasers employed. There have been many reports cataloging the use of various lasers in endoscopic DCR surgery. In an early report Sadiq et al[16] suggested that laser-assisted DCR surgery was a cost-effective, local anesthetic procedure with results comparable to conventional DCRs performed in their unit. Although intranasal laser-assisted DCR has several advantages over endoscopic cold steel DCR surgery, including a shortened operative time, it is associated with lower success rates.[14] Another disadvantage of laser-assisted DCR surgery is the inability to ablate thick bone. This can result in collateral thermal injury with subsequent scarring and adhesion formation.[31]

The complications related to the use of lasers in general are described in detail in other sections of this book.

Lacrimal Sump Syndrome

Lacrimal sump syndrome results as a formation of a kangaroo-like pouch medially in the lower part of the rhinostomy (**Fig. 8.9**). This results in the collection of secretions within the pouch causing a persistent epiphora. The collected secretions are also susceptible to infection. The sump may occur as a result of scarring of the opened sac, of inadequate bone removal, inadequate flap formation and anastomosis, or failure to completely open the sac into the nose.[32]

Sump syndrome can occur despite having an anatomically patent lacrimal system. This is reported to comprise 9% of 90 patients who had persistent epiphora in a series of 837 endoscopic DCR surgeries.[33] Neodymium:yttrium aluminum garnet laser has been successfully used to treat lacrimal sump syndrome following DCR.[34] The nasolacrimal anatomical patency can be assessed using a fluorescein dye disappearance test. Fluorescein placed in the medial conjunctival fornix is cleared rapidly and is seen transiting via the rhinostomy. Key steps to help reduce the incidence of sump syndrome are outlined in **Fig. 8.10**.

Summary

Endoscopic endonasal DCR is a safe and effective technique for the treatment of nasolacrimal duct obstruction. Unlike external DCR surgery it aims to preserve the lacrimal pump mechanism. However, complications can occur and these are summarized in **Fig. 8.11**. To minimize the incidence of complications a thorough knowledge of the relevant anatomy and attention to detail are essential.

---

1. Create large ostium
2. Good exposure of sac

   Adequate bone removal over the frontal process of the maxilla and above the axilla of the middle turbinate to expose the fundus of the sac

   Ensure lower portion of the sac is fully exposed and opened; note that with chronic infection the sac wall may be thickened

   Careful flap design that allows the fundus and lower part of the sac to be exposed
3. Using mucosal flaps to minimize exposed bone and subsequent scarring

---

Fig. 8.10 Prevention and management of lacrimal sump syndrome.

Operative

- Bleeding
- Orbital
  - Fat exposure (breach of lamina papyracea)
  - Minor periorbital bleeding
- Sac trauma (inadvertent drilling)

Early (up to 4 weeks)

- Intranasal adhesions
- Nasal crusting
- Infection
- Rhinostomy
  - Scarring and fibrosis
  - Granulations
- Tube problems
  - Subluxation
  - Displacement into nasal cavity
  - Corneal abrasion
  - Punctual cheese wiring

Late (up to 6 months)

- Rhinostomy scarring and stenosis
- Nasal crusting
- Nasal adhesions
- Lacrimal sump syndrome

Fig. 8.11 Complications associated with dacryocystorhinostomy.

References

1. Tsirbas A, Wormald PJ. Mechanical endonasal dacryocystorhinostomy with mucosal flaps. Br J Ophthalmol 2003;87(1):43–47
2. Tan NC, Rajapaksa SP, Gaynor J, Nair SB. Mechanical endonasal dacryocystorhinostomy—a reproducible technique. Rhinology 2009;47(3):310–315
3. Wormald PJ, Kew J, Van Hasselt A. Intranasal anatomy of the nasolacrimal sac in endoscopic dacryocystorhinostomy. Otolaryngol Head Neck Surg 2000;123(3):307–310
4. Hollsten DA. Complications of lacrimal surgery. Int Ophthalmol Clin 1992;32(4):49–66
5. Cohen NA, Antunes MB, Morgenstern KE. Prevention and management of lacrimal duct injury. Otolaryngol Clin North Am 2010;43(4):781–788
6. Wormald PJ, van Renen G, Perks J, Jones JA, Langton-Hewer CD. The effect of the total intravenous anesthesia compared with inhalational anesthesia on the surgical field during endoscopic sinus surgery. Am J Rhinol 2005;19(5):514–520
7. Schafer AI. Effects of nonsteroidal antiinflammatory drugs on platelet function and systemic hemostasis. J Clin Pharmacol 1995;35(3):209–219
8. Tsirbas A, McNab AA. Secondary haemorrhage after dacryocystorhinostomy. Clin Experiment Ophthalmol 2000;28(1):22–25
9. Bent S, Goldberg H, Padula A, Avins AL. Spontaneous bleeding associated with ginkgo biloba. A case report and systematic review of the literature. J Gen Intern Med 2005;20(7):657–661
10. Fessenden JM, Wittenborn W, Clarke L. Gingko biloba: a case report of herbal medicine and bleeding postoperatively from a laparoscopic cholecystectomy. Am Surg 2001;67(1):33–35
11. Benjamin E, Wong DK, Choa D. 'Moffett's' solution: a review of the evidence and scientific basis for the topical preparation of the nose. Clin Otolaryngol Allied Sci 2004;29(6):582–587
12. Nair S, Collins M, Hung P, Rees G, Close D, Wormald P-J. The effect of beta-blocker premedication on the surgical field during endoscopic sinus surgery. Laryngoscope 2004;114(6):1042–1046
13. Fayet B, Racy E, Assouline M. Cerebrospinal fluid leakage after endonasal dacryocystorhinostomy. J Fr Ophthalmol 2007;30(2):129–134
14. Leong SC, Macewen CJ, White PS. A systematic review of outcomes after dacryocystorhinostomy in adults. Am J Rhinol Allergy 2010;24(1):81–90
15. Sprekelsen MB, Barberán MT. Endoscopic dacryocystorhinostomy: surgical technique and results. Laryngoscope 1996;106(2 Pt 1):187–189
16. Sadiq SA, Hugkulstone CE, Jones NS, Downes RN. Endoscopic holmium:YAG laser dacryocystorhinostomy. Eye (Lond) 1996;10(Pt 1):43–46
17. Dolman PJ. Comparison of external dacryocystorhinostomy with nonlaser endonasal dacryocystorhinostomy. Ophthalmology 2003;110(1):78–84
18. Kallio H, Paloheimo M, Maunuksela EL. Haemorrhage and risk factors associated with retrobulbar/peribulbar block: a prospective study in 1383 patients. Br J Anaesth 2000;85(5):708–711
19. Cionni RJ, Osher RH. Retrobulbar hemorrhage. Ophthalmology 1991;98(8):1153–1155
20. Boezaart AP, van der Merwe J, Coetzee A. Comparison of sodium nitroprusside- and esmolol-induced controlled hypotension for functional endoscopic sinus surgery. Can J Anaesth 1995;42(5 Pt 1):373–376
21. Fayet B, Racy E, Assouline M. Complications of standardized endonasal dacryocystorhinostomy with unciformectomy. Ophthalmology 2004;111(4):837–845
22. Athanasiadis T, Beule AG, Wormald PJ. Effects of topical antifibrinolytics in endoscopic sinus surgery: a pilot randomized controlled trial. Am J Rhinol 2007;21(6):737–742
23. Razavi ME, Eslampoor A, Noorollahian M, O'Donnell A, Beigi B. Non-endoscopic endonasal dacryocystorhinostomy—technique, indications, and results. Orbit 2009;28(1):1–6
24. Simmen D, Jones N. Patient consent and information. In: Manual of Endoscopic Sinus Surgery and its Extended Applications. New York, NY: Thieme Medical Publishers; 2005:146
25. Massegur H, Trias E, Ademà JM. Endoscopic dacryocystorhinostomy: modified technique. Otolaryngol Head Neck Surg 2004;130(1):39–46
26. Valentine R, Athanasiadis T, Moratti S, Hanton L, Robinson S, Wormald PJ. The efficacy of a novel chitosan gel on hemostasis and wound healing after endoscopic sinus surgery. Am J Rhinol Allergy 2010;24(1):70–75
27. Edelstein DR. Revison Endoscopic Dacryocystorhinostomy in Revision Surgery in Otolaryngology. Stuttgart: Thieme; 2009:414
28. Tirakunwichcha S, Aeumjaturapat S, Sinprajakphon S. Efficacy of mitomycin C in endonasal endoscopic dacryocystorhinostomy. Laryngoscope 2011;121(2):433–436
29. Freeman SR, Sivayoham ES, Jepson K, de Carpentier J. A preliminary randomised controlled trial evaluating the efficacy of saline douching following endoscopic sinus surgery. Clin Otolaryngol 2008;33(5):462–465

30. Hollsten DA. Complications of lacrimal surgery. Int Ophthalmol Clin 1992;32(4):49–66
31. Metson R, Woog JJ, Puliafito CA. Endoscopic laser dacryocystorhinostomy. Laryngoscope 1994;104(3 Pt 1):269–274
32. Jordan DR, McDonald H. Failed dacryocystorhinostomy:
the sump syndrome. Ophthal Plast Reconstr Surg 1997;
13(4):281–284
33. Park WH, Kim MJ, Choi YJ, Kim S Jr. Endonasal Dacryocystorhinostomy. J Korean Ophthalmol Soc. 2005;46(7):
1089–1094
34. Migliori ME. Endoscopic evaluation and management of
the lacrimal sump syndrome. Ophthal Plast Reconstr Surg
1997;13(4):281–284

9 Complications in Endoscopic Sinus Surgery

M. A. Tewfik, P.-J. Wormald

Introduction

Despite numerous advances in surgical technique and instrumentation, the risk of serious complication during endoscopic sinus surgery (ESS) is ever present. This is an unavoidable result of the close proximity of various critical structures, such as the orbit, internal carotid arteries, and skull base, to the paranasal sinuses. It is the responsibility of the operating surgeon to minimize the risks through meticulous preoperative preparation, careful operative technique, and diligent postoperative care. Complications in ESS may be subclassified in several ways, including classifications based on anatomical location, severity, and timing. The first two methods are generally considered to be the most relevant in ESS.

With regards to anatomical location, adverse events are categorized according to the site or tissue involved; these include vascular, neurologic, ophthalmic, intranasal wound healing, facial, and packing-related complications. In the severity-based approach, events are broadly divided into major and minor complications. Major ESS complications are those that result in or carry a significant risk of long-lasting or permanent sequelae. Major complications that involve the cranial vault include cerebrospinal fluid (CSF) leak, tension pneumocephalus, meningitis, abscess, intracranial hemorrhage, direct brain injury, and encephalocele formation. Similarly, major complications may involve the eye, such as in medial rectus injury, optic nerve injury, orbital hematoma, and nasolacrimal duct injury, and may result in double vision, loss of vision, and epiphora. Complications that arise from damage to regional blood vessels—including the anterior or posterior ethmoidal, sphenopalatine, or internal carotid arteries—are considered major if the resulting hemorrhage affects cerebral circulation or causes a significant drop in hemoglobin level or requires a transfusion of red blood cells. Other major complications worth mentioning are anosmia and toxic shock syndrome, and complications of ESS may be fatal. Fortunately, all of these complications are quite rare. However, these risks should be disclosed in a thorough preoperative consent procedure due to the serious repercussions that may result.

Minor ESS complications are far more common. They may require surgical correction but generally do not produce any significant long-term adverse outcomes. These may include periorbital emphysema, ecchymosis, and fat herniation through a defect created in the lamina papyracea. A small amount of perioperative bleeding, not requiring transfusion, may be considered minor, as are facial swelling, hyposmia, hypesthesia of the infraorbital nerve or teeth, synechia formation, myospherulosis, atrophic rhinitis, and osteitis.

Finally, complications may be designated as intraoperative, early postoperative, or late postoperative. One example of an intraoperative complication is CSF leak. As with most other intraoperative complications, it is best if the surgeon recognizes the CSF leak at the time of the initial surgery so that an immediate repair can be performed and the risk of serious sequelae such as pneumocephalus, meningitis, or intracranial abscess are minimized. Early postoperative complications may include infection, hemorrhage, or adhesion formation; these may occur anywhere from immediately after surgery to 2 weeks following the procedure. Late complications may include mucocele or mucopyocele formation, and may occur many years after the procedure. It should be noted that all of the above categorizations are artificial and subject to interpretation. They are meant to be used with a degree of common sense and to aid in communication with patients and other clinicians.

Several risk factors exist for the occurrence of complications in ESS;[1] these can be broadly divided into anesthetic, surgeon-related, and disease-related factors. General anesthesia increases the risk of complications through the lack of patient feedback when approaching sensitive structures like the lamina papyracea and the skull base. Also, certain forms of general anesthesia—inhalational in particular—tend to have an adverse effect on intraoperative bleeding and therefore visualization. Surgery on the right side of the nose is a risk factor for a right-handed surgeon because of the angle of the endoscope and instruments, as is left-sided surgery for a left-handed surgeon. Lack of surgeon experience is a risk for the obvious reasons of unfamiliarity with the anatomy and use of instrumentation. Finally, extensive sinus disease, excessive bleeding, and revision surgery, all of which can obscure or distort the sinonasal structures normally encountered during surgery, are important risk factors.

The current chapter seeks to provide a comprehensive and organized discussion of the complications that can occur during or following ESS. Information pertaining to the definition and incidence of the complication will be provided whenever possible. The chapter is subdivided based on the type of complication, and the precise moment during surgery when the complication is at risk of happening will be explained. The management of each complication will be discussed based on the best available evidence, and finally, suggestions for avoiding the complications will also be presented.

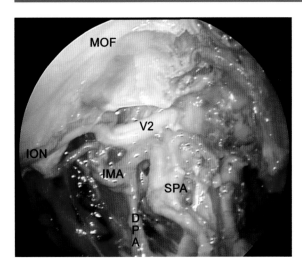

Fig. 9.1 Endoscopic view of cadaver specimen with the posterior wall of the right maxillary sinus removed, illustrating important anatomical relationships relating to the maxillary sinus.
DPA = descending palatine artery; IMA = internal maxillary artery; ION = infraorbital nerve; MOF = medial orbital floor; V2 = maxillary branch of the trigeminal nerve.

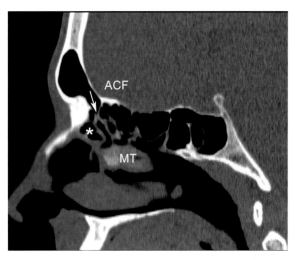

Fig. 9.2 Computed tomography scan of the sinuses, parasagittal cut through the level of the frontal recess (arrow), demonstrating its relationship to the agger nasi (asterisk), middle turbinate (MT), and anterior cranial fossa (ACF).

Special Concerns for Each Sinus

The Maxillary Sinus

The maxillary sinus is the most commonly addressed sinus in ESS. The uncinectomy, with or without an additional antrostomy, is often the first step in the endoscopic sinus procedure. Whether a limited or an extensive procedure is necessary, the maxillary sinus provides a reliable landmark for the initiation of and progression through the steps of ESS. Furthermore, controlling disease within the maxillary sinus is essential to achieving a successful surgical outcome. Although not generally considered a challenging area to operate on, an in-depth understanding of possible complications involving the maxillary sinus and their management is necessary for the above reasons.

Anatomical relationships of importance to maxillary sinus surgery include the orbit superiorly, the nasolacrimal duct anterior to the maxillary ostium, the infraorbital nerve running in or below the roof of the sinus, and the sphenopalatine foramen and artery posterior to the fontanelle of the sinus (**Fig. 9.1**).

The Frontal Sinus

The frontal sinus has long been considered one of the most challenging areas to access and manage surgically. With significant patient-to-patient variability in pneumatization, anatomical complexity, and disease characteristics,

a wide repertoire of surgical techniques is necessary for the sinus surgeon dealing with frontal sinus disease.

The frontal sinus is bounded anteriorly by the thick anterior table of the frontal bone, with its overlying periosteum, facial muscles, galea aponeurotica, soft tissues, and skin; and posteriorly by the much thinner posterior table, and dura of the anterior cranial fossa. Inferiorly are the orbital plates of the frontal bone laterally and the frontal beak medially; and superiorly is the frontal bone as it forms the anterior calvarium. The frontal recess is an hourglass-shaped space connecting the frontal sinus to the ethmoid infundibulum (**Fig. 9.2**). Its boundaries are the skull base posterosuperiorly, the roof and posterior wall of the agger nasi cell anteroinferiorly, the orbit laterally and the middle turbinate medially. The frontal sinus drainage pathway passes through this area and owes its configuration to the fronto-ethmoidal cells that pneumatize into it. A precise understanding of each patient's anatomical variations is essential for the safety and long-term success of their frontal recess dissections.

The Ethmoid Sinuses

The ethmoid sinuses are the most anatomically complex and variable of the paranasal sinuses; nevertheless, many ethmoidal air cells can be identified on preoperative imaging and intraoperatively in a very predictable manner. Adequate removal of the obstructing bony partitions and disease material from within these sinuses is key to the control of chronic rhinosinusitis in medically refractory patients. However, given their location, bordering on the orbit laterally and comprising a significant portion of

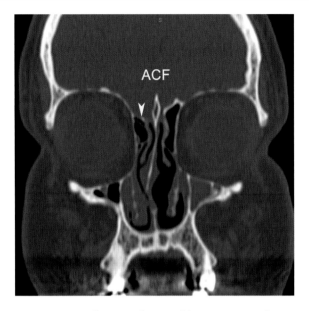

Fig. 9.3 Computed tomography scan of the sinuses, coronal cut through the level of the anterior ethmoid sinuses, showing the close proximity of the anterior cranial fossa (ACF) and the orbits; note that the fovea ethmoidalis is asymmetrical in this patient, being significantly lower on the right (arrowhead) and therefore at greater risk of intraoperative injury.

the anterior cranial fossa floor superiorly, the potential for disastrous complications is particularly present when performing ESS in the region of the ethmoids (**Fig. 9.3**). Furthermore, the majority of iatrogenic CSF leaks are created in the ethmoid region. Preoperative appreciation of high-risk anatomical variants is of particular importance for avoiding complications when performing surgery within the ethmoid region.

The Sphenoid Sinus

The sphenoid sinus is the most posterior of the sinuses, and is the gateway to the sella turcica in endoscopic transsphenoidal approaches to pituitary tumors. Wide sphenoidotomy also allows the operating surgeon to identify with confidence the level of the skull base in ESS procedures, and so it is often performed in more severe cases of chronic rhinosinusitis. Its close relationship to numerous critical structures, such as the brain, the optic nerves, the carotid arteries, the cavernous sinuses and cranial nerves contained therein (**Fig. 9.4**), make it more prone to severe infectious and inflammatory complications in sinonasal disease. For this reason, it is recommended to treat severe sphenoidal disease more aggressively with surgical evacuation and debridement. However, it is also this close anatomical relationship to critical structures that predisposes it to disastrous operative complications, and correspondingly causes many surgeons to shy away from sphenoid surgery.

Vascular Complications

Hemorrhage

Excessive bleeding as a result of ESS may occur during the procedure or in the postoperative period; the majority of bleeding events occur early in the postoperative course. Excessive intraoperative bleeding may significantly affect the operator's visual field, obscuring landmarks and predisposing to further operative complications. At the very least, bleeding may slow the progress of surgery, but in severe cases, it may force the surgeon to abort the

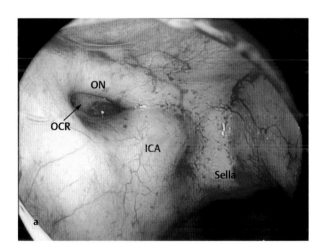

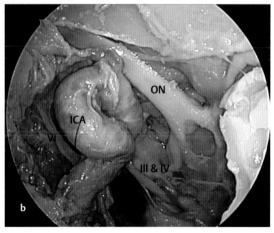

Fig. 9.4a,b

a Endoscopic view of the right lateral sphenoid wall and pituitary sella in a sinus with healthy mucosa. ICA = internal carotid artery; OCR = opticocarotid recess; ON = optic nerve.

b Endoscopic view of cadaver specimen with the lateral wall of the right sphenoid sinus removed, illustrating important anatomical relationships relating to the sphenoid sinus, including cranial nerves III, IV, and VI.

procedure. The reported incidence for epistaxis requiring intervention are 0.6 to 1.6%,[2] and for major hemorrhage requiring transfusion is 0.76%.[3] Causes of bleeding can be surgical/technical or patient related. The bleeding may be diffuse or localized, and if severe enough it may significantly affect the operative visual field and render surgery unsafe.

> **Note**
>
> Any hemorrhage that is severe enough to require a blood transfusion is considered a major complication of surgery.

Risk Factors

Patient factors causing increased surgical bleeding can be broadly divided into local processes such as infection, or systemic comorbidities. The latter must be sought and addressed during the preoperative evaluation. Individuals with underlying hypertension, or peripheral vascular disease should be optimized preoperatively, as controlled hypotension may be more challenging in this group of patients. Liver and renal diseases are important causes of clotting factor deficiency and platelet dysfunction, respectively. Chronic alcohol abuse, malnutrition, and vitamin deficiencies (most notably vitamin K), can also affect coagulation, and must be explored if suspected clinically. Bleeding diatheses, such as hemophilia A or B, and von Willebrand disease, require clotting factor replacement or specialized pharmacotherapy (desmopressin, tranexemic acid, or aminocaproic acid), and must be planned for. Inherited collagen and blood vessel abnormalities, including hereditary hemorrhagic telangiectasias and arteriovenous malformations, are other less common causes of profuse surgical bleeding. Medications that will increase surgical bleeding must be halted before surgery; these include nonsteroidal anti-inflammatory drugs, aspirin, coumadin, heparin, and anti-platelet agents. Several herbal and alternative therapies can affect coagulation pathways, such as ginseng, ginkgo, kava, and fish oil. It is prudent for patients to discontinue all herbal and alternative medicines at least 7 days before surgery.

Important measures for optimizing the visual field in ESS include placing the patient in reverse Trendelenburg positioning, and the application of topical and local vasoconstrictors.[4,5] Furthermore, studies have demonstrated that the ideal mean arterial pressure has been shown to be less than 60 to 75 mmHg and the ideal heart rate to be less than 60 beats/min.[6,7] This is best achieved through the use of total intravenous anesthesia.[6,8] Systemic steroids are helpful in the preoperative period to reduce the size and vascularity of polyps in patients with significant nasal polyposis, so reducing capillary bleeding during functional ESS.[9] The use of perioperative antibiotics in patients with acutely infected and inflamed sinuses may also be beneficial. However, further studies are necessary to clarify the optimal dose, optimal length of treatment, and groups of patients that would benefit from these treatments.

At the end of every ESS procedure, the anesthetist should be asked to restore the patient's blood pressure toward their preoperative level while hemostasis is verified. Thorough saline irrigation and suctioning of blood from within the nose and sinus cavities is performed, followed by careful inspection of the nasopharynx looking for pooling of fresh blood. A suction bipolar instrument is important, as it will allow simultaneous evacuation of blood from the operative field and cauterization of the bleeding points. Most of the mucosal oozing will stop spontaneously after sinus surgery; however, larger blood vessels can result in significant postoperative hemorrhage, especially if these vessels are in spasm during surgery and not dealt with at that time. Common areas of arterial bleeding after ESS that should be attentively examined are the regions supplied by large branches of the sphenopalatine artery and anterior ethmoidal artery. These regions include the posterior rim of an enlarged maxillary antrostomy, the area of the sphenopalatine foramen especially if a middle turbinate resection has been performed; additionally, the anterior face of the sphenoid sinus (which is supplied by the posterior nasal/septal branch) and anterior skull base should be carefully inspected. After appropriately cauterizing the points of bleeding, the nasopharynx is again suctioned and inspected for pooling of fresh blood; this should be the last maneuver performed in any endoscopic sinus procedure.

Nasal packing is not usually necessary after sinus surgery with proper hemostasis; however, some surgeons still employ this practice. Some alternatives to petroleum gauze packing include bioresorbable materials such as Nasopore (Stryker Corp., Kalamazoo, MI, USA), injectable gels, or finger cot dressing (sterile glove fingers stuffed with rolled 5 × 5-cm gauze sponges). These can either be removed in the immediate postoperative period, or left in the patient for later removal in clinic; the length of time they are left is dependent on the material used, with bioresorbables able to stay the longest.

More severe postoperative hemorrhaging may require aggressive management, beginning with attention to the patient's "ABCs." It is exceedingly rare that the patient's airway and breathing require any intervention or protection due to heavy bleeding, but if this is judged to be the case, intubation, sedation and ventilation can be performed. Nasal packing in the postoperative setting is usually traumatic to the fragile healing tissues, and should be avoided when possible. A trial use of an inflatable hemostatic device, such as the Rapid Rhino (ArthroCare ENT, Austin, TX, USA), can be attempted as a temporizing measure until more definite management is undertaken. Depending on the region that is bleeding, ligation of the sphenopalatine or anterior ethmoid arteries may need to be performed. If the former is to be performed, greater palatine foramen infiltration with local anesthetic and epinephrine is helpful.[5] The foramen can be palpated along the posterior hard palate, halfway between the palatal midline and the second molar tooth. A cadaver study performed by the senior author has shown that the successful injection is best achieved by bending a 25-gauge needle through 45° ~ 2.5 cm from the tip of the needle.[10]

Anterior Ethmoidal Artery Injury

The anterior ethmoidal artery (AEA) is a terminal branch of the internal carotid artery, which branches off the ophthalmic artery within the orbit and then heads medially to traverse the lamina papyracea and enter the anterior ethmoid sinus. The AEA usually runs in the skull base along the roof of the ethmoid, just posterior to the anterior face of the bulla ethmoidalis, giving off branches that feed the superolateral nasal wall. It should be visible after thorough clearance of the skull base in this region (**Fig. 9.5**). It then enters the anterior cranial fossa through the lateral wall of the olfactory recess. From there, the artery traverses the cribriform plate to supply the anterior septum. Cadaver studies have shown that the AEA runs in a bony mesentery, hanging below the skull base, in approximately one-third of cases and is amenable to surgical clipping in ~ 20% of cases.[11] Using endoscopic bipolar instruments, however, the artery may be adequately cauterized in a significantly higher percentage of patients.

> **Note**
>
> Bleeding from the anterior artery may cause a significant hemorrhage during surgery, but more importantly, complete transection of the artery may result in retraction of the proximal (lateral) severed end into the orbit. The consequence of this is a rapidly expanding orbital hematoma, which is a surgical emergency; it is covered in more detail below.

The position of the AEA is identified on preoperative imaging before every surgical procedure, to determine whether it is in a bony mesentery or running within the ethmoid roof itself. The artery can be found on a coronal computed tomography (CT) scan as a pinch or "nipple" between the medial rectus and superior oblique muscles (**Fig. 9.6**). Those running in a mesentery tend to be associated with a longer lateral lamella of the olfactory fossa (Keros, type 2 or 3) and a high ethmoid skull base. Care must be taken not to sever the AEA when using the microdebrider to clear polypoid tissue and bone from the ethmoid roof. An important technical point to prevent transection of the artery is to avoid passing the microdebrider blade in a posterior to anterior direction with the tip near the skull base (**Fig. 9.7a**); a safer alternative is to advance

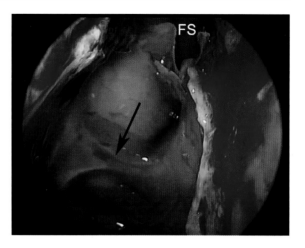

Fig. 9.5 Intraoperative view of a left frontal recess, demonstrating the anterior ethmoid artery (arrow) running in a bony mesentery below the skull base. FS = frontal sinus.

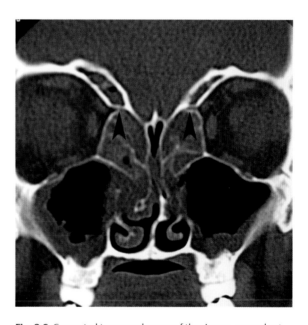

Fig. 9.6 Computed tomography scan of the sinuses, coronal cut at the level of the anterior ethmoid sinuses, showing the anterior ethmoid arteries (arrowheads) running below the skull base bilaterally in bony mesenteries.

and withdraw the tip at an angle tangential to the skull base until the excess tissue and bone have been removed (**Fig. 9.7b**). This will result in a gentle debridement and will avoid the occurrence of a through and through cut of the artery. If necessary, a partial injury to the artery can be easily managed with suction bipolar diathermy. A complete transection of the AEA with retraction of the proximal bleeding end into the orbit should immediately raise concerns for rapid orbital hematoma formation; the management algorithm is presented in **Figure 9.22** in the Orbital hematoma section below.

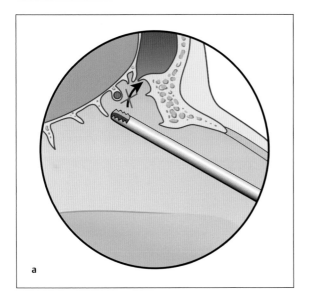
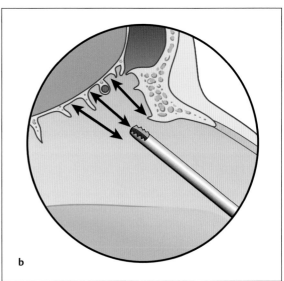

Fig. 9.7a,b Diagram of the nasal cavity in sagittal view.

a Depicting the improper way of using the microdebrider along the skull base, moving from posterior to anterior, placing the anterior ethmoid artery at risk of being severed.

b Depicting the proper method of using the microdebrider along the skull base, moving back and forth toward and away from the skull base.

Sphenopalatine Artery Branch Injury

The sphenopalatine artery supplies a significant portion of the nasal cavity, and is often a source of arterial bleeding during ESS. The branch most often encountered is the posterior nasal artery as it branches off the sphenopalatine artery and runs along the anterior wall of the sphenoid sinus below the sphenoid ostium to eventually become the posterior septal artery (**Fig. 9.8**). It is usually transected if the anterior sphenoid face is removed in a superior to inferior direction starting from the natural ostium with a downward biting instrument. If a wide sphenoidotomy is necessary for severe disease, the use of a sharp Kerrison or Hajek–Koeffler punch leads to a clean transection of the vessel, favoring hemostasis through effective spasm of the vessel after injury. In this way, brisk arterial bleeding may only be seen very briefly as the vessel rapidly goes into spasm; however, the artery may open up again in the early postoperative period and lead to significant hemorrhage. It is therefore recommended that the proximal and distal ends of the transected posterior nasal artery be electrocauterized at the end of surgery whenever a large sphenoidotomy is performed. If the posterior nasal mucosa is excessively traumatized during surgery and the artery is avulsed or partially cut, then arterial spasm will be less effective at achieving hemostasis and immediate cauterization of the bleeding at the time of injury will be necessary.

Because of the proximity of the sphenopalatine artery

main trunk and the presence of feeding branches such as the posterior lateral nasal artery and the inferior turbinate branch,[12] the area of the posterior fontanelle of the maxillary sinus is at risk of significant bleeding during enlargement of antrostomy. Additionally, vessels branch off the sphenopalatine artery as it emerges from the sphenopalatine foramen to supply the inferior and middle turbinates. These vessels are largest at the posterior end of the turbinates and run in the mucosa medial to the bone of the corresponding turbinate (**Fig. 9.8**); it is therefore common to encounter brisk bleeding when performing turbinate reduction or turbinectomy involving these areas. Bipolar diathermy of the posterior ends of the turbinates is recommended whenever damage of these vessels is suspected, even if not actively bleeding at the end of the procedure, to prevent a latent hemorrhage.

Other arteries in the vicinity that may be damaged during surgery of the sphenoid sinus include the posterior ethmoidal artery, as well as the artery of the Vidian canal. Detailed knowledge of the nasal vascular anatomy is helpful in avoiding unwanted and severe operative bleeding.

Internal Carotid Artery Injury

The internal carotid artery is at risk during standard sinus surgery when there is excessive new bone formation and attempts are made to remove the new bone and when intersinus septations are taken down. In a large number of patients the intersinus septum in the sphenoid attaches

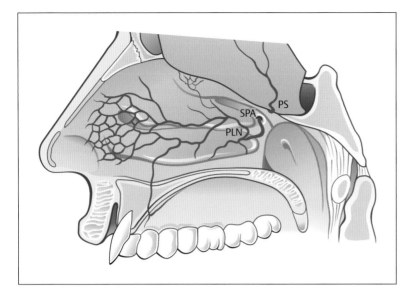

Fig. 9.8 Schematic representation of the posterior lateral nasal wall as well as the septum hinged upward, depicting the anatomy of the sphenopalatine artery (SPA) branches. PLN: posterior lateral nasal branch; PS: posterior septal branch.

to the carotid artery in the lateral wall of the sphenoid sinus. When the septum is taken down care should be taken that the septum is not grasped and rotated as part of the attempt to remove it. This technique can result in a sharp bony base of the septum fracturing, and during rotation of one of these, sharp bony spurs puncturing the carotid. The artery is also at risk if the wall covering the sphenoid protrusion of the carotid is dehiscent. This occurs in ~ 10% of patients and puts the vessel at risk if instruments or microdebriders are used in the sphenoid sinus. A much higher risk of carotid artery injury is present during endoscopic skull base surgery, especially if the tumor involves the carotid. This is commonly seen in pituitary tumors that extend into the cavernous sinus and in skull base tumors of the clivus such as chordomas and meningiomas that may involve the carotid.

Management

If an injury should occur to the carotid, the following steps should be followed and are summarized in **Fig. 9.9**. Help should be called for—both for the anesthetist and for the surgeon. A second surgeon will significantly improve the likelihood of a good outcome for the patient as endoscopic management of this situation usually requires two surgeons. The anesthetist should actively resuscitate the patient and keep the systolic pressure reasonable—this allows for continued contralateral blood flow from the opposite carotid through the cerebral circulation and helps to maintain cerebral perfusion. The surgeon needs to immediately harvest muscle from either the patient's thigh or sternocleidomastoid muscle. This muscle should be ~ 1.5 by 1.5 by 1.5 cm. This muscle should be crushed—usually between two metal kidney dishes, usually available on the scrub nurse's table. Two high-flow suctions are needed. The second surgeon places one suction down

the side where the majority of bleeding appears to be coming from and tries to take as much of the blood flow away as possible. The primary surgeon now places his large volume suction and endoscope down the opposite nostril keeping the surgical field clear as the endoscope is advanced into the region of the bleeding vessel. The first surgeon then places his suction over the bleeding artery

- Help is called for both anesthetist and surgeon
- Anesthetic resuscitation to maintain adequate cerebral perfusion
- Two high-flow suctions used—the second surgeon places one down the side with the majority of bleeding and the primary surgeon places his suction and endoscope down the opposite nostril
- A 1.5 × 1.5 × 1.5 cm piece of muscle is harvested and then crushed
- The crushed muscle patch is held in place by a Blakesleys forceps for 5 to 10 minutes—the pressure should be firm but insufficient to occlude the artery
- A neurosurgical pattie is placed; the Blakesley forceps and pattie are sequentially slowly removed
- A pedicled septal flap is rotated into the sphenoid to cover the muscle patch and is glued into place, covered with Gelfoam and a gentle packing
- The patient is kept intubated and an immediate angiogram is performed to ensure control–stenting or coiling is performed if necessary
- The packing is removed under general anesthesia 5 days later
- The angiogram is repeated at 6 weeks and 3 months to rule out pseudoaneurysm formation

Fig. 9.9 Management of internal carotid injury.

and hovers this suction directly above the site of injury. If his suction is great enough—and one should always be using the strongest possible suction—most of the blood should be attracted to and suctioned up. The primary surgeon now has the lesion in clear vision and can substitute his suction for the crushed muscle patch held by a Blakesley forceps. While the second surgeon keeps the blood flow away from the primary surgeon's side, the primary surgeon slides the muscle patch directly on to the lesion keeping pressure on the patch and lesion during this maneuver. Continued oozing from the lesion is cleared by the second surgeon so that the muscle patch can be seen to be correctly placed on the lesion, the patch should at this stage be controlling the flow from the lesion.

The muscle patch should be held in place for at least 5 but preferably 10 minutes. The second surgeon can now bring a neurosurgical pattie onto the muscle patch and the Blakesley pressure can be slowly lessened. The second surgeon applies gentle pressure to the muscle patch by putting pressure on the pattie and the Blakesley forceps should be able to be withdrawn without the bleeding starting again. Now the pattie is gently removed and the bleeding should have stopped with the muscle patch. A few squares of Surgicel (Ethicon Inc,. Somerville, NJ, USA) are then placed over the patch and if the bleeder is in the sphenoid, a pedicled septal flap is rotated into the sphenoid to cover the muscle patch. This is glued into place and covered with Gelfoam and a pack (ribbon gauze or other) is placed over the flap to allow continued gentle pressure to be applied to the flap and muscle patch.

The patient is kept intubated and asleep and an immediate angiogram is performed to ensure that control has been achieved and to see if there is any ongoing ooze. If there is poor control or continued leakage then endovascular intervention is required and the vessel is either stented or coiled. The pack is then removed under general anesthesia 5 days later. If the initial angiogram was normal this should be repeated at 6 weeks and 3 months to ensure that no pseudoaneurysm has formed.

Neurologic Complications

Intracranial Injury/Cerebrospinal Fluid Leak

The risk of CSF leak is a constant concern in ESS. Most series report a rate between 0.4 and 0.8%,[2,13] although a recent nationwide audit of 40,638 ESS cases in the United States between 2003 and 2007 reported a rate of 0.17%.[3] Transgression of the bone and dura of the skull base will result in a leak of CSF; this can usually be recognized at the time of surgery by a "washout" of clear fluid from the area of the injury, caused by a dilution of the blood covering the surrounding tissues. In instances where there

is an abundance of inflamed tissues and bleeding around the site of injury, the CSF leak may look like a sudden onset of brisk venous bleeding, without any noticeable "washout".[2] A high index of suspicion for CSF leak must be maintained when any sudden increase in bleeding occurs in the vicinity of the skull base. If unrecognized or untreated, the leak of CSF can lead to postoperative pneumocephalus, tension pneumocephalus, meningitis, encephalitis, or epidural or subdural abscess.

Another risk of unrecognized skull base injury at the time of surgery is that of intracranial injury, including damage to cerebral vasculature or to the brain itself. The severity of the injury is dependent on several variables, such as the size and shape of the instrument involved, the type of instrument (powered debrider, electrocautery, cold steel), the depth of penetration, the time lapse between skull base penetration and recognition of the complication by the operating surgeon, and the anatomical structures injured. Depending on the structures affected, the sequelae of intracranial injury may include persistent headache, neurologic deficit, intracranial hemorrhage, and intracranial infection. Meningoencephalocele may occur in the late postoperative setting. Fortunately, these are exceedingly rare occurrences; the reported rates for major intracranial complications in ESS are 0.47 to 0.54%.[2]

A frequent location for iatrogenic CSF leak to occur is along the anterior vertical lamella of the fovea ethmoidalis constituting the lateral wall of the olfactory fossa. This is near the junction of the middle turbinate attachment and the cribriform plate (**Fig. 9.10**). The bone in this area makes up the most medial aspect of the frontal recess dissection, and is the thinnest area of the skull base, measuring as little as 0.1 mm in thickness. It is also perforated by the anterior ethmoid artery. If damaged in this region, electrocautery of this vessel can lead to transmitted thermal injury of the skull base and dura causing an immediate or postoperative CSF leak. This risk is greater with monopolar cautery and can be minimized by using bipolar cautery. Damage to this area can also occur as a result of dissecting instruments being directed toward the olfactory fossa during dissection of the frontal recess. Hence, dissecting instruments such as curettes and probes should be maintained in an upright orientation and used to apply force in a posterior to anterior direction when fracturing bony septations in the frontal recess and along the skull base.

Endoscopic surgery involving the frontal sinus and its drainage pathway is among the most challenging aspects of ESS. As such, surgery in this critical area requires specialized training and expertise. The posterior table of the frontal bone marks the anterior limit of the skull base and anterior cranial fossa, as does the posterosuperior aspect of the frontal recess. The maneuvers in frontal sinus surgery most likely to cause a skull base injury include improper placement of dissecting instruments during the

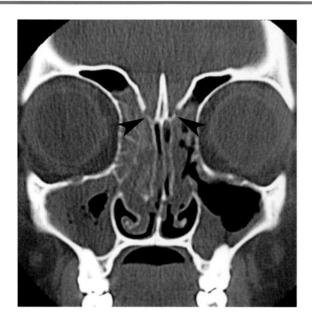

Fig. 9.10 Computed tomography scan of the sinuses, coronal cut at the level of the anterior ethmoid sinuses, showing a particularly deep olfactory recess of the anterior cranial fossa with lateral walls slanted away from the vertical plane and extremely thin lateral lamellae of the fovea ethmoidalis (arrowheads) near the point of penetration of the anterior ethmoid artery. These anatomical features place the patient at higher risk of intraoperative cerebrospinal fluid leak.

removal of obstructing frontoethmoidal cells in the frontal recess. In certain patients, the cell patterns contained within this area can be very complex and confusing, and it is easy for the unprepared surgeon to become disoriented intraoperatively.

Another relatively common area for skull base injury to occur intraoperatively is along the posterior ethmoid roof near the anterior face of the sphenoid sinus. This may occur if the surgeon is unsure of the position of the natural sphenoid ostium and attempts to force an instrument such as a Freer elevator, straight curette, or microdebrider into the ethmoid fovea, under the false impression that the skull base is located more superiorly (**Fig. 9.11**). This can result in CSF leak or, if initially unrecognized, damage to intracranial structures like the brain, arterial blood vessels, or venous sinuses. Given the seriousness of the potential injuries to the skull base, optic nerve, or internal carotid artery, it is strongly advisable not to use powered instrumentation when entering the sphenoid sinus or enlarging the sphenoidotomy.

Alternatively, skull base injury may occur when bringing down the "frontal T" during the frontal drill out (endoscopic modified Lothrop, or Draf III) procedure. As one of the final steps in the drill out, the removal of bone anterior to the olfactory bulb is crucial to maximize the anterior–posterior dimension of the frontal neo-ostium and decrease the chance of postoperative restenosis; this step clearly defines the T-shaped anterior projection of

the cribriform plate (**Fig. 9.12**). The maximum posterior limit is achieved by identifying the first olfactory neuron that forms the anterior boundary of the olfactory fossa. Gradual drilling of this bone should be performed with the aid of image guidance to confirm the anterior limit of the skull base, and extreme care must be taken not to allow the drill to slip above this projection of bone, as the skull base is much thinner in this region.

Prevention

A precise understanding of the anatomy in each individual patient is of utmost importance and preoperative imaging must be carefully reviewed before undertaking surgery. This should allow the surgeon to recognize any high-risk anatomical variants and give an appreciation of the likelihood of skull base injury during the dissection. High-risk variations include a low or asymmetric anterior skull base, a deep olfactory recess (Keros 2 or 3), a slanted lateral lamella of the olfactory groove that is tilted away from the vertical plane (**Fig. 9.10**), as well as any expansile processes such as mucoceles or masses that have caused demineralization and bone loss along the skull base (**Fig. 9.13**).

Careful review of the preoperative CT imaging is also essential to achieve a three-dimensional understanding of the frontal drainage pathway and to create a surgical plan for the frontal recess dissection. In this way, the dissecting instruments can be placed precisely along the elucidated pathway, atraumatically and with minimal resistance, to fracture away the obstructing frontoethmoidal cells in a stepwise fashion that was predetermined by the surgical plan.[14,15] A key principle to safe dissection is that no dissecting instrument should ever be forced through the roof of a frontoethmoidal cell because of the risk of causing a CSF leak; rather, the instrument should be passed either medially or posteriorly to the cell wall according to the position of the frontal drainage pathway. In situations where there is excessive bleeding that is obscuring the surgeon's view in this delicate area, suction instruments such as the Wormald malleable suction curette (Medtronic ENT, Jacksonville, FL, USA) are ideally suited for performing the dissection. The use of powered instruments such as the microdebrider should be minimized in the frontal recess, and if they are to be used, aggressive debriding should only be directed in an anterior direction toward the frontal beak, as this will avoid placing the skull base at risk. Finally, in cases of complex anatomy, exuberant disease, or previous surgery obscuring the drainage pathway intraoperatively, frontal sinus minitrephination (Medtronic ENT) can be helpful. By instilling fluorescein through frontal minitrephines, the frontal sinus drainage pathway is clearly highlighted by a stream of brightly colored fluorescein solution. Dissecting instruments can then be precisely placed into this corridor and the surrounding cells can be fractured away.

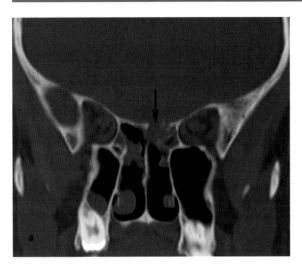

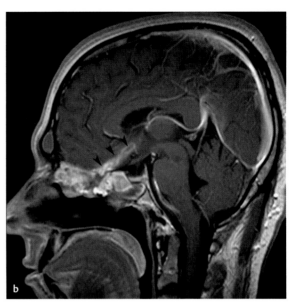

Fig. 9.11a,b Intracranial injuries

a Computed tomography scan of the sinuses, coronal cut at the level of the posterior ethmoid sinuses, showing a traumatic defect in the posterior ethmoid fovea (arrow), an area that is commonly injured in endoscopic sinus surgery.

b T1-weighted magnetic resonance image of the brain with gadolinium enhancement, parasagittal cut, demonstrating a traumatic injury to the gyrus rectus of the frontal lobe following endoscopic sinus surgery.

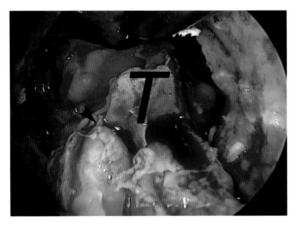

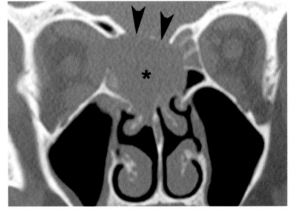

Fig. 9.12 An intraoperative view of the frontal neo-ostium during a Draf type III frontal drill out procedure, demonstrating the frontal "т" made by the floor of the frontal sinus and the superior part of the nasal septum, anterior to the olfactory recess, which needs to be drilled down to the level of the first olfactory neuron (arrowhead) to maximize the diameter of the neo-ostium.

Fig. 9.13 Computed tomography scan of the sinuses, coronal cut at the level of the posterior ethmoid sinuses, showing a mucocele (asterisk) pushing through the nasal septum, skull base (arrowheads) and medial wall of the right orbit.

As mentioned previously, early intraoperative recognition and repair of a CSF leak is important in minimizing the likelihood of serious or long-term sequelae. However, it is also possible that an injury to the skull base goes unrecognized at the time of surgery and that the ensuing CSF leak is diagnosed during the postoperative period. The leak is often diagnosed on a clinical basis, with patients complaining of clear watery rhinorrhea that is salty to taste, and exacerbated on leaning forward or with a Valsalva maneuver. Biochemical confirmation can be achieved with a β_2-transferrin assay; the presence of glucose in the fluid is also suggestive of CSF. Imaging studies that may prove useful include CT cisternography and radionucleotide scanning. Intraoperative localization can be facilitated by intrathecal instillation of fluorescein, which will color the CSF fluorescent green. Our protocol is to withdraw 10 mL of CSF from the lumbar puncture and add 0.1 mL of filtered 10% fluorescein, creating a 0.1% final concentration that is slowly infused intrathecally 30 to 60 minutes before the procedure.

Management

The management in cases of postoperatively detected CSF leak can begin conservatively with bedrest and head elevation, as well as stool softeners to avoid increased intracranial pressure from straining. The use of prophylactic antibiotics is a matter of debate and is discussed in further detail in the Meningitis/Intracranial Abscess section below. However, in our practice, patients are routinely placed on antibiotics after ESS; if there is a CSF leak, the agent of choice is switched to one with better CSF penetration such as a first-generation or second-generation cephalosporin. A lumbar drain may also be placed to decrease the intracranial pressure for a trial of 36 to 48 hours; however, persistent CSF rhinorrhea warrants surgical exploration and repair.

Generally, small skull base injuries can effectively be repaired with a small graft of fat, fascia, or nasal mucosa. Although many methods exist, our preference is to perform the bath-plug technique,[16] whereby a small vicryl suture is tied to one end of an elongated piece of fat, then passed lengthwise through the fat graft to come out the end opposite the knot. The width of the graft should be just thin enough to pass through the dural opening; the ear lobe is an adequate donor site in the majority of patients. After proper preparation of the defect site by clearing a small area of the surrounding mucosa, the fat is carefully fed through the dura using a blunt probe beginning with the knotted end. When the entire piece of fat has been passed intradurally, only the free end of the suture should be coming through the defect. The suture is then gently pulled while using a blunt instrument such as a Freer elevator as a counter-support below the defect; this causes the fat to expand radially and form an effective water-tight plug. The site can then be covered with a small mucosal free graft, or ideally, a small local flap of adjacent mucosa. More sizeable defects can be easily covered with a pedicled nasoseptal flap. Following the operative procedure, the patient should be admitted to hospital for overnight observation and should be placed on CSF precautions (head elevation, stool softeners, etc.). If there is continued CSF rhinorrhea, a 48-hour trial of lumbar drain may be instituted before deciding whether to return to the operating room for a second attempt at repair.

In situations where there has been an intracranial injury, neurosurgery should be consulted. Angiography should be performed if there is suspicion of vascular injury; even if this is normal in the early postoperative period, an angiogram should be performed several weeks postoperatively to rule out the interim development of a aneurysm/pseudoaneurysm.

Pneumocephalus

If a CSF leak is created during ESS, air can make its way intracranially during the postoperative period, resulting in pneumocephalus. Tension pneumocephalus is characterized by a steady increase in intracranial air through a defect in the skull base that acts as a one-way valve; this process is hastened by the use of a lumbar drain to remove CSF in cases of postoperative leak. As the volume of air increases, pressure is placed on the brain tissue vasculature, resulting in decreased cerebral perfusion and in severe cases, herniation through the tentorium. Symptoms of headache, lethargy, or decreased level of consciousness in any patient with a known CSF leak should arouse suspicion for this condition, mandating a CT scan of the head, which provides the definitive diagnosis. Symptoms usually arise within a few hours of surgery or of insertion of a lumbar drain; and as intracranial tension rises, neurologic deficits, including decreased level of consciousness, ataxia and cranial nerve palsies, may become apparent. Although the air may expand into the epidural, subdural, or subarachnoid spaces, a typical radiologic finding is the "Mount Fuji sign," whereby air on either side of the anterior frontal lobes compresses the brain into the shape of a volcano, with twin peaks caused by traction from intact bridging veins, giving the appearance of a midline crater.

The management of pneumocephalus is gauged upon the severity of symptoms, and can begin conservatively with the administration of 100% oxygen inhalation. Most of the gas contained within the pneumocephalus is nitrogen so the oxygen creates a gradient for the absorption of that nitrogen into the bloodstream. In cases where lumbar drain placement is a contributing factor, the drain should be clamped. In more severe cases, the skull base defect should be localized and repaired, which can be done endoscopically in the overwhelming majority of cases. However, neurosurgical consultation should be obtained for possible needle aspiration or craniotomy if unable to evacuate the air from below.

Meningitis/Intracranial Abscess

The spread of bacteria from the sinonasal to the intracranial cavity can occur following ESS when there has been a breach in the skull base. If not treated in a timely fashion, infectious intracranial complications may progress in a stepwise fashion, beginning with meningitis before progressing to encephalitis and abscess formation; all of these conditions are potentially life-threatening. The risk of progression is increased when the skull base violation has gone unnoticed, unrepaired or inadequately repaired at the initial surgery, hence the importance for immediate recognition and management of such injuries. Often, early detection and aggressive treatment of meningitis will prevent progression to encephalitis, abscess, or death.

Symptoms of meningitis include fever, headache, photophobia, neck stiffness, and lethargy. Positive Kernig or Brudzinski signs on physical examination are useful to confirm meningismus. The investigative work-up includes a lumbar puncture for CSF culture and sensitivities, and a contrast-infused CT scan of the head to rule out intracranial abscess. The scan may also identify a skull base defect, which in the presence of active CSF leak, should be repaired endoscopically as soon as the patient is stable enough to undergo general anesthesia. The usual bacteria found in intracranial infections are those infecting the sinonasal cavity and nasopharynx; these include *Streptococcus pneumoniae*, *Haemophilus influenzae*, and occasionally *Moraxella catarrhalis*. *Staphylococcus aureus*, group A streptococcus and anaerobes have also been found but are less common. The choice of antibiotics must be guided by the culture results and should have good CSF penetration.

Because iatrogenic CSF leaks expose the intracranial cavity to potentially pathogenic organisms from the upper respiratory tract, the use of prophylactic antibiotics may be beneficial following skull base injury; however, this remains a topic of controversy. The opponents argue that antibiotic prophylaxis contributes to the development of more serious infections with potentially resistant organisms, and that prophylaxis does not decrease the risk of meningitis. A strong counter argument to this is provided in a meta-analysis by Brodie,[17] which suggested a statistically significant reduction in the incidence of meningitis from using prophylactic antibiotics for CSF leak. The presence of intracranial abscess may require surgical drainage, therefore a neurosurgical consultation must be sought.

Optic Nerve Injury

The optic nerve runs in the optic canal along the superolateral wall of the sphenoid sinus. It travels in a slightly medial direction between the orbital apex anteriorly and the suprasellar cistern where it joins the contralateral nerve to form the optic chiasm. The optic tubercle corresponds to the level of the optic foramen and is often located at the anterior face of the sphenoid sinus. In the absence of excessive mucosal disease, the nerve can usually be clearly seen in the sphenoid sinus (see **Fig. 9.4a**) along with a prominence of the internal carotid artery; these two structures are separated by a depression referred to as the lateral opticocarotid recess, which corresponds to the anterior clinoid process of the lesser sphenoid wing. The thickness of the bone covering the nerve as it travels in the canal is variable and may be dehiscent, predisposing the nerve to injury during instrumentation of the sphenoid sinus. Furthermore, the anterior clinoid process may be pneumatized to a variable degree, and if significant, the optic canal may actually

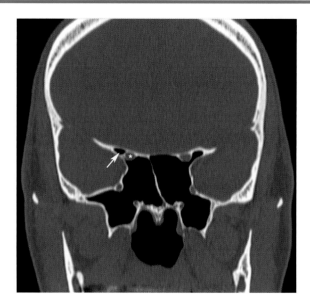

Fig. 9.14 Computed tomography scan of the sinuses, coronal cut at the level of the sphenoid sinus, demonstrating a well pneumatized anterior clinoid process (arrow) corresponding endoscopically to the opticocarotid recess (OCR) and causing the optic nerve (asterisk) to pass through the sinus in a bony mesentery.

run in a mesentery within the sphenoid (**Fig. 9.14**). The potential injury to the optic nerve may be even greater in such circumstances, as a cutting instrument such as a Kerrison rongeur or Hajek–Koefler punch may potentially get around the nerve and transect it as it runs across the roof of the sinus.

Another anatomical variation that places the optic nerve at increased risk of injury is the presence of an Onodi cell. This represents a posterior ethmoid cell that pneumatizes posteriorly along the superolateral aspect of the sphenoid sinus, and therefore harbors the optic nerve in its lateral wall. In such a situation, the optic nerve may be encountered during dissection of the posterior ethmoid sinus rather than the sphenoid as expected. If this anatomical configuration goes unrecognized, the nerve may be injured before the surgeon is aware that they are working near the nerve. In addition, fracturing away the parting wall between the Onodi cell and the sphenoid sinus can injure the nerve if this bony septation inserts on to the optic canal.

For these reasons, Onodi cells must be actively sought and recognized on preoperative imaging before each surgery. This can be done by looking on a CT scan for the first coronal cut demonstrating the complete bony choanal bridge (representing the anterior wall of the sphenoid). Once this is localized, the airspace above it is the sphenoid sinus and if there is a non-vertical septation within the sphenoid, the air cell superior and lateral to that septation represents an Onodi cell (**Fig. 9.15**).

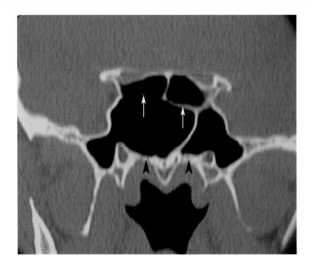

Fig. 9.15 Computed tomography scan of the sinuses, coronal cut at the level of the sphenoid sinus, demonstrating the bony choana (arrowheads) and horizontal septations within the sinus (arrows) indicating the presence of Onodi cells; note that the optic nerve is located superolaterally to the Onodi cells.

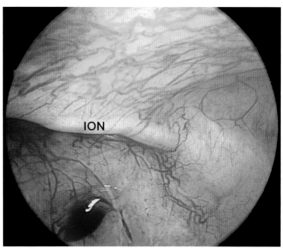

Fig. 9.16 Endoscopic view into the right maxillary antrum using a 70° endoscope, showing a prominent infraorbital nerve (ION) running along the roof of the sinus.

> **Note**
> The best option for optic nerve injury is prevention, as little can be done to reverse the visual loss associated with transection of the nerve.

If the nerve suffers a contusion from blunt injury during sinus surgery, the nerve can be decompressed endoscopically to make room for the injured area to expand until the resolution of swelling. Whether injury to the optic nerve is recognized or not, the patient will complain of decreased ipsilateral vision and may exhibit a relative afferent pupillary defect on swinging flashlight test. Such a situation should prompt an immediate ophthalomologic consultation. Nasal packings if present should be promptly removed. If there are no medical contraindications, the patient should be given high-dose corticosteroids. The decision to take the patient back to the operating room for an exploration or decompression should be made in collaboration with the ophthalmologist based on a poor response to steroid treatment, and corroborated by evidence of optic nerve injury on postoperative CT or magnetic resonance imaging. It should be stated however that neither steroid therapy nor surgical decompression are considered standard care, as they have not been demonstrated to be superior to observation alone.[18]

Infraorbital Nerve Injury

The infraorbital nerve is a terminal branch of the trigeminal nerve V2 that innervates the skin of the cheek; transient or permanent paresthesias may result from its injury. Injury to the infraorbital nerve is truly rare in routine endoscopic surgery of the maxillary sinus. However, the course of the nerve along the roof of the sinus makes it susceptible to surgical trauma during instrumentation of the sinus. This is particularly true if it is low lying or running within a mesentery in the sinus antrum (**Fig. 9.16**). This may consist of an avulsion injury, or partial or complete disruption of the nerve.

Injury of the nerve is a particular risk during clearance of disease from the roof of the maxillary sinus, as well as during removal of the back wall of the maxillary sinus to gain access to the infratemporal fossa as part of an expanded endoscopic approach. Prevention is best achieved by identifying a low V2 nerve on the preoperative CT scan, localizing the location of an aberrant nerve in surgery through the use of a 70° scope directed laterally or an image-guidance system when available, and minimizing instrumentation along the roof of the sinus. Once the injury occurs, the management is conservative; if the nerve has not been completely transected, the patient can expect a possible slow return of sensation over several months. However, the patient must be warned that the paresthesia may be permanent.

Ophthalmic Complications

Orbital Injury

Orbital injury may occur anywhere along the orbital walls that partition the orbital contents from the sinonasal cavity. The lamina papyracea of the ethmoid bone makes up the lateral border of the ethmoid sinuses and constitutes a large portion of the medial orbital wall. It lies superior to the natural ostium of the maxillary sinus and can easily be injured during the maxillary antrostomy. A fine periosteal layer, also referred to as the periorbita, lies immediately lateral to the lamina papyracea and sheathes the orbital contents. The orbital cavity can be divided grossly into an extraconal compartment, containing mostly fat, as well as an intraconal compartment, which in addition to fat, contains the extraocular muscles, optic nerve, and ocular globe. The boundaries of this "cone" run along the plane of the extraocular muscles, which originate at the annulus of Zinn posteriorly and insert on the sclera anteriorly. It should be noted that the medial rectus runs in a plane that is slightly tangential to the plane of the lamina, so that the body of the muscle posteriorly is in close approximation to the bone, and therefore at much greater risk of injury in ESS than the anterior part of the muscle, which is separated from the lamina by a thicker layer of fat (**Fig. 9.17**).

Recognized risk factors for orbital injury include surgeon disorientation, excessive surgical bleeding, scarring from previous surgery, and pre-existing medial wall abnormality. Certain anatomical variants may also predispose to orbital penetration such as an excessively medialized lamina papyracea relative to the lateral nasal wall (**Fig. 9.18**), or an underdeveloped middle turbinate. The former variant may be encountered in association with an underdeveloped or atelectatic maxillary sinus, or in silent sinus syndrome. An abnormally small middle turbinate may lead the inexperienced surgeon to believe that the maxillary ostium is more superior than it actually is, resulting in orbital penetration by the surgeon when they are attempting to probe the natural ostium.

There are several possible mechanisms for injury to the orbit in ESS, including direct penetration, thermal injury from the transmission of heat from electrocautery or radiofrequency ablation near the orbit,[19] but it is the use of powered instrumentation such as the microdebrider that has the greatest potential of severe and long-lasting sequelae. The combination of suction and rapid tissue removal allows for tissue to be resected from within the orbit even through very limited lamina defects. As a result, these injuries are often irreparable because of the large volumes of tissue lost.[20] Consequently, early recognition of lamina papyracea dehiscence is critical in the prevention of medial rectus injury and its long-term effects including severe disabling diplopia.

Orbital injury may occur during the uncinectomy, or when initially attempting to probe the natural ostium, or during enlargement of the antrostomy superiorly toward the medial orbital floor. Variable degrees of injury to the intraorbital structures may occur, depending on the type of instrument used and the depth of penetration into the orbit. Fat prolapse may be the only indication of a breach of the periorbita (**Fig. 9.19a**); alternatively, muscle injury with or without diplopia, optic nerve or ocular globe injury with loss of vision may occur.

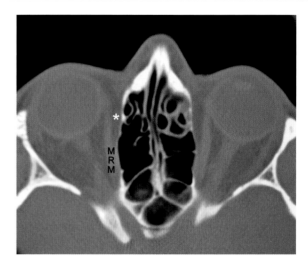

Fig. 9.17 Computed tomography scan of the sinuses, axial cut through the level of the orbits, illustrating the close relationship between the medial rectus muscle (MRM) and the lamina papyracea, which are in close apposition posteriorly, but become separated by a layer of orbital fat (asterisk) more anteriorly.

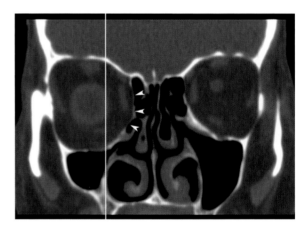

Fig. 9.18 Computed tomography scan of the sinuses, coronal cut at the level of the maxillary ostia in a patient with a particularly underdeveloped right maxillary sinus causing the medial orbital wall (arrowheads) to lie in a plane much more medial than the lateral nasal wall (white line).

> **Note**
> Powered instruments have the greatest potential for serious injury because of the rapidity with which they remove tissue.

When performing surgery on the frontal sinuses, the risk to the orbit is particularly present along the lateral limit of the frontal recess, and rarely, along the floor of the frontal sinus itself. Although this is quite rare, with a reported overall incidence for serious orbital complications in ESS of 0.07 to 0.12%,[2,3] this can occur when attempting to maximize the lateral extent of the frontal

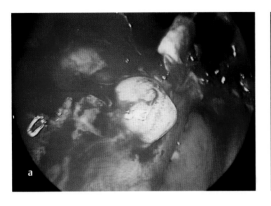
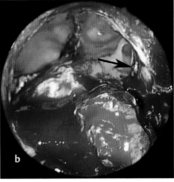

Fig. 9.19a,b Orbital injuries.

a Endoscopic view of orbital fat protruding through a traumatic defect in the right lamina papyracea.

b Endoscopic view of the frontal neo-ostium during a Draf type III frontal drill out procedure, showing an area of exposed periorbita and injury of the trochlea of the left orbit.

recess dissection. Similarly, the orbit may be inadvertently entered when maximizing the anterolateral area of the frontal neo-ostium during the frontal drill out procedure (**Fig. 9.19b**), placing the trochlear ligament and tendon of the superior oblique muscle at risk of injury. Care must be exercised whenever these areas are approached in any surgical procedure.

Prevention

Measures to avoid orbital injury include the careful review of imaging in the preoperative setting, with attention to the lamina papyracea bilaterally along its entire length. The surgeon must actively seek to identify high-risk anatomical variants such as dehiscences or orbital fat protrusion into either the ethmoid or maxillary sinuses (**Fig. 9.20**), or an excessively medialized position relative to the lateral nasal wall, particularly in cases of atelectasis of the maxillary sinus (**Fig. 9.18**). These situations must be recognized before surgery because they increase the likelihood of orbital penetration. Intraoperatively, care must also be taken never to direct dissecting instruments or probes toward the orbit, and never to apply pressure on the lamina papyracea itself. Instead, dissecting probes or curettes should always be oriented in a superior direction, keeping the tip of the instrument clearly in the surgeon's visual field. Bony lamellae should only be fractured and removed by applying pressure in a posterior to anterior direction.

In a study aiming to compare techniques for performing the uncinectomy in terms of safety and efficacy,[21] with 636 procedures per arm, the senior author found the rate of orbital penetration to be 0.94% using the traditional sickle knife technique and 0% using the swing-door technique. The latter technique was created with the aim of achieving a complete removal of the midportion of the uncinate process and exposing the natural ostium of the maxillary sinus. A sickle knife is used to perform a superior cut in the uncinate horizontally just under the axilla of the middle turbinate, where the risk of penetration of the orbit is extremely small. Next the pediatric backbiter is used for the inferior horizontal cut in the uncinate process. The midportion of the uncinate process

is fractured anteriorly using the right-angled ball probe, and upturned 45° through-biting Blakesley forceps are used to cut the uncinate flush with the lateral nasal wall. The mid-portion of the uncinate can now be removed in one piece.

The use of the microdebrider is discouraged for removal of the vertical portion of the uncinate. To remove the uncinate flush with the frontal process of the maxilla, the microdebrider blade needs to be pushed firmly against the orbital wall. This significantly increases the risk of orbital penetration and damage to the medial rectus muscle. If the microdebrider blade is used only very gently against the frontal process, inevitably a variable amount of uncinate will remain and this will make identification of the natural ostium more difficult. In addition even gentle use of the microdebrider blade on this portion of the lamina papyracea may be sufficient to penetrate the orbit. The thinnest and therefore the most dangerous region of the lamina papyracea is the region directly behind the frontal process of the maxilla and may in fact be dehiscent in some patients. This is usually evident with ballottement of the eye, and therefore this maneuver should be used frequently when operating near the lamina papyracea. Removal of the midportion of the uncinate is easily and cleanly achieved with cold steel instruments without significant risk to the orbit, so this is the recommended technique. Removal or trimming of the horizontal section of the uncinate is often performed using the microdebrider with the direction of the blade inferior and away for the lamina papyracea, therefore not putting this area at risk.

When initially entering the maxillary ostium following the uncinectomy, it is also important to orient the right-angle ball probe or short curved suction probe with the tip rotated 45° inferior to the horizontal plane. In general, probes and dissecting instruments should not be directed toward the orbit, and pressure should never be applied on the lamina because of the risk of orbital penetration. Similarly, when performing revision surgery on the maxillary sinus, it is critically important to look for any evidence of orbital dehiscence, both on preoperative imaging and with ballottement of the globe during surgery.

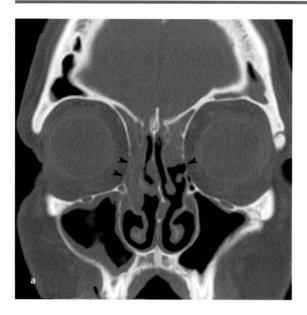

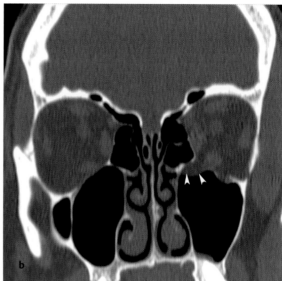

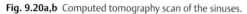

Fig. 9.20a,b Computed tomography scan of the sinuses.

a Coronal cut at the level of the anterior ethmoid sinuses in a patient with extremely thinned areas of the lamina papyracea (arrowheads), placing the orbit at increased risk of injury during ESS.

b Coronal cut at the level of the posterior ethmoid sinuses demonstrating a defect in the medial floor of the left orbit with protrusion of orbital fat (arrowheads).

Unplanned transgression of the bony wall of the orbit can result in various degrees of orbital injury. In its mildest form, asymptomatic exposure of periorbita or orbital fat may occur at the site of the bony breach; in its most severe form, damage to one or more extraocular muscles results in severe diplopia. In the advent of a mild injury, without any evidence of damage to the orbital contents, it is recommended to leave the area of breach alone and not to explore the injury. It is wise not to use suction or any form of powered instrumentation in the vicinity of such a defect. A bedside assessment of vision and extraocular muscle function is warranted in the immediate postoperative period, as is an examination looking for discoloration, periorbital swelling or emphysema, or proptosis. It is crucially important to instruct the patient not to blow their nose in the weeks following surgery, until adequate healing has taken place, for fear of blowing air or infected material into the orbit.

> **Note**
>
> The exact location, nature and severity of the injury should be clearly documented in the patient's hospital chart for future reference by other surgeons, as an unrecognized dehiscence in the orbital wall may lead to more severe injury during a subsequent surgical procedure.

Management

If the postoperative examination yields any abnormal findings, or if there is any evidence of more significant intraorbital injury at the time of surgery, then an urgent ophthalmology consultation is warranted. An intraoperative forced duction test may be performed to evaluate ocular range of motion and to rule out extraocular muscle entrapment. A thorough ophthalmologic examination is necessary in the postoperative period to detect diplopia, assess extraocular movement, and determine visual acuity and ocular pressure. The patient should also be monitored for signs of retrobulbar hematoma such as pain, proptosis, and periorbital ecchymosis (**Fig. 9.21**). The management of hematoma is discussed below.

Damage to the superior oblique muscle or trochlea can lead to an iatrogenic Brown syndrome, with severe diplopia. Several distinct processes affecting the structural integrity or function of the trochlea can lead to Brown syndrome, which has the clinical hallmark of impaired upward gaze and adduction of the ocular globe with resultant diplopia. There are several published reports of iatrogenic Brown syndrome occurring following external approaches to the sinuses,[22,23] but it can occur during ESS as well.[24] In a published case description that occurred during a frontal drill out (Draf type III) procedure, periostium was exposed in the area of the orbital roof and the posterior table of the frontal sinus. The operating surgeon did not recognize this until a strand of periosteum

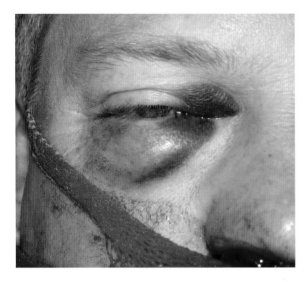

Fig. 9.21 Lid edema and periorbital ecchymosis in a patient with a medial rectus injury.

was sucked into the suction port of the 70° diamond bur and became wrapped solidly around the shaft of the bur. Marked bradycardia and loss of the blood pressure reading occurred immediately thereafter, but normalized after release of the bur from the hand-piece of the debrider.

Extraocular Muscle Injury

As stated above, injury to the lamina papyracea may occur during the clearance of bony ethmoid septations off the medial wall of the orbit. Fortunately, the incidence of extraocular muscle injury is extremely low. In a multicenter series, 30 cases were identified with a reported incidence of 0.0014%.[25] The medial rectus is the most common extraocular muscle involved, followed by the inferior rectus.[26] Several patterns of injury have been described, including muscle transection, contusion or hematoma, oculomotor nerve branch injury, and muscle entrapment.[25] All of these patterns are associated with variable amounts of exotropia and ocular adduction deficits, except for entrapment, which is characterized by an abduction deficit.

Prevention

Prevention is best achieved by careful history and physical examination, meticulous scrutiny of the preoperative CT imaging, as well as continuous vigilance during the operative procedure. Dehiscence of the medial orbital wall should be considered if there is a history of previous surgery, maxillofacial trauma, sinonasal neoplasm, an expansile inflammatory process, or primary orbital pathology. The configuration and integrity on the lamina papyracea is best assessed while viewing coronal sections of the preoperative CT scan in bony windows. The lamina

is visually scanned on each side while scrolling through cuts from anterior to posterior, paying particular attention for areas of bony fracture, remodeling or dehiscence, or prolapse of orbital contents into the ethmoid cells (**Figs. 9.18 and 9.20**). Sinonasal pathology that may cause demineralization of the orbital wall includes mucocele, mucopyocele, severe polyposis, and fungal disease.

Intraoperatively, frequent ballottement of the eye is performed routinely upon approaching the lamina, including after performing the uncinectomy and after entering the bulla ethmoidalis. Applying pressure onto the globe of the eye in the presence of a bony defect along the medial orbital wall will cause transmitted movement of the orbital contents at the site of the breach, alerting the surgeon to the increased risk of orbital injury. Care must be taken to avoid directing any dissecting instruments (probes, curettes, or other sharp instruments) toward the lamina papyracea; rather, they must be kept in a vertical orientation parallel to the plane of the lamina and used to fracture septations in a posterior to anterior direction. Pressure must never be applied in the direction of the orbit for the risk of penetration. Hajek–Koefler or Kerrison punches are safe options to remove ethmoid septations inserting onto the lamina; even so, it is good practice to repeatedly verify its integrity by balloting the globe.

The use of powered instruments, such as the microdebrider, directly on the lamina papyracea should be avoided, particularly in oscillating mode because this results in more aggressive removal of soft tissues. The microdebrider is ideally kept several millimeters medial to the lamina, allowing edematous and polypoid tissues to be gently aspirated by the instrument. It is also good practice to keep the instrument moving using gentle sweeping motions along the edges of bony septations; "parking" the activated instrument in one spot for several seconds increases the risk of a significant orbital injury should it be placed near an unrecognized orbital wall dehiscence. Finally, it is useful to note that the microdebrider can be used in forward mode (i.e., non-oscillating mode) when approaching sensitive areas like the medial orbital wall, as this will be less aggressive on soft tissues while preferentially removing bony septations.

Management

Once a suspected extraocular muscle injury has occurred, immediate management is centered on ruling out the possibility of associated severe but reversible complications that threaten the patient's vision. Immediate ophthalmologic consultation must be obtained including tonometry and fundoscopic examination to ensure perfusion of the optic nerve and retina.[20] Once elevated intraocular pressure has either been ruled out or appropriately managed, the focus of management becomes the muscle injury. Gadolinium-enhanced magnetic resonance imaging is the imaging modality of choice to precisely determine the site, extent, and pattern of extraocular muscle injury. Depending on the amount of tissue loss, primary surgical reanastomosis, interposition grafting, or the use of adjustable sutures may be attempted. In addition, the use of Botox injection in the ipsilateral lateral rectus muscle may be a useful adjunct in the first few weeks after repair to reduce tension across the anastomosis site.[27]

Orbital Hematoma

Orbital hematoma consists of a collection of blood inside the orbit that occurs as a consequence of bleeding from local blood vessels. Two mechanisms for orbital hematoma formation have been proposed:[28] one occurs as a result of slow bleeding, from veins or capillaries running along the lamina papyracea, and the other occurs as a result of rapid arterial bleeding. The most commonly recognized mechanism for orbital hematoma formation during ESS is by transection of the anterior ethmoid artery, with subsequent retraction of the proximal bleeding artery into the orbit. As discussed above, this often occurs while clearing disease from the anterior skull base, and can occur whether periorbita is injured or not.

The most dreaded consequence of orbital hematoma is blindness. This can arise because the orbit is a confined bony space with tight fascial attachments holding the globe at its anterior edge. The occurrence of bleeding within this space therefore causes intraorbital pressure to increase rapidly, resulting in ischemic injury to the retina or optic nerve. In venous retrobulbar hematomas, the retina may tolerate elevated pressure for perhaps 60 to 90 minutes; however, in fast arterial hematomas, the immediate high pressure on the optic nerve must be reduced in 15 to 30 minutes to avoid blindness.[28] Permanent damage to the retina in animals has been noted after ~ 100 minutes of ischemia.[29] Timely recognition and management of this complication is therefore critical in preventing long-term visual loss, and an acute awareness of this possibility is essential for any otolaryngologist operating near the orbit.

Arterial bleeding results in a more rapid evolution of clinical signs and symptoms than venous bleeding. Signs include proptosis, lid edema and ecchymosis (**Fig. 9.21**), chemosis, subconjunctival hemorrhage, mydriasis, and afferent pupillary defect; symptoms in an awake patient may include orbital pain, diplopia, loss of color vision or visual acuity, and eventually irreversible blindness.

Prevention

At the beginning of surgery, the eyes are lubricated with ointment and left uncovered so that they may be examined regularly during the procedure. Alternatively, the eyes can be kept closed with laterally placed clear tape, if there is a particular concern that the lids will remain

open and lead to exposure keratitis. The globes should be periodically inspected and balloted as a rough gauge of intraorbital pressure and to endoscopically search for areas of dehiscent lamina papyracea. The possibility of hematoma formation should be considered intraoperatively if the medial orbit is penetrated, orbital fat is visualized, or significant bleeding occurs along the skull base near the lamina or posterior frontal recess. If in the postoperative period, the patient reports pain, diplopia, periorbital ecchymosis, or edema, or loss of acuity or color vision, orbital hemorrhage must be suspected.

Management

It is best to establish a clear plan to deal with this complication, and to review it regularly given the relative rarity of its occurrence. One proposed algorithm is presented in **Fig. 9.22**. Once the diagnosis of orbital hematoma is suspected, an ophthalmology consult should be urgently obtained, and serial examination must be initiated looking for the above signs. The nasal cavity must be immediately cleared of any packing material. Orbital massage has been suggested to redistribute intraocular and extraocular fluids, decreasing pressure on the globe, and possibly even arresting intraorbital bleeding.[28] A more efficacious maneuver may in fact be to apply four-finger pressure to the affected globe to apply transmitted pressure to the bleeding vessel. This is done with the aim of arresting the bleed before the resulting hematoma completely fills the confined space within the orbit and runs out of room to expand. However, it must be emphasized that this applied pressure should be stopped if the globe becomes rock-hard. Care must also be exercised in patients who have undergone ocular surgery previously, as orbital massage is contraindicated in such cases. If this occurs during surgery, the procedure should be stopped until a hematoma is either ruled out, or appropriately managed.

The ophthalmologic examination should include tonometry to detect elevated intraocular pressure, as determined by a pressure exceeding 21 mmHg. The retinal examination should look for pallor caused by decreased central retinal artery perfusion; under such circumstances, the macula may appear as a "cherry red spot". Based on the ophthalmologist's assessment or the clinical evolution as assessed by the surgeon, the decision of whether to attempt conservative medical management or to initiate surgical decompressive maneuvers must be made.

Several medical therapies may be tried to decrease intraorbital pressure. Mannitol (20%, 1 to 2 g/kg over 20 minutes) administered intravenously has a rapid onset of effect. High-dose intravenous steroids such as Decadron (8 to 10 mg every 8 hours) may also act rapidly. Acetazolamide 500 mg intravenously, and Timolol drops (0.5%, one or two drops topically twice daily) may be administered, but have a slow onset of action because

- Suspected orbital hematoma: any pain, proptosis, afferent pupillary defect, vision loss, or high intraocular pressures?
  - If no: observe
  - If yes: urgent ophthalmology consultation
- Remove any packings and suction at bleeding site
- Apply four-finger digital pressure to the globe if the eye is soft
- Orbital massage (controversial)
- Initiate treatment
  - Medical treatment:
    - Mannitol 1–2 g/kg in 20% intravenous infusion (100 g in 500-mL bag) over 20 minutes
    - Decadron 8–10 mg intravenously 8-hourly for three to four doses
    - Acetazolamide 500 mg intravenously 4-hourly as required
    - Timolol 0.5% ophthalmic drops (only if slow bleed)
  - Surgical treatment:
    - Lateral canthotomy/cantholysis (for acute decompression if in the recovery room)
    - Subsequent orbital decompression is required for definitive treatment
    - Endoscopic decompression, or
    - Medial external decompression via Lynch incision ± anterior ethmoidal artery ligation

Fig. 9.22 Management of orbital hematoma.

they act to decrease aqueous humor production; they may therefore only be useful in slow venous bleeds. Persistently elevated pressures, or poor clinical evolution may warrant surgical intervention.

If the patient is still under general anesthesia, it is best to proceed directly to an endoscopic orbital decompression in the operating room. Briefly, the technique consists of clearing the lamina papyracea of ethmoid septation, delicately fracturing away the bony lamina to uncover the periorbita, and incise the periorbita to tease out orbital fat and achieve adequate decompression. If the patient is in the recovery room or on the ward and the hematoma is progressing rapidly despite the initial measures, relief of intraorbital pressure can be achieved with lateral canthotomy and inferior cantholysis (**Fig. 9.23**). This can buy time until the patient can be brought to the operating theater for an endoscopic decompression. This is achieved by cutting the lateral canthus between the upper and lower lids in a lateral direction using sharp iris scissors, and then cutting the attachment of the lateral canthal tendon to Whitnall tubercle, located 5 mm posterior to the orbital rim. Canthotomy and cantholysis can be expected to provide 14 to 30 mmHg of pressure relief, and decompression an additional 10 mmHg.

Because the anterior and posterior ethmoid arteries arise from the internal carotid artery through the ophthalmic branch, embolization is not recommended because of the elevated risks of blindness and stroke. If needed, these arteries may be ligated through a transcutaneous approach to the orbit, via a Lynch incision. The AEA is found on the medial orbital wall along the frontoethmoidal suture line 24 mm back from the anterior lacrimal crest. The posterior ethmoidal artery is located another 12 mm posteriorly, and the optic foramen another 6 mm posteriorly.

Nasolacrimal Duct Injury

The nasolacrimal duct lies only 3 to 6 mm anterior to the natural maxillary ostium, and enters the inferior meatus via the Hasner valve, within 1 cm from the anterior end of the inferior turbinate. The duct may be uncovered of its protective lacrimal bone or injured during the middle meatal antrostomy. Injury to the duct and the subsequent scarring may result in partial or complete obstruction to the flow of tears between the nasolacrimal sac and the inferior meatus, resulting in varying degrees of epiphora.

An early published report found the incidence of occult nasolacrimal duct injury to be 15%,[30] but in a retrospective comparison, the incidence of injury with the swing-door technique was 0.62%, and 0% with the traditional sickle knife technique.[21] Even though intraoperative injury to the lacrimal drainage system in ESS may be common, the clinical sequelae are rare, as the duct tends to heal spontaneously or create a patent drainage system between the violated duct and the middle meatus.[30] The incidence of epiphora after injury has been reported to be 0.14 to 1.7%.[31–33] Based on a report of eight patients with epiphora after ESS by Serdahl et al,[34] it appears that if patients are going to develop clinical sequelae, the symptoms usually manifest immediately or within 2 weeks after surgery.

Injury usually occurs during the uncinectomy, specifically during the removal of the vertical middle portion on the uncinate process. If the backbiter is used too aggressively, the instrument may cut anteriorly beyond the attachment of the uncinate to the lacrimal bone and through the nasolacrimal duct, which lies just lateral to the bone. Usually, three bites of the backbiter are necessary before the lacrimal bone is reached, but this may vary from patient to patient and be considerably less in patients with a retrocurved uncinate. With the third bite, the backbiter is rotated upward from the horizontal plane until it is angled at 45° so that the tooth when closed passes medial to the nasolacrimal duct. This maneuver reduces the risk of injury to the nasolacrimal duct. It should be noted that transection of the duct is expected in certain procedures such as the endoscopic medial maxillectomy. In such instances, the duct should be cut

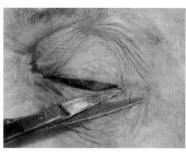
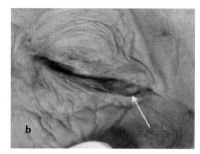
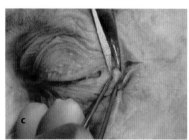
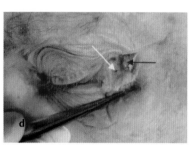

Fig. 9.23a–d Lateral canthotomy.

a Lateral canthotomy performed with straight sharp scissors.

b View of the inferior canthal tendon (arrow) after the lateral canthotomy.

c Cutting of the inferior canthal tendon to complete the cantholysis.

d Medial (white arrow) and lateral (black arrow) ends of the cut inferior canthal tendon.

sharply and splayed open if possible to allow the duct to heal in an open configuration.

Given the rarity of epiphora after injury to the duct, observation alone is recommended. If epiphora develops, a complete ophthalmologic examination should be performed. Even if the cause of symptoms is presumed to be surgical trauma, other causes should be excluded. Follow-up of these patients is recommended for several months, because the epiphora may resolve as postoperative intranasal inflammation resolves. Persistent epiphora can be treated with an endoscopic dacryocystorhinostomy with the expectation of complete symptom resolution.

Intranasal Wound Healing Complications

Middle Turbinate Lateralization

Lateralization of the middle turbinate is one of the most common complications of ESS, and probably the most common surgical cause of ESS failure. Several series have looked at the causes of postsurgical persistent or recurrent disease requiring revision ESS, and have found that middle meatal scarring and lateralization of the middle turbinate[35,36] were the most common findings. This occurs as an early postoperative complication in situations where the middle turbinate is destabilized or partially resected, allowing opposing mucosal surfaces between the turbinate and lateral nasal wall that have been injured, abraided, or stripped to come into contact and form an adhesion (**Fig. 9.24**). The middle turbinate may become destabilized during the frontal recess dissection with over-zealous removal of the medial aspects

of the agger nasi or frontoethmoidal cells, as these often form the anterior attachment of the turbinate. This may also occur with excessive manipulation of the turbinate itself as it is medialized before performing the middle meatal antrostomy.

A lateralized middle turbinate can cause obstruction of the osteomeatal complex and frontal recess drainage pathway. This leads to poor aeration of the affected sinuses as well as suboptimal access of topical therapies to the sinus mucosa. These facts in turn lead to worsening of mucosal inflammation, mucus accumulation, and infection. Late postoperative complications include acute or recalcitrant chronic frontal sinusitis, mucocele, and mucopyocele. Obstruction of the sinuses also interferes

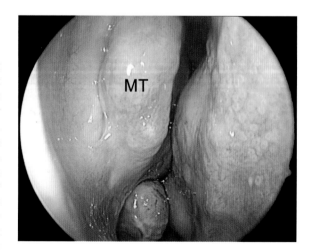

Fig. 9.24 Endoscopic view of a lateralized middle turbinate (MT), with adhesions formed between the inferior aspect of the turbinate and the lateral nasal wall.

with the surgeon's ability to perform debridement, and disease surveillance.

Prevention

Measures to prevent middle turbinate lateralization are best performed at the time of surgery. Several technical points for the dissection may help to prevent scarring beginning in the axilla of the middle turbinate: where care should be taken not to apply excessive force (especially force directed laterally) to the turbinate to preserve its stability. The axillary flap (**Fig. 9.25**) provides both a spacer between the turbinate and the lateral nasal wall, as well as a mucosal lining that covers the bare bone, which is inevitably exposed during the removal of the anterior wall and floor of the agger nasi during the frontal sinusotomy.[14]

If the turbinate does become unstable, or "floppy," then a stabilizing maneuver must be performed before the conclusion of surgery. Several alternative techniques exist: some authors advocate suturing the turbinates to the septum; in the event of a simultaneous septoplasty, our preferred technique is to used a running mattress stitch of 4–0 vicryl rapide with a knot tied into one end. The suture is passed through the one middle turbinate, the septum and through the contralateral turbinate. The suture is then passed from side to side in a posterior to anterior direction to eventually encompass the anterior septal incision and is tied inside the nasal vestibule just deep to the columella. Alternatively, controlled scarring can be encouraged between the medial surface of the

turbinate and the septum, in a technique that has come to be known as "Bolgerization".[37] Stenting of the middle meatus in the early postoperative period is a principle that has gained popularity, and there is currently a wide variety of absorbable and nonabsorbable materials to choose from. A few popular options include nonresorbable barriers such as silicon elastomer sheeting and surgical glove finger cots. Alternatively, bioresorbable dressings can be used, such as hyaluronic acid, carboxy methyl cellulose, and Nasopore (Polyganics, Groningen, the Netherlands). Gelfoam should be avoided because of its propensity to cause scar formation. Some authors even advocate the removal of an unstable middle turbinate; while this may be necessary in patients where there is extensive polypoid degeneration with significant demineralization of the turbinate bone, there are several potential pitfalls to this practice: over-resection can damage or remove olfactory epithelium worsening hyposmia, lead to headache or atropic rhinitis, and under-resection of the anterior end of the turbinate can itself predispose to lateralization.[35]

If lateralization is noted at the first postoperative visit, lysis of the adhesions may be attempted in clinic, but this can lead to significant discomfort in the patient and is rarely successful if no barrier is placed. The likelihood of success is increased if a spacer is placed in the middle meatus following adhesiolysis. Surgical revision in the operating room with the placement of Silastic sheets (Dow Corning, Midland, MI, USA) may be necessary.

Frontal Recess Scarring

Frontal recess scarring refers to the obstruction of a previously operated frontal drainage pathway as a result of cicatricial contracture, and not simply as a result of recurrent inflammatory or polypoid disease. This generally occurs as a late postoperative complication because scar tissue tends to form gradually after surgery. Several studies have reported on this phenomenon after the endoscopic modified Lothrop procedure;[38–43] it has been demonstrated that the frontal neo-ostium contracts an average of 33% within the first year after surgery.[41] The size of the ostium tends to stabilize after 12 to 18 months[38] as the fibrous tissue thins and ceases remodeling.

Scarring tends to occur in instances where circumferential mucosal injury is created at the time of surgery, or when extensive areas of mucosal stripping result in denuded bone within the frontal recess. The osteitis that ensues causes an intensive fibrotic reaction that can lead to scarring and obstruction of the frontal drainage pathway (**Fig. 9.26**). Risk factors for this include narrow frontal recess anatomy, as assessed by the distance between the frontal beak and skull base on parasagittal cuts of preoperative CT imaging. Other factors include a previous failed Draf type IIA procedure, middle turbinate lateralization from previous surgery, polypoid disease, and thick osteoneogenesis in the region of the frontal recess. It is also

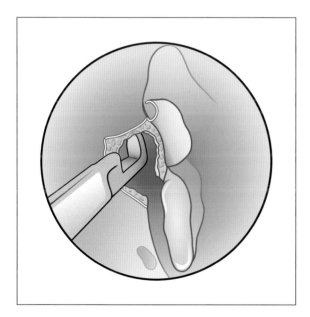

Fig. 9.25 Schematic view of the axilla of the left middle turbinate, demonstrating the position of the axillary flap, which is elevated before frontal recess dissection.

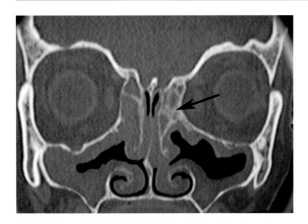

Fig. 9.26 Computed tomography scan on the sinuses, coronal cut at the level of the maxillary antrostomies demonstrating osteoneogenesis in the anterior ethmoid region due to chronic osteitis after a previous endoscopic sinus surgery.

believed that excessive bleeding during and after surgery can also predispose to scarring. Blood clots that remain in the area of the frontal recess act as a scaffold for fibroblast migration and scar formation, and therefore thorough postoperative debridement is thought to be important in preventing this from occurring.

Varying degrees of sinus outflow obstruction are possible as a result of scarring. Mild or asymptomatic restenosis can be observed, whereas severe or complete restenosis can cause late postoperative complications, including mucocele, mucopyocele, acute or recalcitrant chronic frontal sinusitis, necessitating an intervention. The management of these complications will be detailed below.

Prevention

The prevention of frontal recess scarring is best achieved by taking into account all of the above risk factors. The proper selection of patients requiring frontal recess work, preoperative identification of narrow or complex frontal drainage pathway anatomy, a clear understanding of each individual patient's frontal recess anatomy, and the establishment of a surgical plan for performing the dissection are all helpful measures. Dissecting instruments must be precisely and atraumatically introduced into the frontal drainage pathway allowing obstructing frontoethmoidal cells to be fractured away while minimizing mucosal injury. In cases of complex anatomy, exuberant disease, or pre-existing local scarring from previous surgery, frontal sinus minitrephination (Medtronic ENT) and fluorescein instillation can help to highlight the drainage pathway. With judicious use, the angled microdebrider blade can be extremely useful in clearing the frontal recess pathway; however, care must be exercised to avoid circumferential trauma or excessive removal of mucosa within this narrow region. Also, because of the intense fibrotic

reaction that may occur, the authors recommend avoiding the use of a drill on a unilateral frontal beak within the frontal recess unless a maximally large opening is performed in the form of a complete frontal drill out (Draf type III or endoscopic modified Lothrop procedure).

Surgical failure in the form of symptomatic frontal sinus obstruction or local disease recurrence in the setting of frontal recess scarring requires revision surgery. This can consist of either a revised frontal recess dissection, or a drill out procedure. Placement of long-term silastic stents[44] and the topical application of Mitomycin C[45] have been suggested for the prevention of restenosis after revision surgery.

Maxillary Ostial Stenosis

As with the frontal recess, obstruction of the maxillary ostium can occur as a late postoperative complication, particularly if a circumferential mucosal injury is created during the antrostomy procedure. This is usually a result of scarring causing concentric narrowing of the ostium over time; however, mucosal edema or polyp recurrence can also result in postoperative ostial obstruction. In addition, lateralization of the middle turbinate can contribute to obstruction of the osteomeatal complex in general. In series looking at the causes of postsurgical persistent or recurrent sinus disease, middle meatal antrostomy stenosis was found to represent 27 to 39% of cases.[36,46]

Any one of the above causes can contribute to promoting acute or ongoing chronic infection, recalcitrant inflammatory sinus disease, and rarely mucocele formation. Prevention of ostial stenosis begins intraoperatively by avoiding the contributing factors mentioned above: these include the creation of a circumferential mucosal injury (particularly if the final middle meatal antrostomy dimension is small), mucosal stripping around the ostium causing bone exposure and osteitis, excessive bleeding and clotting, and an unstable middle turbinate.

Prevention

Determining what is the adequate size for the maxillary antrostomy is still a matter of controversy. Cadaveric studies have shown that a minimum ostial size of 4 mm is necessary for good penetration of postoperative topical therapies into the sinus.[47] If there exists any pathology within the sinus requiring instrumentation of the sinus at the time of surgery, then enlargement of the antrostomy into the fontanelle is necessary. A reasonable approach to this question is to tailor the extent of surgery to the disease burden of the maxillary sinus as assessed intraoperatively. In the setting of mild mucosal disease or a history of recurrent acute infections, simple uncinectomy with preservation of posterior and superior mucosa of the natural ostium is likely to be sufficient. Whenever possible, it is preferable to leave mucosal edges in close

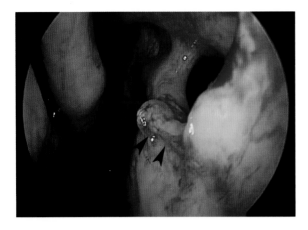

Fig. 9.27 Intraoperative view of directly apposing mucosal edges (arrowheads) following uncinectomy, favoring primary intention healing in the postoperative period.

approximation, allowing healing by primary intention (**Fig. 9.27**). If inspection of the maxillary antrum reveals small to medium-size polyps, mucus retention cysts, or submucosal abscesses, then it is possible to enlarge the antrostomy posteriorly into the fontanelle. This will allow the introduction of curved instruments into sinus for thorough clearance of pathology. If large polyps or thick eosinophilic mucus is found in surgery, then a maximal antrostomy—with or without an adjunct procedure like the canine fossa trephination—may be the best option for clearing the inflammatory tissues intraoperatively and controlling the disease postoperatively.

Meticulous hemostasis at the end of surgery, securing of unstable middle turbinates, copious postoperative saline irrigations, and thorough debridement of blood clots in clinic are additional measures that may help to prevent middle meatal stenosis. If stenosis occurs in the setting of symptomatic recalcitrant sinus disease, a revision middle meatal antrostomy should be performed.

Mucocele Formation

A mucocele is a benign, expansile process filled with mucus and bordered by respiratory mucosa. It arises when an obstructed sinus becomes filled with mucous that is secreted on an ongoing basis by the sinus mucosa, exerting outward pressure and causing bony remodeling of the sinus walls. The mucus may become infected, forming a mucopyocele, and can extend into adjacent structures like the orbit or the cranial vault. It is suspected on CT when there is a smooth, round enlargement of a completely opacified sinus with associated bony remodeling and thinning (**Fig. 9.28**).

Due to its narrow anatomical outflow pathway, the frontal sinus is particularly susceptible to this complication, and so is often the target of revision sinus surgery. It most commonly arises as a late postoperative

complication following an external approach to the frontal sinus, such as the osteoplastic flap with sinus obliteration; however, it can also arise following endoscopic procedures. In the setting of endoscopic orbital decompression for Graves orbitopathy, a mucocele can arise if the decompressed orbital fat obstructs the frontal sinus outflow tract (**Fig. 9.29**). To prevent this, care must be exercised not to remove the lamina papyracea too high anteriorly near the frontal recess. Conversely, mucoceles arising from the maxillary sinus are relatively infrequent, accounting for less than 10% of all paranasal sinus mucoceles.[48,49] The most common circumstances leading to the development of mucoceles in this area is following Caldwell–Luc procedures, where the mucosa of the sinus has been stripped.

> **Note**
>
> Key concepts for avoiding mucocele formation are similar to those for avoiding frontal recess scarring, as this is often a requisite first step in mucocele formation. Another important point is to avoid stripping mucosa within the frontal sinus, which is also a risk factor.

As with many other local pathologies, it is useful to follow a graded approach to frontal sinus mucoceles. If the mucocele is very medial or extends into the frontal recess, then simple endoscopic marsupialization from below with or without stenting can be performed. If the pathology is situated more laterally within the sinus, then either the endoscopic modified Lothrop or osteoplastic flap are useful options.

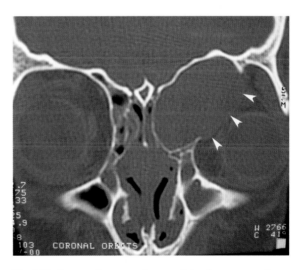

Fig. 9.28 Computed tomography scan of the sinuses, coronal cut at the level of the anterior ethmoid sinuses in a patient with a large fronto-ethmoidal mucocele eroding into the left orbit (arrowheads).

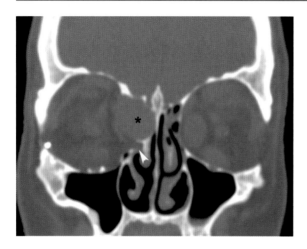

Fig. 9.29 Computed tomography scan of the sinuses, coronal cut at the level of the anterior ethmoid sinuses in a patient with a right fronto-ethmoidal mucocele (asterisk) complicating a previous endoscopic orbital decompression (arrowhead) for Graves orbitopathy.

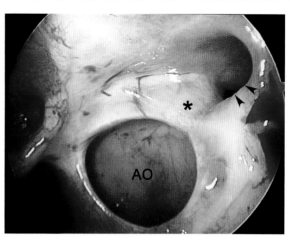

Fig. 9.30 Endoscopic view of a "missed ostium sequence" with a large iatrogenic accessory ostium (AO) in the fontanelle region, the natural maxillary ostium anteriorly (arrowheads), and a bridge of tissue (asterisk) separating the two, predisposing the patient to mucus recirculation.

Missed Ostium Sequence/ Mucus Recirculation

The missed ostium sequence was initially described by Parsons et al[50] and occurs when there is incomplete removal of the most anterior portion of the uncinate process, obscuring the position of the natural maxillary sinus ostium. This prevents the middle meatal antrostomy from communicating with the natural ostium, resulting in a recirculation phenomenon (**Fig. 9.30**). Mucociliary flow causes mucous to exit the natural ostium, pass over the intervening bridge of mucosa and re-enter the sinus via the iatrogenic accessory ostium created in the area of the fontanelle. This causes a functional obstruction of the maxillary sinus and continued sinus disease. A frequent complaint is abundant postnasal drip in the supine position as the recirculation leads to an accumulation of mucus within the maxillary sinus, which drains when the patient lies down to sleep.

The missed ostium sequence can be prevented by paying particular attention to ensuring a complete uncinectomy at the time of surgery, as well as employing a 30° endoscope to visualize the natural ostium in every case. In this way, one can ensure that the middle meatal antrostomy is in direct communication with the natural maxillary sinus ostium.

The treatment for this problem, as with mucus recirculation due to an accessory maxillary sinus ostium, is to resect the intervening tissue between the two ostia; this removes the bridge generating the recirculation. A 70° endoscope is ideally suited to examine these regions and to ensure that there is no residual uncinate or scarring present.

Other Complications

Skin Injury

Damage to the facial skin can occur with the use of powered instruments, such as the microdebrider or drill, during the frontal drill out procedure. This is because one of the initial steps in the frontal drill out is the exposure of skin over the nasal pyramid as the lateral extent of the frontal neoostium. Damage from powered instruments may be mechanical or thermal. Because a cutting bur may perforate the skin if applied to an area for several seconds, it is advisable to continually move the bur around the area of bone being drilled. Hence, if an area of exposed skin goes initially unrecognized, the chances of creating a perforation are dramatically reduced. Similarly, copious irrigation is recommended to dissipate heat generated by the bur and prevent thermal injury to the skin.

Electrocautery can also cause skin injury but this is less likely with the use of bipolar cautery. The use of monopolar cautery should be kept to a minimum. Any injury of the skin should be managed with local wound care measures to promote the best possible healing result. Scar revision at a later date is reserved for those that heal poorly.

Subcutaneous Emphysema

Subcutaneous emphysema refers to the presence of gas or air below the skin. In the setting of ESS, emphysema can occur in the periorbital region when there has been violation of the lamina papyracea, even if the fracture was minor and not recognized at the time of surgery. This is manifested by swelling and crepitus to palpation of the periorbital tissues—most often involving the lower eyelid—and may be accompanied by ecchymosis.

For air to make its way into the subcutaneous tissues, it must first be forced through the break in the lamina papyracea and then disperse through the periorbital soft tissues. This usually occurs as a result of nose blowing by the patient following the operation; so it is important to instruct patients not to blow their noses during the first 2 weeks after surgery. This would allow any breaks or surgically induced weaknesses in the orbital wall to heal over. Other mechanisms that can force air into the soft tissues include aggressive bagging by the anesthetic team, and sneezing or straining by the patient in the early postoperative period.

In general, subcutaneous emphysema is a benign and self-limited condition, and patients can be reassured that the air will resorb within 7 to 10 days. However, given that penetration of the orbit carries a risk of associated bleeding, observation for orbital hematoma is recommended with serial bedside examinations.

> **Note**
> Orbital hemorrhage may, in rare instances, occur in a delayed fashion. Patients should be advised to look out for any worrisome symptoms of eye pain, swelling, bruising or visual change after discharge from hospital, and to immediately return to the emergency room in such circumstances.

Anosmia/Hyposmia

This complication is defined as a postoperative loss or reduction in olfactory ability. One obvious mechanism for this alteration is surgical damage to the olfactory mucosa; however, the olfactory baseline in patients with chronic rhinosinusitis is often already stifled by acute and chronic inflammation, infection, or obstruction to airflow from polyps, further complicating the situation. The olfactory epithelium is distributed along the roof of the olfactory cleft within the nasal cavity, just below the cribriform plate of the ethmoid bone, as well as variable amounts of the superior septum and middle turbinate mucosa. Mucosal stripping or injury to any of these areas, or overaggressive resection of the middle turbinates, can adversely affect the patient's postoperative olfactory ability, so special attention must be paid to avoiding these occurrences. Furthermore, the postoperative formation of intranasal adhesion that occurs as a result of excessive mucosal injury may also interfere with olfaction, both by scarring of the sensory epithelium and by obstruction of airflow in the olfactory cleft.

The prognosis of olfactory loss depends on the mechanism of injury (conductive versus sensorineural).

- Conductive loss stems from scarring between the middle turbinate and the nasal septum, acting as an obstruction to airflow into the olfactory cleft and preventing odorants from reaching receptors in the olfactory neuroepithelium. This type of olfactory loss may improve with lysis of adhesions and optimization of the nasal airflow.
- Sensorineural loss results from damage to the olfactory neuroepithelium itself, consisting of mucosal injury, denudement, or high middle turbinate resection. This type of olfactory loss tends to be irreversible.

As previously stated, there is a high prevalence of anosmia and hyposmia in patients with chronic rhinosinusitis before surgery, and so the underlying disease itself confounds a poor postoperative olfactory outcome. Our experience is that 54% of patients undergoing a complete ESS including frontal recess dissection will have improved olfactory function postoperatively, 36% will have no change and 10% will worsen (unpublished data).

> **Note**
> Maneuvers that threaten the integrity of the olfactory neuroepithelium should be avoided if possible; these include working medial to the middle turbinate, and excessive resection of the middle turbinates. Any patient presenting with anosmia, resulting from surgery or not, should be cautioned about the dangers of food poisoning and faulty smoke detectors at home.

Toxic Shock Syndrome

Toxic shock syndrome is a severe disease characterized by fever, shock and multiple organ involvement, and is mediated by *Staphylococcus aureus* exotoxin. Symptoms may include malaise, headaches, high fever, chills, hypotension, nausea, vomiting diarrhea, multi-organ failure (usually kidneys and liver), and a generalized erythematous rash that leads to desquamation of the palms and soles. This condition is usually associated with nasal packing after surgery but has also been noted to occur in the presence of excessive crusts without packing, as long as 5 weeks after surgery.[51]

Management includes intravenous antibiotics, aggressive fluid resuscitation and supportive measures in an intensive care setting. Preventative treatment mandates antibiotic coverage targeting *Staphylococcus aureus* whenever nasal packing is used.

> **Note**
> Although, toxic shock syndrome may be rapidly fatal if untreated, patients usually recover with appropriate and timely management.

Myospherulosis

Myospherulosis is a rare idiopathic foreign body reaction to the petroleum component in ointments used in packing or as an antibiotic coating for stenting material at the end of surgery. The term was originally coined as a result of the histopathologic appearance of affected muscle or subcutaneous tissues, which resembled pseudocysts or "myospherules".[52] The occurrence of this condition tends to adversely affect healing by promoting the formation of adhesions.[53] For this reason, and because petroleum-based ointments are not absorbable within the sinonasal cavity, it is advisable to minimize their use at the conclusion of surgery; water-based creams are a more favorable choice for antibiotic agents to be used on stenting material within the nasal cavity.

Conclusion

Endoscopic sinus surgery is an essential element in the continuum of management of medically refractory chronic rhinosinusitis. Constant refinements in endoscopic technique are allowing an expanded range of applications and a lower rate of complications for this kind of surgery. However, the potential for devastating complications is always present. The sinus surgeon must always be aware of this fact; actively seeking to identify high-risk situations preoperatively, employing careful surgical technique to minimize the risk of complications, and having a clear emergency plan to deal with their inevitable occurrence. In the end, the sinus surgeon must recognize his or her own limitations, and select surgical cases that are commensurate with his or her level of expertise.

References

1. Stankiewicz JA. Complications of sinus surgery. In: Bailey BJ Johnson JT, Newlands SD, eds. Head & Neck Surgery—Otolaryngology. 4th ed. Philadelphia: Lippincott Williams & Wilkins; 2006:477–491
2. May M, Levine HL, Mester SJ, Schaitkin B. Complications of endoscopic sinus surgery: analysis of 2108 patients—incidence and prevention. Laryngoscope 1994;104(9):1080–1083
3. Ramakrishnan VR, Kingdom TT, Nayak JV, Hwang PH, Orlandi RR. Nationwide incidence of major complications in endoscopic sinus surgery. Int Forum Allergy Rhinol 2012;2(1):34–39
4. Cohen-Kerem R, Brown S, Villaseñor LV, Witterick I. Epinephrine/Lidocaine injection vs. saline during endoscopic sinus surgery. Laryngoscope 2008;118(7):1275–1281
5. Wormald PJ, Athanasiadis T, Rees G, Robinson S. An evaluation of effect of pterygopalatine fossa injection with local anesthetic and adrenalin in the control of nasal bleeding during endoscopic sinus surgery. Am J Rhinol 2005;19(3):288–292
6. Wormald PJ, van Renen G, Perks J, Jones JA, Langton-Hewer CD. The effect of the total intravenous

anesthesia compared with inhalational anesthesia on the surgical field during endoscopic sinus surgery. Am J Rhinol 2005;19(5):514–520
7. Athanasiadis T, Beule AG, Wormald PJ. Effects of topical antifibrinolytics in endoscopic sinus surgery: a pilot randomized controlled trial. Am J Rhinol 2007;21(6):737–742
8. Eberhart LH, Folz BJ, Wulf H, Geldner G. Intravenous anesthesia provides optimal surgical conditions during microscopic and endoscopic sinus surgery. Laryngoscope 2003;113(8):1369–1373
9. Sieskiewicz A, Olszewska E, Rogowski M, Grycz E. Preoperative corticosteroid oral therapy and intraoperative bleeding during functional endoscopic sinus surgery in patients with severe nasal polyposis: a preliminary investigation. Ann Otol Rhinol Laryngol 2006;115(7):490–494
10. Douglas R, Wormald PJ. Pterygopalatine fossa infiltration through the greater palatine foramen: where to bend the needle. Laryngoscope 2006;116(7):1255–1257
11. Floreani SR, Nair SB, Switajewski MC, Wormald PJ. Endoscopic anterior ethmoidal artery ligation: a cadaver study. Laryngoscope 2006;116(7):1263–1267
12. Lee HY, Kim HU, Kim SS, et al. Surgical anatomy of the sphenopalatine artery in lateral nasal wall. Laryngoscope 2002;112(10):1813–1818
13. Bumm K, Heupel J, Bozzato A, Iro H, Hornung J. Localization and infliction pattern of iatrogenic skull base defects following endoscopic sinus surgery at a teaching hospital. Auris Nasus Larynx 2009;36(6):671–676
14. Wormald PJ. The axillary flap approach to the frontal recess. Laryngoscope 2002;112(3):494–499
15. Wormald PJ, Chan SZ. Surgical techniques for the removal of frontal recess cells obstructing the frontal ostium. Am J Rhinol 2003;17(4):221–226
16. Wormald PJ, McDonogh M. The bath-plug closure of anterior skull base cerebrospinal fluid leaks. Am J Rhinol 2003;17(5):299–305
17. Brodie HA. Prophylactic antibiotics for posttraumatic cerebrospinal fluid fistulae. A meta-analysis. Arch Otolaryngol Head Neck Surg 1997;123(7):749–752
18. Levin LA, Beck RW, Joseph MP, Seiff S, Kraker R. The treatment of traumatic optic neuropathy: the International Optic Nerve Trauma Study. Ophthalmology 1999;106(7):1268–1277
19. Bhatti MT, Schmalfuss IM, Mancuso AA. Orbital complications of functional endoscopic sinus surgery: MR and CT findings. Clin Radiol 2005;60(8):894–904
20. Graham SM, Nerad JA. Orbital complications in endoscopic sinus surgery using powered instrumentation. Laryngoscope 2003;113(5):874–878
21. Wormald PJ, McDonogh M. The 'swing-door' technique for uncinectomy in endoscopic sinus surgery. J Laryngol Otol 1998;112(6):547–551
22. Blanchard CL, Young LA. Acquired inflammatory superior oblique tendon sheath (Brown's) syndrome. Report of a case following frontal sinus surgery. Arch Otolaryngol 1984;110(2):120–122
23. Rosenbaum AL, Astle WF. Superior oblique and inferior rectus muscle injury following frontal and intranasal sinus surgery. J Pediatr Ophthalmol Strabismus 1985; 22(5):194–202
24. Leibovitch I, Wormald PJ, Crompton J, Selva D. Iatrogenic Brown's syndrome during endoscopic sinus surgery with powered instruments. Otolaryngol Head Neck Surg 2005;133(2):300–301
25. Huang CM, Meyer DR, Patrinely JR, et al. Medial rectus muscle injuries associated with functional endoscopic sinus surgery: characterization and management. Ophthal Plast Reconstr Surg 2003;19(1):25–37
26. Thacker NM, Velez FG, Demer JL, Wang MB, Rosenbaum AL. Extraocular muscle damage associated with endoscopic

sinus surgery: an ophthalmology perspective. Am J Rhinol 2005;19(4):400–405

27. Hong S, Lee HK, Lee JB, Han SH. Recession–resection combined with intraoperative botulinum toxin A chemodenervation for exotropia following subtotal ruptured of medial rectus muscle. Graefes Arch Clin Exp Ophthalmol 2007;245(1):167–169

28. Stankiewicz JA, Chow JM. Two faces of orbital hematoma in intranasal (endoscopic) sinus surgery. Otolaryngol Head Neck Surg 1999;120(6):841–847

29. Hayreh SS, Kolder HE, Weingeist TA. Central retinal artery occlusion and retinal tolerance time. Ophthalmology 1980;87(1):75–78

30. Bolger WE, Parsons DS, Mair EA, Kuhn FA. Lacrimal drainage system injury in functional endoscopic sinus surgery. Incidence, analysis, and prevention. Arch Otolaryngol Head Neck Surg 1992;118(11):1179–1184

31. Davis WE, Templer JW, Lamear WR, Davis WE Jr, Craig SB. Middle meatus anstrostomy: patency rates and risk factors. Otolaryngol Head Neck Surg 1991;104(4):467–472

32. Freedman HM, Kern EB. Complications of intranasal ethmoidectomy: a review of 1,000 consecutive operations. Laryngoscope 1979;89(3):421–434

33. Kennedy DW, Zinreich SJ, Shaalan H, Kuhn F, Naclerio R, Loch E. Endoscopic middle meatal antrostomy: theory, technique, and patency. Laryngoscope 1987; 97(8 Pt 3, Suppl 43):1–9

34. Serdahl CL, Berris CE, Chole RA. Nasolacrimal duct obstruction after endoscopic sinus surgery. Arch Ophthalmol 1990;108(3):391–392

35. Chu CT, Lebowitz RA, Jacobs JB. An analysis of sites of disease in revision endoscopic sinus surgery. Am J Rhinol 1997;11(4):287–291

36. Musy PY, Kountakis SE. Anatomic findings in patients undergoing revision endoscopic sinus surgery. Am J Otolaryngol 2004;25(6):418–422

37. Bolger WE, Kuhn FA, Kennedy DW. Middle turbinate stabilization after functional endoscopic sinus surgery: the controlled synechiae technique. Laryngoscope 1999;109 (11):1852–1853

38. Schlosser RJ, Zachmann G, Harrison S, Gross CW. The endoscopic modified Lothrop: long-term follow-up on 44 patients. Am J Rhinol 2002;16(2):103–108

39. Casiano RR, Livingston JA. Endoscopic Lothrop procedure: the University of Miami experience. Am J Rhinol 1998;12(5):335–339

40. Georgalas C, Hansen F, Videler WJ, Fokkens WJ. Long terms results of Draf type III (modified endoscopic Lothrop) frontal sinus drainage procedure in 122 patients: a single centre experience. Rhinology 2011;49(2):195–201

41. Tran KN, Beule AG, Singal D, Wormald PJ. Frontal ostium restenosis after the endoscopic modified Lothrop procedure. Laryngoscope 2007;117(8):1457–1462

42. Rajapaksa SP, Ananda A, Cain T, Oates L, Wormald PJ. The effect of the modified endoscopic Lothrop procedure on the mucociliary clearance of the frontal sinus in an animal model. Am J Rhinol 2004;18(3):183–187

43. Samaha M, Cosenza MJ, Metson R. Endoscopic frontal sinus drillout in 100 patients. Arch Otolaryngol Head Neck Surg 2003;129(8):854–858

44. Weber R, Mai R, Hosemann W, Draf W, Toffel P. The success of 6-month stenting in endonasal frontal sinus surgery. Ear Nose Throat J 2000;79(12):930–932, 934, 937–938 passim

45. Amonoo-Kuofi K, Lund VJ, Andrews P, Howard DJ. The role of mitomycin C in surgery of the frontonasal recess: a prospective open pilot study. Am J Rhinol 2006;20(6):591–594

46. Ramadan HH. Surgical causes of failure in endoscopic sinus surgery. Laryngoscope 1999;109(1):27–29

47. Grobler A, Weitzel EK, Buele A, et al. Pre- and postoperative sinus penetration of nasal irrigation. Laryngoscope 2008;118(11):2078–2081

48. Caylakli F, Yavuz H, Cagici AC, Ozluoglu LN. Endoscopic sinus surgery for maxillary sinus mucoceles. Head Face Med 2006;2:29

49. Har-El G. Endoscopic management of 108 sinus mucoceles. Laryngoscope 2001;111(12):2131–2134

50. Parsons DS, Stivers FE, Talbot AR. The missed ostium sequence and the surgical approach to revision functional endoscopic sinus surgery. Otolaryngol Clin North Am 1996;29(1):169–183

51. Younis RT, Lazar RH. Delayed toxic shock syndrome after functional endonasal sinus surgery. Arch Otolaryngol Head Neck Surg 1996;122(1):83–85

52. McClatchie S, Warambo MW, Bremner AD. Myospherulosis: a previously unreported disease? Am J Clin Pathol 1969;51(6):699–704

53. Sindwani R, Cohen JT, Pilch BZ, Metson RB. Myospherulosis following sinus surgery: pathological curiosity or important clinical entity? Laryngoscope 2003; 113(7):1123–1127

10 Complications in Endoscopic Skull Base Surgery

B. A. Otto, D. de Lara, L. F. S. Ditzel Filho, R. Cadore Malfado, D. M. Prevedello, A. B. Kassam, R. L. Carrau

Introduction

Recent technologic advances and a greater understanding of the intricate anatomy of the human skull base have fostered exponential growth of endoscopic skull base surgery (ESBS) to treat a large variety of benign and malignant conditions of the skull base. Over the past decade, neurosurgeons and otolaryngologists, working in accord, have transformed ESBS from its initial alternative role to that of standard of care for many pathologic processes involving the skull base.

As with any other paradigm shift in medicine, ESBS has faced some criticism and disbelief. Cerebrospinal fluid (CSF) leaks, nasal flora contamination and risk of postoperative infections, inability to comfortably reach or fully resect complex lesions and the steep learning curve necessary to master these techniques were but a few of the obstacles that the emerging field had to overcome. Slowly but consistently, most of these issues were addressed and resolved. Recent outcome studies have demonstrated that, although not perfect, endoscopic techniques are safe and effective when practiced by experienced hands in carefully selected patients.[1-4] Nonetheless, as in traditional skull base surgery, the complex nature of skull base anatomy and diversity of diseases that affect the region leads to a certain degree of risk of surgery-related morbidity and mortality.

The aim of this chapter is to provide an overview of the complications related to ESBS. As with any surgical procedure, potential for treatment-related or disease-related complications exists in all phases of patient care (i.e., presurgical, intraoperative, and postoperative). Although discussion of presurgical complications is beyond the objectives of this chapter, consideration of potential treatment-related complications begins with the initial patient encounter. Likewise, risk reduction strategies and prevention of intraoperative and postoperative complications begin in the preoperative phase.

Scope of the Problem

The established complication rate for skull base surgery is variable because of the heterogeneity of conditions treated and the various approaches necessary to access lesions of the skull base. Most contemporary literature regarding surgical resection of malignant skull base tumors reports complication and mortality rates ranging from 30 to 50% and 0 to 7%, respectively.[5,6] A recent international multi-institutional study aimed at identifying predictors of morbidity and mortality related to craniofacial resection for a variety of skull base lesions identified respective rates of 36.3% and 4.7% in a study population of 1,193 patients. In that study, the presence of comorbid medical conditions was a significant predictor of mortality, and comorbid medical conditions, previous radiation treatment, dural invasion, and brain invasion were significant predictors of postoperative complications.[5]

> **Note**
> The overall complication rate related to ESBS is not as well established, but appears comparable or even favorable to traditional techniques.[1]

While most of the same hurdles of traditional surgical approaches hold for ESBS, there are some differences, mainly because the sinonasal cavity serves as the corridor. In addition, ESBS is still in its infancy relative to traditional approaches. Techniques and protocols are not universal among the community of physicians treating skull base diseases. Furthermore, within institutions, the complication rates will undoubtedly fluctuate as techniques are mastered. In a recent review, Kassam et al[1] reported on 800 ESBS cases performed for a variety of skull base diseases. Barring CSF leaks, the overall rate of complications related to ESBS was 9.3%. In their review, there was an overall CSF leak rate of 15.9%. However, as noted above, the postoperative CSF leak rate was dynamic, and with the introduction of pedicled flaps, the CSF leak rate was brought to less than 5%.[7]

Complication Avoidance

> **Note**
> Comprehensive complication management starts with risk reduction and avoidance.

First and foremost, the surgical team should be appropriately trained in both endoscopic and traditional open techniques. Although otolaryngologists are generally comfortable with endoscopic endonasal surgery, challenges arise when first attempting two-surgeon, three-handed or four-handed surgery. Accordingly, teams should mature by progressing from less complex to more complex cases as experience leads.

Anatomic Corridors in Endoscopic Endonasal Approaches

Endoscopic endonasal approaches may be organized as modules based on anatomical corridors in the sagittal and coronal planes:

- Sagittal plane modules use corridors medial to the lamina papyracea and internal carotid artery (ICA) and include transcribriform, transplanum, transtuberculum, transsellar, transclival, and transodontoid approaches.
- Coronal plane approaches are divided into anterior, mid, and posterior modules.

Anterior Plane Modules

Anterior plane modules provide both extraconal and intraconal access to the orbits. Orbital decompression for Grave disease is one example of an extraconal approach. Intraconal approaches generally use the corridor between the medial and inferior rectus muscles to address lesions medial to the optic nerve.

Midcoronal and Posterior Coronal Planes

The midcoronal and posterior coronal planes are divided into seven anatomical zones based on their relationship to the ICA. The "infrapetrous" and "suprapetrous" planes referred to in this discussion pertain to the plane to the petrous ICA, not necessarily the petrous bone. The seven anatomical zones are as follows:

- Zone 1: the anterior petrous apex.
- Zone 2: the midbody of the petrous bone below the level of the horizontal segment of the petrous carotid.
- Zone 3: the suprapetrous region consisting of the *quadrangular space.* The quadrangular space is defined medially by the paraclival ICA, inferiorly by the horizontal segment of the petrous ICA, laterally by the second division of the trigeminal nerve, and superiorly by the course of the sixth cranial nerve within the cavernous sinus. Through this approach the Meckel cave and the gasserian ganglion can be reached.
- Zone 4: the superior lateral cavernous sinus, representing the region through which the oculomotor (III), trochlear (IV), first division of the trigeminal (V), and abducens (VI) nerves traverse.
- Zone 5: the transpterygoid/infratemporal space with direct access to the middle fossa.
- Zone 6: the region of the condyle, the paramedian region located immediately lateral to the inferior third of the clivus and foramen magnum. It is anterolaterally bound by the eustachian tube and fossa of

Table 10.1 Suggested levels of training

Level 1	Sinonasal surgery
Level 2	Traumatic or spontaneous cerebrospinal fluid leaks Intrasellar or limited extrasellar lesions
Level 3 (Extradural)	Median approaches to the ventral skull base where the dura is not entered Trans-odontoid approach
Level 4 (Intradural)	Normal tissue separates the lesion from vascular structures Lesion adjacent or adhered to vascular structures
Level 5 (Vascular)	Paramedian approaches (dissection of the internal carotid artery) Lesions invading or surrounding vascular structures.

Rosenmuller, which mark the parapharyngeal ICA laterally. Superiorly it has its limit on the petroclival synchondrosis. Lesions in this region can involve the hypoglossal canal.

- Zone 7: the region lateral to the parapharyngeal ICA. The approach for this region extends along the floor of the maxillary sinus and contains the lateral pterygoid plate and attached soft tissue. Most importantly, this region contains the jugular foramen posteriorly.[8–11]

A systematic approach to training, based on graduated mastery of approaches with progressive levels of difficulty has been recommended (**Table 10.1**).[4] The levels of difficulty depicted in **Table 10.1** are important, as this stratification has significant implications on the potential complications that one may encounter in the perioperative period.

Principles of Endoscopic Endonasal Surgery

The specific techniques germane to endoscopic endonasal skull base surgery have been described extensively in the literature and will not be detailed in this chapter.[3,4,8–13] However, there are certain key principles that should be consistently adhered to:

- Choosing the correct corridor and creating sufficient room for unhindered three-handed or four-handed dissection
- Meticulous dissection of the tumor or lesion
- Minimizing trauma to surrounding neurovascular structures
- Adequate reconstruction of the skull base to separate the intracranial and sinonasal cavities.

> **Note**
> The sinonasal cavity should be respected, as inadvertent mucosal trauma may lead to unnecessary sinonasal morbidity.

Surgical Planning

Beyond surgical training, the surgical team should incorporate a regular, standardized approach to surgical planning. Preoperative imaging should be obtained in advance of the procedure. In our program, we review imaging as a team at least weekly. Likewise, any available pathology should be reviewed. When not contraindicated by prolapse of meninges or tumor vascularity, neoplasms involving the sinonasal cavity should be biopsied either in the office or operative suite before definitive resection. This allows the surgeon to best inform the patient of the expected extent of resection, expected morbidity and potential risks based not only on size and location of tumor, but on pathology. Referral to appropriate medical services and/or anesthesiology allows for risk stratification and medical optimization.

> **Note**
> In cases where significant blood loss is anticipated, blood products should be made available.

Intraoperative Steps

Depending on the pathology, extent of disease, planned procedure, and medical comorbidities, further steps may be taken to avoid, or at least optimally treat, complications or intraoperative hurdles. Computer-assisted stereotactic navigation is widely used in ESBS. It is important to review the available imaging studies to ensure that they were performed with the appropriate protocol for use with these systems when needed.

Neurophysiologic monitoring, including somatosensory evoked potentials and surveillance of cranial nerves at risk during dissection, is used routinely at our institution. In addition to feedback regarding nearby cranial nerves, neurophysiologic monitoring of somatosensory evoked potentials may serve as a general indicator of cortical perfusion during management of carotid artery injury.

In cases where the carotid artery is encased in tumor, or where extensive dissection around the artery is necessary, preoperative imaging, including magnetic resonance angiography or computed tomography angiography, can be performed to gain an understanding of the intracranial vasculature. These studies can be used for computer-assisted stereotactic navigation. Additionally, angiography provides an accurate anatomical assessment of tumor vascularity, intracranial circulation and collateral circulation. However, to best determine if there is sufficient collateral flow to withstand occlusion of the ICA, angiography balloon occlusion xenon computed tomography is recommended.[14]

Intraoperative Complications

> **Note**
> The majority of intraoperative complications and the major sources of morbidity in skull base surgery relate to intraoperative neural or vascular injury. As might be expected, the incidence of neural and vascular complications is higher in more complex cases, specifically Level IV and V procedures.

Bleeding and Vascular Injury

Intraoperative bleeding remains one of the most significant challenges to safe resection of skull base tumors. As in any approach, the location, size, and vascularity of the tumor, the length of the case, and any systemic factors leading to a bleeding diathesis contribute to blood loss. In ESBS, the sinonasal corridor may present a significant factor in overall blood loss because of the vascularity of sinonasal mucosa.

Bleeding Classification

In general, bleeding may be categorized based on two factors; the source (venous or arterial) and the rate (low flow or high flow):
- Low-flow venous bleeding is most commonly encountered as diffuse mucosal oozing, whereas an example of high-flow venous bleeding is that which occurs from the cavernous sinus.
- Low-flow arterial bleeding occurs from small vessels, such as perforating vessels, whereas high-flow arterial bleeding includes medium to large vessels, such as the sphenopalatine or internal maxillary arteries, as well as the ICA.

Generally, this categorization will allow the surgeon to determine the most appropriate method to achieve hemostasis. However, the choice is also influenced by factors such as the type of tissue (mucosa, bone, or tumor); the proximity of neurovascular structures; and the area (extradural or intradural) of dissection.[12]

Low-Flow Venous Bleeding

Low-flow venous oozing is commonly encountered during the dissection and development of the sinonasal corridor.

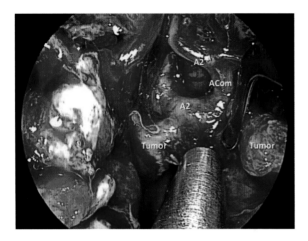

Fig. 10.1 Intraoperative endoscopic view of a transcribriform approach for resection of an olfactory groove meningioma. Meticulous dissection of the underlying vascular structures is paramount to preventing cerebrovascular complications. A2 = A2 segment of the anterior cerebral artery; ACom = anterior communicating artery.

In our experience, warm saline irrigation is quite effective in addressing this type of bleeding. A recommended temperature for irrigation is 40 to 42°C.[12] Especially during lengthy cases, it is important to keep an account of the irrigation used to maintain an accurate assessment of blood loss. For persistent focal low-flow venous bleeding, or in some cases of more brisk venous bleeding, such as that which occurs from focal cavernous sinus exposure, application of hemostatic agents, such as Floseal (Baxter International Inc.; Deerfield, IL, USA) or Avitene (Ethicon Inc., Johnson and Johnson; Somerville, NJ, USA), is frequently successful.

Arterial Bleeding

Although the rate of arterial bleeding is generally proportional to the size of the vessel, the neurologic consequences of arterial damage are not necessarily size dependent. This fact underscores the need to respect arterial vessels of all sizes, practicing meticulous dissection with judicious use of cautery (**Fig. 10.1**).

Small arterial damage is generally encountered during dissection of tumor from the surrounding neurovascular bed. In appropriately selected patients in whom there is no significant cortical cuff or critical neurovascular structure (i.e., optic nerve) between the tumor and sinonasal corridor, endoscopic endonasal approaches allow resection of tumor with minimal brain retraction or dissection. Nonetheless, the interface between the tumor and the underlying neurovascular stroma must be respected and dissection at the interface should be meticulous. In the anterior cranial fossa, frontal polar arteries are encountered during dissection of tumors such as olfactory neuroblastoma or olfactory groove meningioma. Similarly, in

the middle and posterior cranial fossae, small perforating vessels supplying the brainstem and optic chiasm must be preserved to prevent potentially catastrophic deficits.[15]

In the aforementioned review of 800 cases, Kassam et al[1] reported a total of seven major intraoperative vascular complications that encompassed 0.9% of cases. In one patient, avulsion of a P1 perforator resulted in severe, but transient dysphasia. There were three patients with significant permanent deficits resulting from intraoperative vascular injury: one patient was rendered quadriplegic by a pontine bleed, one patient developed hemiparesis following an internal maxillary artery laceration, and one patient developed unilateral lower limb paresis following a frontopolar avulsion. In one patient, an ophthalmic artery avulsion occurred, but there were no sequelae as the patient was already blind in that eye.

In general, injury to small or medium-sized vessels, such as those mentioned here, are encountered during exposure or dissection of the lesion. Control of bleeding from these vessels depends not only on the flow rate, but also on adjacent anatomy. Bipolar electrocautery is quite effective and efficient. When appropriate, it is the authors' method of choice. However, thermal damage to adjacent structures may preclude the use of bipolar electrocautery. In this situation, application of hemostatic agents, such as Floseal or Avitene are efficacious, especially when the surrounding anatomy is amenable to the application of gentle pressure to these agents to form a "seal" at the site of the defect.

Internal Carotid Artery Injury

Perhaps the most feared vascular complication in ESBS is ICA injury. Of the seven (0.9%) cases of intraoperative vascular injury noted above, two involved the ICA. Neither patient had a permanent deficit. Comprising up to 12.8% of all intracranial aneurysms, cavernous ICA aneurysms are not infrequent and may be more prevalent in patients with pituitary adenoma. In a review of a case series involving ICA injury, 6 of 111 cases occurred in the setting of unrecognized preoperative ICA aneurysm.

> **Note**
>
> Anatomical risks for intraoperative ICA injury include carotid dehiscence, sphenoid septal attachment to the ICA, and medialized ICA. Other risks include revision surgery, previous radiotherapy, previous bromocriptine treatment, and acromegaly.[16]

As the highest of high-flow arterial bleeding generally encountered in ESBS, an emergent, efficient, coordinated team approach is key to successful management. Because many tasks must occur simultaneously, every member of the operating team must be ready to act in the event of a carotid injury. In addition to repairing the injury, steps must also be taken to prevent collateral deleterious

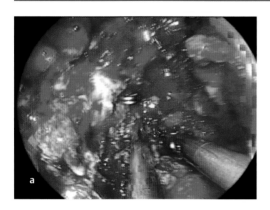
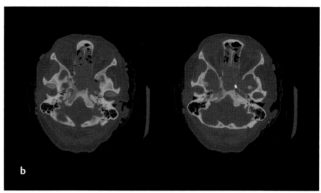

Fig. 10.2a,b Aneurysm clip.

a Intraoperative endoscopic view of an aneurysm clip placed to control a left internal carotid artery injury.

b Postoperative computed tomography scan demonstrating the aneurysm clip used to repair the left internal carotid artery.

effects. Cerebral perfusion pressure must remain adequate. For this reason, controlled hypertension is desired to maintain cerebral perfusion; hypotensive anesthesia is contraindicated. Neurophysiologic monitoring is vital in this situation, as it offers a reflection of cerebral perfusion. Additionally, the patient should be anticoagulated. In the setting of carotid injury, anticoagulation theoretically has minimal effect on overall blood loss. However, it may help to prevent embolic phenomena during and after repair of the vessel. Additional medical resuscitation and administration of blood products must be an ongoing, dynamic process coordinated by anesthesia and support staff.

Although compression of the ipsilateral cervical carotid artery may diminish proximal flow, it will generally be insufficient because of collateral flow leading to increased distal bleeding and incomplete closure by compression. Successful immediate control and repair should be directed on the defect. A two-surgeon, four-hand approach is critical in this situation, allowing for bimanual repair of the defect by one surgeon with simultaneous evacuation of blood from the cavity and dynamic control and cleansing of the scope by the other surgeon.

Based on an animal model of carotid artery damage, Valentine and Wormald[17] evaluated various techniques used during control of carotid artery rupture. Based on their experience, seamless, coordinated teamwork and the ability to maintain visualization are paramount to controlling the surgical field. Strategies for maintaining visualization include the use of lens-cleaning devices, use of larger bore suctions (12-Fr or larger) and strategic endoscope navigation through the nasal cavity with less blood flow. Frequently, the posterior septal margin shields one nasal cavity from the stream of blood, rendering it more favorable for endoscopic navigation. Once adequate visualization is achieved, the view is maintained by using the suction tip to direct the stream of blood while the repair

is accomplished. While using suction and gentle pressure with a cottonoid, the defect is exposed and repaired. In some cases, surrounding bone must be removed to fully access the defect. Repair options include bipolar electrocauterization of the vessel to "weld" the defect or to induce thrombosis of the vessel; direct compression; compressive packing; suture repair; reconstruction using aneurysm clips (**Fig. 10.2**); and circumferential ligation or clipping of the vessel.[15] Application of a crushed muscle patch is also an effective option;[17] if the thigh or abdomen is prepped for the harvest of fascia, then muscle can usually be obtained quickly by an additional surgeon if available.

Once the bleeding is controlled, the patient should undergo endovascular assessment followed by completion of the definitive repair. It should be noted that if the dura is opened, compressive packing should be avoided to prevent bleeding into the subdural space. Although in most cases the carotid is ultimately sacrificed, it is possible to preserve patency via the use of covered stents.[18] Intraoperative preservation of the vessel may be best achieved using aneurysm clips or lumen-sparing Sundt–Keyes clips.

Neurologic Injury

Incidence of significant neural injury related to ESBS ranges from 0 to 33%, and is dependent mainly on the level of difficulty of the cases presented.[1,19,20] Based on a previous report, the rate of neural injury is 1.8%, with 0.5% of all patients experiencing permanent cranial neuropathy, 0.8% a transient cranial neuropathy and 0.5% transient hemiparesis. The permanent deficits included cranial nerve VI (two patients), cranial nerves IX and X (one patient), and cranial nerves IX, X, and XII (one patient). The transient deficits included cranial nerve III (two patients), V3 motor (one patient), cranial nerve VI (three patients), and hemiparesis (four patients).[1] When

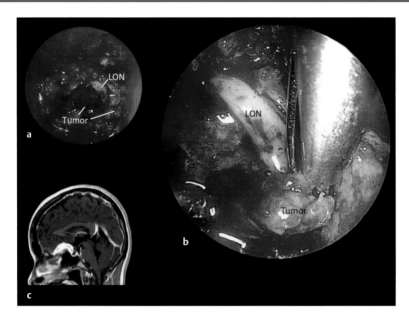

Fig. 10.3a–c Intraoperative endoscopic view of a transplanum approach for resection of a planum sphenoidale meningioma.

a Olfactory nerve is encased by the tumor. LON: left olfactory nerve.

b Dissecting the tumor from the nerve with direct visualization.

c Preoperative sagittal T1-weighted magnetic resonance image.

stratified based on levels of difficulty, Level IV and V procedures were demonstrated to be predictors of neurologic injury. When considering extrasellar surgery alone, the rate of intraoperative neural injury is 2.4% (1% permanent deficit), which is favorable, or at least comparable, to microscopic transsphenoidal surgery or traditional skull base surgical resection of tumors.[1] In addition to the cases noted above, there was a 1.9% rate of delayed postoperative neural deficit, with 0.6% representing permanent deficits. Nonetheless, the overall rate of permanent neurologic deficit was less than 1%.[1]

Abducens Palsy (Cranial Nerve VI)

The most common cranial neuropathy encountered is cranial nerve VI palsy.[1,21] Injury to the abducens nerve compromises the function of the lateral rectus muscle, resulting is diplopia. At the level of the clivus and cavernous sinus, the abducens nerve is the most ventrally situated cranial nerve. The nerve is particularly at risk during transclival and paramedian approaches. Tumors or other skull base diseases may compress the nerve resulting in preoperative palsy, and those occupying the prepontine cistern may displace the nerve in any direction, increasing intraoperative risk. A thorough understanding of normal anatomy, coupled with a prediction of the origin of the lesion to be addressed may give insight into expected variations in the course of the nerve.[21,22]

As described by Barges-Coll et al,[21] identifying key anatomical landmarks can help to prevent injury to cranial nerve VI during dissection. During a transclival approach, the vertebrobasilar junction is used as a landmark for the dural opening. Other useful landmarks include the lacerum segment of the ICA for the medial petrous apex approach, and cranial nerve V2 for the Meckel's cave

approach. V2 serves as a landmark to determine the maximum height of the quadrangular space that can be dissected. It should be remembered that the approaches mentioned above require significant dissection around the ICA, and represent advanced procedures. While the ICA provides a useful landmark for cranial nerve VI, it also poses increased risk not only to the ICA itself, but also to the vasa nervorum of cranial nerve VI via injury of the inferolateral trunk.[21]

As noted previously, neurophysiologic monitoring should be used in any case where cranial nerves are at risk. Meticulous, unhindered dissection, made possible by an adequate sinonasal corridor, is required when dissecting lesions from surrounding cranial nerves (**Fig. 10.3**). Unless removal of a segment of a cranial nerve or extensive dissection along the nerve is necessary to meet a more significant priority, protection of the surrounding cranial nerve should be a top priority during dissection. Poor tolerance of manipulation mandates that the corridor should not cross the plane of a given cranial nerve. Therefore, the use of multiple corridors (either lateral or anterior) should be implemented when necessary. When a paralysis is noted postoperatively, especially when unexpected, imaging studies may assist in ruling out postoperative etiologies such as compression from hematoma. Additionally, other sources of compression should be addressed, such as nasal packing compressing the optic nerves resulting in postoperative visual loss.[1]

Postoperative Complications

Major complications directly related to surgery generally involve disruption of the skull base reconstruction with associated CSF leak or pneumocephalus; infection, manifesting as meningitis and/or abscess; delayed intracranial bleeding, delayed neurologic deficit, such as visual loss or hemiplegia; or systemic complications, such as deep venous thrombosis or pneumonia.

Complications Related to Skull Base Reconstruction

The major goal of skull base reconstruction following ESBS is complete separation of the intracranial and sinonasal cavities. When this goal is not met, the clinical consequence is generally manifested as a CSF leak, which in and of itself is little more than a nuisance. However, the potential sequelae or concomitant conditions associated with CSF leaks mandates prompt attention to those patients identified postoperatively. For example, clinical evidence of CSF leak in a patient with acute mental status changes should prompt an investigation into and treatment of possible tension pneumocephalus. Similarly, the association of meningitis with CSF leaks further supports prompt treatment to avoid this life-threatening associated complication.

Cerebrospinal Fluid Rhinorrhea

One of the hurdles in the evolution of ESBS has been the prevention of postoperative CSF leak. Although several options for skull base reconstruction exist, the introduction of the Hadad–Bassagaisteguy nasoseptal flap revolutionized ESBS and has since become the workhorse of skull base reconstruction for endoscopic approaches. Since the introduction of the nasal septal flap, other local intranasal flaps have been described, including middle turbinate, inferior turbinate, anterior and posterior pedicle lateral nasal wall mucosal flaps. Additionally, locoregional flaps such as pericranial, temporalis, buccal, and palatal flaps have been described; however, these are generally only considered when intranasal flaps are not possible or are insufficient to cover the defect.

> **Note**
>
> Since the routine use of vascularized flaps, with the overwhelming majority comprising nasoseptal flaps, the postoperative CSF leak rate is less than 5%, down from over 40% initially.[7]

The main physiologic advantage of flaps is the maintenance of nutrients to the tissues, as opposed to mucosal grafts that rely on imbibition for nutrients, or acellular material that requires mucosalization of the defect to complete the healing process. Accordingly, one of the most important technical aspects related to the use of intranasal flaps is preservation of the neurovascular pedicle. This point is especially salient in light of the fact that in most cases, the pedicle must be fully dissected and freed up from the underlying bed to rotate and

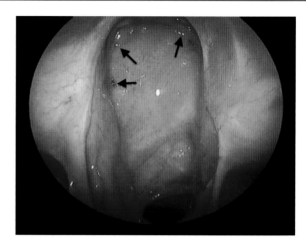

Fig. 10.4 Postoperative endoscopic view of the sinonasal cavity following endoscopic endonasal transcribriform resection of an olfactory neuroblastoma. U-clips (dark arrows) that were used to help secure the nasoseptal flap during reconstruction can be visualized.

advance the flap into position. In fact, full dissection of the pedicle is a critical step in obtaining the "reach" and arc of rotation necessary to fill some defects. To prevent desiccation of the pedicle and flap failure, underlying tissue must support the pedicle. In some situations, the reconstruction must be modified to achieve this requisite while simultaneously shortening the distance the flap must travel to reach the distal limit of the defect. For example, transcribriform resection of anterior cranial fossa tumors may leave a defect extending anteriorly to the frontal sinus. In this situation, the nasoseptal flap is generally not long enough to reach the anterior limit of the defect when the pedicle is draped along the sphenoid. A fat graft placed into the sphenoid sinus, after removal of mucosa, shortens the path necessary to reach the posterior table of the frontal sinus and provides a bed on which the pedicle is supported. Although this is frequently all that is required to sufficiently support the flap, in some cases additional measures may be taken to secure the flap. For example, placement of U-clips (Medtronic, Inc.; Minneapolis, MN, USA) along the anterior limit of the flap may help to prevent dehiscence along the anterior limit of the reconstruction during healing and contraction of the flap (**Fig. 10.4**). Finally, the recipient bed must be optimized before flap placement. Although in many cases, the underlying bed of the entire flap surface has been denuded, it has been demonstrated that the minimal requirement is circumferential removal of all mucosa from the bed immediately surrounding the defect.[23]

In our program, local flaps are used when possible as part of a multilayered closure. Before flap placement, the dural defect is covered with a resorbable collagen matrix graft (Duragen Dural Graft Matrix; Integra LifeSciences Corporation; Plainsboro, NJ, USA). It is the preference of the authors to place this as an inlay graft when possible. Next, the flap is placed into position, and full coverage of the defect is confirmed. When the flap is insufficient to fill the entire defect, the reconstruction can be modified to fill the gaps. As discussed above, fat placed in the sphenoid sinus may allow for a more efficient flap positioning to cover anterior defects. Gaps along the sides of the flap or in central defects may be closed using fascia, fat, or acellular dermis materials. Next, the flap must be supported in the initial healing phase. Our preference is to support the flap with synthetic glue (DuraSeal; Covidien; Mansfield, MA, USA), followed by a combination of absorbable/degradable packing and removable bolster. The removable bolster commonly consists of various combinations of nasal packing or balloon catheters. It is important to remember that no one material is perfect in every situation. The critical component of any supporting material is that it allows the flap to conform to the underlying defect along its edges with enough pressure to prevent egress of CSF while preserving perfusion of the flap tissue. The placement of absorbable or degradable materials between the flap and bolster helps to eliminate flap displacement during removal of the latter. The timing of removal is dependent on the size of the defect and nature of the leak. High-flow leaks and larger defects may require 5 to 7 days.

Taken together, the measures discussed above will optimize the chances of a successful closure. Nonetheless, there still exists a definite risk of postoperative CSF leak. In their review of 150 patients for whom the nasoseptal flap was used to reconstruct the skull base, Patel et al[7] identified six patients (4%) with a postoperative leak. Of this group, 59 patients had high-flow intraoperative leaks and four (6.7%) experienced a postoperative CSF leak. In the patients with low-flow intraoperative leaks, the postoperative CSF leak rate was 2.1% (2/91). When a leak is identified postoperatively, steps should be taken to repair the leak as quickly as possible to prevent associated tension pneumocephalus or meningitis. Options for repair include revision of the reconstruction under anesthesia or placement of a lumbar shunt. Although placement of a lumbar shunt may successfully resolve low-flow postoperative CSF leaks,[7] operative assessment and repair allows the surgeon to assess the defect, optimize position of grafts or flaps, and bolster the reconstruction with new tissue, such as abdominal fat, when necessary. In postoperative CSF leak cases where an intraoperative high-flow leak was noted, or when the placement of the flap is deemed to be sufficient, CSF diversion with a lumbar drain may improve the ability to resolve postoperative leaks. Similarly, expedient placement of ventriculoperitoneal shunts may help to decrease delayed postoperative CSF leaks in patients who have intracranial hypertension and concomitant skull base defects. For example, our postoperative protocol for a patient presenting with idiopathic CSF rhinorrhea and a clinical suspicion of idiopathic intracranial hypertension includes a lumbar tap and measurement of intracranial pressure 36 to 48 hours after repair of the skull base defect. If the pressure is greater than 25 mmHg, we offer the patient a ventriculoperitoneal shunt.

Tension Pneumocephalus

Tension pneumocephalus is a potentially life-threatening complication that results as a consequence of a skull base defect that acts as a one-way valve. Although intracranial air is frequently demonstrated on postoperative imaging following ESBS, the natural course is marked by slow, steady resolution of the air. Tension pneumocephalus differs in that the one-way valve causes continued ingress of air, resulting in increased intracranial pressure and compression of the brain. Air trapped in the intracranial cavity frequently compresses the frontal lobes, resulting in the "Mount Fuji Sign", a symmetrical cone-shaped appearance of the frontal lobes (**Fig. 10.5**).[24]

Treatment for tension pneumocephalus involves releasing the trapped air and repairing the skull base defect. The most expedient way of achieving these goals simultaneously is to return emergently to the operating suite. The reconstruction should be taken down and air should be allowed to exit. The skull base defect should then be meticulously replaced, augmenting any identified defects with grafts or other material as necessary. Maintaining adequate blood pressure and administering

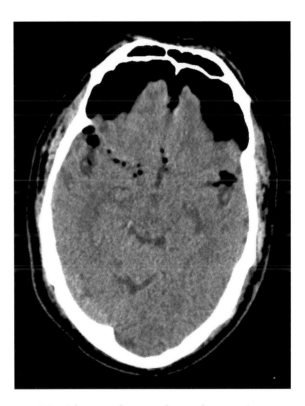

Fig. 10.5 Axial computed tomography scan demonstrating the "Mount Fuji" sign, that is characterized by symmetrical cone-shaped effacement of the frontal lobes caused by trapped intracranial air.

supplemental oxygen may help to maintain perfusion or even assist in absorption of air, but surgical evacuation of air is the most important factor in resolving tension pneumocephalus.[24,25] Similar to patients with postoperative CSF leak, the skull base defect that leads to tension pneumocephalus may be a risk factor for meningitis. Consideration should be made to continuing antibiotic prophylaxis in these patients for at least 24 to 48 hours following repair.

Infectious Complications

Meningitis

One of the more feared neurosurgical complications, acute bacterial meningitis is an infection of the meninges that often causes hearing loss and is fatal in 5 to 40% of children and 20 to 50% of adults despite adequate antibiotic administration.[26] The rate of meningitis following traditional transsphenoidal surgery ranges from 0.7 to 3.1%.[27–29] For open craniotomy the rate of meningitis ranges from 0.9 to 2.5%,[30–32] whereas for skull base procedures specifically, the rate ranges from 2.0 to 4.8%.[33,34] In a review of 1,000 cases, Kono et al[2] reported a 1.8% incidence of meningitis. Noted risk factors included male sex, history of surgery (craniotomy or endonasal surgery), procedures with higher levels of complexity (level IV or V), the placement of an external ventricular drain or a ventriculoperitoneal shunt before hospitalization, and postoperative CSF leakage. The most important risk factor was a postoperative CSF leak, with an intracranial infection occurring in 13 (9.3%) of 140 patients who experienced a postoperative CSF leak. Other studies have demonstrated this same correlation.[35,36]

ESBS procedures are generally "clean–contaminated" procedures, assuming the absence of acute bacterial rhinosinusitis at the time of the procedure. Because of the increased pathologic bacterial load associated with acute bacterial rhinosinusitis, we routinely abort any procedure where purulence is encountered during the approach. Other authors[37] have suggested that chronic inflammation related to chronic sinusitis may not be a contraindication to endoscopic endonasal pituitary surgery, as long as the patient has not recently experienced an acute infectious exacerbation. However, the timing of an elective surgery should be optimized and any infection should be treated before the skull base is transgressed. This is especially relevant if the resection will extend intradurally where seeding of bacteria has immediate life-threatening consequences.

Currently, there is no antibiotherapy that safely sterilizes the nasal cavity. Perioperative antibiotic prophylaxis has been evaluated previously, although randomized controlled studies specific to ESBS are lacking. The use of broad-spectrum prophylactic antibiotics has been evaluated for traditional skull base surgery, with an overall trend toward decreased wound infections with the use of perioperative antibiotics.[36,38] However, the efficacy of prophylactic antibiotics in preventing meningitis and brain abscess is controversial, as not all studies have demonstrated benefit.[36] In the review by Kono et al,[2] where a meningitis rate of less than 2% was noted, the standard antibiotic prophylaxis regimen used was ceftriaxone or cefepime. Vancomycin and aztreonam were administered to β-lactam-allergic patients. If the operation crossed the dura and the CSF was penetrated, antibiotic therapy was continued until the postoperative nasal packing was removed. Patients who had nasal packing without penetration of the dura received ampicillin–clavulanic acid or alternative antibiotics until the packing was removed. Antibiotics were discontinued after surgery for patients who did not receive nasal packing. Although more work is needed to clarify the role of perioperative prophylactic antibiotics, the current rate of meningitis related to ESBS remains low.

Nonetheless, adherence to strict aseptic techniques, preparation of the external nose and nasal aperture, and copious irrigation are routinely used at our institution. Before beginning the surgery, povidone–iodine solution is used to prepare the skin overlying the nose, adjacent midface and glabellar region. Care is taken to prevent entry of the solution into the eyes. If any additional approach is needed, the preparation is extended as indicated. We do not routinely place povidone–iodine posterior to the nasal vestibule. However, before intracranial exposure, we copiously irrigate the sinonasal cavity with saline. Nasal irrigation theoretically reduces the bacterial load of the sinonasal cavity and may be an important factor in reducing the overall microbial load of the sinonasal cavity and corridor before intracranial entry.

Regardless of the low rate of meningitis associated with ESBS, every case poses a risk to the patient. Patients should be educated regarding the symptoms of meningitis and instructed to report any concerns immediately. Clinical diagnosis of meningitis should prompt consultation of the infectious disease service, transfer to a monitored bed, and administration of broad-spectrum antibiotics. The addition of corticosteroids to the regimen may reduce the risk of neurologic sequelae of meningitis, including sensorineural hearing loss. However, there does not appear to be a significant survival benefit to the addition of corticosteroids.[26]

Systemic Complications

Systemic complications related to ESBS occur in 2.9% of cases overall, but range from 1.6 to 6.7% depending on the level of complexity of a given case. Risk factors such as age over 60 years, Cushing disease, and postoperative CSF leak have been shown to predict postoperative systemic complications.[1,39] As in any other surgical procedure, cardiopulmonary, peripheral vascular, renal, gastrointestinal, endocrine, or other systemic complications can be a hurdle to a successful outcome. Presurgical risk stratification and medical optimization may help to clear some of these hurdles. Nonetheless, these complications remain a real risk for anyone undergoing surgery. As in any complication, management of the problem, with consultation to appropriate specialists should be completed as quickly as possible. If indicated, transfer to a more acute setting may help to prevent a snowballing of unwanted events. In addition to routine postoperative monitoring and care related to any systemic complications, proper nutrition is paramount. If a feeding tube must be placed, this should be accomplished by the otolaryngology service under direct visualization to prevent inadvertent intracranial placement of the tube.

Conclusion

ESBS is a dynamic, evolving field. The techniques employed have given surgical teams new opportunities to treat skull base disease in a potentially less invasive manner. Although more work is needed, ESBS appears safe when performed by experienced teams. Nonetheless, ESBS has associated risks that parallel those of traditional approaches, at least qualitatively. Understanding the potential risks associated with a given case should allow for preoperative optimization to reduce the chance of complications. Experienced teams that prepare for catastrophes and expeditiously address intraoperative and postoperative complications likely have the best chance of preventing, or at least minimizing, the long-term effects of those complications.

References

1. Kassam AB, Prevedello DM, Carrau RL, et al. Endoscopic endonasal skull base surgery: analysis of complications in the authors' initial 800 patients. J Neurosurg 2011;114(6):1544–1568
2. Kono Y, Prevedello DM, Snyderman CH, et al. One thousand endoscopic skull base surgical procedures demystifying the infection potential: incidence and description of postoperative meningitis and brain abscesses. Infect Control Hosp Epidemiol 2011;32(1):77–83
3. Lund VJ, Stammberger H, Nicolai P, et al. European position paper on endoscopic management of tumours of the nose, paranasal sinuses and skull base. Rhinol Suppl 2010;(22):1–143
4. Snyderman CH, Carrau RL, Kassam AB, et al. Endoscopic skull base surgery: principles of endonasal oncological surgery. J Surg Oncol 2008;97(8):658–664
5. Ganly I, Patel SG, Singh B, et al. Complications of craniofacial resection for malignant tumors of the skull base: report of an International Collaborative Study. Head Neck 2005;27(6):445–451
6. Kryzanski JT, Annino DJ Jr, Heilman CB. Complication avoidance in the treatment of malignant tumors of the skull base. Neurosurg Focus 2002;12(5):e11
7. Patel MR, Stadler ME, Snyderman CH, et al. How to choose? Endoscopic skull base reconstructive options and limitations. Skull Base 2010;20(6):397–404
8. Kassam A, Snyderman CH, Mintz A, Gardner P, Carrau RL. Expanded endonasal approach: the rostrocaudal axis. Part I. Crista galli to the sella turcica. Neurosurg Focus 2005;19(1):E3
9. Pirris SM, Pollack IF, Snyderman CH, et al. Corridor surgery: the current paradigm for skull base surgery. Childs Nerv Syst 2007;23(4):377–384
10. Kassam AB, Gardner PA, Snyderman CH, Carrau RL, Mintz AH, Prevedello DM. Expanded endonasal approach, a fully endoscopic transnasal approach for the resection of midline suprasellar craniopharyngiomas: a new classification based on the infundibulum. J Neurosurg 2008;108(4):715–728
11. Kassam AB, Vescan AD, Carrau RL, et al. Expanded endonasal approach: vidian canal as a landmark to the petrous internal carotid artery. J Neurosurg 2008;108(1):177–183
12. Kassam A, Snyderman CH, Carrau RL, Gardner P, Mintz A. Endoneurosurgical hemostasis techniques: lessons learned from 400 cases. Neurosurg Focus 2005;19(1):E7
13. Hadad G, Bassagasteguy L, Carrau RL, et al. A novel reconstructive technique after endoscopic expanded endonasal approaches: vascular pedicle nasoseptal flap. Laryngoscope 2006;116(10):1882–1886
14. Snyderman CH, Carrau RL, deVries B. Carotid artery resection: Update on preoperative evaluation. In: Johnson JT, Derkay CS, Mandell-Brown MK, Newman RK, eds. AAO-HNS Instructional Courses. Alexandria (VA): American Academy of Otolaryngology–Head and Neck Surgery 1993;341–346
15. Solares CA, Ong YK, Carrau RL, et al. Prevention and management of vascular injuries in endoscopic surgery of the sinonasal tract and skull base. Otolaryngol Clin North Am 2010;43(4):817–825
16. Valentine R, Wormald PJ. Carotid artery injury after endonasal surgery. Otolaryngol Clin North Am 2011;44(5):1059–1079
17. Valentine R, Wormald PJ. Controlling the surgical field during a large endoscopic vascular injury. Laryngoscope 2011;121(3):562–566
18. Lippert BM, Ringel K, Stoeter P, Hey O, Mann WJ. Stent-graft-implantation for treatment of internal carotid artery injury during endonasal sinus surgery. Am J Rhinol 2007;21(4):520–524
19. de Divitiis E, Cappabianca P, Cavallo LM, Esposito F, de Divitiis O, Messina A. Extended endoscopic transsphenoidal approach for extrasellar craniopharyngiomas. Neurosurgery 2007; 61:(5, Suppl 2):219–227, discussion 228
20. de Divitiis E, Cavallo LM, Esposito F, Stella L, Messina A. Extended endoscopic transsphenoidal approach for tuberculum sellae meningiomas. Neurosurgery 2008; 62(6, Suppl 3):1192–1201
21. Barges-Coll J, Fernandez-Miranda JC, Prevedello DM, et al. Avoiding injury to the abducens nerve during expanded endonasal endoscopic surgery: anatomic and clinical case studies. Neurosurgery 2010;67(1):144–154, discussion 154
22. Esposito F, Becker DP, Villablanca JP, Kelly DF. Endonasal transsphenoidal transclival removal of prepontine epidermoid tumors: technical note. Neurosurgery 2005;56(2 Suppl):E443; discussion E443
23. Bleier BS, Wang EW, Vandergrift WA III, Schlosser RJ. Mucocele rate after endoscopic skull base reconstruction using vascularized pedicled flaps. Am J Rhinol Allergy 2011;25(3):186–187
24. Michel SJ. The Mount Fuji sign. Radiology 2004;232(2):449–450

25. Schirmer CM, Heilman CB, Bhardwaj A. Pneumocephalus: case illustrations and review. Neurocrit Care 2010;13(1):152–158
26. Brouwer MC, McIntyre P, de Gans J, Prasad K, van de Beek D. Corticosteroids for acute bacterial meningitis. Cochrane Database Syst Rev 2010;9:CD004405
27. van Aken MO, de Marie S, van der Lely AJ, et al. Risk factors for meningitis after transsphenoidal surgery. Clin Infect Dis 1997;25(4):852–856
28. van Aken MO, Feelders RA, de Marie S, et al. Cerebrospinal fluid leakage during transsphenoidal surgery: postoperative external lumbar drainage reduces the risk for meningitis. Pituitary 2004;7(2):89–93
29. Dumont AS, Nemergut EC II, Jane JA Jr, Laws ER Jr. Postoperative care following pituitary surgery. J Intensive Care Med 2005;20(3):127–140
30. Korinek AM; Service Epidémiologie Hygiène et Prévention. Risk factors for neurosurgical site infections after craniotomy: a prospective multicenter study of 2944 patients. The French Study Group of Neurosurgical Infections, the SEHP, and the C-CLIN Paris-Nord. Neurosurgery 1997;41(5):1073–1079, discussion 1079–1081
31. Korinek AM, Golmard JL, Elcheick A, et al. Risk factors for neurosurgical site infections after craniotomy: a critical reappraisal of antibiotic prophylaxis on 4,578 patients. Br J Neurosurg 2005;19(2):155–162
32. Korinek AM, Baugnon T, Golmard JL, van Effenterre R, Coriat P, Puybasset L. Risk factors for adult nosocomial meningitis after craniotomy: role of antibiotic prophylaxis. Neurosurgery 2006;59(1):126–133, discussion 126–133
33. Donald PJ. Complications in skull base surgery for malignancy. Laryngoscope 1999;109(12):1959–1966
34. Kryzanski JT, Annino DJ, Gopal H, Heilman CB. Low complication rates of cranial and craniofacial approaches to midline anterior skull base lesions. Skull Base 2008; 18(4):229–241
35. Harvey RJ, Smith JE, Wise SK, Patel SJ, Frankel BM, Schlosser RJ. Intracranial complications before and after endoscopic skull base reconstruction. Am J Rhinol 2008; 22(5):516–521
36. Horowitz G, Fliss DM, Margalit N, Wasserzug O, Gil Z. Association between cerebrospinal fluid leak and meningitis after skull base surgery. Otolaryngol Head Neck Surg 2011;145(4):689–693
37. Heo KW, Park SK. Rhinologic outcomes of concurrent operation for pituitary adenoma and chronic rhinosinusitis: an early experience. Am J Rhinol 2008;22(5):533–536
38. Carrau RL, Snyderman C, Janecka IP, Sekhar L, Sen C, D'Amico F. Antibiotic prophylaxis in cranial base surgery. Head Neck 1991;13(4):311–317
39. Semple PL, Laws ER Jr. Complications in a contemporary series of patients who underwent transsphenoidal surgery for Cushing's disease. J Neurosurg 1999;91(2):175–179

11 External Approaches to the Paranasal Sinuses and Skull Base

A. Janjua, I. J. Witterick

Introduction

External approaches to the sinuses were largely employed before the introduction of endoscopy. In the setting of inflammatory sinus disease, external approaches facilitated open visualization of the sinus mucosal lining, removal of diseased sinus lining and the creation of dependent (and presumed functional) drainage pathways from the sinus cavities into the nose. The introduction of rod lens technology and advances in clinicians' understanding of the physiologic pattern of sinus drainage have largely led to the replacement of external approaches with endoscopic techniques, which preserve mucosal lining and restore the patency of the natural drainage pathways of the sinuses (toward which the cilia direct mucous outflow from the sinuses).

More recently, external approaches have continued to be employed when open access to the sinuses is required for the surgical removal of sinonasal tumors. Despite the development of endoscopic techniques in the 1970s and 1980s to address inflammatory sinus disease,[1–6] the removal of nasal and sinus tumors continued to occur through external approaches. Only recently has the superiority of en bloc tumor resection been challenged,[7] and the development of advanced endoscopic instrumentation allowed for endoscopic removal of nasal and sinus tumors.

Still, endoscopic approaches have some limitations and external approaches to the sinuses may be required (and, indeed, superior) in situations where substantially wider exposure to the sinuses is required;[8] although, several authors have described more extensive endoscopic exposures to tackle these situations.[9–11] Nonetheless, modern advanced endoscopic nasal surgery requires specialized and costly endoscopic instruments and technologies, to which some institutions may not have access. As such, all rhinologists should be familiar with external approaches to the paranasal sinuses. Due to decreased instruction regarding external approaches during surgical training, it is important that rhinologists understand their potential pitfalls and complications, and the preventive steps that may be taken to minimize them.

As with any surgery, bleeding that obscures visualization may lead to intraoperative complications, so minimizing intraoperative hemorrhage is essential. In each of the approaches described in this chapter, key steps to prevent intraoperative blood loss and avoid poor surgical visualization will be described (**Fig. 11.1**).

A detailed review of the patient's preoperative status and imaging is paramount in identifying potential complications and so minimizing their occurrence. Careful review of preoperative computed tomography scans to evaluate the integrity and height of the skull base is crucial, particularly for preventing intracranial complications. As the surgeon proceeds posteriorly, the skull base is not parallel to the hard palate; rather, it slopes inferiorly. The degree of the slope can be ascertained from preoperative imaging and this can alert the surgeon to the potential for violation of the cranial base posteriorly.

It is also prudent to review the patient's ophthalmologic history, and document gross visual acuity and ocular range of motion. If abnormalities are suspected, a formal ophthalmologic consultation should take place. May and colleagues[12] reported that the only significant difference between their analysis of complications during traditional sinus surgery versus functional endoscopic sinus surgery techniques was orbital complications, particularly retrobulbar hematoma. In their series of 2,108 patients, they reported minor and major orbital complication rates of 1.7% and 0.05%, respectively.

With the above issues taken into consideration preoperatively, complications may thereby be minimized. Still, the surgeon's experience with open sinus surgical techniques may be the most crucial factor in determining the risk and type of complications that may ensue during external sinus surgery.

External Approaches to the Maxillary Sinus

Introduction

George Caldwell and Henri Luc first described an anterior approach to the maxillary sinus in the late 1800s. Their initial description was that of an upper gingivobuccal sulcus incision, entrance to the maxillary sinus via the canine fossa, complete stripping of the maxillary sinus mucosa and creation of an inferior meatal antrostomy.[13] More recently, the term Caldwell–Luc is generally used to describe any form of access to the maxillary sinus via an upper gingivobuccal sulcus incision and entrance via the anterior wall of the maxillary sinus.

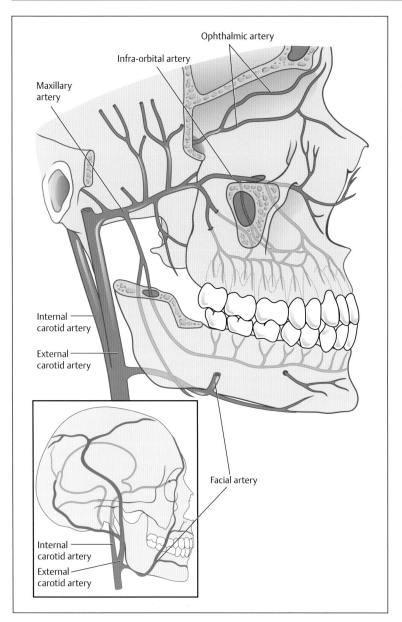

Fig. 11.1 Schematic depiction of the paranasal sinuses and the surrounding major vascular anatomy. Depicted are the infra-orbital artery between the roof of the maxillary sinus and orbit and the course of the facial artery supplying the external midface. The ophthalmic artery gives rise to the anterior and posterior ethmoid arteries which traverse the roof of the ethmoid sinuses (not shown).

Indications

External approaches to the maxillary sinus are indicated under the following conditions:
- Septated or lateral inflammatory disease within the maxillary sinus that is either refractory to endoscopic techniques or difficult to access transnasally
- The necessity for wide exposure of the posterior wall of the maxillary sinus (i.e., in juvenile angiofibroma resection, pterygopalatine fossa or infratemporal fossa exploration, and tumor resection)
- For exposure of the orbital floor during transantral repair of orbital floor fractures

- To facilitate instrumentation of the anterior wall of the maxillary sinus via endoscopic techniques (i.e., during removal of a mass lesion involving the anterior wall mucosa)
- For direct closure of select oroantral fistulas (although the majority of these may be resolved via endoscopic creation of an unimpeded drainage pathway from the maxillary sinus into the nasal cavity and simple intra-oral fistula closure with oral mucosal rotation flap techniques)
- For transantral ligation of the maxillary artery in the setting of refractory epistaxis; however, this approach has largely been replaced by transnasal endoscopic sphenopalatine artery ligation.

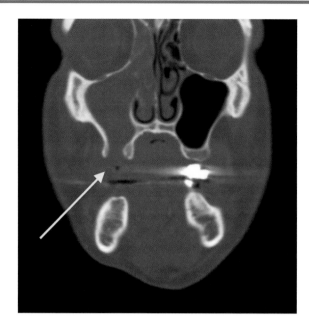

Fig. 11.2 Computed tomography of oroantral fistula (arrow) and chronic maxillary sinusitis.

Complications: Prevention and Management

Oroantral Fistulas

A persistent communication between the maxillary antrum and the maxillary alveolus (or gingivobuccal sulcus) may result following access to the maxillary sinus via an incision in this location. The reported incidence of an oroantral fistula is 1.0% (**Fig. 11.2**).[14]

Prevention of postoperative fistulas may be achieved by the creation of a low-resistance drainage pathway from the maxillary sinus into the nose (most commonly via middle meatal antrostomy), to ensure adequate postoperative intranasal sinus drainage and to avoid excessive pressure or tension on the incision line. Resection of the fistula tract (if longstanding and subsequently epithelially lined) and utilization of maxillary sinus and/or oral mucosal flaps to interpose tissue over the fistula site should be performed. Planning an incision that preserves at least 5 mm of buccal mucosa away from the sulcus allows for adequate closure and good mucosal approximation, thereby minimizing the risk of fistula. Saline solution or other nonalcoholic mouth rinses are indicated for 1 to 2 weeks after surgery, to keep the area clean and to prevent postoperative infection.

Maxillary Artery Injury

The maxillary artery lies in close proximity to the posterior wall of the maxillary sinus. Avoiding violation of the posterior wall prevents the significant hemorrhage that can occur as the result of injury to this artery. Delayed hemorrhage following cauterization of the artery can occur, albeit rarely, and may result in significant postoperative epistaxis. Furthermore, posterior extension of a middle meatal antrostomy may result in injury to the sphenopalatine artery (the terminal branch of the maxillary artery) as it enters the nose immediately posterior to the crista ethmoidalis.

Infraorbital Nerve (V2) Dysesthesia

Dental numbness, facial pain and local hypoesthesia may occur as the result of injury to the infraorbital nerve or its superior alveolar branches. Surgical exposure involves reflection of soft tissue from the face of the maxillary sinus. The periosteum is incised and elevated to provide adequate exposure to the bony anterior maxillary sinus wall. During elevation, care must be taken to identify the infraorbital nerve and prevent injury or division. The pupil is an approximation in the sagittal plane where the infraorbital nerve exits the surface of the facial skeleton. The use of cautery in close proximity to the nerve, or failure to avoid excessive retraction of the cheek soft tissues overlying the nerve, will result in postoperative nerve dysfunction. Excessive removal of the anterior bony wall of the maxillary sinus is routinely complicated by anterior superior alveolar nerve dysfunction.

Injury to the infraorbital nerve may also occur as a result of instrumentation or violation of the superior wall of the maxillary sinus. Care must be taken when using instruments in this area or when stripping mucosa from the roof of the maxillary sinus, as the nerve may or may not have a bony covering in this location. The nerve may simply be hanging in a soft tissue mesentery within the roof of the maxillary sinus, making careful instrumentation of the area essential.

Violation or removal of the posterior wall of the maxillary sinus provides exposure of the pterygopalatine fossa and may also lead to injuries of the descending palatine branches from the maxillary nerve, resulting in numbness of the ipsilateral soft and hard palate.

Localized numbness of the upper lip resulting from cutting through the direct cutaneous sensory nerves when performing the gingivobuccal sulcus incision occurs frequently; however, it is usually temporary and resolves following healing and sensory nerve reinnervation. During healing, patients often complain of a numb and achy sensation along their ipsilateral maxillary dentition for several months postoperatively, and should be counseled appropriately preoperatively. Long-term facial numbness or paresthesia has been reported in ~ 9.0% of patients (**Fig. 11.3**).[14]

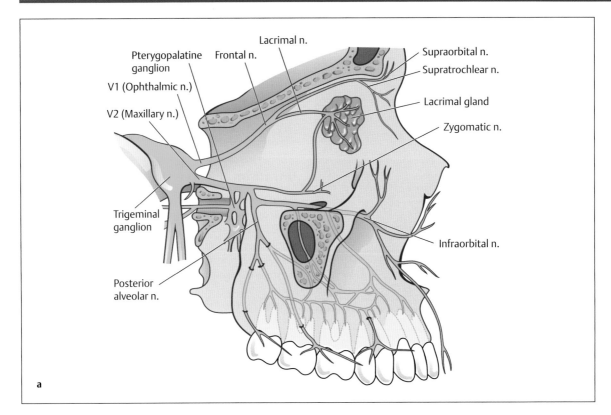

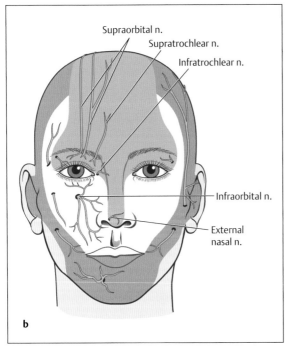

Fig. 11.3 Schematic depiction of the paranasal sinuses and surrounding sensory nerves as well as the associated cutaneous distributions.

a Sagittal view of the first and second divisions of the trigeminal nerve and their proximity to the sinuses.

b Illustration of the cutaneous distribution of the three major branches of the trigeminal nerve. The cutaneous branches of V1 and V2 that are at particular risk during external approaches to the sinuses are labelled.

Epiphora

The creation of a pathway for postoperative ventilation and drainage of the maxillary sinus occurs either via inferior meatal antrostomy or, more commonly, middle meatal antrostomy. Care must be exercised when creating either form of maxillary antrostomy to avoid injury to the nasolacrimal duct (NLD) or significant scarring, which may result in epiphora. Inadvertent lacrimal system injury occurs frequently, however, the exact incidence and prevalence is not known. Most injuries are believed to heal spontaneously, often without resultant symptomatic epiphora.

During inferior meatal antrostomy, avoidance of the anterior/superior region of the inferior meatus (the area of Hasner's valve) minimizes this risk. Planning an inferior meatal antrostomy in the posterior two-thirds of the inferior meatus is prudent to avoid this complication.

During middle meatal antrostomy, the risk of injury to the NLD may be minimized by ensuring that the maxillary antrostomy is not extended too anteriorly along the lateral nasal wall. Should damage to the NLD occur, intubation of the lacrimal apparatus via the lacrimal puncta with temporary silicone tubing may be performed to stent the NLD during the healing phase; however, this procedure is rarely necessary.

In recurrent, severe or refractory cases of scarring of the lacrimal drainage apparatus, a formal dacryocystorhinostomy may be performed to allow lacrimal drainage superiorly in the nose, proximal to the area of NLD stenosis. This may be achieved endoscopically or through an open approach. Mucosa of the anterior lateral wall of the nose is elevated over the superior segment of the bony nasolacrimal canal. The medial wall of this bony canal is removed (often with a fine drill) and the NLD is entered medially and marsupialized to allow for free lacrimal flow. Once again, temporary silicone tubing may be placed during the healing phase and removed postoperatively in the office setting. Alternatively, a permanent glass Lester Jones tube may be inserted, should permanent stenting be required to ensure long-term patency.

Intranasal Crusting

Intranasal crusting usually results from postoperative exposure of bone or cartilage following stripping of the overlying mucosa. An intraoperative technique that minimizes removal of mucosal lining—and so does not expose the underlying bone or cartilage—significantly minimizes this complication. Frequent postoperative saline irrigation may minimize excessive crusting and promote more rapid mucosalization in the event that inadvertent mucosal stripping occurs or when pathologic mucosal lining must be removed. Intranasal crusting is associated with a foul odor; if crusting does occur, an intensified saline irrigation regimen, frequent debridement, and systemic antibiotics may be required.

Packing-Related Complications

It is usually not necessary to insert packing into a maxillary sinus following surgery. Should packing be required, either dissolvable or formal nasal packing may be used. The advantage of resorbable nasal packing is that it does not need to be removed postoperatively, a process which may be quite uncomfortable for the patient. Should the surgeon elect to use formal, nondissolving packing, care must be taken to ensure that all packing is secured, but easily removable from the nose, such that migration and aspiration of the packing cannot occur and no packing is inadvertently retained. Regardless of the type of nasal packing used, appropriate postoperative antibiotic coverage should be provided to prevent secondary infection. Of note, when packing is placed, early postoperative saline lavage may not be performed; rather, lavage should be initiated following packing removal.

Toxic Shock Syndrome

Toxic shock syndrome is a rare and potentially fatal infectious complication related to nasal packing. Most cases result from the release of an exotoxin produced by *Staphylococcus aureus*. Diagnostic criteria from the U.S. Centers for Disease Control and Prevention include a fever > 102°F (39°C), diffuse macular rash, desquamation, and hypotension; in addition, at least three organs must be involved. The presentation usually occurs within 48 hours of packing placement and has been associated with various types of nasal packing. Although antibiotics are commonly recommended for the prevention of toxic shock syndrome and other infectious complications, their efficacy is subject to debate.[15-17] Treatment includes packing removal, nasal cultures, debridement of necrotic or infected tissue, resuscitation of blood pressure, and the administration of antistaphylococcal antibiotics.

Hyperostotic Bone Formation

Following Caldwell–Luc approaches, substantial bony changes frequently occur along the violated anterior wall or concentrically within the maxillary sinus. This complication is more pronounced following mucosal stripping, but is not limited to this procedure. Hyperostotic bone formation may cause difficulty with respect to interpreting postoperative imaging and render subsequent access to the sinus difficult.

Cheek Edema

Cheek edema is a common occurrence following Caldwell–Luc approaches to the maxillary sinus, and is seen in 89% of patients.[14] Postoperative icing for 24 to 48 hours and head elevation may minimize its severity.

Facial Cellulitis/Abscess

Secondary infection of the nasal vestibule or facial soft tissues overlying the maxillary area, most commonly caused by *Staphylococcus aureus*, may occur following external approaches to the maxillary sinus (**Fig. 11.4**). Subsequent abscess collection may also occur (**Fig. 11.5**). Patients should be given perioperative antibiotics to minimize the risk of these complications.

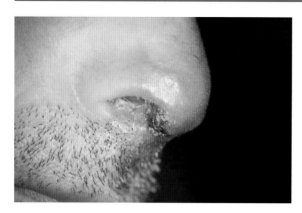

Fig. 11.4 Nasal vestibulitis following Caldwell–Luc approach to the maxillary sinus.

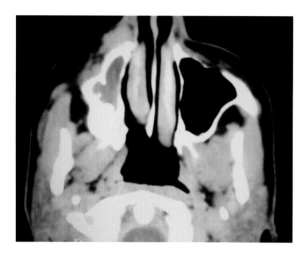

Fig. 11.5 Computed tomography displaying signs of right facial cellulitis/abscess following a Caldwell–Luc approach.

Facial Asymmetry

Excessive removal of the anterior bony wall of the maxillary sinus may result in various alterations in facial cosmesis. Excessive removal of the medial vertical maxillary buttress may result in depression or collapse of the lateral aspect of the lower lateral cartilage; the visual appearance is that of flattening of the lateral aspect of the nasal ala.

Excessive removal or weakening of the lateral maxillary buttress is further thought to lead to an increased potential for lateral facial asymmetry. It has been suggested that this risk may be minimized by leaving intact the bony wall lateral to the midpupillary line.[18] The reported rate of asymmetry following resolution of postoperative facial swelling is 2 to 3%.[19]

Dental Complications

Injury to the maxillary tooth roots (most commonly the molars, as theirs roots project further into the maxillary sinus) may occur during surgical entrance to the maxillary sinus via its anterior wall, or during removal of the sinus mucosal lining in the setting of maxillary tooth roots that project superiorly into the sinus. Care must be taken to avoid low entrance into the maxillary sinus or removal of excessive bone inferiorly (along the anterior wall of the maxilla) when making the bony window for visualization within the maxillary sinus. Preoperative imaging may identify tooth roots that project into the maxillary sinus, and so are at increased risk. In a series of 670 Caldwell–Luc procedures, the rate of devitalized dentition was reported to be 0.4% ($n = 2$).[14] These patients required root canal work to resolve the dental symptoms.

External Ethmoidectomy

The surgical technique for external ethmoidectomy was first described in 1933 by Ferris Smith.[20] Since then, several modifications have been described, which include the use of a variety of facial incisions along the nasal sidewall. Typically, a curvilinear incision is made midway between the nasion and the medial canthus. Incisions may be extended superiorly or laterally to address concomitant frontal sinus pathology.

Currently, ethmoid surgery is generally accomplished by endoscopic techniques, which offer superior visualization of anatomical detail compared with headlight surgery through a small incision.

Indications

Indications for the utilization of external ethmoidectomy include the following:

- To address chronic inflammatory sinus disease involving the ethmoid and frontal sinuses
- For anterior and posterior ethmoid artery ligation
- For transethmoid approaches to the sphenoid sinus and sella
- Drainage of subperiosteal or orbital abscess; an external approach is routinely faster than an endoscopic approach. Moreover, endoscopic approaches may be further complicated by difficulty in visualization and endoscopic dissection of the ethmoids in the setting of acute sinus infection
- Orbital decompression
- In the setting of benign tumors with extension from the ethmoids into the medial orbit (e.g., osteoma). By using an external incision, the surgeon is able to protect the orbital contents by directly visualizing and retracting the periorbita laterally, and subsequently dissecting medially through the lateral nasal wall and into the ethmoid air cells

- External approaches have also been used to provide wider access to the anterior cranial base and cribriform region to address cerebrospinal fluid (CSF) leak repairs, dermoid excisions, meningoencephalocele repairs, and tumor (e.g., esthesioneuroblastoma) resections.[8]

Technique

External access to the ethmoid sinuses occurs via a curvilinear incision extending inferiorly from the medial end of the eyebrow, along the nasal sidewall midway between the medial palpebral line and the nasal dorsum. This incision usually heals well, leaving an inconspicuous scar. However, in some patients hypertrophy or webbing of the scar can occur. Gentle tissue handling and careful closure can minimize scarring. A zigzag or running "W-plasty" may be used to further camouflage the facial scar and may be particularly useful to prevent hypertrophic scarring in prone individuals. The angular vessels in this area are ligated with bipolar cauterization. The dissection should be extended down to the periosteum. Care must be taken to avoid injury to the supraorbital and supratrochlear neurovascular bundles that lie further laterally along the orbital rim. The periosteum is incised anterior to the anterior lacrimal crest, and it is elevated off the lacrimal bone. The medial canthal ligament should be elevated cleanly off the underlying bone. In doing so, the medial canthal ligament attachment remains intact and the lacrimal apparatus may be elevated out of its bony groove and retracted laterally with the orbit. The medial canthal ligament is returned to its native site at the conclusion of the procedure to restore aesthetic facial symmetry. The ligament is commonly fixed in placed with a nonabsorbable braided suture through a small drill hole made in the adjacent nasal bone and then through the ligament to reapproximate the proper position of the medial canthus.

During dissection further posteriorly, care must be taken to avoid damage to the trochlea of the superior oblique muscle, and the periosteum in this region must be elevated cleanly off the bone to avoid postoperative diplopia. Elevation further posteriorly reveals the lamina papyracea, frontoethmoidal suture line, anterior and posterior ethmoid arteries, and the optic nerve. The ethmoid air cells may be entered by traversing the lamina papyracea. The entire lamina, or the portion of the lamina required for appropriate exposure of the anterior and posterior ethmoid air cells based on the indication, may be removed. The importance of understanding the inferior slope of the ethmoid roof as one progresses further posteriorly warrants repeating. The surgeon must understand this anatomy and maintain orientation within the posterior orbit/ethmoids to avoid inadvertent entry into the intracranial cavity. During the entirety of the procedure, globe retraction should be gentle and released on occasion to prevent retinal ischemia.

Complications: Prevention and Management

Bleeding and Blindness

Bleeding from the superficial angular vessels may obscure visualization and cause difficulty during deeper dissection. Bipolar cautery should be used for optimal hemostatic control. Effective cauterization of these vessels will significantly minimize postoperative periorbital ecchymosis. Ligation with ties may result in postoperative subcutaneous thickening in this thin-skinned area. Similarly, ligation with clips should be avoided.

Bleeding from the anterior or posterior ethmoid arteries may result in significant retrobulbar hemorrhage, which may in turn result in vision loss. Knowledge of the location of these arteries may prevent injury. The anterior ethmoid artery is located within the frontoethmoidal suture line, 20 to 26 mm posterior to the anterior lacrimal crest. The posterior ethmoid artery is located ~ 10 to 12 mm posterior to the anterior ethmoid artery. The optic nerve is in close proximity to the posterior ethmoid artery (range: 2 to 8 mm posterior to the posterior ethmoid artery).[21] Control of these arteries should occur via clipping or bipolar cauterization. Many surgeons will elect to ligate at least the anterior ethmoid artery prophylactically such that further manipulation will not inadvertently transect it, resulting in an orbital hematoma. It may be safer to prophylactically ligate this artery because the consequences of an intraorbital hematoma are substantial. The posterior ethmoid artery does not need to be routinely ligated unless further lateralization of the orbit is required for greater posterior exposure. Should the posterior ethmoid artery be ligated, extra care must be taken to avoid injury to the optic nerve, given the close proximity of the optic nerve immediately posterior to the posterior ethmoid artery.

Injury of either of the ethmoid arteries may be complicated by retraction of the vessel into the orbital fat and subsequent retrobulbar hemorrhage and hematoma formation. Rapid proptosis may occur with brisk retroorbital bleeds. Less rapid bleeds may be heralded by signs such as lid edema, ecchymosis, proptosis, and an afferent pupillary defect. Intraoperatively, the eyes should be exposed so that these signs may be recognized early. Postoperatively, regardless of whether this occurs intraoperatively or postoperatively, blindness may result after a brief duration (60 to 90 minutes) of retinal ischemia. Ophthalmologic consultation should occur immediately.

If proptosis occurs intraoperatively, steps should be taken to normalize intraocular pressure. This may be serially monitored with an ocular tonometer. The periorbita may be incised to allow egress of the blood collecting in the retro-orbital space. If visible, the cut end of the artery should be identified and controlled with cautery or clips; however, if the cut end of the artery is not visible, further dissection into the orbital fat to visualize the severed artery is not advised, as it may lead to further orbital injury. Removal of any remaining lamina allows for decompression of the orbital contents into the nasal cavity, thereby reducing intraocular pressure.[22]

Proptosis may only become apparent postoperatively, either in the setting of an occult anterior or posterior ethmoid artery injury that progresses rapidly in the recovery room following an episode of coughing/straining, or over a protracted period of time as the result of a slowly progressing venous bleed. In all cases of suspected intraoperative disruption of the orbital blood supply, tight packing and postoperative nose blowing are prohibited. Careful postoperative monitoring for ecchymosis, firmness of the globe and a differential globe compressibility compared with the contralateral normal eye should be undertaken. Intraocular pressures of 40 mmHg and an afferent pupillary defect may occur. Arterial or venous bleeds leading to progressive increases in intraocular pressure and deterioration in vision represent surgical emergencies, and require a return to the operating room to surgically decompress the orbit (either as above or endoscopically). Several steps may be undertaken immediately while awaiting assessment by ophthalmology and/or return to the operating theater (see Chapter 9, Figure 9.22 for the emergency management of orbital hematoma). Any ipsilateral nasal packing left in place should be removed. Lateral canthotomy (cutting laterally from the lateral lid commissure; the endpoint is the lateral orbital rim) and inferior cantholysis can be performed rapidly at the bedside to allow expansion of the orbital contents anteriorly and a return of blood flow. The inferior tarsal plate may be identified and divided sharply. A small portion of tarsus should be left laterally to allow subsequent reapposition following resolution of this emergency situation.

The optic nerve is prone to injury during dissection within a posteriormost ethmoid air cell that pneumatizes around the optic nerve (the Onodi cell). In this situation, lateral dissection within this ethmoid air cell may result in optic nerve injury and resultant visual dysfunction or blindness. Optic nerve injury results in decreased visual acuity and visual field defects. Guidelines for the optimal management of optic nerve trauma are lacking. The use of high doses of intravenous steroids remains controversial. When optic nerve injury is confirmed, common protocols suggest the administration of intravenous dexamethasone with an initial loading dose of 1 mg/kg followed by 0.5 mg/kg every 6 hours thereafter.[23] If vision improves, therapy is continued for a further 5 days. If vision fails to improve within 36 hours, or initially improves but then deteriorates, optic nerve decompression should be considered. However, in the International Optic Nerve Trauma Study, a comparative interventional study of 133 patients, investigators failed to demonstrate a difference in outcomes when comparing steroid therapy, surgical optic nerve decompression, and observation in patients with traumatic optic neuropathy.[24] They concluded that neither steroids nor surgical decompression should be considered the standard of care and that, in many cases, no intervention may suffice as management of a terminal traumatized optic nerve.

Significant lateral retraction of the orbital contents to improve visualization may also result in impaired blood flow to the retina and other orbital structures. Delicate and careful retraction, with frequent removal of retraction pressure, is recommended to facilitate blood flow to the orbit.

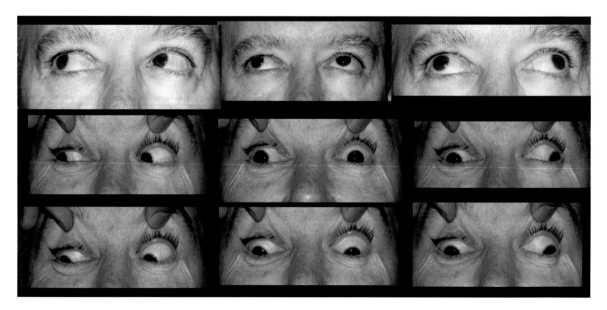

Fig. 11.6 Injury to the right medial rectus muscle and subsequent alteration in eye movements.

Violation of Periorbita

Care must be taken during dissection and lateralization of the orbit to preserve the periorbita, as violation of the periorbita allows medial herniation of orbital fat. This may obscure visualization (particularly of the posterior ethmoids and orbital apex).

Herniation of orbital fat may also cause mild postoperative enophthalmos as the orbital fat displaces into the adjacent surgically aerated ethmoid complex. This may also contribute to, or worsen, the temporary diplopia that may occur following external ethmoidectomy. The herniated contents and fat may also obstruct the frontal sinus drainage pathway and result in secondary, iatrogenic frontal sinus chronic inflammatory disease. This may be prevented by limiting bone removal anteriorly and superiorly along the medial orbital wall, or by stenting the frontal sinus drainage pathway during healing.

Medial rectus muscle injury may occur as a result of instrumentation within the orbital fat, causing temporary or permanent diplopia (**Fig. 11.6**). Immediate ophthalmologic consultation is advised in the setting of medial rectus injury, although few immediate solutions exist. Complete transection of the medial rectus muscle may be managed with surgical reapposition, although often a portion of the muscle is missing, rendering the procedure difficult and often unsuccessful. In the setting of partial mechanical injury or thermal injury (via cautery), steps may be taken to minimize scarring and fibrosis of the muscle, including the delivery of direct steroid injections or systemic steroids. Furthermore, botulinum toxin type A (Botox©) injection of the lateral rectus muscle may be used to weaken the unopposed lateral pull on the globe.[25]

Intracranial Complications

The frontoethmoidal suture line should serve as an approximate landmark for the level of the cribriform plate. As such, medial bone removal superior to this suture line may result in entry into the anterior cranial fossa and potential subsequent CSF leakage or intracranial hemorrhage. CSF leaks should be repaired intraoperatively.[26]

Intracranial hemorrhage from injury to an intracranial artery may represent an acute, life-threatening emergency and necessitates immediate neurosurgical and/or neuroradiologic consultation and treatment.

Sensory Dysesthesia

Injury to the supraorbital or supratrochlear neurovascular bundles results in bleeding or dysesthesia in the supratrochlear and supraorbital nerve distributions of the ipsilateral scalp. Care must be taken when dissecting superiorly along the medial orbital rim. The supratrochlear notch may be palpated externally. As an anatomical

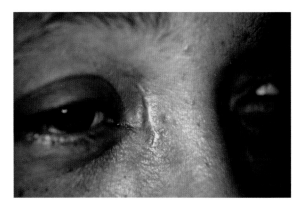

Fig. 11.7 Scarring following a medial canthal incision.

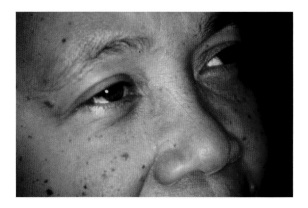

Fig. 11.8 Improvement in postoperative hypertrophic scarring of a medial canthal incision following three steroid injections.

reference, if the length of the orbit from the medial palpebral line to the lateral palpebral line is divided into thirds, the neurovascular bundle lies along the supraorbital rim in a line dividing the medial third and the lateral two-thirds of the orbit. Further note should be made that retraction and thermal injury may result in temporary nerve dysfunction (see **Fig. 11.3**).

Packing-Related Complications

Ethmoid cavities have classically been packed following external ethmoidectomy. Packing is believed to prevent scarring within the ethmoid complex and maintain long-term aeration of the ethmoids, thereby preventing recurrent inflammatory disease. Packing has the same disadvantages alluded to above with respect to the maxillary sinus (i.e., infection risk, inability to immediately deliver saline mists or rinses). Furthermore, it must be noted that without the medial orbital wall, excessive packing—or swelling of packing—may result in direct pressure on the orbital contents, with the potential for ischemia of the optic nerve and retina.

Medial Canthal Scarring/Subcutaneous Thickening

Using a zigzag skin incision may minimize hypertrophic or keloid scarring of the medial canthal incision. As noted above, using bipolar cautery for hemostasis of the subcutaneous tissues may limit the need for suture material and clips, which may cause thickening in this thin-skinned area (**Fig. 11.7**). Postoperative hypertrophic scarring may be managed with intradermal steroid injections (**Fig. 11.8**).

Medial Canthal Rounding and Hypertelorism

The periosteum should be formally reapproximated at the conclusion of the dissection to re-establish the medial pull of the medial canthal ligament. This may be achieved

via direct suture techniques or by drilling a hole into the remaining nasal bone to place a permanent suture from the medial canthal tendon through the hole to reapproximate the medial canthal tendon. Failure to do so may result in medial canthal rounding and hypertelorism.

Epiphora

Epiphora results from injury to the superior or inferior canaliculi or lacrimal sac. This may occur during lateralization of the periosteum of the medial orbital wall, through instrumentation during elevation of the lacrimal apparatus, or during reapposition. This may be avoided with careful soft tissue handling. Should injury to the lacrimal apparatus occur, temporary or permanent stents may be used as described previously.

Ethmoid Mucocele Formation

Following an external excision to access the nasal cavity and ethmoid sinuses, care must be taken not to trap mucosal epithelium within the soft tissue or bony closure. Inadvertent trapping of mucosa without the ability for it to drain intranasally may result in mucocele formation within the incision line (**Fig. 11.9**). This may occur several years after the initial surgery (**Fig. 11.10**). The patient may experience intermittent swelling along the previous incision line if this non-draining mucosal tissue becomes inflamed (i.e., during an upper respiratory tract infection), and may potentially develop an abscess in this location.

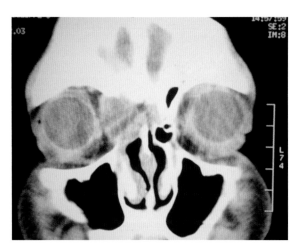

Fig. 11.9 Coronal computed tomography scan demonstrating a right ethmoid mucocele that developed 7 years after a lateral rhinotomy to access the nasal cavity.

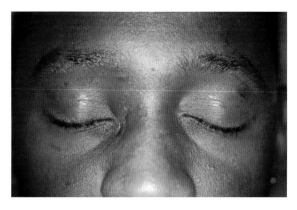

Fig. 11.10 Visible swelling in the right medial canthal area from an ethmoid mucocele 7 years after a lateral rhinotomy to access the nasal cavity.

External Approaches to the Frontal Sinus

The anterior/superficial location of the frontal sinuses affords several options for surgical access via external approaches. In the early phase of endoscopic approaches to the paranasal sinuses, the unavailability and lack of experience with angled endoscopes necessitated the continued use of external approaches for a significant proportion of frontal sinus pathologies. Several advances in angled instrumentation have broadened the ability of clinicians to access the frontal sinus endoscopically, although there remain clinical circumstances for which endoscopic approaches are not appropriate.[27]

Indications

Indications for the utilization of external approaches to the frontal sinus include the following:
- When lateral access within the frontal sinus is required: access to the lateral extension of the frontal sinus (further than one-half of the width of the orbit) can be difficult via endoscopic techniques

- To address large Kuhn type III or type IV frontal sinus cells resulting in recalcitrant frontal sinus disease
- CSF leak repairs superiorly on the posterior table of the frontal sinus
- Intracranial or intraorbital complications of frontal sinusitis
- Repair of frontal sinus fractures
- Lack of tools or expertise to perform endoscopic frontal sinus procedures
- Failed endoscopic approaches
- Obliteration/cranialization of the frontal sinus.

Technique

The frontal sinuses may be accessed via several external approaches. These include direct frontal sinus access via either an external incision similar to that used to access the ethmoid sinuses, a gull-wing incision across the superior aspects of both eyebrows and across the glabella, or a direct "brow" incision (typically through an existing horizontal skin crease). In addition, various external bicoronal incisions may be used for an osteoplastic flap approach to the frontal sinus. These bicoronal incisions may be made over the vertex of the scalp or either just in front of (pretrichial) or just behind (posttrichial) the hairline.

When determining which type of incision should be made to approach the frontal sinuses, both the visibility of the incision and resultant scalp sensory disturbance should be considered. As the sensory supply to the scalp comes from the supraorbital and supratrochlear nerves, the lower the incision, the more resultant numbness of the scalp. Furthermore, although the lower incisions (i.e., gull-wing, brow) may provide more direct access to the frontal sinuses, they often result in very poor cosmesis with an incision that is quite noticeable. For this reason, gull-wing and direct brow incisions may be less favorable choices for most patients, compared with bicoronal incisions. Men with receding hairlines or thinning hair may achieve better cosmesis with a true vertex bicoronal incision versus pretrichial or posttrichial incisions, which may become more noticeable with time. Women may also prefer a true vertex bicoronal incision, because there is less scalp hypesthesia with a bicoronal incision placed further posteriorly; this issue pertains especially to women who blow-dry their hair, as they may become unaware of excessive heat that may be delivered to the scalp, which can result in cutaneous burns to the hypesthetic areas. As such, the true vertex bicoronal incision is the most used of the various incisions to access the frontal sinuses.

Once access to the frontal sinuses is gained, appropriate instrumentation of the sinus is based on indication (i.e., resection of a tumor within). Following surgical access to the frontal sinus, a decision must be made regarding closure. Simple closure may be undertaken as long as postoperative ventilation and drainage of the

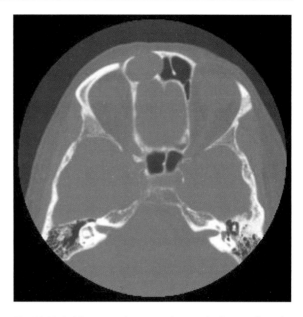

Fig. 11.11 Axial computed tomography scan displaying a frontal sinus mucocele. Note the erosion of the anterior and posterior table of the frontal sinus caused by progressive mucocele expansion.

sinus via the nasal cavity is ensured; otherwise, development of a mucocele may ensue. Alternatively, others have described frontal sinus obliteration or cranialization in appropriate circumstances.

General Complications

Lack of Resolution of Symptoms and Mucocele Formation

Most frontal sinus procedures performed entirely via external incisions do not adequately address the frontal recess; as such, if the aim is to maintain a functional frontal sinus postoperatively, they have been associated with high failure rates.[28] Failure to address the frontal sinus drainage pathway may result in persistent poor ventilation and drainage, and subsequent frontal mucocele formation. Combining an external approach with an endoscopic dissection of the frontal recess minimizes the risk of failure and mucocele formation. Stenting of narrow frontal sinus outflow tracts and meticulous postoperative debridement should be undertaken to minimize stenosis and maintain long-term patency.

Obliteration of the frontal sinus is prone to frontal mucocele formation if careful attention is not paid to ensuring that all frontal sinus mucosa is stripped before sinus obliteration and obstruction of the frontal recess. One potential area for remaining mucosa is the bilateral foramina of Breschet (small venules that drain sinus mucosa into the dural vein), which are located along the posterior wall of the frontal sinus. Furthermore, in the setting of bony erosion of the posterior table of the frontal sinus and the supraorbital roof, it is extremely difficult to completely remove mucosa sitting directly on the dura and periorbita. In this setting, obliteration of the frontal sinus should be avoided because the risk of mucocele formation is great (**Fig. 11.11**).[29]

Intracranial Complications

Entry into the anterior cranial fossa must be avoided, to prevent such complications as CSF leakage and intracranial hemorrhage. Identification of the dimensions of the frontal sinus previously occurred via 6-foot Caldwell radiographs or transillumination.[30] Image-guidance systems have routinely replaced these techniques to ensure safe entrance into the frontal sinus during removal of bone of the anterior table within the confines of the frontal sinus margins.[31]

Care must be taken during instrumentation of the posterior wall of the frontal sinus when dissection within the sinus is undertaken, as violation of the posterior wall will result in exposure of the dura and potential CSF leakage.

Complications Due to Specific External Approaches

Trephination

Trephination may be used as an adjunct to endoscopic frontal sinus surgery in several surgical situations.[32] Commercially available 'mini-trephination' kits include an indwelling injection port for irrigation. Irrigation may be useful in the setting of acute frontal sinusitis or as an adjunct to safely localize the frontal sinus drainage pathway during endoscopic dissections. When using the mini-trephination technique, the surgeon instills saline with or without diluted fluorescein into the trephine nail to aid in identification of the frontal sinus drainage pathway endoscopically. During saline instillation, the surgeon should monitor endoscopically to ensure that the saline is discharging from either the ipsilateral or (surprisingly, in some cases) the contralateral frontal sinus outflow tract. If the fluid cannot be seen, the surgeon must consider the possibility of intracranial penetration before too much fluid is pushed into the intracranial cavity.

A larger "true" trephination of the frontal sinus may be made with a drill for various indications, including drainage of acute infection, direct endoscopic visualization, or for direct instrumentation within the frontal sinus. Complications during trephination include injury to the supraorbital and supratrochlear neurovascular bundles, inadvertent intracranial entry, and scarring and alopecia at the incision site.

The incision should be placed within the medial brow and beveled parallel to the hair follicle shafts to prevent alopecia. In addition, the incision should terminate medial to the supraorbital notch to obviate the potential for supraorbital nerve injury. Furthermore, advantage can be taken of the laxity of the skin in this area to pull upward above the orbital rim, before entry into the sinus. This positioning has the advantage of allowing for surveillance of the entire sinus, rather than the drainage pathway only (frontal recess), when placed low in the medial portion of the frontal sinus. This is balanced by the fact that theoretically, entry through the floor of the sinus carries less risk of osteomyelitis than entry through the diploic bone of the anterior wall. The dimensions of the frontal sinus are highly variable and as such, the mandatory review of preoperative computed tomography imaging is essential. An image-guidance system may be used to minimize the risk of inadvertent trephination outside the confines of the frontal sinuses.[33]

Frontoethmoidectomy

Several procedures in which the anterior wall and floor of the frontal sinus are removed have been described in the literature. These walls may be exposed by superior or lateral extension of the external ethmoidectomy incision. Similar complications to those that occur during external ethmoidectomies should be considered; however, the potential for supraorbital and supratrochlear neurovascular injury is more pronounced.

The Reidel procedure involves complete removal of the floor and anterior wall of the frontal sinus. Its aim is to collapse the soft tissue of the forehead and orbit into the frontal sinus and so obliterate it. Unfortunately, this procedure is quite disfiguring, as removal of the entire anterior wall and the floor of the frontal sinus (including the supraorbital rim) results in a very noticeable cosmetic forehead defect. Killian described a modification of the Riedel procedure in which the supraorbital rim was preserved. Although this technique improved cosmesis, it often did not obliterate the portion of the sinus behind the orbital rim and so led to increased failures (including an increased rate of mucocele and mucopyocele formation).

The Lynch procedure combined an external ethmoidectomy with removal of only the floor of the frontal sinus. More recent modification of the Lynch procedure advocates preservation of as much mucosa as possible and parallels the mucosal preservation concepts championed in modern endoscopic frontal sinus surgery. Of note, removal of the medial and superior walls of the anterior orbit may be associated with herniation of the orbital contents into the drainage pathway of the frontal sinus and hence postoperative failure. Stenting may be required to prevent this from occurring.

The most common complications of all of these procedures are cosmetic deformities and frequent failure.

Osteoplastic Flap

The majority of external approaches to the frontal sinus have been largely replaced by advanced endoscopic techniques; however, the osteoplastic flap is a robust procedure still used for frontal sinus pathologies that require improved ability for instrumentation and manipulation within the frontal sinus (i.e., CSF leakage, fractures, tumors) or to access areas that are not amenable to endoscopic instrumentation (i.e., far laterally within the frontal sinus). This approach is additionally employed as salvage for failed endoscopic attempts at aeration.[34]

Technique

The osteoplastic flap operation may be approached via either a gull-wing incision, a direct brow incision, a hairline (either trichial or pretrichial) bicoronal incision, or a classic vertex bicoronal incision. As previously mentioned, the gull-wing and direct brow incisions are not favorable with respect to cosmetic outcome and sensory deficits, and as such are not frequently employed.

When comparing the hairline and classic vertex incisions, the hairline approaches are complicated by more extensive numbness of the scalp (posterior/superior to the incision line). In both cases, the skin of the scalp is reflected anteriorly in a plane superficial to the pericranium. Care must be taken at this stage to avoid direct injury to the frontalis muscle or injury to the temporal branches of the facial nerve, which innervates the frontalis muscle. The temporal branches of the facial nerve travel in the temporoparietal fascia until they reach the undersurface of the frontalis muscle, ~ 1 cm lateral to the brow.

The consequence of either of these injuries is paralysis of the forehead musculature. To prevent damage to the temporal branch, the dissection should be taken down to the superficial layer of the deep temporal fascia. The plane can be identified as the layer directly adherent to the temporalis muscle. Cutting through this dense white fascia will reveal the temporalis muscle. Staying in the correct plane under direct visualization will help to minimize damage to the temporal branches of the facial nerve.

Following anterior reflection of the scalp soft tissues, the pericranium is incised and elevated off the frontal bone, with the exception of the periostium directly overlying the frontal sinuses. Identification of the margins of the frontal sinuses (as described previously) allows the pericranium to remain in continuity with the anterior table of the frontal bone (which overlies the frontal sinuses and forms its anterior wall). This maneuver maintains the blood supply to the bone flap and provides direct postoperative vascularization to minimize the risk of bone flap necrosis.

The most common intraoperative complication during removal of the bone flap is entry into the intracranial

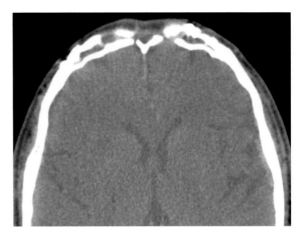

Fig. 11.12 Axial computed tomography scan demonstrating necrosis of the anterior table of the frontal bone following an osteoplastic flap procedure.

cavity and subsequent CSF leak. The rate of CSF leakage is ~ 3%. This may occur if the margins of the frontal sinuses are incorrectly identified or followed, or via injury to the posterior wall of the frontal sinus during osteotomies of the anterior table and bone flap elevation. Beveling of the osteotomies through the anterior table of the frontal sinus, within the boundaries of the frontal sinus, minimizes the risk of CSF leakage. Should this occur, the dura can be reapproximated directly with sutures and covered with a fascia flap (i.e., temporalis fascia).

This technique provides wide access to the frontal sinus for several indications (listed previously). Once completed, the operation is completed by replacing and securing the bone flap and closure of the overlying soft tissues of the scalp.

Postoperative Complications

Bony Cosmetic Defects and Bone Flap Nonunion

The most troublesome complication following osteoplastic flap surgery is nonunion of the bone flap (**Fig. 11.12**). This is a rare occurrence, even when the attachment of the periosteum cannot be maintained, because of the very good vascularity of the scalp. During replacement of the flap, it is important to carefully secure the bone flap, to minimize the risk of nonunion. In the past, sutures or wires were used to secure the flap. More recently, rigid fixation with mini-plates is used routinely and probably leads to less frequent nonunion of the bone flap.

Furthermore, bony cosmetic defects of the forehead may occur if the surgeon miscalculates on the original osteotomies and is required to subsequently drill away more bone (usually laterally). This may result in large bony gaps between the bone flap and the native frontal bone laterally. This may also occur if the anterior bone

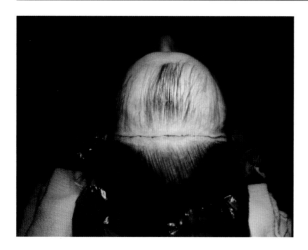

Fig. 11.13 Placement of the bicoronal incision far posteriorly results in good cosmesis and limits sensory hypoesthesia.

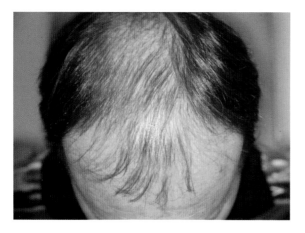

Fig. 11.14 Careful beveling of the bicoronal incision parallel to the hair follicle and limited use of cautery results in a very good cosmetic outcome.

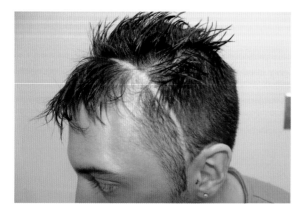

Fig. 11.15 Failure to bevel the bicoronal incision or excessive use of cautery may result in significant alopecia at the incision line.

plate is fractured during osteotomy, and is more likely to occur in the setting of a frontal sinus mucocele that has thinned out the anterior table preoperatively. In these situations, the surgeon may use titanium "manhole" covers (akin to those used by neurosurgeons following bur holes) or bone substitute to help cover and smooth out these bony defects.

Alopecia

Temporary hair loss is common at the incision site and in the surrounding 1 cm. Permanent alopecia may be avoided by beveling the bicoronal incision parallel to the hair follicles and avoiding using excessive cauterization (**Figs. 11.13, 11.14, 11.15**). Alopecia may be minimized by the avoidance of monopolar cautery during the bicoronal incision and judicious use of bipolar cautery on the undersurface of the scalp, to minimize thermal damage. Elevating the flap in the avascular subgaleal plane deep to the hair follicles is also essential.[35]

Hematoma/Seroma Formation and Superficial Skin Infections

Postoperatively, osteoplastic flap procedures can be complicated by hematoma and seroma formation; suction drains are routinely placed beneath skin incisions to avoid these complications. Secondary complications include infection leading to abscess and surrounding cellulitis. Perioperative antibiotics are routinely used to minimize these risks. Lastly, abscess collection must be surgically addressed to evacuate the collection and avoid necrosis of the underlying bone flap. Skin infection and skin necrosis in the absence of an infected hematoma or seroma are rare, given the thickness of the flap and the excellent blood supply of the supraorbital and supratrochlear vessels.

Incision-line Dehiscence with Osteoplastic Flap

Wound closure under tension may lead to incision-line dehiscence, which can usually be avoided with multiple deep absorbable sutures in the galea, followed by skin staples or the use of another strong, nonabsorbable material that should be left in place for a minimum of 10 days. If dehiscence occurs, the edges should be freshened with reapproximation of the hair-bearing skin. If healing by secondary intention is allowed to occur, a patch of alopecia will likely result.

Sensory Deficits (Scalp Hypoesthesia)

Patients undergoing bicoronal incisions should be counseled to expect hypoesthesia posterior to the incision, which may last for 3 or more months. The supraorbital and supratrochlear sensory nerves are at significant risk where they exit from the foramina in the mediosuperior orbit during elevation of the flap near the supraorbital rims. The nerves should be directly visualized by turning down the coronal flap. In up to 10% of patients, these nerves may arise from foramina 1 to 2 cm superior to the supraorbital rim and so can be injured without visualization.[36]

External Approaches to the Sphenoid Sinus

The location of the sphenoid sinus, combined with the proximity of several vital surrounding structures (carotid arteries, V1 and V2 branches of the trigeminal nerves, cavernous sinuses, optic nerves, nerves of extraocular movement [oculomotor, trochlear, and abducens cranial nerves], sella) underscores the difficulty and danger associated with its exposure via external incision. Because of its location posteriorly and superiorly within the nose, endoscopy has proved to be a superior method for visualization of the sphenoid sinus.

Transsphenoidal approaches to the sella have employed the use of an operating microscope in conjunction with external approaches since the early 1970s.[37,38] This substantially improved the visualization of structures within and surrounding the sphenoid. However, these approaches are associated with a limited field of view and cumbersome maneuverability within the operative field.[39] The purported advantage of a microscopic approach to the sella is that it allows for two-handed dissection.

More recently, the development of advanced endoscopic instrumentation, as well as collaboration between otolaryngology and neurosurgery to form Advanced Endoscopic Skull Base Surgery teams, has allowed for "four-handed" endoscopic approaches to a variety of parasphenoidal and anterior cranial base pathologies.

Indications

Indications for the use of external approaches to the sphenoid sinus include the following:
- Chronic inflammatory sinus disease involving the sphenoid sinus
- Sphenoid CSF leak repairs
- Repair of sphenoid meningoencephaloceles
- Neurosurgical access to the sella and parasellar areas (which allows for two-handed dissection).

Complications

The main difficulty with an open approach to the sphenoid is that despite an external incision, visualization is still poor because of the depth of the sinus from the skin surface. This results in a narrow corridor via which to visualize the sphenoid and its surrounding structures,

as well as limited ability to instrument within. Further complexity exists because of significant anatomical variability within the sphenoid sinus. This includes:
- Variable pneumatization: extensive pneumatization may leave vital structures "floating" in the sinus cavities and so relatively unprotected by surrounding bony walls. Several anatomical and radiologic studies have shown that the rates of dehiscence of the carotid artery and the optic nerve within the sphenoid are between 4.8 and 14.4% and between 0 and 24.0%, respectively[40]
- The presence of variable intersinus septa, which routinely extend posteriorly onto the internal carotid arteries
- The presence of supraorbital ethmoid cells (also known as Onodi cells), which pneumatize superiorly and laterally to the sphenoid sinus and can complicate exposure of the sphenoid and subsequent dissection within. The structure most at risk during dissection within an Onodi cell is the optic nerve.

General Complications

Complications arising from external approaches to the sphenoid sinus occur during access to the sphenoid or during dissection within the sphenoid. These general complications that may occur with any approach to the sphenoid are discussed below. This is followed by a discussion of specific complications based on the different external approaches to the sphenoid sinus.

Entry into the sphenoid sinus via its anterior face may be complicated by significant bleeding from the posterior nasal branch of the sphenopalatine artery. The posterior nasal branch traverses the anterior face of the sphenoid sinus horizontally between the superior margin of the choana and the natural ostium of the sphenoid sinus. Injury to this artery may be controlled via suction, monopolar cautery, or bipolar cautery. Of note, the posterior nasal artery continues medially and turns anteriorly to supply the posterior septal mucosa. In this location it is known as the posterior septal artery.

During intrasphenoidal dissection, injury to the roof of the sphenoid may occur, resulting in a CSF leak or pneumocephalus. Furthermore, damage to the anterior wall of the sella may result in injury to the pituitary gland. In addition, injury to the vital structures along the lateral wall of the sphenoid, including those within the cavernous sinus, may occur. These include: the internal carotid artery, the nerves of extraocular movement (oculomotor, trochlear and abducens nerves), the optic nerve and the first two branches of the trigeminal nerve (the ophthalmic and maxillary nerves).

Injury to the carotid artery can be exceedingly difficult to manage intraoperatively because of limited exposure and difficulty in formally ligating the artery. Often, this requires packing and emergent involvement of the neurovascular and neuroradiologic teams. Valentine and Wormald[41] recently investigated various materials to control carotid artery bleeding using a sheep model. A crushed muscle patch placed over the bleeding carotid artery was found to be an effective hemostatic agent that maintained vascular patency.

Leaks of CSF should be identified intraoperatively and sealed appropriately with an underlay or overlay technique. Postoperative use of a lumbar drain may be considered.

Packing following sphenoid surgery may result in obstruction of drainage from the sinus and resultant infection of the static mucoid contents. Due to the location of the sphenoid, meningitis may result and patients should receive antibiotic prophylaxis while packing is in place. Furthermore, if a significant amount of the bony posterior, superior, or lateral walls of the sphenoid has been removed, excessive packing or expansion of packing may result in the significant transmission of pressure intracranially and to the cavernous sinus. This may result in increased intracranial pressure or visual compromise (either ophthalmoplegia from dysfunction of the nerves of extraocular movement or vision loss from compression of the optic nerve and resultant impairment of retinal blood supply). Careful monitoring for signs of such dysfunction is required postoperatively and initial management should involve removal of the packing.

Complications Related to Specific External Approaches

External Ethmoidectomy Approach to the Sphenoid Sinus

Complications include those outlined above, as well as those discussed in the "External Ethmoidectomy" section of this chapter.

Transantral Approach to the Sphenoid Sinus

Complications include those described above, as well as those described in the "External Approaches to the Maxillary Sinus" section of this chapter. Using this approach requires particular attention to the vasculature behind the posterior wall of the maxillary sinus. Visualization of the sphenoid may require removal of the medial portion of the posterior wall of the maxillary sinus. In this location, care must be taken to avoid or formally ligate the maxillary artery. Furthermore, bleeding from the descending palatine artery may occur in this location and should be cauterized. This approach, and cauterization of these vessels, may also result in numbness of the ipsilateral palate.[42]

Transseptal Approach to the Sphenoid Sinus

All transseptal approaches are complicated by the risk of postoperative septal deviation, including caudal

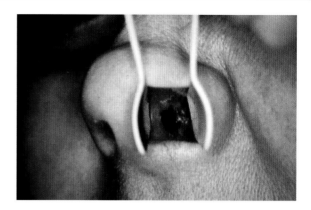

Fig. 11.16 Septal perforation. (Image courtesy of Michael Hawke, MD, University of Toronto.)

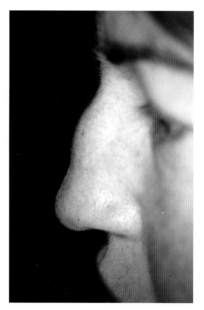

Fig. 11.17 Saddle nose deformity.

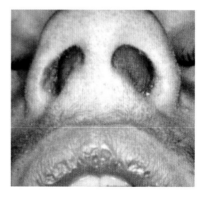

Fig. 11.18 Septal hematoma.

dislocations of the septum. There is additionally a risk of tears along the septal mucosa and a subsequent potential for postoperative septal perforation (**Fig. 11.16**). If substantial cartilage is removed without ensuring that dorsal and caudal septal struts remain, the patient may be predisposed to a future saddle nose deformity or nasal tip ptosis (**Fig. 11.17**). Postoperative collection of blood between the septal flaps may result in a septal hematoma with the potential for secondary infection leading to a septal abscess (**Fig. 11.18**). Care should be taken to limit the dead space between the septal mucosal flaps, either via septal quilting sutures or bilateral nasal packing.

Other complications from transseptal approaches depend upon the choice of access to space beneath septal mucosal flaps. If a sublabial incision is used for access to the septum, many of the complications associated with sublabial access to the maxillary sinus may occur, including lip edema, numbness, and the potential for fistula formation. If a transcolumellar incision is made to access the septum, various nasal cosmetic complications may occur, most notably a columellar scar or nasal tip ptosis. Should an intranasal mucosal incision be used to access the septum, minor complications seem to result, the most frequent of which is intranasal synechia formation. However, this approach yields the most limited corridor for visualization.

A direct transnasal approach to the natural sphenoid ostium may be undertaken; however, the depth of the sphenoid and the difficulty with intranasal visualization and dissection render this approach challenging without the use of an endoscope.

References

1. Draf W. The endoscopy of paranasal sinuses. Diagnostic and therapeutic possibilities (author's transl). [Article in German] Laryngol Rhinol Otol (Stuttg) 1975;54(3):209–215
2. Draf W. Therapeutic endoscopy of the paranasal sinuses. Endoscopy 1978;10(4):247–254
3. Stammberger H. Endoscopic endonasal surgery—concepts in treatment of recurring rhinosinusitis. Part II. Surgical technique. Otolaryngol Head Neck Surg 1986; 94(2):147–156
4. Stammberger H. Nasal and paranasal sinus endoscopy. A diagnostic and surgical approach to recurrent sinusitis. Endoscopy 1986;18(6):213–218
5. Stammberger H. Personal endoscopic operative technic for the lateral nasal wall—an endoscopic surgery concept in the treatment of inflammatory diseases of the paranasal sinuses. [Article in German] Laryngol Rhinol Otol (Stuttg) 1985;64(11):559–566
6. Messerklinger W. Background and evolution of endoscopic sinus surgery. Ear Nose Throat J 1994;73(7):449–450
7. Lund VJ, Stammberger H, Nicolai P, et al. European position paper on endoscopic management of tumours of the nose, paranasal sinuses and skull base. Rhinol Suppl 2010;(22):1–143
8. Murr AH. Contemporary indications for external approaches to the paranasal sinuses. Otolaryngol Clin North Am 2004;37(2):423–434
9. Kassam A, Snyderman CH, Mintz A, Gardner P, Carrau RL. Expanded endonasal approach: the rostrocaudal axis. Part I. Crista galli to the sella turcica. Neurosurg Focus 2005;19(1):E3
10. Kassam A, Snyderman CH, Mintz A, Gardner P, Carrau RL. Expanded endonasal approach: the rostrocaudal axis. Part II. Posterior clinoids to the foramen magnum. Neurosurg Focus 2005;19(1):E4
11. Kassam AB, Gardner P, Snyderman C, Mintz A, Carrau R. Expanded endonasal approach: fully endoscopic, completely transnasal approach to the middle third of the clivus, petrous bone, middle cranial fossa, and infratemporal fossa. Neurosurg Focus 2005;19(1):E6
12. May M, Levine HL, Mester SJ, Schaitkin B. Complications of endoscopic sinus surgery: analysis of 2108 patients—incidence and prevention. Laryngoscope 1994;104(9):1080–1083
13. Macbeth R. Caldwell, Luc, and their operation. Laryngoscope 1971;81(10):1652–1657
14. DeFreitas J, Lucente FE. The Caldwell–Luc procedure: institutional review of 670 cases: 1975-1985. Laryngoscope 1988;98(12):1297–1300
15. Kaygusuz I, Kizirgil A, Karlidağ T, et al. Bacteremia in septoplasty and septorhinoplasty surgery. Rhinology 2003;41(2):76–79
16. Finelli PF, Ross JW. Endocarditis following nasal packing: need for prophylaxis. Clin Infect Dis 1994;19(5):984–985
17. Mäkitie A, Aaltonen LM, Hytönen M, Malmberg H. Postoperative infection following nasal septoplasty. Acta Otolaryngol Suppl 2000;543:165–166
18. Kim E, Duncavage JA. Prevention and management of complications in maxillary sinus surgery. Otolaryngol Clin North Am 2010;43(4):865–873
19. Cutler JL, Duncavage JA, Matheny K, Cross JL, Miman MC, Oh CK. Results of Caldwell–Luc after failed endoscopic middle meatus antrostomy in patients with chronic sinusitis. Laryngoscope 2003;113(12):2148–2150
20. Duvvuri U, Carrau RL, Lai SY. External approaches in sinus surgery. In: Bailey BJ, Johnson JT, eds. Head and Neck Surgery—Otolaryngology, 4th ed. Philadelphia, PA: Lippincott Williams & Wilkins; 2006:365–76
21. Buus DR, Tse DT, Farris BK. Ophthalmic complications of sinus surgery. Ophthalmology 1990;97(5):612–619
22. Patel ZM, Govindaraj S. The prevention and management of complications in ethmoid sinus surgery. Otolaryngol Clin North Am 2010;43(4):855–864
23. Levine M. Ophthalmologic complications of endoscopic sinus surgery. In: Levine HL, Clemente MP, eds. Sinus Surgery: Endoscopic and Microscopic Approaches. New York: Thieme; 2004:285–289
24. Levin LA, Beck RW, Joseph MP, Seiff S, Kraker R. The treatment of traumatic optic neuropathy: the International Optic Nerve Trauma Study. Ophthalmology 1999;106(7):1268–1277
25. Dutton JJ. Orbital complications of paranasal sinus surgery. Ophthal Plast Reconstr Surg 1986;2(3):119–127
26. Schnipper D, Spiegel JH. Management of intracranial complications of sinus surgery. Otolaryngol Clin North Am 2004;37(2):453–472, ix
27. Close LG, Stewart MG. Looking around the corner: a review of the past 100 years of frontal sinusitis treatment. Laryngoscope 2009;119(12):2293–2298
28. Javer AR, Alandejani T. Prevention and management of complications in frontal sinus surgery. Otolaryngol Clin North Am 2010;43(4):827–838
29. Bockmühl U, Kratzsch B, Benda K, Draf W. Paranasal sinus mucoceles: surgical management and long term results. [Article in German] Laryngorhinootologie 2005; 84(12):892–898
30. Melroy CT, Dubin MG, Hardy SM, Senior BA. Analysis of methods to assess frontal sinus extent in osteoplastic flap surgery: transillumination versus 6-ft Caldwell versus image guidance. Am J Rhinol 2006;20(1):77–83
31. Sindwani R, Metson R. Impact of image guidance on complications during osteoplastic frontal sinus surgery. Otolaryngol Head Neck Surg 2004;131(3):150–155

32. Hahn S, Palmer JN, Purkey MT, Kennedy DW, Chiu AG. Indications for external frontal sinus procedures for inflammatory sinus disease. Am J Rhinol Allergy 2009; 23(3):342–347

33. Zacharek MA, Fong KJ, Hwang PH. Image-guided frontal trephination: a minimally invasive approach for hard-to-reach frontal sinus disease. Otolaryngol Head Neck Surg 2006;135(4):518–522

34. Isa AY, Mennie J, McGarry GW. The frontal osteoplastic flap: does it still have a place in rhinological surgery? J Laryngol Otol 2011;125(2):162–168

35. Lee JM, Palmer JN. Indications for the osteoplastic flap in the endoscopic era. Curr Opin Otolaryngol Head Neck Surg 2011;19(1):11–15

36. Isse NG. Endoscopic facial rejuvenation. Clin Plast Surg 1997;24(2):213–231

37. Hardy J, Vezina JL. Transsphenoidal neurosurgery of intracranial neoplasm. Adv Neurol 1976;15:261–273

38. Hardy J. The transsphenoidal surgical approach to the pituitary. Hosp Pract 1979;14(6):81–89

39. Isolan GR, de Aguiar PH, Laws ER, Strapasson AC, Piltcher O. The implications of microsurgical anatomy for surgical approaches to the sellar region. Pituitary 2009;12(4):360–367

40. Unal B, Bademci G, Bilgili YK, Batay F, Avci E. Risky anatomic variations of sphenoid sinus for surgery. Surg Radiol Anat 2006;28(2):195–201

41. Valentine R, Wormald PJ. Carotid artery injury after endonasal surgery. Otolaryngol Clin North Am 2011;44 (5):1059–1079

42. Cavallo LM, Messina A, Gardner P, et al. Extended endoscopic endonasal approach to the pterygopalatine fossa: anatomical study and clinical considerations. Neurosurg Focus 2005;19(1):E5

12 Complications of Adenotonsillectomy

A. Elmaraghy

Introduction

Adenotonsillectomy is a commonly performed procedure, with over 300,000 completed annually in the United States.[1] Most adenotonsillectomies are not technically difficult and are performed by otolaryngologists at various levels of training and experience (**Fig. 12.1**). Despite its commonality, adenotonsillectomy can be fraught with both minor and major complications.

Post-tonsillectomy Hemorrhage

Hemorrhage following adenotonsillectomy (**Fig. 12.2**) occurs at a rate of 2 to 3%[2] and can be defined as a primary bleed, which occurs within the first 24 hours, or a secondary hemorrhage, which occurs after 24 hours. Primary hemorrhage is thought to occur from inadequate hemostasis during the procedure. The incidence of primary hemorrhage has been reported to be ~ 0.2 to 1%.[3]

Inspecting the tonsillar fossa in a systematic fashion is paramount to avoid primary hemorrhage. Special attention should be paid to the inferior pole area because of the high concentration of blood vessels in that region (**Fig. 12.3**). As a routine, release of the mouth gag or nasopharyngeal catheter to reduce tension on the fossae with reinspection will often reveal bleeding sites that were not obvious.

Secondary hemorrhage is more difficult to avoid. Use of electrocautery or radiofrequency creates an eschar in

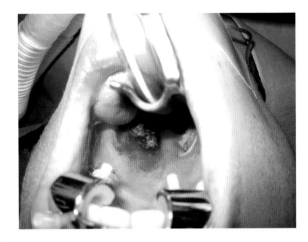

Fig. 12.2 Clot in left tonsillar fossa.

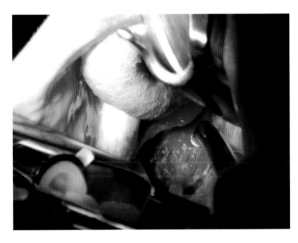

Fig. 12.3 Bleeding in inferior pole.

the tonsillar fossa and loss of this eschar, which occurs 5 to 7 days after tonsillectomy, is thought to contribute to the etiology (**Fig. 12.4**). Maintaining the plane between pharyngeal constrictor muscle and tonsillar capsule without violation of the muscle may prevent exposure of larger caliber vessels. Maintaining the airway is the critical first step during a severe hemorrhage. Rapid sequence intubation is preferred as the patients have often swallowed a great deal of blood and are at aspiration risk. Bronchoscopy equipment should be available if blood is aspirated and ventilation becomes difficult. A ventilating bronchoscope with suction port and large caliber tracheal suction would be necessary should this scenario arise (**Fig. 12.5**). Following control of the hemorrhage, it is important to

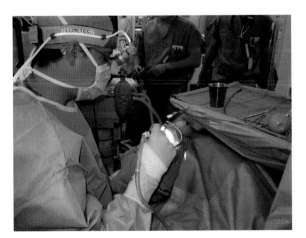

Fig. 12.1 Otolaryngologist performing adenotonsillectomy.

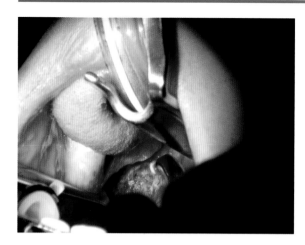

Fig. 12.4 Eschar in tonsillar fossa following cauterization.

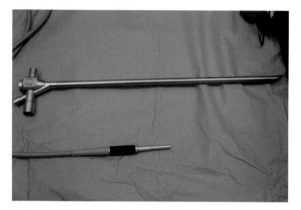

Fig. 12.5 Ventilating bronchoscope.

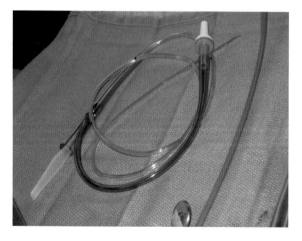

Fig. 12.6 Orogastric tube.

pass an orogastric tube to evacuate the swallowed blood to prevent postoperative emesis (**Fig. 12.6**).

Although bleeding is the most common complication of adenotonsillectomy, patients are typically not screened for a bleeding diathesis unless a family history for a bleeding disorder exists or a personal history of easy bleeding or bruising is present. Hemophilia A or B does not typically present in an insidious fashion and is usually diagnosed before presentation to an otolaryngologist. However, some bleeding disorders are discovered following a bleeding episode resulting from adenotonsillectomy. Von Willebrand disease may be present in up to 1.3% of the population and is often discovered in this manner.[4] Type 1 and 2 are inherited in an autosomal dominant fashion and the first manifestation of the disease may be posttonsillectomy hemorrhage. Patients with von Willebrand disease have a higher risk of bleeding following surgery and their postoperative management should include consultation with hematologists. Use of intranasal desmopressin preoperatively and postoperatively and aminocaproic acid orally may help to prevent bleeding. Despite these measures, the rate of postoperative bleeding in patients with von Willebrand disease may be as high as 13 to 17%.[5] No consensus exists as to the ideal technique for performing the surgery but the general principle is one of meticulous dissection and intraoperative hemostasis, which is used in all adenotonsillectomies. Counseling of patients with coagulopathies, and their parents, on these risks is imperative. Weighing the potential benefits of surgery against the rate of bleeding must be done in a clear manner.

Rarely, bleeding may not be controlled transorally. In these cases, ligation of the external carotid may be necessary. This has been reported in cases of massive hemorrhage or repeated hemorrhages following tonsillectomy.[6] Aberrant vasculature in the posterior pharynx or medialized carotids may present a risk factor for catastrophic bleeding. Patients with velocardiofacial syndrome or 22q11 are at risk for medialized carotid arteries and special caution is needed. Aberrant arteries have been reported in the nasopharynx as well.[7] Major vessel injury can be fatal and use of interventional radiology may be necessary. Entry into the parapharyngeal space during tonsillectomy may cause carotid pseudoaneurysm formation. Patients with repeated severe hemorrhage, or hemorrhage later than 14 days following surgery, may need thorough work-up including a pseudoaneurysm as part of the differential diagnosis. Diagnosis involves angiography, which could include embolization of the offending vessel.

Postoperative Respiratory Distress

The incidence of respiratory distress following adenotonsillectomy is rare in patients without medical comorbidities and the expected rate is ~ 1.3%.[8] Obstructive sleep apnea is the most common risk factor for postoperative respiratory issues. The range of incidence of respiratory events following adenotonsillectomy in obstructive sleep apnea is 6 to 21%.[9] They may manifest as increased oxygen requirement, but may also present as fulminant respiratory failure, precipitated by pulmonary edema or hypoventilation due to the narcotic sensitivity of obstructive sleep apnea patients.

Risk Factors

Polysomnography may be predictive for postoperative respiratory distress. Pediatric obstructive sleep apnea associated with an apnea–hypopnea index greater than 5 and oxygen saturation nadir of less than 80% are independent predictors of respiratory events.[10] Children under the age of 4 undergoing adenotonsillectomy for obstructive symptoms may also have a higher incidence of respiratory complications and caution should be taken if the surgery is carried out in a same-day surgery setting.[11]

In addition to obstructive sleep apnea, the presence of other medical comorbidities can increase the chance of a respiratory event. Patients with asthma have an increased rate of respiratory complications following adenotonsillectomy.[12] Prevention of exacerbation of the asthma requires coordination among anesthesia, pulmonary, and otolaryngology services. Caution should be exerted in people with asthma who have a history of recent exacerbations.

Obesity is another independent risk factor for respiratory problems following adenotonsillectomy. Obesity, defined as body mass index (weight in kg/height in m^2) greater than 30, increases the need for supplemental oxygen following surgery and increases the chance of postoperative upper airway obstruction.[13] Patients with obesity may need overnight observation because of the increase in respiratory issues.

Patients with neuromuscular disorders are also at increased risk for respiratory difficulties following adenotonsillectomy. Effects of postoperative oropharyngeal edema, increased secretions, pain, and dysphagia may be magnified in patients with neuromuscular problems. The incidence of complications in this group of patients can be as high as 20 to 25% leading to reintubation in 13% of these patients.[14] Prevention of serious complications involves recognizing the need for intensive monitoring of this patient population, maintaining adequate analgesia, and respiratory physiotherapy to assist with clearing of secretions.

Airway Fire

Use of electrical devices during adenotonsillectomy present the possibility of fire during the procedure.[15] For a fire to occur, combustible material, an ignition source, and an oxidizing agent must be present. In adenotonsillectomy, combustible materials include the endotracheal tube, nasopharyngeal catheter, tonsil pack, or tissue. The ignition source is the electrocautery or electrical device and the oxidizing agent is the supplemental oxygen or nitrous oxide. Prevention of airway fire requires keeping the supplemental oxygen lower than 40%. This requires direct communication with anesthesia staff and awareness of when a higher percentage of inspired oxygen is necessary. Use of appropriate endotracheal tubes is critical as well. A cuffless tube with a large leak increases the oxygen concentrations at the operative site; therefore, keeping the leak to a minimum with an appropriately sized tube is important. Limiting the power on electrocautery is another factor and the minimum power level should be used to complete hemostasis. Excessive charring may create organic gases, which may become combustible.

Perioral Burns

Use of electrocautery may pose a burn risk to the perioral region. The true incidence of this complication is unknown as there are few cases reported in the literature. One institution reported an incidence of 0.16% and a survey conducted reported the incidence to be 0.01 to 0.04%.[16] Burns occur from contact with a conducting region of the electrical instrument. This can occur with inadvertent activation of the device or from exposure of the cautery coupling area between the handpiece and the insulated region.

Minor burns respond to local care but more severe burns can cause scarring, deformities, and functional issues. Severe burns in close proximity to the oral commissure may lead to problems such as microstomia. Prevention of this complication requires diligence in ensuring that the electrocautery tip is completely inserted without any exposure of the conducting portion. Use of guarded tips with a shielded, insulated area to prevent contact of the conducting portion is also prudent. Some surgeons use cheek retractors to protect the perioral region. Treatment of perioral burns may require consultation with the burn team, use of topical antibiotics, possible steroid injections, stenting, or commissuroplasty.

Cervical Complications Following Adenotonsillectomy

Complications involving the cervical region are rare but important to recognize because their implications may be serious. One of the more commonly encountered issues following adenotonsillectomy involving the cervical region is atlantoaxial subluxation or Grisel syndrome. Because this is not frequently reported, the true incidence is unknown. Patients typically present with painful torticollis beginning several days after the procedure.

The subluxation may be minor or severe and is thought to be a result of hematogenous spread of infection from the pharynx to the cervical spine with resultant destabilization of atlantoaxial ligaments and subluxation. At particular risk for this are people with Down syndrome, who have a 15% incidence of postoperative atlantoaxial instability.

Recognition of this complication is important because severe neurologic sequelae such as spinal cord compression, quadriplegia, and, potentially, death may ensue. Diagnosis involves computed tomography to detail the bony anatomy and magnetic resonance imaging to diagnose the ligamentous inflammation. Prevention of this complication may involve obtaining flexion–extension radiographs in patients with Down syndrome before adenotonsillectomy with referral to Orthopedic or Neurosurgical services in patients with abnormal films. Treatment involves systemic antibiotics, bed rest, muscle relaxants, nonsteroidal anti-inflammatory agents, cervical stabilization with soft-collar for minor cases, and potentially cervical traction with stiff collar or halo fixation.[17]

Velopharyngeal Insufficiency Following Adenotonsillectomy

Postoperative voice changes are common following adenotonsillectomy. Removal of large tonsils will typically change the voice quality and there are some data to suggest improvement in acoustic parameters;[18] however, velopharyngeal insufficiency with postoperative hypernasality is troublesome, albeit uncommon. In one series, up to 53% of patients with persistent hypernasality following adenotonsillectomy required surgical intervention.[19] This is traditionally a result of aggressive adenoidectomy. Patients with cleft palate or submucous cleft palate are at particular risk for this complication. A partial adenoidectomy for this group of patients is wise with sparing of the inferior adenoid pad. Transient hypernasality may be more common but its true incidence is unknown. The basis for the hypernasality is typically loss of the nasopharyngeal seal created by articulation of the soft palate with the inferior adenoid pad. Prevention involves palpating the hard palate to screen for occult submucous cleft and avoiding overaggressive adenoidectomy. Surgical treatment may involve posterior pharyngeal augmentation or pharyngeal flap.

Nasopharyngeal Stenosis

Nasopharyngeal stenosis is a rare condition following adenotonsillectomy that is heralded by the return of snoring and obstructive symptoms several weeks to months following surgery. Scarring between the tonsillar pillars, soft palate, and posterior pharynx may result from overaggressive resection of the posterior pillar with subsequent scar formation to the posterior pharynx. Patients also at risk are those with history of keloids, surgery in the presence of severe inflammation such as peritonsillar abscess, or concomitant uvulopalatopharyngoplasty with adenoidectomy. Its incidence has been reported to be as high as 3.5% following uvulopalatopharyngoplasty.[20] Diagnosis of nasopharyngeal stenosis requires postoperative endoscopy in patients who present with obstructive symptoms following adenotonsillectomy. The cicatricial scar may need treatment if the patient exhibits obstructive sleep apnea. Correction of nasopharyngeal stenosis may require stents, local flaps, free tissue transfer, or use of mitomycin C or steroid injection.

References

1. Hall M, Lawrence L. Ambulatory surgery in the United States, 1996. Advance data from vital and health statistics; no. 300. Hyattsville, MD: National Center for Health Statistics, 1998
2. Evans AS, Khan AM, Young D, Adamson R. Assessment of secondary haemorrhage rates following adult tonsillectomy—a telephone survey and literature review. Clin Otolaryngol Allied Sci 2003;28(6):489–491
3. Abou-Jaoude PM, Manoukian JJ, Daniel SJ, et al. Complications of adenotonsillectomy revisited in a large pediatric case series. J Otolaryngol 2006;35(3):180–185
4. Jiménez-Yuste V, Prim MP, De Diego JI, et al. Otolaryngologic surgery in children with von Willebrand disease. Arch Otolaryngol Head Neck Surg 2002;128(12):1365–1368
5. Statham MM, Myer CM III. Complications of adenotonsillectomy. Curr Opin Otolaryngol Head Neck Surg 2010;18(6):539–543
6. Windfuhr JP. Excessive post-tonsillectomy hemorrhage requiring ligature of the external carotid artery. Auris Nasus Larynx 2002;29(2):159–164
7. Hofman R, Zeebregts CJ, Dikkers FG. Fulminant post-tonsillectomy haemorrhage caused by aberrant course of the external carotid artery. J Laryngol Otol 2005;119 (8):655–657
8. Richmond KH, Wetmore RF, Baranak CC. Postoperative complications following tonsillectomy and adenoidectomy—who is at risk? Int J Pediatr Otorhinolaryngol 1987;13(2):117–124
9. Brown KA, Morin I, Hickey C, Manoukian JJ, Nixon GM, Brouillette RT. Urgent adenotonsillectomy: an analysis of risk factors associated with postoperative respiratory morbidity. Anesthesiology 2003;99(3):586–595
10. Jaryszak EM, Shah RK, Vanison CC, Lander L, Choi SS. Polysomnographic variables predictive of adverse respiratory events after pediatric adenotonsillectomy. Arch Otolaryngol Head Neck Surg 2011;137(1):15–18
11. Brigger MT, Brietzke SE. Outpatient tonsillectomy in children: a systematic review. Otolaryngol Head Neck Surg 2006;135(1):1–7
12. Kalra M, Buncher R, Amin RS. Asthma as a risk factor for respiratory complications after adenotonsillectomy in children with obstructive breathing during sleep. Ann Allergy Asthma Immunol 2005;94(5):549–552
13. Fung E, Cave D, Witmans M, Gan K, El-Hakim H. Postoperative respiratory complications and recovery in obese

children following adenotonsillectomy for sleep-disordered breathing: a case–control study. Otolaryngol Head Neck Surg 2010;142(6):898–905

14. Manrique D, Sato J, Anastacio EM. Postoperative acute respiratory insufficiency following adenotonsillectomy in children with neuropathy. Int J Pediatr Otorhinolaryngol 2008;72(5):587–591

15. Mattucci KF, Militana CJ. The prevention of fire during oropharyngeal electrosurgery. Ear Nose Throat J 2003; 82(2):107–109

16. Nuara MJ, Park AH, Alder SC, Smith ME, Kelly S, Muntz H. Perioral burns after adenotonsillectomy: a potentially serious complication. Arch Otolaryngol Head Neck Surg 2008;134(1):10–15

17. Richter GT, Bower CM. Cervical complications following routine tonsillectomy and adenoidectomy. Curr Opin Otolaryngol Head Neck Surg 2006;14(6):375–380

18. Subramaniam V, Kumar P. Impact of tonsillectomy with or without adenoidectomy on the acoustic parameters of the voice: a comparative study. Arch Otolaryngol Head Neck Surg 2009;135(10):966–969

19. Fernandes DB, Grobbelaar AO, Hudson DA, Lentin R. Velopharyngeal incompetence after adenotonsillectomy in non-cleft patients. Br J Oral Maxillofac Surg 1996; 34(5):364–367

20. Katsantonis GP, Friedman WH, Krebs FJ III, Walsh JK. Nasopharyngeal complications following uvulopalatopharyngoplasty. Laryngoscope 1987;97(3 Pt 1):309–314

III A Surgery of the Oral Cavity and Oropharynx

13 Complications of Obstructive Sleep Apnea Surgery

A. F. Lewis, R. J. Soose

Introduction

Obstructive sleep apnea (OSA) can be treated by multiple medical and surgical methods. Continuous positive airway pressure (CPAP), oral appliances, and weight loss serve as the foundation of medical therapy for most patients. For those patients who are unable to tolerate or unable to achieve treatment success with medical therapy options, surgical therapy can be beneficial—successfully improving symptoms and quality of life as well as reducing cardiovascular risks. Surgery for OSA can be used as an adjunct to improve adherence and success with medical device therapy (CPAP or oral appliance). Surgery can also be employed as a sole treatment strategy, most commonly as a staged multilevel plan.

Most OSA surgical procedures are aimed at enlarging and stabilizing the narrow and collapsible portions of the upper airway. Proper airway phenotyping, thorough examination and endoscopy techniques, and proper procedure selection are critical to successful surgical therapy and are beyond the scope of this chapter. In general terms, OSA surgery encompasses procedures of the nasal airway, pharynx, and craniofacial skeleton. Bariatric surgery, hypoglossal nerve stimulation, and tracheotomy also fall under the category of surgical therapy for OSA. This chapter focuses specifically on the soft tissue surgical procedures of the pharynx and the associated perioperative complications, whereas nasal surgery and craniofacial procedures are discussed elsewhere (**Figure 13.1**) Complications associated with office-based procedures for nonapneic snoring or mild OSA are also described, as well as the perioperative management of any patient with OSA undergoing general anesthesia.

Palatal Surgery

Since its introduction by Fujita in 1981, uvulopalatopharyngoplasty (UPPP) has been one of the most commonly performed operations for the treatment of OSA.[1] Incidence and severity of some complications have changed with modifications of the procedure; however, the most commonly reported complications specific to UPPP remain bleeding, velopharyngeal insufficiency, nasopharyngeal stenosis, and globus sensation. As with any surgical therapy for OSA, airway obstruction/respiratory compromise, vascular complications, and persistent OSA are also potential risks.

Complications in the Perioperative Period

Anatomical factors and comorbidities associated with OSA predispose patients to complications in the perioperative patient. Incidence of serious complications following UPPP in the early postoperative period, however, is relatively low in most studies.[2–7] Most of the data come from case series with a limited number of patients and varying descriptions of the complications. Kezirian et al[2] prospectively collected data on the incidence of serious complications and 30-day mortality rate in over 3,000 adults undergoing inpatient UPPP from the national Veterans' Affairs database from 1991 to 2001 and found an overall incidence of only 1.5%. This included death,

---

Surgeries included

- Palatal surgeries
  - Uvulopalatopharyngoplasty
  - Transpalatal advancement pharyngoplasty
  - Expansion pharyngoplasty
  - Anterior palatoplasty
- Hypopharyngeal surgery
  - Volumetric reduction procedures
  - Radiofrequency of the base of tongue
  - Tongue-base suspension
  - Hyoid suspension
- Snoring procedures
  - Palatal implants
  - Snoreplasty
  - Radiofrequency of the palate

Surgeries not included

- Skeletal procedures
  - Genioglossus advancement
  - Mandibular advancement
  - Maxillary advancement
- Nasal surgery
- Tracheotomy

Fig. 13.1 Sleep surgeries discussed in the chapter.

respiratory; cardiovascular, including cardiac arrest, myocardial infarction, cerebrovascular accidents, pulmonary embolism, hemorrhage greater than 3 units of packed erythrocytes, coma, wound infection, systemic sepsis, deep venous thrombosis, and renal failure.

The most common and potentially severe complication is respiratory compromise. The severity of respiratory compromise varies and may include oxygen desaturation, reintubation, pneumonia, prolonged ventilation (> 48 hours), emergent tracheotomy, or pulmonary edema. The incidence of respiratory compromise varies widely between studies, with reported rates between 1.1% and 11%.[2,8]

Studies evaluating whether UPPP can be safely performed as an outpatient procedure showed that serious airway complications including airway obstruction and postoperative pulmonary edema occurred in the immediate postoperative period, usually evident in the recovery room within the first few hours after surgery. Oxygen desaturation may occur at any time during the postoperative period, but because oxygen desaturation is part of the underlying disease process, it may be difficult to distinguish between the disease itself and a postoperative respiratory complication. Riley et al[7] reported that six of 182 patients had desaturation to the upper 80% range in the first two postoperative days. In a retrospective review by Hathaway and Johnson,[8] 3% of patients undergoing UPPP with or without septoplasty had oxygen desaturation in the recovery room. Studies have shown that postoperative oxygen desaturation is comparable to that observed during preoperative polysomnography. The polysomnography, as well as patients' body mass index, cardiopulmonary status, and other clinical factors, should be considered when choosing patients who can safely have surgery as an outpatient.[8,9]

Careful patient selection and postoperative monitoring for several hours, avoids perioperative cardiopulmonary complications in most situations, even if the surgery is performed as an outpatient procedure. Reports of risk factors for serious complications following UPPP are conflicting in the literature. Haavisto and Suonpaa[4] found that previous cardiac disease contributed. Esclamado et al[3] suggested that weight, apnea–hypopnea index and lowest oxygen saturation on the polysomnogram, and preoperative narcotics were all associated with perioperative risks. Concurrent nasal procedures may temporarily worsen sleep-disordered breathing in the immediate postoperative period, particularly if nasal packing is used, by interfering with the nasal receptor-mediated control of breathing.[3–5] More recently, Kezirian et al[10] analyzed the records of 3130 veterans and concluded that apnea–hypopnea index, body mass index, medical comorbidities, and concurrent tongue-base procedures were each associated with an increased risk of serious complications.

Hemorrhage and Wound Dehiscence

Bleeding following UPPP has been estimated between 2 and 14% and appears to be similar to the bleeding rates following adult tonsillectomy.[9,11] One cohort study showed that the incidence of a substantial hemorrhage (> 4 units packed red blood cells) was 0.3%.[2] Bleeding may occur in the immediate postoperative period and likely represents a technical error. More commonly, bleeding after palatal surgery, with or without tonsillectomy, occurs in a delayed fashion and can occur anytime in the first 2-weeks after surgery.[12] Delayed or secondary hemorrhage is likely related to wound healing factors, including granulation tissue formation, the inflammatory process, and eschar disruption. Although the data are conflicting, dietary and activity restrictions as well as postoperative medical therapy to reduce secondary inflammation and promote mucosalization, such as corticosteroids and topical sucralfate, may reduce the risk of postoperative bleeding. Exposed muscle in the tonsillar fossa may also contribute to the bleeding risk. Typically, the tonsils are removed concomitantly, and the tonsillar pillars are closed. Tension on the closure often leads to dehiscence of the closure, particularly at the tonsillar poles, leading to exposed muscle and potential for bleeding.

Velopharyngeal Insufficiency

Velopharyngeal insufficiency (VPI) is the inability of the velopharyngeal sphincter to sufficiently separate the oropharynx and nasopharynx during swallowing or speech. Closure of the velopharynx depends on the musculus uvula and the action of the levator palatine muscles.

Following traditional UPPP with aggressive resection of the uvula and velum, temporary postoperative VPI is common; however, more permanent or long-term VPI may also occur with potentially devastating impact on quality of life. Some studies have reported that up to 10 to 24% of patients continued to complain of intermittent nasopharyngeal regurgitation 1 year after surgery.[4,13] In his survey of 72 centers over 9 years, however, Fairbanks reported only a small number of patients with this complication.[14]

The amount of soft palate that can be safely resected varies among patients because the point of contact of the elevating palate and posterior pharyngeal wall varies, as does palatal length. A traditional resection of 1 to 2 cm will compromise the velopharyngeal function in some patients. Preoperative evaluation of the kneepoint, which corresponds to the distal point of the levator sling, is important. Intraoperatively it can be evaluated by retroplacement of the velum to the posterior pharyngeal wall. Surgical resection should not violate the levator sling. Extensive cautery and subsequent scarring can further shorten the palate and decrease velopharyngeal function.[13,15]

As VPI has potentially serious, long-term consequences, the best treatment of VPI is avoidance. VPI is best avoided altogether by employing current reconstructive procedures that preserve mucosa, uvular structure and function; rather than destructive or excisional, palatal procedures. Surgical correction of VPI is difficult because of shortening of the palate and scarring. It also carries the risk of worsening OSA. A superior pharyngeal flap or sphincter palatoplasty has been reported to result in improvement. Palatal pushback procedures, obturators, and Teflon paste injections have also been described.[16-18]

Nasopharyngeal Stenosis

Nasopharyngeal stenosis (NPS) is the partial or complete obstruction between the nasopharynx and oropharynx due to concentric scar contracture of the tonsillar pillars and posterior pharyngeal wall (**Figs. 13.2** and **13.3**).[19] NPS can cause nasal airway obstruction, hyponasal speech, rhinorrhea, and worsening of OSA. Fortunately, it is a rare problem estimated to be less than 1%.[20] In the prevention of nasopharyngeal stenosis, it is important to avoid forming a contiguous raw surface about the nasopharyngeal isthmus.[15] Technical errors that have been shown to increase the incidence of NPS include excessive removal or cauterization of the posterior tonsillar mucosa or undermining the posterior pharyngeal wall mucosa, as well as closure under tension. A concomitant adenoidectomy should also be avoided.[13,21]

As with VPI, the best treatment of NPS is avoidance by using UPPP modifications that maximally preserve mucosa of the velopharyngeal isthmus. Once it has occurred, the treatment of NPS is difficult.[21] Krespi and Kacker[22] reported 18 patients with NPS following UPPP. All patients were treated with the CO_2 laser with or without a nasopharyngeal obturator resulting in adequate nasopharyngeal lumens following treatment. Though severity ranged from mild to severe, it should be noted that results are typically better in less severe forms of stenosis. Jones et al had success with treatment of patients with laser followed by Mitomycin C and an obturator.[23] Other treatment options include dilation, scar revision with or without skin grafting, scar excision with maxillofacial prosthesis, local flaps, pedicled flaps, and free-tissue transfer.[23-28]

Hypogeusia

Though most of the above complications of UPPP have been well documented and studied, less attention has been given to postoperative taste disturbances. A review of the literature revealed a reported rate of 7 to 10%.[29,30] A longitudinal intervention study designed specifically to investigate taste disturbances following UPPP revealed a

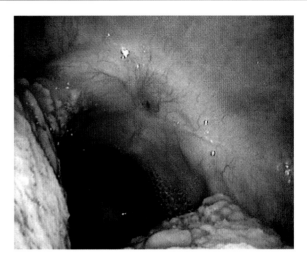

Fig. 13.2 Nasopharyngeal stenosis: a transoral preoperative view of a patient with a wide, thick scar band obliterating the soft palate and leaving only a pinpoint nasopharyngeal dimple. (Image courtesy of Prof. M. Gerek, MD.)

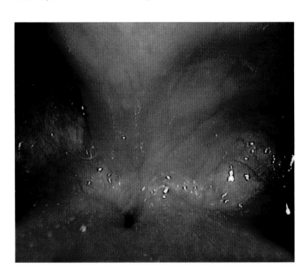

Fig. 13.3 Nasopharyngeal stenosis: a transnasal view, using flexible fiberoptic laryngoscopy, of a patient with pinpoint stenosis at the soft palate. (Image courtesy of Prof. M. Gerek, MD.)

4.6% rate 3 months after surgery. Nine months after the operation all but one of five patients had a restoration of their taste sensation. Gustatory function tests showed that deficiency of sweet sense was the most common type of taste disturbance.[31] Following lateral pharyngoplasty, which is discussed further in a following section, Cahali[32] also noted one patient with a taste loss for chocolate, which recovered after 6 months.

Causes of taste dysfunction may include damage to the lingual branch of the glossopharyngeal nerve in the tonsillar fossa, excision of taste receptors on the soft palate, or mechanical pressure on the tongue. It is speculated that the decreased use of electrocautery for tonsillectomy, particularly at the inferior tonsillar pole region, may decrease the incidence of taste dysfunction. The palate receives its taste sensation from the geniculate ganglion via the great petrosal nerve. Sweet sensation is the most sensitively perceived taste of the palate. In the study by Li et al,[29] the incidence of taste disturbances was significantly higher for patients with electrocautery used during development of the uvulopalatal flap. Avoiding excision of the soft palate during palatopharyngeal surgery and decreasing the use of electrocautery on the soft palate may further decrease postoperative hypogeusia, particularly to sweet tastes.[29-31]

Voice Disturbances

The results of voice disturbances following UPPP have varied in the literature. Powell pointed out that interpretation of speech problems are difficult; he suggested that the redundant mucosa may have led to abnormal speech patterns before surgery. Van Lierde et al[33] performed a prospective study of nasalance, nasality, voice, and articulation of 26 patients after UPPP and found that there was no impact on nasality, voice, and articulation. Regarding nasalance, the only change that occurred involved the sound "i".

Brosch et al[34] prospectively studied patients undergoing muscle sparing UPPP and tonsillectomy and found a significant raising of the fundamental frequency. Tewary and Cable[35] found that the fundamental frequency was lower in patients undergoing UPPP compared with those undergoing tonsillectomy. Most patients will not notice such changes, but professional voice users should be counseled preoperatively.

Globus Sensation

Though often considered minor when compared with the other reported complications of UPPP, globus, or a foreign body sensation, has been the most commonly reported complaint following UPPP. It has been reported in 22 to 31% of patients after 1 year and up to 60% of patients after 3 years. Some patients even complain of persistent long-term discomfort. This potentially very bothersome complication may result from scarring of the soft palate and excision of the uvula. The uvula contains the highest concentration of serous glands in the oral cavity/oropharynx and plays an important role in lubricating the posterior pharyngeal wall, which explains why removal of the glands may result in pharyngeal dryness and globus sensation.[15,36-38]

Therefore, preservation of the uvula may substantially reduce the incidence of this complication. Kwon et al[39] designed a study to evaluate the postoperative effect of uvular-preserving palatopharyngoplasty on OSA and globus sensation. Using a VAS, they showed no change in globus sensation following surgery compared with

preoperative values. No treatment has been shown to be curative, but injection of scarred tissue with depot corticosteroids in the intermediate postoperative period has been attempted. For long-term treatment, oral lubricants may provide modest symptomatic relief.

Complications Related to Specific Palate Procedures

The following procedures have not been as widely researched, and the actual incidence of the complications is not known. The reported rates of complications, as well as the potential complications, and avoidance and treatment strategies are discussed that have been reported in the literature.

Transpalatal Advancement Pharyngoplasty

This technique was first described in the literature in 1993 and was developed to address the limitations of traditional UPPP techniques. This technique enlarges the velopharynx and retropalatal segment by excising a portion of the posterior hard palate and advancing the soft palate anteriorly. Like most mucosa-sparing reconstructive techniques, the overall incidence of complications, particularly VPI, NPS, and globus sensation, may be dramatically reduced compared with traditional UPPP. However, the transpalatal advancement pharyngoplasty, with its osteotomy technique, introduces the possibility of a new complication: oronasal fistula.

In the literature, the fistula rate increased when the technique was modified and the tensor tendon was incised to increase mobilization. The largest series to date showed the occurrence of an oronasal fistula in 12.7% (6 of 47 patients). Subsequent modifications have led to a reduction in fistula rates. Shine and Lewis[40] compared effectiveness of the procedure using two incision types, traditional Gothic arch incision and a modified propeller incision. They noted decreased fistula rates in the patients who had undergone the propeller soft tissue approach.

Fistulas are successfully treated with occlusive oral splints and suture reapproximation of the soft tissues in the office during the postoperative period.[41,42]

Expansion Sphincter Pharyngoplasty

Lateral pharyngeal wall collapse has been demonstrated to be an important component of OSA and is not addressed by standard UPPP techniques. In 2003, Cahali[32] first described the lateral pharyngoplasty, which involved sectioning of the superior pharyngeal constrictor muscle and creating a laterally based flap. In addition, a palatopharyngeal Z-plasty was performed. After the procedure most patients reported dysphagia especially to dry, solid foods lasting from 8 to 70 days, with a median time 14.5 days. Pharyngeal swallow returned without further treatment.

The expansion sphincter pharyngoplasty (ESP) was developed, as a modification of the lateral pharyngoplasty, to enlarge the lateral dimension of the retropalatal space in patients with a large lateral wall component. Bilateral rotation flaps comprising the palatopharyngeus muscles characterize the ESP. In a prospective controlled trial comparing ESP with traditional UPPP, ESP provided more effective treatment of the OSA and was not associated with any significant complications.[43]

Anterior Palatoplasty

For patients with a primarily anterior–posterior pattern of palatal collapse at the level of the levator sling and velum, anterior palatoplasty may provide successful management of the palatal flutter and obstruction while limiting complications by preserving the structure and function of the uvula and free edge of the soft palate. In this technique, a strip of mucosa and submucosal tissue is removed from the proximal soft palate followed by closure of the horizontal defect and anterior advancement of the soft palate. In a prospective series of 77 patients, there was no VPI, NPS, or other reported complications.[44]

Oropharyngeal/ Hypopharyngeal Procedures

A variety of oropharyngeal/hypopharyngeal procedures are available for the treatment of OSA. Although genioglossus advancement, other skeletal procedures, and hypoglossal nerve stimulation address this portion of the airway as well, this section focuses on the soft tissue procedures only. These procedures primarily involve either (1) volumetric reduction or (2) advancement/suspension of the tongue base.

Hypopharyngeal procedures carry the risk of significant perioperative complications, which may be more difficult to treat because of their location lower in the airway. Identification and control of hemorrhage and airway obstruction may be more challenging, and potentially dangerous, complications in this area. Data suggest that most of these patients should be kept overnight though the perioperative complications following hypopharyngeal surgery have not been as well studied as those following UPPP. In the study by Kezirian et al,[2] they showed an increased risk of perioperative morbidity when performing tongue-base procedures with UPPP, though it was not possible to separate the cumulative risk versus the individual risk of the procedures.

Volumetric Reduction Procedures

Midline Glossectomy

Glossectomy involves decreasing the size of the soft tissues of the tongue base and hypopharynx. Initially, this procedure was associated with a high morbidity as the result of aggressive resections.[45–47] Submucosal minimally invasive lingual excision (SMILE), transoral submucosal endoscopy-assisted glossectomy, and lingual tonsillectomy have all been described as modifications developed to treat tongue-base-associated airway obstruction in adult and pediatric patients. The SMILE technique and transoral endoscopy-assisted glossectomy both involve removal using a plasma-mediated radiofrequency device (coblation) while sparing the taste buds and mucosa.[47,48] Potential complications include bleeding, hypoglossal nerve injury, edema, and airway compromise.[49] Actual incidence of complications with the transoral endoscopy-assisted glossectomy technique is not known, as there is little in the literature, but surgeon reports are rare.

SMILE

Using the SMILE technique Maturo and Mair[48] noted no incidences of significant bleeding in their series of patients, though Friedman et al[49] reported two cases of damage to the lingual artery in their retrospective analysis of 48 patients. Temporary hypoglossal nerve injury occurred in 4 out of 48 patients and resolved spontaneously. There was only 1 out of 48 with permanent unilateral hypoglossal injury. Knowledge of the anatomy is key to avoiding the hypoglossal lingual nerve vascular bundle. Through anatomical dissections, it has been found that keeping the path of the coblator wand roughly within 1 to 2 cm of the foramen cecum in the posterior tongue base is preventive (**Fig. 13.4**).[50] Posterior to the foramen cecum, the course of the lingual artery and nerve are more lateral, ~ 2.5 cm from the foramen cecum.

Other Measures

Other preventive measures taken are endoscopic visualization of the lingual cavity and preoperative ultrasound to map the location of the artery. Most cases of bleeding are minimal and can be controlled with direct pressure and epinephrine. Floseal (Baxter, Deerfield, IL, USA) can also be placed in the lingual cavity. For more serious cases of bleeding, bipolar cautery under direct visualization may be necessary. One of the two cases of bleeding reported by Friedman et al[49], required ligation of the lingual artery through an external neck excision.[48,49]

Though there were no reported airway complications in the studies reviewed, there is a risk of airway compromise following the SMILE procedure due to formation of

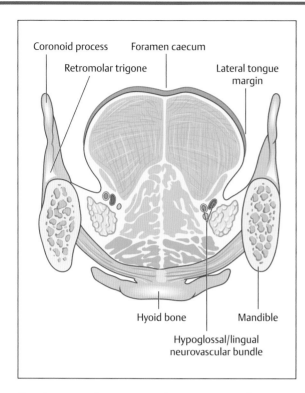

Coronoid process   Foramen caecum

Retromolar trigone

Lateral tongue margin

Hyoid bone   Mandible

Hypoglossal/lingual neurovascular bundle

Fig. 13.4 Tongue-base neurovascular anatomy: coronal section through the tongue showing location of lingual artery and nerve bundle ~ 1–2 cm lateral and 2.5 cm inferior to the foramen cecum (From Maturo and Mair, 2007.[48] Reproduced with permission from Sage Publications.)

seromas. The surgery results in the creation of dead space in the tongue-base region without a route for fluid escape (**Fig. 13.5**). This is a very serious complication that should be treated with drainage. A tracheotomy may be needed depending on the degree of obstruction.

Lingual tonsillectomy using bipolar cautery uses a malleable instrument for more precise removal, and the addition of an angled rod lens scope improves visualization. Risks of the procedure include bleeding, dysphagia, airway obstruction, and changes in taste. In a small series of 18 patients reported by Robinson et al[51] there were no reactive or secondary bleeds and no airway complications. Only three patients had a change in taste, which resolved spontaneously within 3 months.[47]

Radiofrequency Ablation of the Tongue Base

This is a minimally invasive technique that uses radiofrequency energy to induce submucosal thermal injury in the submucosal tissues of the tongue base and so cause volumetric reduction to address hypopharyngeal obstruction. The radiofrequency needle electrode is used to deliver a set amount of energy to a specific site at a controlled temperature. Typically one to three lesions are created per session.[52–55]

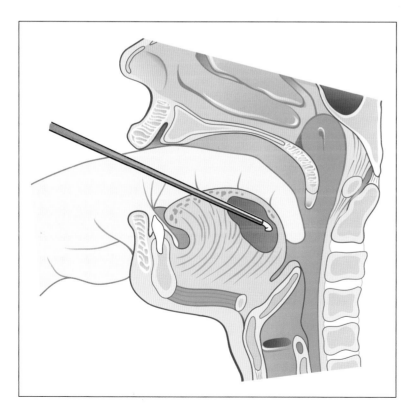

Fig. 13.5 SMILE technique (submucosal minimally iinvasive lingual excision): coblation wand is introduced through the incision and advanced toward the vallecula. Submucosal tissue excision is guided by palpation with the nondominant hand. (Reprint with permission from Friedman M, Soans R, Gurpinar B, et al. Evaluation of submucosal minimally invasive lingual excision technique for treatment of obstructive sleep apnea/hypopnea syndrome. Otolaryngol Head Neck Surg 2008;139:378–384.)

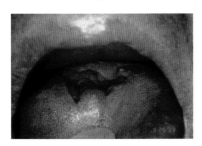

Fig. 13.6 Tongue-base abscess: midline tongue base abscess 3 weeks after tongue-base radiofrequency ablation.

Bleeding and Nerve Injury

In the studies reviewed, there were no cases of significant bleeding. The incidence of tongue-base neuralgias reported in the literature ranges from 0 to 16% with a spontaneous burning sensation lasting for up to 3 months.[53,54] Friedman et al[49] also report one case of partial hypoglossal nerve paralysis in their report of 48 patients that resolved spontaneously within 1 month. The lateral aspect of the tongue is not treated to prevent injury to the neurovascular bundle.[50,52,53]

Infections and Tongue-Base Abscesses

Tongue-base abscesses are one of the more serious complications associated with radiofrequency ablation of the tongue base (**Figs. 13.6 and 13.7**). The reported incidence has varied in the literature from 0 to 8%. As a result of these infections, avoidance strategies have

been recommended: antibiotics for 10 days and steroids for 5 days. Troell et al[52] recommend not treating with more than 750 J at any one focus and pretreatment with chlorhexidine oral rinses. Patients with persistent complaints of dysphagia, globus, or pain lasting longer than 1 week should undergo physical examination and possible computed tomography scan. Treatment requires hospital admission with incision and drainage, airway monitoring, and intravenous antibiotics. Tracheotomy has been necessary in several patients.[53]

Edema and Airway Compromise

Pazos and Mair[53] reported 2 out of 25 patients with severe edema of the floor of the mouth, but they also used up to 1000 J per treatment site. This is higher than reported by most studies, which have limited the amount of radiofrequency energy, as recommended above, to reduce potential airway obstructing tongue edema. Posttreatment airway protection for a minimum of 5 days with nasal continuous positive airway protection is recommended (**Table 13.1**).[52]

Tongue-Base Suspension

Tongue-base suspension involves placement of a bone screw in the lingual cortex of the mandibular symphysis. An attached suture is then looped through the tongue base and tied anteriorly to prevent collapse of the retrolingual

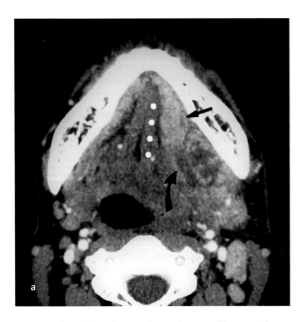

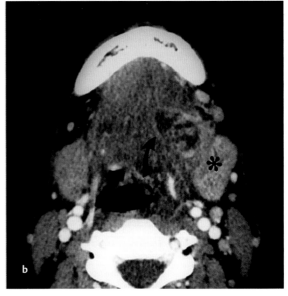

Fig. 13.7a,b Sublingual space abscess. (From Mukherji SK, Chong V. Atlas of Head and Neck Imaging. 1st ed. New York: Thieme, 2003.)

a Axial contrast-enhanced computed tomography shows a mixed attenuation abscess in the left sublingual space (curved arrow). Note the enlargement of the left sublingual gland (straight arrow) and displacement of the left genioglossus (asterisks) to the contralateral side.

b Axial contrast-enhanced computed tomography shows that abscess extends inferiorly into the left submandibular space (curved arrow) abutting and slightly displacing the left submandibular gland (asterisk).

Table 13.1 Summary of complications of radiofrequency ablation

RFA complications	Number	Type	Severity	Onset	Notes
Palatal RFA (n = 13)	11	Superficial mucosal ulceration	Mild	2–7 days	No significant deviation from clinical course in all patients
	2	Uvular slough	Moderate	4–7 days	Loss of uvula with increased pain × 1 week. No VPI
Tongue-base RFA (n = 8)	4	Tongue neuralgia	Moderate	> 1 week	"Burning" sensation with slow resolution over weeks
	2	Floor of mouth edema	Severe	Within 24 hours	Airway compromise; requires hospital admission, intravenous antibiotics, steroids, and airway monitoring for 24 hours
	2	Tongue abscess	Severe	3–4 weeks	Airway compromise; requires hospital admission, intravenous antibiotics, incision and drainage, and airway monitoring

RFA, radiofrequency ablation; VPI, velopharyngeal insufficiency.

Reprinted with permission from Pazos and Mair, 2001.[53]

airway. Complication rates reported in the literature are between 15 and 26% and include the following.[56–59]

Sialadenitis and Infection

This complication has been one of the most commonly reported (9 to 11%) and is usually associated with an intraoral approach. It can occur as a result of direct injury to the Wharton duct during the procedure or from edema. The screw should be placed posterior to Wharton duct orifices and care should be taken when passing the suture. Most cases are delayed, and all have responded to conservative treatment with oral antibiotics. A sterile submental approach and screw placement may significantly reduce the incidence of sialadenitis and infection. Preoperative and postoperative broad-spectrum antibiotics and steroids have been recommended to further reduce the risk of infection.[56,57]

Suture Migration, Extrusion, and Breakage

The suture is tightened based on the surgeon's discretion by palpating the tongue base where an indentation is felt. It is difficult to determine the exact amount of tightness needed to prevent collapse but not strangulate or place too much tension on the tissues. Overtightening also increases postoperative pain and edema. Tongue movements also increase tension on the suture. With time the suture can migrate and reduce effectiveness. Cases of extrusion and breakage have also been reported commonly in the literature, although the exact incidence is unknown.[56–58]

Dysarthria and Dysphagia

Most patients undergoing the procedure experience dysarthria, dysphagia, and odynophagia typically lasting from 7 to 21 days. The postoperative pain typically contributes to the dysphagia. Rarely, the postoperative dysphagia is severe enough to require intravenous hydration.[56]

Dental Injury

Few cases have been reported though it is a risk due to the screw placement in the mandibular symphysis. The screw should be placed below the level of the incisor tooth roots. The typical location is 1 cm from the inferior border of the mandible. If injury is suspected, the patient should be referred to a dental specialist for evaluation of vitality of the tooth. Endodontic treatment or dental extraction may be needed.[60]

Hypoglossal or Lingual Neurovascular Injury

The incidence of this complication is not known, though it appears to be rare. To avoid injury, care is taken not to pass the needle too far laterally when placing the suture, usually only 1 to 1.5 cm from midline.[60]

Hyoid Suspension

Hyoid suspension involves advancement and stabilization of the hyoid bone to increase the retrolingual/retroepiglottic space. Two techniques have been studied: suspension of the hyoid (1) anterosuperiorly to the inferior border of the anterior mandible and (2) anteroinferiorly to the thyroid cartilage.[61–65] With both techniques dysphagia is the most common postoperative complication and is generally expected following surgery. Most report dysphagia lasting only for a few days, though it may last up to 4 weeks.[62,66] Dysphagia may result from several factors: edema, change in the anatomy, and nerve injury. Edema related to surgical dissection is felt to cause the initial transient dysphagia.[65]

Increase in the pharyngeal dimensions may make airway protection more difficult. Neruntarat[63] recorded a transient aspiration rate of 9.3% though this is higher than most of the other studies discussed in this section. It resolved in all patients within 3 weeks. Damage to the internal branch of the superior laryngeal nerve, which supplies sensation to the supraglottic airway, and overly aggressive suspension may also lead to aspiration.[65,67] Injury can also occur to the hypoglossal nerve, but in most patients the paralysis resolves spontaneously.[64] All patients with persistent dysphagia should be evaluated endoscopically to rule out nerve injury or edema.

Other potential complications include suture breakage, seromas/infections, and pharyngocutaneous fistulas. Overall, the rate of seromas and infections reported has been less than 2%.[63] Most authors recommend a passive or active suction drain for at least 1 to 2 days to prevent seromas and hematomas.[66,68] In their study, Richard et al.[64] noted that the patients who had infections or abscesses had not received prophylactic antibiotics; perioperative antibiotics are therefore recommended for prevention. Treatment involves simple drainage and culture-directed antibiotics, although removal of hardware may be necessary in some patients.

Tschopp[69] showed that in a computed tomography scan the mean distance between the hyoid and pharynx is only 3 mm. This distance is depicted in the schematic representation shown in **Fig. 13.8**. This explains how fistulization or violation of the pharyngeal mucosa can easily occur from the passage of the suture or wire around the hyoid bone.[69] A persistent fistula may require removal of the suture.

Office-based Procedures for Nonapneic Snoring

For patients with nonapneic snoring, particularly those who have failed other conservative therapy such as weight loss, positional therapy, or treatment of nasal congestion, palatal stiffening techniques can be beneficial to reduce or eliminate palatal flutter and to improve symptoms. Procedures to stiffen the soft palate include pillar palatal implants, injection snoreplasty, and radiofrequency. Although these procedures are primarily used for the treatment of snoring, they may be used in select cases of mild OSA, particularly when combined with other procedures as part of a multilevel surgery.

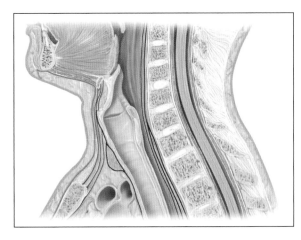

Fig. 13.8 Fascial relationships in the neck. Left lateral view. This midsagittal section shows that the deepest layer of the deep cervical fascia, the prevertebral layer, directly overlies the vertebral column in the median plane and is split into two parts. With tuberculous osteomyelitis of the cervical spine, for example, a gravitation abscess may develop in the "danger space" along the prevertebral fascia (retropharyngeal abscess). This fascia encloses muscles laterally and posteriorly. The carotid sheath is located further laterally and does not appear in the midsagittal section. From Schuenke M, Schulte E, Schumacher U, Voll M, Wesker KH. Thieme Atlas of Anatomy, Neck and Internal Organs, 2nd ed. Stuttgart: Thieme; 2009.

Pillar Implants

Extrusion is the most common complication with rates reported from 4 to 20%.[70–75] Risk factors include a thin palate and placement under general anesthesia. Extrusion rates have been higher in women, particularly those who had implants placed in the operating room (**Table 13.2, Fig. 13.9**). This is felt to be a result of the thinner palates in women and inversion of the device in the surgeon's hand.[73] Following implant placement, flexible nasopharyngoscopy should be performed to evaluate for posterior placement through the soft palate. If extrusion occurs, the implant should be removed. It is typically recommended that the wound is allowed to heal and the implant is replaced.[74]

Globus sensation is a rare complaint. In many cases, patients who complained of globus sensation have been found to have a partial extrusion that required removal.[74] We recommend evaluation for extrusion in any patient complaining of lasting discomfort or a foreign body sensation. Fistulas have not been reported in the literature.

Injection Snoreplasty

Infection, fistula, VPI, and mucosal breakdown are all potential complications of this procedure though complications have been rare. Mucosal breakdown has been the most commonly reported complication with rates up to 22% in one of only two studies in the literature. All

Table 13.2 Pillar implant-related complications

	Complication rate	*p*-value
Event		
Patients with implant extrusion	10/79 (12%)	
Patients with poor placement	6/79 (8%)	
Total	16/69 (20%)	
Implant number		
Number of first 3 implants causing complications	16/237 (6.8%)	0.74
Number of 4th/5th implants causing complication	2/50 (4%)	
Gender		
Females with complication	8/14 (57%)	0.001
Males with complication	8/65 (8.3%)	
Sedation level		
Nonsedated	7/58 (12%)	0.009
General anesthesia	9/21 (43%)	
p-values were calculated with Fisher exact test.		

Reprinted with permission from Gillespie et al, 2009.[73]

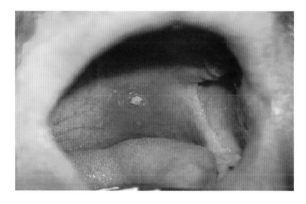

Fig. 13.9 Partial extrusion of palatal implant. (Image courtesy of Prof. K. Hörmann.)

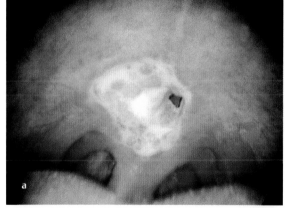

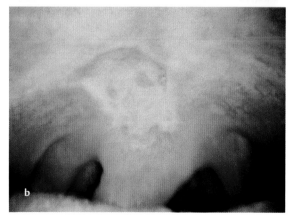

Fig. 13.10a,b Palatal fistula after injection snoreplasty. ▷
(With kind permission from Brietzke SE, Mair EA. Injection snoreplasty: extended follow-up. Otolaryngol Head Neck Surg 2003;128(5):605–615).

a Palatal fistula in a 120-lb, female patient who had received a single midline injection of 3% sodium tetradecyl sulfate. Two weeks post-injection. Note healing granulation tissue. Patient complained of mild pain only.

b Three weeks after injection. Fistula completely closed with supportive treatment only. No antibiotics were given.

cases resolved with conservative treatment (**Fig. 13.10**). To prevent VPI and fistulas, the procedure should not be performed in patients with a thin or short soft palate.[76,77]

Radiofrequency of the Soft Palate

Though not as likely to cause complications as radiofrequency of the tongue base, complication rates have been variable in the literature. They have been divided between minor (8.1%) and major (0.1%) complications. Complications include ulceration, hemorrhage, fistula, and VPI. Mucosal breakdown or ulceration (12.5%) has been the most common complication in most studies, and all cases resolved uneventfully with conservative treatment. The procedure can be performed by temperature-controlled radiofrequency or plasma-mediated ablation. In those using radiofrequency, they noted a higher incidence of complications when delivering 800 J in the middle of the soft palate compared with 550 J.[52,53,78]

General Anesthesia in Patients with OSA

Many studies have shown that the complex nature of respiratory management of patients with OSA during and after anesthesia have contributed to increased perioperative complications. In addition, obstructive sleep apnea is also associated with other comorbidities, which also increase the perioperative complication rate. Patients with OSA undergoing general anesthesia for any surgery have an increased risk of cardiovascular and pulmonary complications.[79-81] Awareness of this increased risk, preventive/precautionary measures, and close clinical observation are fundamental to avoiding such complications in the perioperative period.

Preoperative Recommendations

Preoperative planning is critical and these patients should be screened regarding their OSA risk factors. In the absence of a sleep study, OSA should be suspected in patients with loud snoring, daytime sleepiness, increased neck circumference, hypertension, obesity, or other symptoms, examination findings, or clinical history suggestive of sleep-disordered breathing. The patient may be managed based on clinical criteria alone or a sleep study may be obtained based on the anesthesiologist and surgeon's discretion. Preoperative treatment with CPAP and other forms of OSA therapy, such as smoking cessation and weight loss, as well as optimization of the patient's general medical condition may substantially lower the patient's anesthetic risk. Although preoperative diagnosis and management of OSA are recommended, the specific risk reduction associated with preoperative CPAP use is unclear and likely varies greatly between patients.[82-84]

Intraoperative Management

The surgeon should be in the operating room during both intubation and extubation. In addition, difficult airway equipment, such as a glidescope, fiberoptic endoscopes, and a tracheotomy tray, should always be readily available. Riley et al[85] described difficult intubations in 18.6% of 182 patients undergoing UPPP. The method of intubation or choice of anesthetic should be decided before intubation. In the guidelines outlined by the American Society of Anesthesiology, local anesthetics and nerve blocks are preferred when relevant. General anesthesia with a secured airway is preferable to moderate or deep sedation when undergoing procedures of the upper airway. Benzodiazepines should be limited or even avoided if possible. If moderate sedation is used, monitoring should include capnography and one should consider administering CPAP.

Patients should be extubated while awake and full reversal of neuromuscular agents should verified.[82,86] "Deep extubation" is a risk for loss of the airway as well as postobstructive pulmonary edema. Reversing volatile anesthetics reduces the risk of immediate postoperative complications and expedites discharge from the postanesthesia care unit by 35%.[87]

Postoperative Management

A much higher percentage of patients with OSA suffer postoperative complications and require transfer to the ICU. Most complications occur within the first 24 hours and are felt to be related to sedatives, narcotics, and anesthetic agents.[88] Opioids should be limited, and alternative pain medications should be considered. The use of postoperative oxygen in patients with OSA is not well studied though supplemental oxygen is often used to limit the degree of hypoxemia. Head of bed elevation and the use of CPAP are recommended in the postoperative setting and have been shown to decrease respiratory events even in the setting of postoperative narcotics, though there is little in the literature to support this finding. Prolonged observation in the recovery room is also recommended with some advocating a monitored setting for 3 hours longer than their non-OSA counterparts and for 7 hours after the last episode of airway obstruction or hypoxemia while breathing room air.[82,83] There is considerable debate in the literature as to which patients should be kept in the hospital for overnight observation. Recommendations for discharge versus hospital admission must be individualized to each patient based on a multitude of factors including the type and duration of anesthesia, the surgical procedure itself, OSA severity, obesity, cardiopulmonary status, and other patient factors.

References

1. Fujita S, Conway W, Zorick F, Roth T. Surgical correction of anatomic abnormalities in obstructive sleep apnea syndrome: uvulopalatopharyngoplasty. Otolaryngol Head Neck Surg 1981;89(6):923–934

2. Kezirian EJ, Weaver EM, Yueh B, et al. Incidence of serious complications after uvulopalatopharyngoplasty. Laryngoscope 2004;114(3):450–453

3. Esclamado RM, Glenn MG, McCulloch TM, Cummings CW. Perioperative complications and risk factors in the surgical treatment of obstructive sleep apnea syndrome. Laryngoscope 1989;99(11):1125–1129

4. Haavisto L, Suonpää J. Complications of uvulopalatopharyngoplasty. Clin Otolaryngol Allied Sci 1994;19(3):243–247

5. Mickelson SA, Hakim I. Is postoperative intensive care monitoring necessary after uvulopalatopharyngoplasty? Otolaryngol Head Neck Surg 1997;117:648–652

6. Harmon JD, Morgan W, Chaudhary B. Sleep apnea: morbidity and mortality of surgical treatment. South Med J 1989;82(2):161–164

7. Riley RW, Powell NB, Guilleminault C, Pelayo R, Troell RJ, Li KK. Obstructive sleep apnea surgery: risk management and complications. Otolaryngol Head Neck Surg 1997;117(6):648–652

8. Hathaway B, Johnson JT. Safety of uvulopalatopharyngoplasty as outpatient surgery. Otolaryngol Head Neck Surg 2006;134(4):542–544

9. Spiegel JH, Raval TH. Overnight hospital stay is not always necessary after uvulopalatopharyngoplasty. Laryngoscope 2005;115(1):167–171

10. Kezirian EJ, Weaver EM, Yueh B, Khuri SF, Daley J, Henderson WG. Risk factors for serious complication after uvulopalatopharyngoplasty. Arch Otolaryngol Head Neck Surg 2006;132(10):1091–1098

11. Demars SM, Harsha WJ, Crawford JV. The effects of smoking on the rate of postoperative hemorrhage after tonsillectomy and uvulopalatopharyngoplasty. Arch Otolaryngol Head Neck Surg 2008;134(8):811–814

12. Windfuhr JP, Chen YS. Incidence of post-tonsillectomy hemorrhage in children and adults: a study of 4,848 patients. Ear Nose Throat J 2002;81(9):626–628, 630, 632 passim

13. Croft CB, Golding-Wood DG. Uses and complications of uvulopalatopharyngoplasty. J Larnygol Otol 1990;104(11):871–875

14. Fairbanks DN. Uvulopalatopharyngoplasty complications and avoidance strategies. Otolaryngol Head Neck Surg 1990;102(3):239–245

15. Colman MF, Rice DH. A method of determining the correct amount of palatal resection in palatopharyngoplasty. Laryngoscope 1985;95(5):609–610

16. Jackson IT, Kenedy D. Surgical management of velopharyngeal insufficiency following uvulopalatopharyngoplasty: report of three cases. Plast Reconstr Surg 1997;99(4):1151–1153

17. Altermatt HJ, Gebbers JO, Sommerhalder A, Vrticka K. Histopathologic findings in the posterior pharyngeal wall 8 years after treatment of velar insufficiency with Teflon injection. [Article in German] Laryngol Rhinol Otol (Stuttg) 1985;64(11):582–585

18. Furlow LT Jr, Williams WN, Eisenbach CR 2nd, Bzoch KR. A long term study on treating velopharyngeal insufficiency by teflon injection. Cleft Palate J 1982;19(1):47–56

19. Stevenson EW. Cicatricial stenosis of the nasopharynx. Laryngoscope 1969;79(12):2035–2067

20. Hathaway B, Johnson J. Complications of palatal approaches. In: Kountakis SE, Onerci M, eds. Rhinologic

and Sleep Apnea Surgical Techniques. New York, NY: Thieme Medical Publishers;2007:391–395

21. Katsantonis GP, Friedman WH, Krebs FJ 3rd, Walsh JK. Nasopharyngeal complications following uvulopalatopharyngoplasty. Laryngoscope 1987;97(3 Pt 1):309–314

22. Krespi YP, Kacker A. Management of nasopharyngeal stenosis after uvulopalatoplasty. Otolaryngol Head Neck Surg 2000;123(6):692–695

23. Jones LM, Guillory VL, Mair EA. Total nasopharyngeal stenosis: treatment with laser excision, nasopharyngeal obturators, and topical mitomycin-c. Otolaryngol Head Neck Surg 2005;133(5):795–798

24. Van Duyne J, Coleman JA Jr. Treatment of nasopharyngeal inlet stenosis following uvulopalatopharyngoplasty with the CO2 laser. Laryngoscope 1995;105(9 Pt 1):914–918

25. Cotton RT. Nasopharyngeal stenosis. Arch Otolaryngol 1985;111(3):146–148

26. Stepnick DW. Management of total nasopharyngeal stenosis following UPPP. Ear Nose Throat J 1993;72(1):86–90

27. Ingrams DR, Spraggs PD, Pringle MB, Croft CB. CO2 laser palatoplasty: early results. J Laryngol Otol 1996;110(8):754–756

28. Kazanjian VH, Holmes EM. Stenosis of the nasopharynx and its correction. Arch Otolaryngol 1946;44:261–273

29. Li HY, Lee LA, Wang PC, et al. Taste disturbance after uvulopalatopharyngoplasty for obstructive sleep apnea. Otolaryngol Head Neck Surg 2006;134(6):985–990

30. Kamel UF. Hypogeusia as a complication of uvulopalatopharyngoplasty and use of taste strips as a practical tool for quantifying hypogeusia. Acta Otolaryngol 2004;124(10):1235–1236

31. Hagert B, Wikblad K, Odkvist L, Wahren LK. Side effects after surgical treatment of snoring. ORL J Otorhinolaryngol Relat Spec 2000;62(2):76–80

32. Cahali MB. Lateral pharyngoplasty: a new treatment for obstructive sleep apnea hypopnea syndrome. Laryngoscope 2003;113(11):1961–1968

33. Van Lierde KM, Van Borsel J, Moerman M, Van Cauwenberge P. Nasalance, nasality, voice, and articulation after uvulopalatopharyngoplasty. Laryngoscope 2002;112(5):873–878

34. Brosch S, Matthes C, Pirsig W, Verse T. Uvulopalatopharyngoplasty changes fundamental frequency of the voice—a prospective study. J Laryngol Otol 2000;114(2):113–118

35. Tewary AK, Cable HR. Speech changes following uvulopalatopharyngoplasty. Clin Otolaryngol Allied Sci 1993;18(5):390–391

36. Hagert B, Wikblad K, Odkvist L, Wahren LK. Side effects after surgical treatment of snoring. ORL J Otorhinolaryngol Relat Spec 2000;62(2):76–80

37. Goh YH, Mark I, Fee WE Jr. Quality of life 17 to 20 years after uvulopalatopharyngoplasty. Laryngoscope 2007;117(3):503–506

38. Back GW, Nadig S, Uppal S, Coatesworth AP. Why do we have a uvula? Literature review and a new theory. Clin Otolaryngol Allied Sci 2004;29(6):689–693

39. Kwon M, Jang YJ, Lee BJ, Chung YS. The effect of uvula-preserving palatopharyngoplasty in obstructive sleep apnea on globus sense and positional dependency. Clin Exp Otorhinolaryngol 2010;3(3):141–146

40. Shine NP, Lewis RH. Transpalatal advancement pharyngoplasty for obstructive sleep apnea syndrome: results and analysis of failures. Arch Otolaryngol Head Neck Surg 2009;135(5):434–438

41. Woodson BT, Toohill RJ. Transpalatal advancement pharyngoplasty for obstructive sleep apnea. Laryngoscope 1993;103(3):269–276

42. Woodson BT, Robinson S, Lim HJ. Transpalatal advancement pharyngoplasty outcomes compared with

uvulopalatopharyngoplasty. Otolaryngol Head Neck Surg 2005;133(2):211–217

43. Pang KP, Woodson BT. Expansion sphincter pharyngoplasty: a new technique for the treatment of obstructive sleep apnea. Otolaryngol Head Neck Surg 2007;137(1):110–114

44. Pang KP, Tan R, Puraviappan P, Terris DJ. Anterior palatoplasty for the treatment of OSA: three-year results. Otolaryngol Head Neck Surg 2009;141(2):253–256

45. Mickelson SA, Rosenthal L. Midline glossectomy and epiglottidectomy for obstructive sleep apnea syndrome. Laryngoscope 1997;107(5):614–619

46. Woodson BT, Fujita S. Clinical experience with lingualplasty as part of the treatment of severe obstructive sleep apnea. Otolaryngol Head Neck Surg 1992;107(1):40–48

47. Woodson BT. Innovative technique for lingual tonsillectomy and midline posterior glossectomy for obstructive sleep apnea. Otolaryngol Head Neck Surg 2007;18:20–28

48. Maturo SC, Mair EA. Submucosal minimally invasive lingual excision (SMILE): technique for tongue base reduction. Operative Techniques in Otolaryngol 2007;18:29–32

49. Friedman M, Soans R, Gurpinar B, Lin HC, Joseph N. Evaluation of submucosal minimally invasive lingual excision technique for treatment of obstructive sleep apnea/hypopnea syndrome. Otolaryngol Head Neck Surg 2008;139(3):378–384, discussion 385

50. Lauretano AM, Li KK, Caradonna DS, Khosta RK, Fried MP. Anatomic location of the tongue base neurovascular bundle. Laryngoscope 1997;107(8):1057–1059

51. Robinson S, Ettema SL, Brusky L, Woodson BT. Lingual tonsillectomy using bipolar radiofrequency plasma excision. Otolaryngol Head Neck Surg 2006;134(2):328–330

52. Troell RJ, Li KK, Powell NB, et al. Radiofrequency tongue base reduction in sleep-disordered breathing. Operative Techniques in Otolaryngol 2000;11(1):47–49

53. Pazos G, Mair EA. Complications of radiofrequency ablation in the treatment of sleep-disordered breathing. Otolaryngol Head Neck Surg 2001;125(5):462–466, discussion 466–467

54. Kezirian EJ, Powell NB, Riley RW, Hester JE. Incidence of complications in radiofrequency treatment of the upper airway. Laryngoscope 2005;115(7):1298–1304

55. Riley RW, Powell NB, Li KK, Weaver EM, Guilleminault C. An adjunctive method of radiofrequency volumetric tissue reduction of the tongue for OSAS. Otolaryngol Head Neck Surg 2003;129(1):37–42

56. Woodson BT. A tongue suspension suture for obstructive sleep apnea and snorers. Otolaryngol Head Neck Surg 2001;124(3):297–303

57. Miller FR, Watson D, Malis D. Role of the tongue base suspension suture with The Repose System bone screw in the multilevel surgical management of obstructive sleep apnea. Otolaryngol Head Neck Surg 2002;126(4):392–398

58. Omur M, Ozturan D, Elez F, Unver C, Derman S. Tongue base suspension combined with UPPP in severe OSA patients. Otolaryngol Head Neck Surg 2005;133(2):218–223

59. DeRowe A, Gunther E, Fibbi A, et al. Tongue-base suspension with a soft tissue-to-bone anchor for obstructive sleep apnea: preliminary clinical results of a new minimally invasive technique. Otolaryngol Head Neck Surg 2000;122(1):100–103

60. Kühnel TS, Schurr C, Wagner B, Geisler P. Morphological changes of the posterior airway space after tongue base suspension. Laryngoscope 2005;115(3):475–480

61. Riley RW, Powell NB, Guilleminault C. Obstructive sleep apnea and the hyoid: a revised surgical procedure. Otolaryngol Head Neck Surg 1994;111(6):717–721

62. Bowden MT, Kezirian EJ, Utley D, Goode RL. Outcomes of hyoid suspension for the treatment of

obstructive sleep apnea. Arch Otolaryngol Head Neck Surg 2005;131(5):440–445

63. Neruntarat C. Hyoid myotomy with suspension under local anesthesia for obstructive sleep apnea syndrome. Eur Arch Otorhinolaryngol 2003;260(5):286–290

64. Richard W, Timmer F, van Tinteren H, de Vries N. Complications of hyoid suspension in the treatment of obstructive sleep apnea syndrome. Eur Arch Otorhinolaryngol 2011;268(4):631–635

65. Li KK. Hyoid suspension/advancement. In: Fairbanks DNF, Mickelson SA, Woodson BT, eds. Snoring and OSA. 3rd ed. Philadelphia: Lippincott Williams & Wilkins; 2003:178–182

66. Hormann K, Baisch A. Hyoid Suspension. In: Kountakis SE, Onerci M, eds. Rhinologic and Sleep Apnea Surgical Techniques. New York, NY: Thieme Medical Publishers;2007:355–360

67. Riley RW, Powell NB, Li KK, Troell RJ, Guilleminault C. Surgery and obstructive sleep apnea: long-term clinical outcomes. Otolaryngol Head Neck Surg 2000;122(3):415–421

68. Hörmann K, Baisch A. The hyoid suspension. Laryngoscope 2004;114(9):1677–1679

69. Tschopp KP. Modification of the Hörmann technique of hyoid suspension in obstructive sleep apnoea. J Laryngol Otol 2007;121(5):491–493

70. Ho WK, Wei WI, Chung KF. Managing disturbing snoring with palatal implants: a pilot study. Arch Otolaryngol Head Neck Surg 2004;130(6):753–758

71. Nordgård S, Wormdal K, Bugten V, Stene BK, Skjøstad KW. Palatal implants: a new method for the treatment of snoring. Acta Otolaryngol 2004;124(8):970–975

72. Catalano P, Goh YH, Romanow J. Additional palatal implants for refractory snoring. Otolaryngol Head Neck Surg 2007;137(1):105–109

73. Gillespie MB, Smith JE, Clarke J, Nguyen SA. Effectiveness of Pillar palatal implants for snoring management. Otolaryngol Head Neck Surg 2009;140(3):363–368

74. Romanow JH, Catalano PJ. Initial U.S. pilot study: palatal implants for the treatment of snoring. Otolaryngol Head Neck Surg 2006;134(4):551–557

75. Friedman M, Schalch P, Joseph NJ. Palatal stiffening after failed uvulopalatopharyngoplasty with the Pillar Implant System. Laryngoscope 2006;116(11):1956–1961

76. Brietzke SE, Mair EA. Injection snoreplasty: how to treat snoring without all the pain and expense. Otolaryngol Head Neck Surg 2001;124(5):503–510

77. Brietzke SE, Mair EA. Injection snoreplasty: extended follow-up and new objective data. Otolaryngol Head Neck Surg 2003;128(5):605–615

78. Kania RE, Schmitt E, Petelle B, Meyer B. Radiofrequency soft palate procedure in snoring: influence of energy delivered. Otolaryngol Head Neck Surg 2004;130(1):67–72

79. Dart RA, Gregoire JR, Gutterman DD, Woolf SH. The association of hypertension and secondary cardiovascular disease with sleep-disordered breathing. Chest 2003;123(1):244–260

80. Hung J, Whitford EG, Parsons RW, Hillman DR. Association of sleep apnoea with myocardial infarction in men. Lancet 1990;336(8710):261–264

81. Lavie P, Herer P, Peled R, et al. Mortality in sleep apnea patients: a multivariate analysis of risk factors. Sleep 1995;18(3):149–157

82. Gross JB, Bachenberg KL, Benumof JL, et al. Practice guidelines for the perioperative management of patients with obstructive sleep apnea: a report by the American Society of Anesthesiologists Task Force on Perioperative Management of patients with obstructive sleep apnea. Anesthesiology 2006;104(5):1081–1093

83. Johnson JT, Braun TW. Preoperative, intraoperative, and postoperative management of patients with obstructive

sleep apnea syndrome. Otolaryngol Clin North Am 1998;31(6):1025–1030

84. Rennotte MT, Baele P, Aubert G, Rodenstein DO. Nasal continuous positive airway pressure in the perioperative management of patients with obstructive sleep apnea submitted to surgery. Chest 1995;107(2):367–374

85. Riley RW, Powell NB, Guilleminault C, Pelayo R, Troell RJ, Li KK. Obstructive sleep apnea surgery: risk management and complications. Otolaryngol Head Neck Surg 1997;117(6):648–652

86. Meoli AL, Rosen CL, Kristo D, et al. Upper airway management of the adult patient with obstructive sleep apnea in the perioperative period—avoiding complications. Sleep 2003;26(8):1060–1065

87. Katznelson R, Minkovich L, Friedman Z, Fedorko L, Beattie WS, Fisher JA. Accelerated recovery from sevoflurane anesthesia with isocapnic hyperpnoea. Anesth Analg 2008;106(2):486–491

88. Gupta RM, Parvizi J, Hanssen AD, Gay PC. Postoperative complications in patients with obstructive sleep apnea syndrome undergoing hip or knee replacement: a case-control study. Mayo Clin Proc 2001;76(9):897–905

III A Surgery of the Oral Cavity and Oropharynx

14 Complications in Cleft Lip and Palate Surgery

R. Brusati, G. Colletti

Introduction

Cleft lip and palate (CLP) and cleft palate alone (CP) are some of the most frequent craniofacial malformations, and in Europe affect ~ 1 in 700 newborns. It is therefore an epidemiologically relevant disease, and its consequences can be severely impairing. For these reasons, it is considered of considerable medical and social importance. Treatment of CLP and CP is essentially surgical, along with orthodontists and speech pathologists, and requires several subsequent steps during the life of the patient. Most often, the treatment is completed only at the end of the patient's puberty.

During each of these surgical sessions, complications can potentially occur, which will be examined separately in this chapter. Complications after the following will be discussed: cheilorhinopalatoplasty, gingivoperiosteoplasty and cleft alveolar bone grafting, maxillary osteotomy and maxillary distraction osteogenesis, and velopharyngoplasty. For each phase, we will describe the immediate and late complications as well as unfavorable results.

Cheilorhinoplasty, Palatoplasty

Primary treatment of CLP is not uniformly coded. The ideal period to treat the cleft of the lip and of the palate is still debated. Different centers often adopt nonhomogeneous protocols that differ greatly in terms of timings, which must be considered when describing the frequency of complications and unfavorable results. Surgery of the lip when performed at 4 to 6 months of age (as in our center) is associated with an exceptionally low frequency of early complications.

Hemorrhage is extremely rare and infection is even rarer (short-term antibiotic treatment is administered prophylactically). Hemorrhage during the preparative phase, namely during flap sculpting and lip–nasal and maxillary undermining, usually come from the lip coronary artery and are easily managed with bipolar cautery.[1] However, in the literature there are reports of substantial perioperative hemorrhage needing blood transfusions.[2]

Lip Surgery

Lip wound infection is also exceptionally rare,[2,3] but can lead to dehiscence with delayed healing and secondary retracted scars. According to some recent investigations, patients with van der Woude syndrome may be more prone to wound infection. Infection at the tip of the nose after primary rhinoplasty is also very rare.[4] Infection and dehiscence must be treated conservatively with cleansing and disinfection. If a secondary deformity occurs, this should be treated with a secondary correction, waiting at least 6 months after the previous surgery. In surgical correction of bilateral CLP, necrosis of the central cutaneous flap containing the prolabium as the result of incorrect dissection with disruption of the nourishing vascular network has been described. As a consequence, there is poor reconstruction of the central part of the upper lip and of the columella (**Fig. 14.1**).

Late complications of lip surgery are essentially hypertrophic scars or keloids. These conditions are often the result of the patient's biological response and are therefore difficult to cure. Treatment relies essentially on the use of local steroids and compressive silicone sheets. Unfavorable results consist of residual deformities affecting the lip, the nose (**Fig. 14.2**) or the septum (**Fig. 14.3**). These should be addressed individually.

Cleft Surgery

Corrective surgery for CP can be performed with various techniques. If the cleft is very large (and always with some techniques), lateral releasing incisions must be performed (**Fig. 14.4**). However, these are associated with a

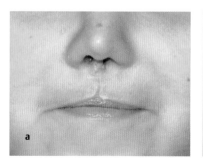
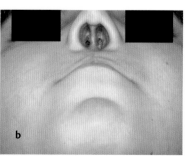

Fig. 14.1 Poor results after improper reconstruction of lip **(a)** and columella **(b)** in a patient with cleft lip and palate.

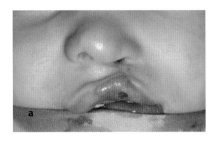 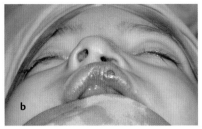 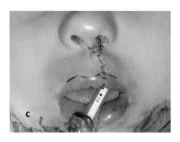

Fig. 14.2a–c Severe deformities of the lip and nose after incorrect primary treatment of a unilateral complete cleft lip and palate, operated on at another institution.

a, b Clinical view.
c Immediate postoperative result after early secondary correction.

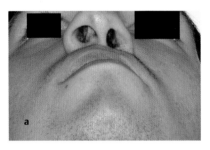 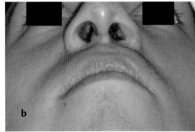

Fig. 14.3a,b Right septal deviation after primary cleft lip and palate correction.

a Clinical view.
b Result after septoplasty and LeFort I osteotomy.

definite risk of tearing the palatine vessels and hemorrhages are therefore more likely. Releasing incisions are frequently filled with hemostatic gauze. In any case, the overall risk of bleeding or infection is very low, especially if one takes care to seek and minimally cauterize bleeding at the level of the lateral releasing incisions at the end of the intervention.

If bleeding complicates a palatoplasty, this normally produces a self-limiting hematoma. Conversely, if bleeding continues, there is the need to revise the site to look for the bleeding source so that it can be cauterized. Finally, a bulky palatal or pharyngeal hematoma can impede breathing and therefore must be promptly evacuated.

Complete wound breakdown can occur on occasion (**Fig. 14.5**). This is devastating and must be addressed secondarily with a new palatoplasty.

Conversely, in any palatoplasty there is a risk of developing a residual fistula or velopharyngeal incompetence.[5,6] The main problem with fistulas after palatoplasty is that they have an extremely high chance of relapse. Accordingly, every effort should be directed toward preventing them by meticulously suturing the nasal, muscular, and oral layers avoiding tension and using atraumatic horizontal mattress stitches. The correction of fistulas relies on local flaps (**Fig. 14.6**) or, sometimes, on a lingual flap (wide, anterior fistulas). Velopharyngeal incompetence can be a complication of incorrect muscular reconstruction or may simply be due to suboptimal results. The most troublesome consequence is altered speech. The timing for correction of velopharyngeal incompetence is critical—late corrections bear the highest chance of leaving definitive speech impairment.[7]

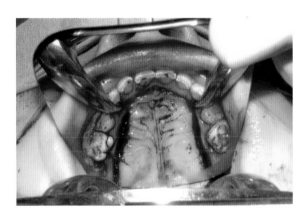

Fig. 14.4 Lateral releasing incisions in a palatoplasty.

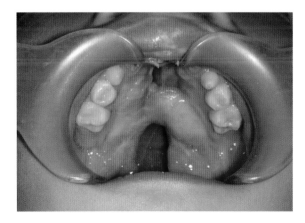

Fig. 14.5 Complete wound breakdown after a primary palatoplasty treated at another institution.

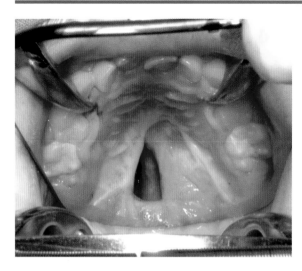
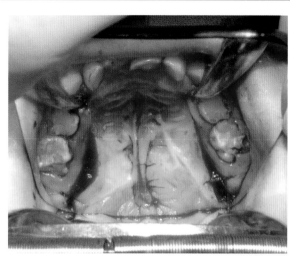
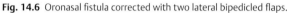

Fig. 14.6 Oronasal fistula corrected with two lateral bipedicled flaps.

Gingivoalveoloplasty and Cleft Bone Grafting

Gingivoperiosteoplasty (or gingivoalveoloplasty, GAP) and bone grafting in the cleft alveolus share the same objective, namely of creating bone continuity to permit tooth eruption. Additionally, in bilateral cases bony continuity is essential to obtain skeletal stability in the premaxilla, which is otherwise mobile. Long-term results are discussed in the literature, an issue that is beyond the scope of the present chapter. GAP is a technically demanding procedure but it gives excellent results,[8] and consists of rebuilding the periosteal lining of the cleft alveolus with mucoperiosteal flaps. Early (intraoperative) complications are tooth bud injury with subsequent eruptive disturbances, failure to restore a complete mucoperiosteal lining (more often of the nasal plane), and fracture or devascularization of the premaxilla. This last should be highly feared when performing GAP in bilateral cases. Hemorrhages and infections are exceptionally uncommon in this procedure.

Considering potentially unfavorable results, GAP can adversely affect maxillary growth. This may be particularly true if the procedure is performed early (primary GAP). This has been debated in the literature, but there is some agreement on the fact that, to avoid growth disturbance, the procedure should be performed at 18 to 24 months of age (early secondary GAP). Another unfavorable result of the procedure is insufficient bone formation in the cleft alveolus, which in our case series has been observed in 0.75% of patients (**Fig. 14.7**).

When GAP is not performed, alveolar bone grafting will be needed. The bone graft is routinely harvested from the ilium and positioned at the level of the bony alveolar cleft. The risks in this procedure are common to all oral bone grafting techniques, and are relative to donor site morbidity and graft infection.

The complications of ilium bone harvesting are anesthesia in the lateral thigh as a consequence of injury to the lateral femorocutaneous nerve, retroperitoneal hematoma, and ilium infection or fracture.[9] The last of these, generally rare, is exceptionally uncommon in cleft grafting because of the extremely small quantity of bone harvested. Graft infection, in contrast, is possible and can lead to partial or total loss of the grafted bone. It is managed conservatively with antibiotics and irrigation, but complete healing is often obtained only when the infected graft is removed.

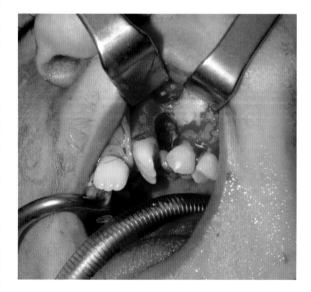

Fig. 14.7 Insufficient ossification after gingivoalveoloplasty.

Maxillary Osteotomy and Maxillary Distraction Osteogenesis

Maxillary hypoplasia is infrequent in cleft patients (10 to 50% of cases). It becomes noticeable during growth and is overt by the end of puberty. Its severity generally correlates with the initial severity of the cleft and is worsened by early timing of surgery and by some surgical techniques. Maxillary hypoplasia is corrected surgically by maxillary osteotomy or maxillary distraction osteogenesis. Without entering into details, osteotomy is the preferred technique in the majority of patients, whereas distraction is reserved for more severe hypoplasia (> 10 mm) or for pediatric patients. The complications of maxillary osteotomy in cleft patients can be severe and are the consequence of an altered maxillary perfusion owing to the malformation itself and to the scars of previous surgical interventions. Early complications are profuse bleeding,[10] oral–nasal and oral–antral lacerations with consequent fistulas, and (although extremely rare) visual complications such as injury to the abducens nerve and loss of vision.[11] Sustained bleeding should be prevented with intraoperative hypotension, and formation of fistulas should be avoided by being particularly delicate during osteotomy (paramedian osteotomy carries a greater risk), and while dissecting and elevating the soft tissues. Late complications are fistulas and tooth injury. This typically takes the form of a root reabsorption, but an entire tooth can be lost, especially if an osteotomy in two or more fragments is performed. Other late complications are periodontal disturbances and rare but disastrous partial or total necrosis (**Fig. 14.8**) of the osteotomized fragment caused by vascular impairment.[12] Lastly, another rare complication is malunion. Distraction osteogenesis, if performed with internal devices, can present troublesome control on distraction vectors,[13] and this mandates surgical repositioning of the device, otherwise the maxilla will end up in an incorrect position. In contrast, if an external device is used (**Fig. 14.9**), local infection, pin loosening or skull penetration by the pins can occur.[14]

If bone grafts are used to bridge bony gaps during osteotomies, the same complications cited for cleft bone grafting hold true (donor site morbidity and graft exposure or infection).

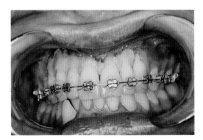

Fig. 14.8 Complete necrosis of the maxilla after a LeFort I osteotomy performed at another institution.

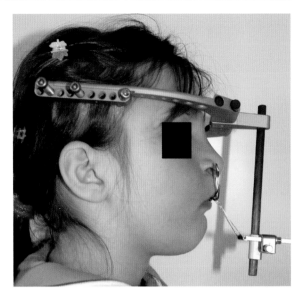

Fig. 14.9 Placement of an external maxillary distraction or rigid external device.

Unfavorable results of osteotomy and distraction are relapse of the hypoplasia and velopharyngeal incompetence. Skeletal relapse can occur in any patient who undergoes maxillary osteotomy. The vertical dimension is particularly delicate, and maxillary lowering is therefore even more prone to relapse then maxillary advancement. Velopharyngeal incompetence can occur as a consequence of a maxillary advancement, and this must be considered during surgical planning. Patients who are preoperatively borderline are more prone to develop velopharyngeal incompetence.

Distraction osteogenesis was adapted to the maxilla to overcome such unfavorable results, namely, relapse and velopharyngeal incompetence. Moreover, it spares the need for bone grafting in major advancements and lowering. Unfortunately, even distraction can be complicated by relapse and velopharyngeal incompetence, as well as nonunion.[15]

Velopharyngoplasty

As previously stated, some patients with CP may suffer from a variable degree of velopharyngeal incompetence. If the anteroposterior defect is moderate (3 to 4 mm), a new palatoplasty (e.g., according to Furlow) can be used to address the issue. However, if the defect is greater than 4 to 5 mm a velopharyngoplasty must be performed. This can be performed using various techniques, but most rely on elevating and translating flaps (superiorly or inferiorly based) from the posterior pharyngeal wall and suturing them to the posterosuperior end of the soft palate (**Fig. 14.10**). Harvesting a flap from the posterior pharyngeal wall is a delicate procedure associated with definite

Section III   Complications of Head and Neck Surgery

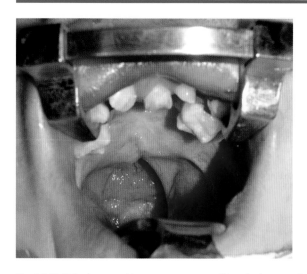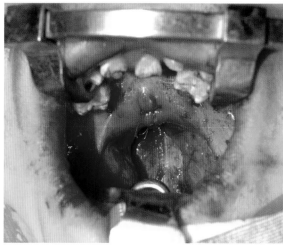

Fig. 14.10 Velopharyngeal incompetence treated by velopharyngoplasty (superior pedicle).

morbidity. The most feared intraoperative complication is hemorrhage, which is normally caused by minor vessels and is therefore easily managed in superiorly based flaps. Nonetheless, in some patients affected by 22q11 deletion syndrome (or velocardiofacial syndrome or Shprintzen syndrome) some anatomical variations make the procedure particularly risky. In these patients, in fact, the internal carotid artery can be tortuous and have an anomalous medial course at the level of the posterior pharyngeal wall. This syndrome must always be taken into account, because ~ 8% of patients presenting with CP (overt or submucous) will suffer from it.[16]

Postoperative hemorrhage, which normally occurs during the first 3 to 4 postoperative days, requires new anesthesia for its management, and can cause aspiration pneumonia.[17] Another complication of velopharyngoplasty is donor site infection. This is almost always uncomplicated, superficial, and localized, but very rarely the process reaches the vertebral bodies to cause vertebral osteomyelitis.[18] This can happen even if the donor site is sutured, and for this reason many authors prefer to leave it unsutured.

Unfavorable results can arise from the difficult balance between residual incompetence and results from hyponasality up to obstructive syndrome. Nonetheless, a true obstructive syndrome is very rare and some have asserted that it is more frequent after a velopharyngoplasty than following a Furlow palatoplasty.[19]

Complications after inserting a tracheal tube into the donor site where the former was forced submucously into the mediastinum during an emergency procedure early in the postoperative period are very rare. The same complication could theoretically occur while positioning a gastric tube. Attention must be given to directly visualize where a tube is being led to avoid these severe complications.

References

1. Demey A, Vadoud-Seyedi J, Demol F, Govaerts M. Early postoperative complications in primary cleft lip and palate surgery. Eur J Plast Surg 1997;20(2):77–79
2. Lees VC, Pigott RW. Early postoperative complications in primary cleft lip and palate surgery—how soon may we discharge patients from hospital? Br J Plast Surg 1992;45(3):232–234
3. Reinish JF, Sloan GM. Complications of cleft lip repair. In: Bardach J, ed. Multidisciplinary Management of Cleft Lip and Palate. Philadelphia: Saunders; 1990:247–252
4. Alef M, Irwin C, Smith D, et al. Nasal tip complications of primary cleft lip nasoplasty. J Craniofac Surg 2009;20(5):1327–1333
5. Sullivan SR, Marrinan EM, LaBrie RA, Rogers GF, Mulliken JB. Palatoplasty outcomes in nonsyndromic patients with cleft palate: a 29-year assessment of one surgeon's experience. J Craniofac Surg 2009;20(Suppl 1):612–616
6. Andersson EM, Sandvik L, Semb G, Abyholm F. Palatal fistulas after primary repair of clefts of the secondary palate. Scand J Plast Reconstr Surg Hand Surg 2008;42(6):296–299
7. Rohrich RJ, Love EJ, Byrd HS, Johns DF. Optimal timing of cleft palate closure. Plast Reconstr Surg 2000;106(2):413–421, quiz 422, discussion 423–425
8. Meazzini MC, Rossetti G, Garattini G, Semb G, Brusati R. Early secondary gingivo-alveolo-plasty in the treatment of unilateral cleft lip and palate patients: 20 years experience. J Craniomaxillofac Surg 2010;38(3):185–191
9. Schaaf H, Lendeckel S, Howaldt HP, Streckbein P. Donor site morbidity after bone harvesting from the anterior iliac crest. Oral Surg Oral Med Oral Pathol Oral Radiol Endod 2010;109(1):52–58
10. Van de Perre JP, Stoelinga PJ, Blijdorp PA, Brouns JJ, Hoppenreijs TJ. Perioperative morbidity in maxillofacial orthopaedic surgery: a retrospective study. J Craniomaxillofac Surg 1996;24(5):263–270
11. Bendor-Samuel R, Chen YR, Chen PKT. Unusual complications of the Le Fort I osteotomy. Plast Reconstr Surg 1995;96(6):1289–1296, discussion 1297
12. de Mol van Otterloo JJ, Tuinzing DB, Greebe RB, van der Kwast WA. Intra- and early postoperative complications of the Le Fort I osteotomy. A retrospective study on 410 cases. J Craniomaxillofac Surg 1991;19(5):217–222

13. Jeblaoui Y, Morand B, Brix M, Lebeau J, Bettega G. Maxillary distraction complications in cleft patients. Rev Stomatol Chir Maxillofac 2010;111(3):e1–e6
14. Cai M, Shen G, Wang X, Fang B. Intracranial fixation pin migration: a complication of external Le Fort III distraction osteogenesis in Apert syndrome. J Craniofac Surg 2010;21(5):1557–1559
15. He D, Genecov DG, Barcelo R. Nonunion of the external maxillary distraction in cleft lip and palate: analysis of possible reasons. J Oral Maxillofac Surg 2010;68(10):2402–2411
16. Shprintzen RJ, Siegel-Sadewitz VL, Amato J, Goldberg RB. Retrospective diagnoses of previously missed syndromic disorders among 1,000 patients with cleft lip, cleft palate, or both. Birth Defects Orig Artic Ser 1985;21(2):85–92
17. Canady JW, Cable BB, Karnell MP, Karnell LH. Pharyngeal flap surgery: protocols, complications, and outcomes at the University of Iowa. Otolaryngol Head Neck Surg 2003;129(4):321–326
18. Bardach J, Salyer KE, Jackson IT. Pharyngoplasty. In: Bardach J, Salyer KE, eds. Surgical Techniques in Cleft Lip and Palate. 2nd ed. Toronto: Mosby Year Book; 1991:274
19. Liao YF, Noordhoff MS, Huang CS, et al. Comparison of obstructive sleep apnea syndrome in children with cleft palate following Furlow palatoplasty or pharyngeal flap for velopharyngeal insufficiency. Cleft Palate Craniofac J 2004;41(2):152–156

III A Surgery of the Oral Cavity and Oropharynx

15 Pull Through, Visor Flap, and Transmandibular Surgery

L. G. T. Morris, J. P. Shah

General Considerations

When oral cavity or oropharyngeal tumors cannot be satisfactorily approached through the open mouth, due to size, location, local extension, or proximity to the mandible or maxilla, an access procedure becomes necessary. This chapter will focus on the prevention and management of complications arising from access procedures, including mandibulotomy, mandibular lingual release or "pull-through", and lower cheek flap and visor flap approaches.

Selecting the Correct Approach: Patient and Tumor Factors

In cases of tumors requiring enhanced access with one of these procedures, the first step in avoiding complications is to ensure that the chosen approach is appropriate given oncologic, functional, and aesthetic considerations. For example, intraoperative recognition of a need for segmental mandibulectomy, or substantial marginal mandibulectomy, after performing an access mandibulotomy, will place the patient at risk of unplanned extension of the operative procedure, without adequate reconstructive support, leading to poor wound healing and suboptimal functional outcome. Therefore, detailed and accurate preoperative evaluation is necessary for surgical planning. This includes a thorough head and neck examination and appropriate imaging, commonly computed tomography scan and panoramic dental X-rays, to evaluate the relationship of the tumor to the bone, and the status of the teeth.[1–4] Preoperative dental evaluation is essential, and some authors have underscored the importance of optimizing oral hygiene preoperatively to reduce the risk of bacterial translocation.[5]

Risk Factors for Complications

The risk factors for wound infection after surgery for oral cavity and oropharyngeal tumors are readily identifiable. Diabetes, impaired nutritional status, and blood transfusion are all significant independent predictors of postoperative wound infection on multivariate analysis.[6]

The first two conditions underscore the importance of medically and nutritionally optimizing patients in the preoperative and perioperative periods. Risks associated with blood transfusion are likely to be attributable to the escalated extent of surgery signified by the need for transfusion; however, blood transfusion does have immunosuppressive sequelae and it is prudent to optimize hemostasis during surgery.[7] In addition, poor dental hygiene, with grossly infected teeth, and previous exposure to radiation, also contribute to the risk of infection. Risks specifically associated with mandibular plating can be inferred from the mandibular trauma literature, which has established tobacco and alcohol use as a strong independent predictor of infectious complications or bony nonunion.[8–12]

Because oral cavity or oropharyngeal surgery requiring enhanced access is clean-contaminated surgery, prophylactic antibiotics (a first-generation cephalosporin and metronidazole, or clindamycin) should be given before skin incision and continued for 24 to 48 hours.[1] Contemporary research has not confirmed any effectiveness for extended antibiotic use beyond the perioperative period in decreasing rates of infection.[13] Therefore extended antibiotic use is usually limited to high-risk patients.

Mandibulotomy

The lip-splitting mandibulotomy was first described by Roux in 1839,[14] and was subsequently described by others, including Sedillot[15] and Trotter.[16] Although the mandibulotomy fell out of favor during the era of composite mandibular resection, it was later understood that mandibular resection is not universally required in all patients in whom a tumor is encroaching on the mandible.[4,17] Subsequently, interest in the mandibulotomy was rekindled by Spiro and colleagues at Memorial Hospital in New York in the 1980s.[18–21] Compared with the pull-through or visor flap approaches, the lip-splitting mandibulotomy affords unparalleled exposure to the posterior oral cavity and oropharynx, although it was initially viewed by many as a disfiguring operation, subject to frequent complications. Technical refinements supported by contemporary outcomes data confirm that this technique can be performed with favorable aesthetic and functional outcomes, and with a low risk of morbidity.

Complications after Mandibulotomy: Historical Data

The safety of mandibulotomy in radiated patients was once controversial. However, the consensus of contemporary evidence is now that there is no escalated risk of complications after mandibulotomy, either in patients with a history of radiation therapy or in patients who go on to receive postoperative radiation therapy.[22–24] There is extensive literature describing the incidence and nature of complications after mandibulotomy. The largest series of mandibulotomies for oral or oropharyngeal cancers consists of 313 patients from Memorial Hospital, reviewed by Dubner and Spiro[18] in 1991. A total of 44% of patients experienced minor or major complications: 19% developed hardware exposure, 14% developed soft tissue wound infections, and 11% developed cardiac or pulmonary complications. The majority of local complications were minor and resolved with conservative measures such as drainage or wound packing. Other series have confirmed comparable rates of wound infection, ranging from 5 to 42%, and rates of fixation failure ranging from 0 to 26%.[22] Recent data drawn from 220 patients at the University of Alberta revealed a 7.7% rate of wound infection, and 2.7% rate of fixation failure.[22,25] These historical data can be challenging to interpret, as they reflect a variety of different surgical techniques, in addition to significant advances in plating and radiation therapy techniques over the past 30 years. This section will focus on technical refinements focused on preventing complications related to the incision, osteotomy, and bone fixation.

Incision Design

Skin Incision

The mandibulotomy typically necessitates a lip-splitting incision. Several authors have described the technique for paramedian mandibulotomy using only a cervical incision and no lip-splitting incision, mainly to enhance transcervical access to the parapharyngeal space, without swinging the mandible laterally.[26,27] Although this approach offers the potential benefits of avoiding a facial incision and tracheotomy, it provides very limited exposure, because of the minimal mobility of the divided segment of the mandible, and does not enhance access to the oral cavity or oropharynx. For access to these areas, a lip-splitting incision and mandibular swing are necessary parts of the mandibulotomy approach. However, the lip-splitting incision need not be aesthetically disfiguring, if carefully planned and meticulously closed.

The facial incision can be designed in one of four ways: midline,[14,16] lateral,[28] midline with a circummental extension,[29,30] or midline with a chevron in the mentolabial sulcus[31] (**Fig. 15.1**). These approaches were compared in 60 patients by Rapidis et al[32] from Athens. The lateral incision was associated with the poorest outcomes, both cosmetic and functional, notably a high rate of oral incompetence with food and saliva because of facial nerve and mental nerve transection. Midline incisions avoided these sequelae and achieved favorable cosmetic outcomes as rated by both patients and physicians. Similar results were reported by Dziegielewski et al[25] from Alberta, who administered validated scar and functional

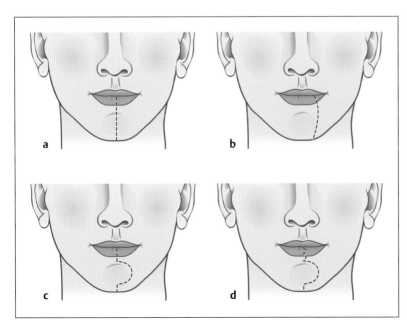

Fig. 15.1 Lip-splitting incisions for mandibulotomy (from left to right: lateral, median, circummental extension, chevron). (From Rapidis Valsamis S, Anterriotis DA, Skouteris CA. Functional and aesthetic results of various lip-splitting incisions: a clinical analysis of 60 cases. J Oral Maxillofac Surg 2001;59(11):1292–1296. Reproduced with permission from WB Saunders.)

quality-of-life instruments to patients undergoing either midline lip-splitting mandibulotomy or peroral resection. Levels of scar satisfaction and functional outcome after lip-splitting mandibulotomy were equivalent to those in patients undergoing peroral resection, confirming that meticulous closure of the midline lip incision results in good aesthetic outcome. To reduce the possibility of linear scar contracture, several authors have advocated placement of a chevron, either in the labiomental sulcus or the submental region.[22,31,33] Rapidis, Hayter and McGregor's groups have advocated the circumferential extension, to avoid scar contracture and loss of chin pad contour, and to respect the chin aesthetic subunit.[29-32] Although Rapidis et al[32] did not observe a significant advantage of any modifications to the straight midline incision, these incision designs may have utility in patients at risk of hypertrophic scarring. To facilitate precise closure of the vermilion border of the lip, a stair-step or chevron incision can sometimes be helpful, although this is not strictly necessary. We prefer a straight midline lip-splitting skin incision. Precise repair aligning the vermilion border, sublabial, mental, and submental skin creases, gives an excellent aesthetic result.

Mucosal Incision

Before making the paralingual mucosal incisions, care should be taken to preserve at least a 1-cm cuff of gingival mucosa for closure, to minimize salivary leakage, hardware exposure, infection, and possible fistula formation. Meticulous closure of the trifurcation in the vestibule at the junction of the midline lip and marginal mucosal incisions is necessary, as this overlies the osteotomy and is a frequent location for wound breakdown.[34]

Incision Closure

At closure, the stumps of the divided mylohyoid muscle should be reapproximated: although this closure is imprecise, it helps to obliterate the dead space.[1] Before skin closure, the orbicularis oris muscle should be carefully reapproximated to best preserve oral competence. A mentalis-tacking stitch, to anchor the mental soft tissues over the midline chin, may help to maintain chin contour and protect the inferior aspect of the osteotomy site.[21] Before closing the skin, a single interrupted nylon stitch is first used to precisely align the vermilion border of the lip, as a disparity as small as 1 mm will be evident to the eye.[1,35] The skin should be closed meticulously with fine permanent suture.

Osteotomy

Location

There is a significant range of surgeon preference with respect to design of the mandibular osteotomy. Osteotomy sites can be either midline,[5,14,36] paramedian,[1,4,5] or lateral (through the body or angle of the mandible). The lateral osteotomy is not recommended because of a high rate of complications, attributable to transection of the inferior alveolar nerve, disruption of blood supply to a large segment of distal mandible, unequal muscle pull on the lateral and medial bone segments, and placement of the osteotomy site within radiation fields. The midline mandibulotomy avoids these problems, but it places the roots of both central incisors at risk, unless one is extracted. In general, dental extraction at the time of mandibulotomy should be avoided because the empty socket becomes an additional possible focus of infection. Furthermore, midline mandibulotomy requires division of the geniohyoid and genioglossus from the genial tubercle, delaying rehabilitation of swallowing and chewing function. The genioglossus muscle draws the tongue inferiorly, reducing its convexity, and channeling fluids posteriorly. The geniohyoid muscle pulls the hyoid bone and tongue anteriorly, facilitating swallowing. For these reasons, a paramedian osteotomy, located between the lateral incisor and canine, or between the canine and first premolar, is the preferred site. This location permits preservation of muscle insertion at the genial tubercle (except for the mylohyoid, which is divided with minimal functional consequence), and remains anterior to the mental nerve, permitting its preservation. There is a greater angle of divergence, and wider horizontal distance, between the roots of the canine and lateral incisor than between the roots of the two central incisors, meaning that osteotomy is less likely to injure teeth if placed in the paramedian location.[5]

After incising the periosteum by the midline, care must be taken to minimize elevation of periosteum off the surface of the mandible, as this compromises periosteal blood supply to the anterior mandible. The mental nerve must be identified and preserved in its foramen to minimize the likelihood of postoperative oral incompetence. Depending on the size of plate chosen, the contralateral periosteum may not need to be elevated to the contralateral mental nerve.

> **Note**
>
> It is helpful to adapt plates to the mandible contour, drill holes, and measure depth for screw lengths before the osteotomy, to facilitate restoration of the mandible to its native orientation after tumor resection. This minimizes the probability of postoperative malocclusion.

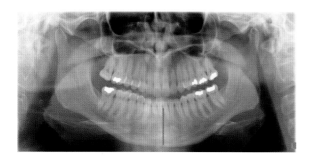

Fig. 15.2 Depiction of midline mandibulotomy (red line), demonstrating the necessity of extracting one central incisor, to avoid injury to both tooth roots.

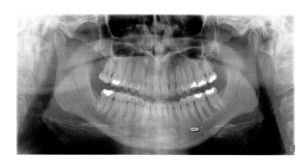

Fig. 15.3 Depiction of lateral mandibulotomy (red line), demonstrating placement posterior to the mental foramen (blue oval), necessitating division of the inferior alveolar nerve.

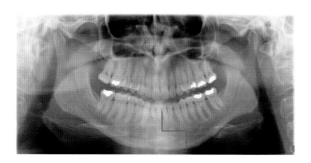

Fig. 15.4 Depiction of midline stair-step mandibulotomy (red line), necessitating removal of a central incisor, but providing increased rotational stability and lengthened healing surface.

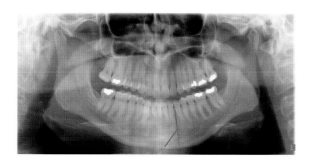

Fig. 15.5 Depiction of paramedian mandibulotomy (red line), between the lateral incisor and the canine. At this location, the tooth roots are divergent, leaving space for the osteotomy. The osteotomy can be angled toward the mental symphysis (solid red line), increasing stability and length of the healing surface, or alternatively can be carried straight down (dashed red line), preserving the attachments of the muscles at the genial tubercle.

Design

Osteotomy shape has been described as straight, dovetailed, stair-stepped, or notched (**Figs. 15.2, 15.3, 15.4, 15.5**). Although none of these configurations counteracts the unequal muscular pull on the medial and lateral aspects of the mandible, which will tend to distract the anterior mandible downward and the lateral mandible upward and medially,[5] the mandible can be adequately stabilized if the principles of rigid fixation are adhered to. A low rate of complications has been reported with the straight osteotomy.[36] The stair-step and angled configurations, although more time consuming to cut, do offer some potential advantages, including greater vertical stability, rotational stability, and a broader healing surface.[1,22] Care should be taken to keep the upper portion of the osteotomy straight, to avoid injury to the tooth roots. A powered saw with an ultra-thin blade minimizes the bone gap, and bone cuts should be made with ample irrigation to prevent thermal injury to bone.

Bone Fixation Technique

Bone fixation techniques have evolved significantly with the advent of osseointegrated titanium plating systems, which have essentially replaced the need for stainless steel wire. These two techniques were first directly compared by Shah et al[37] in 1993, establishing comparable rates of nonunion and wound infection with either technique in patients undergoing mandibulotomy. Parallel advances in our understanding of bone healing have also come from the craniomaxillofacial trauma literature. The sine qua non of bone fixation is that the fixation must be stable. In the *Arbeitsgemeinschaft für Osteosynthesefragen* (AO) philosophy of rigid fixation, inferred from knowledge of long bone fixation, it is argued that even subtle movement of the bone fragments, in any direction, will risk nonunion and subsequent wound infection.[35] In partial contrast, the philosophy espoused by Champy and Michelet argues that micromotion is acceptable, actually facilitating bone union, and that fixation need only be rigid along lines of stress.[38] The particular plating technique should be tailored to the surgeon's experience and comfort. The AO philosophy traditionally requires a locking reconstruction plate and tension band, whereas the Champy philosophy relies on two miniplates at the osteotomy: one on the anterior surface of the mandibular symphysis, and one along the inferior rim. Reliable results have been reported with both approaches. The Memorial Sloan-Kettering experience with mandibulotomy has established the feasibility of rigid fixation using two four-hole or six-hole titanium miniplates, one with monocortical screws and one with bicortical screws (**Fig. 15.6**). In most cases, the difference between these two plating philosophies is moot as few patients undergoing mandibulotomy will be chewing in the immediate postoperative period. Provided that stable fixation can be achieved with plating, there is no need to place patients in intermaxillary fixation after mandibulotomy.

> **Note**
> - Care should always be taken when drilling holes to avoid devitalizing the teeth, meaning that bicortical screws should only be placed well below the tooth roots.
> - Irrigation during drilling is necessary to avoid thermal injury to bone and to minimize the likelihood of loose screws.
> - Screws found to be loose at the time of surgery should not be left in place, and should be either replaced with a "safety screw," or relocated to another location.

Treatment of Complications

While meticulous surgical technique will prevent many complications, the literature confirms that a small percentage of patients will inevitably experience complications, generally minor and self-limiting, after mandibulotomy. These are generally related to infection or failed bone fixation. Despite the lateral swing of the mandible, temporomandibular joint complications are not seen after this procedure.[39] Wound infection can result from a devitalized tooth, poor oral hygiene, or inadequate fixation leading to excessive movement at the osteotomy site. Teeth should be extracted if they are fractured or have significant mobility.[8] When infection or wound breakdown develops, local wound care with irrigation and packing should be initiated. If abscesses develop, they should be drained and treated with appropriate antibiotics. Hardware exposure and local infection do not universally require removal of hardware, provided that the plate and screws remain stable. However, the development of infection in the context of a mobile bone segment, loose plate or loose screw, does necessitate hardware removal, thorough washout, and remedial plating. Nonunion results when there is persistent motion at the site of fixation, and necrotic or fibrous tissue fills the bone gap. In this case, the intervening fibrous tissue must be curetted, and the fresh bone edges must be rigidly fixated. A small percentage of patients will develop late symptoms attributable to hardware, commonly pain or temperature sensitivity, which can be remedied with hardware removal once bone healing is stable.[40]

Pull-Through Procedure

The mandibular–lingual releasing procedure, or "pull-through" was first described by Ward and Robben in 1951[41] and later popularized by Bradley and Stell in the UK,[42] and Stanley in the United States,[43] in the 1980s. This technique releases the entire floor of the mouth from the mandible, delivering the tongue into the neck, and affording access to the oral tongue and base of tongue. A lip-splitting incision and mandibular osteotomy are avoided, although a tracheotomy is still necessary, as in mandibulotomy. Although this technique provides adequate exposure for bulky lesions of the anterior and middle third of the tongue, exposure decreases as one moves posteriorly. Before choosing this approach, the surgeon must also be confident that a marginal or segmental mandibular resection will not be needed.

If this procedure is chosen, preventing complications requires careful design of incisions and meticulous, layered repair of the floor of the mouth. Because the entire floor of mouth diaphragm is released, it is essential that it be appropriately resuspended. The entire mandibular-lingual release should be performed in a subperiosteal plane. At the time of neck dissection, the superior subplatysmal flap is elevated to the lower border of the mandible, taking care to preserve the marginal mandibular branches of the bilateral facial nerves. Intraoral mucosal

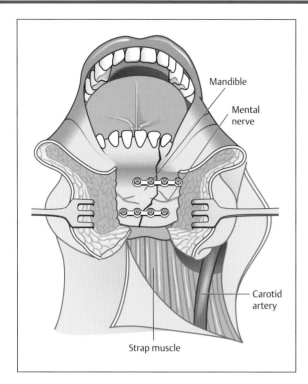

Fig. 15.6 Optimal placement of miniplates for fixation after mandibulotomy.

reported. There was no aesthetic advantage, based on ratings by patients, laypersons, or physicians, to either approach, even though the pull-through avoids a lip-splitting incision. However, patients undergoing lingual release had significantly poorer speech, swallowing, and chewing outcomes on the University of Washington quality-of-life instrument. The authors concluded that, despite meticulous reattachment of the floor of mouth musculature, the integrity of the oral diaphragm was significantly compromised by the lingual release. Unlike the mandibular swing procedure, the pull-through procedure requires division of bilateral genioglossus and geniohyoid muscles. In an effort to better preserve the integrity of these muscles, these authors now advocate avoiding muscle division by performing a genial osteotomy. Using a fine saw, an inferior rectangle of bone at the mental symphysis, encompassing the genial tubercle, is detached from the mandible, and left pedicled upon the genioglossus and geniohyoid musculature. The lingual release is then completed without dividing these muscles. The bone fragment is then reattached to the mandible at the conclusion of the case with miniplates or lag screws.[45] By preserving genioglossus and geniohyoid muscle integrity, this technique has been noted to ameliorate the swallowing dysfunction associated with the pull-through procedure (Merrick, personal communication).

incisions are then made, from glossopalatine fold to glossopalatine fold, leaving a cuff of attached gingiva for closure. A mucoperiosteal flap is raised along the lingual surface of the mandible down to the level of the floor of mouth musculature. A corresponding mucoperiosteal flap is raised from the lower border of the mandible upward. Complete bilateral division of the mylohyoid, geniohyoid, and genioglossus muscles is necessary. After tumor resection, the key to minimizing complications in this approach is meticulous layered closure, starting with posterior mucosal closure through the open mouth. Then, the intraoral edge of the mucoperiosteal flap is closed. This is most easily secured in the edentulous patient, as it can be sutured to remaining periosteum over the alveolar crest. In the dentate patient, durable closure to remaining periosteum can be difficult. Suspension of the mucoperiosteum via mattress sutures tied around the teeth can be helpful in supporting the closure.[43] Then, working through the neck, the floor of mouth muscles are reapproximated to the mandible. This repair is further supported by closing the elevated periosteum along the lower border of the mandible. Optimal closure of these layers will decrease the likelihood of salivary contamination and fistula formation.

Devine et al[44] from Glasgow compared functional and aesthetic outcomes in 150 patients undergoing either the lip-splitting mandibulotomy or pull-through procedures for oral cancer. Rates of wound complications were not

Lower Cheek and Visor Flaps

When a composite resection, with either segmental or marginal mandibulectomy, is indicated, a lower cheek flap or visor flap is usually necessary to provide adequate exposure to the mandible and oral cavity. The visor flap offers exposure to tumors in the anterior oral cavity, although exposure to the middle or posterior oral cavity remains inadequate. The primary distinction between the two approaches is that the visor flap obviates the need for a lip-splitting incision, but requires sacrifice of both mental nerves. The key to minimizing postoperative sequelae is appropriate choice of approach. In most cases, there is no functional consequence to a lip-splitting incision, whereas the morbidity of bilateral mental nerve sacrifice and its attendant lip and chin anesthesia can be disabling in elderly patients.[1] However, if the inferior alveolar nerves are going to be sacrificed due to mandibulectomy, a visor flap may be a reasonable alternative to a lip-splitting incision and lower cheek flap. A hemi-visor flap, which preserves the contralateral mental nerve when exposure of the anterolateral mandible and oral cavity is needed, has been advocated.[46,47] As in the other approaches, meticulous closure is key to the avoidance of complications. This requires careful preservation of a cuff of gingival mucosa at the time of flap elevation, and meticulous approximation of the vermilion border of the lip. The incorporation of a chevron into the lip-splitting incision may be useful in patients who form hypertrophic scars. As in other approaches, wound complications are generally self-limited with conservative management.

References

1. Shah JP, Johnson NW, Batsakis JG. Oral Cancer. London New York, NY: Martin Dunitz; 2003:496. Distributed in the United States by Thieme New York

2. Shah JP. Color Atlas of Operative Techniques in Head and Neck Surgery: Face, Skull, and Neck. Orlando, New York: Grune & Stratton; Harcourt Brace Jovanovich. 1987:256

3. Shah JP, Patel SG, and American Cancer Society. Cancer of the Head and Neck. American Cancer Society Atlas of Clinical Oncology. Hamilton, Ont.: BC Decker. 2001:484

4. Shaha AR. Mandibulotomy and mandibulectomy in difficult tumors of the base of the tongue and oropharynx. Semin Surg Oncol 1991;7(1):25–30

5. Dai TS, Hao SP, Chang KP, Pan WL, Yeh HC, Tsang NM. Complications of mandibulotomy: midline versus paramidline. Otolaryngol Head Neck Surg 2003;128(1):137–141

6. Liu SA, Wong YK, Poon CK, Wang CC, Wang CP, Tung KC. Risk factors for wound infection after surgery in primary oral cavity cancer patients. Laryngoscope 2007;117(1):166–171

7. Fergusson D, Khanna MP, Tinmouth A, Hébert PC. Transfusion of leukoreduced red blood cells may decrease postoperative infections: two meta-analyses of randomized controlled trials. Can J Anaesth 2004;51(5):417–424

8. Bui P, Demian N, Beetar P. Infection rate in mandibular angle fractures treated with a 2.0-mm 8-hole curved strut plate. J Oral Maxillofac Surg 2009;67(4):804–808

9. Seemann, R, Lauer, G, Poeschl, PW, et al. CROOMA, complication rates of operatively treated mandibular fractures, paramedian and body. Oral Surg Oral Med Oral Pathol Oral Radiol Endod 2011;111(4):449–454

10. Seemann R, Perisanidis C, Schicho K, et al. Complication rates of operatively treated mandibular fractures—the mandibular neck. Oral Surg Oral Med Oral Pathol Oral Radiol Endod 2010;109(6):815–819

11. Seemann R, Schicho K, Wutzl A, et al. Complication rates in the operative treatment of mandibular angle fractures: a 10-year retrospective. J Oral Maxillofac Surg 2010;68(3):647–650

12. Furr AM, Schweinfurth JM, May WL. Factors associated with long-term complications after repair of mandibular fractures. Laryngoscope 2006;116(3):427–430

13. Kyzas, PA. Use of antibiotics in the treatment of mandible fractures: a systematic review. J Oral Maxillofac Surg 2011;69(4):1129–1145

14. Butlin HT, Spencer WG. Diseases of the Tongue. New enlarged ed. London: Cassell. 1900

15. Sedillot A. La chirugie par voie de mandibulotomie. Gazette d'hopital 1844;17:83

16. Trotter, W. A Method of Lateral Pharyngotomy for the Exposure of Large Growths of the Epilaryngeal Region. Proc R Soc Med 1920;13(Laryngol Sect):196–198

17. Marchetta FC, Sako K, Murphy JB. The periosteum of the mandible and intraoral carcinoma. Am J Surg 1971;122(6):711–713

18. Dubner S, Spiro RH. Median mandibulotomy: a critical assessment. Head Neck 1991;13(5):389–393

19. Spiro RH, Gerold FP, Shah JP, Sessions RB, Strong EW. Mandibulotomy approach to oropharyngeal tumors. Am J Surg 1985;150(4):466–469

20. Spiro RH, Gerold FP, Strong EW. Mandibular "swing" approach for oral and oropharyngeal tumors. Head Neck Surg 1981;3(5):371–378

21. Tollefsen HR, Spiro RH. Median labiomandibular glossotomy. Ann Surg 1971;173(3):415–420

22. Dziegielewski PT, Mlynarek AM, Dimitry J, Harris JR, Seikaly H. The mandibulotomy: friend or foe? Safety outcomes and literature review. Laryngoscope 2009;119(12):2369–2375

23. Davidson J, Freeman J, Gullane P, Rotstein L, Birt D. Mandibulotomy and radical radiotherapy: compatible or not? J Otolaryngol 1988;17(6):279–281

24. Eisen MD, Weinstein GS, Chalian A, et al. Morbidity after midline mandibulotomy and radiation therapy. Am J Otolaryngol 2000;21(5):312–317

25. Dziegielewski PT, O'Connell DA, Rieger J, Harris JR, Seikaly H. The lip-splitting mandibulotomy: aesthetic and functional outcomes. Oral Oncol 2010;46(8):612–617

26. Teng MS, Genden EM, Buchbinder D, Urken ML. Subcutaneous mandibulotomy: a new surgical access for large tumors of the parapharyngeal space. Laryngoscope 2003;113(11):1893–1897

27. Baek CH, Lee SW, Jeong HS. New modification of the mandibulotomy approach without lip splitting. Head Neck 2006;28(7):580–586

28. Robson MC. An easy access incision for the removal of some intraoral malignant tumors. Plast Reconstr Surg 1979;64(6):834–835

29. McGregor IA. Symphyseal mandibular osteotomy in the approach to sublingual dermoid cyst. Br J Plast Surg 1991;44(7):544–545

30. McGregor IA, MacDonald DG. Mandibular osteotomy in the surgical approach to the oral cavity. Head Neck Surg 1983;5(5):457–462

31. Hayter JP, Vaughan ED, Brown JS. Aesthetic lip splits. Br J Oral Maxillofac Surg 1996;34(5):432–435

32. Rapidis AD, Valsamis S, Anterriotis DA, Skouteris CA. Functional and aesthetic results of various lip-splitting incisions: a clinical analysis of 60 cases. J Oral Maxillofac Surg 2001;59(11):1292–1296

33. Rudolph R, Goldfarb P, Hunt RG. Aesthetic aspects of composite oromandibular cancer resection and reconstruction. Ann Plast Surg 1985;14(2):128–134

34. Cilento BW, Izzard M, Weymuller EA, Futran N. Comparison of approaches for oral cavity cancer resection: lip-split versus visor flap. Otolaryngol Head Neck Surg 2007;137(3):428–432

35. Papel ID. Facial Plastic and Reconstructive Surgery. 3rd ed. New York: Thieme. 2009:xxi, 1174

36. Amin MR, Deschler DG, Hayden RE. Straight midline mandibulotomy revisited. Laryngoscope 1999;109(9):1402–1405

37. Shah JP, Kumaraswamy SV, Kulkarni V. Comparative evaluation of fixation methods after mandibulotomy for oropharyngeal tumors. Am J Surg 1993;166(4):431–434

38. Champy M, Lodde JP. Mandibular synthesis. Placement of the synthesis as a function of mandibular stress. [Article in French] Rev Stomatol Chir Maxillofac 1976;77(8):971–976

39. Christopoulos E, Carrau R, Segas J, Johnson JT, Myers EN, Wagner RL. Transmandibular approaches to the oral cavity and oropharynx. A functional assessment. Arch Otolaryngol Head Neck Surg 1992;118(11):1164–1167

40. Bakathir AA, Margasahayam MV, Al-Ismaily MI. Removal of bone plates in patients with maxillofacial trauma: a retrospective study. Oral Surg Oral Med Oral Pathol Oral Radiol Endod 2008;105(5):e32–e37

41. Ward GE, Robben JO. A composite operation for radical neck dissection and removal of cancer of the mouth. Cancer 1951;4(1):98–109

42. Bradley PJ, Stell PM. Surgeon's workshop: a modification of the "pull through" technique of glossectomy. Clin Otolaryngol Allied Sci 1982;7(1):59–62

References

43. Stanley RB. Mandibular lingual releasing approach to oral and oropharyngeal carcinomas. Laryngoscope 1984;94(5 Pt 1):596–600

44. Devine JC, Rogers SN, McNally D, Brown JS, Vaughan ED. A comparison of aesthetic, functional and patient subjective outcomes following lip-split mandibulotomy and mandibular lingual releasing access procedures. Int J Oral Maxillofac Surg 2001;30(3):199–204

45. Merrick GD, Morrison RW, Gallagher JR, Devine JC, Farrow A. Pedicled genial osteotomy modification of the mandibular release access operation for access to the back of the tongue. Br J Oral Maxillofac Surg 2007;45(6):490–492

46. Cantù G, Bimbi G, Colombo S, et al. Lip-splitting in trans-mandibular resections: is it really necessary? Oral Oncol 2006;42(6):619–624

47. LaFerriere KA, Sessions DG, Thawley SE, Wood BG, Ogura JH. Composite resection and reconstruction for oral cavity and oropharynx cancer. A functional approach. Arch Otolaryngol 1980;106(2):103–110

16 Intubation Injuries and Airway Management

K. Sandu, P. Monnier

Introduction

Otolaryngologists are frequently asked to evaluate patients who are endotracheally intubated and remain difficult to extubate or have voice or airway complaints after being extubated. Translaryngeal intubation may result in damage to the glottis, the subglottic segment, or the trachea itself. It usually follows periods of prolonged intubation with a translaryngeal cuffed tube in an intensive care setup for ventilation support. It has been observed that intubation injuries are less frequent but more severe in infants and children than adults, probably because children are more likely to have congenital anatomical abnormalities combined with a small airway or are commonly subject to improper tube selection for intubation.

> **Note**
>
> Any physician being asked to evaluate a patient having dyspnea and/or dysphonia after extubation should be aware of both the acute and long-term intubation complications and understand their diagnosis, management, and prevention.

Historical Note

The first endotracheal intubation was performed as early as AD 1000. In 1878, MacEwen first described orotracheal intubation using a brass tube for the administration of anesthesia. Annandale, in 1889, designed a tube fabricated of rubber. Later, Guedel and Waters added an inflatable cuff to such a rubber tube.[1,2] In 1964, the first polyvinylchloride tube with an integrated inflatable cuff was marketed. High-volume, low-pressure cuffs were introduced in 1970. Polyvinylchloride has the advantage of being less traumatic because it softens slightly at body temperature compared with room temperature, whereas rubber becomes more rigid and has a greater possibility of inducing mucosal injury. Furthermore, rubber endotracheal tubes (ETT) do not have high-volume, low-pressure cuffs.

Mechanism of Intubation Injury

Intubation injuries can be broadly classified into immediate and late. Immediate or acute injuries are those that occur during the initial intubation. These can occur during a traumatic on-site intubation when airway visualization is difficult due to severe upper airway bleeding or due to inadequate instrumentation or an inexperienced staff. Injuries in this type of intubation include mucosal abrasion, vocal cord hematoma, laryngotracheal tears and dislocation of the cricoarytenoid joint space.

Once the patient has been intubated, the most important consideration is of the airway mucosal capillary perfusion.[3] It is important to note that the glottic shape is triangular, being broad at the posterior commissure and narrow at the anterior commissure. The ETT exerts pressure in the posterior larynx at four main sites (**Fig. 16.1**):

- medial surface and the vocal processes of the arytenoid cartilages and cricoarytenoid joints
- posterior glottis consisting of the interarytenoid region
- subglottis, which is more vulnerable in infants and small children because the cricoid ring is relatively small compared with that of the adults
- trachea at the site of the ETT cuff.

In a patient with prolonged intubation, an ETT with circular cross-section occupies the interarytenoid space of the triangular glottis. If such a patient is not adequately sedated, the vocal process of the arytenoid cartilages is traumatized during their adductive movements, causing mucosal abrasion. Prolonged intubation causes pressure necrosis and mucosal ischemia leading to congestion, edema and ulceration leading to perichondritis and potential chondral necrosis (**Fig. 16.2**). The final stage of a laryngeal "bedsore" is reached when there is necrosis of the cricoarytenoid joint and the cricoid cartilage. All of these events, along with fibrocicatrization, lead to laryngeal stenosis.

Factors Contributing to Intubation Trauma

Patient-related Factors

- *Difficult anatomy*—as in obese, short-necked individuals, protruding anterior teeth, retrognathic mandible, and restricted mouth opening
- *Difficult intubation* of congenitally malformed larynges (webbing, cartilagenous stenosis)
- *Bleeding in the upper airway*, which makes the intubation difficult and risky
- *Oropharyngolaryngeal tumors*

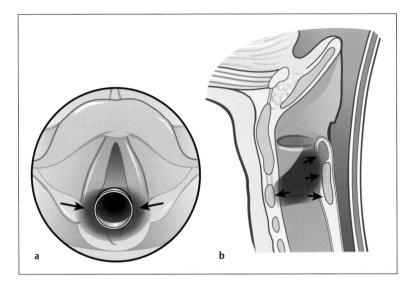

Fig. 16.1a,b Diagram of the potential sites of pressure-induced endotracheal tube injuries in the larynx:

a Maximum pressure is exerted on the medial aspect of the arytenoid cartilages (arrows).

b Other sites of predilection for pressure-induced necrosis include the posterior laryngeal commissure and the posterolateral and circumferential subglottis (arrows).

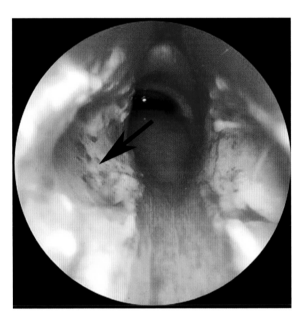

Fig. 16.2 Posterolateral deep ulceration in the v-shaped upper portion of the cricoid with exposure of the cartilage.

- *Severely inflamed larynges* are more prone to injury, as in acute laryngotracheobronchitis where the inflammatory response already present within the larynx makes the mucosa more susceptible to pressure necrosis

- *Acute or chronic diseased status* (altered consciousness, poor tissue perfusion, diabetes mellitus). Medical conditions associated with decreased tissue perfusion increase the likelihood of tissue necrosis and ulceration. These conditions include head trauma, congestive heart failure, liver failure, hypoxemia, and anemia. Gaynor and Greenberg[4] noted a very high incidence of severe complications in patients with insulin-dependent diabetes mellitus. Immunosuppressed patients

are more prone to bacterial infection of the airway mucosal ulcerations and should be closely monitored for the development of chronic chondronecrosis and its sequelae.

- *Gastroesophageal reflux and aspiration* are common in critically ill patients. This repetitive bathing of the laryngeal structures with gastric acid causes a chemical irritation that adds to local injury from the ETT. It may be beneficial to use H2-blockers or proton-pump inhibitors to minimize reflux in critically ill and intubated patients.

- The presence of a *nasogastric tube* increases the likelihood of reflux. Nasogastric tubes may also cause irritation and ulceration in the postcricoid region causing cricoid ulcers. Injury caused by nasogastric tubes may occur with or without endotracheal tubes, and the concurrent presence of both may worsen the insult.

Procedure-related Factors

- Intubation by novice in-training resident doctor, repeated intubations

- *Duration of intubation* is an important factor contributing toward intubation sequelae. Normally intubation side effects can be seen within about 5 to 7 days in an adult and 7 to 14 days in children, noting here that infants do not have a specific time limit of intubation and could undergo continued intubation for 2 to 3 months if required, without performing a tracheotomy; however, this certainly invites a high risk of long-term intubation problems.[2] Patients who undergo surgeries of long duration are at increased risk of developing intubation injury sequelae.

- *Physical characteristics of the tubes*, i.e., size and type, are also important in determining intubation injuries. Large-size, rigid or rubber tubes are more traumatic and hence siliconized smooth-walled less irritating tubes are preferred. During an elective endotracheal intubation, recommended ETT norms are a 6.5-size (outer diameter 8.8 mm maximum) for an adult female and 7.5-size tube (outer diameter 10.2 mm maximum) for an adult male.[5] In infants and children less than 8 years old an uncuffed tube with a diameter that allows an air leak in the subglottic space with a ventilating pressure of 20 cmH$_2$O is preferred.[6] High-volume, low-pressure cuff has an additional advantage of reducing pressure-induced mucosal ischemia.

- The *ETT cuff* may still induce excessive trauma if it is inflated too high within the larynx. Even with an appropriately sized ETT, excessive motion of the tube may induce repeated mucosal trauma. This may occur as a result of inadequate patient sedation, transmitted movements from the ventilator or manipulations during suctioning.

Patient Evaluation

History

The evaluation of a patient with suspected intubation injury begins with a thorough history, and the following points should be carefully noted:

- The reason for intubation and any coexisting illnesses
- The date of initial intubation, failed attempts at extubation, and total duration of intubation
- The mode of intubation, i.e., fiberoptic/rigid broncho-scopy-assisted/blind. Needless to say that more initial airway damage can be expected of a blind awake intubation
- The place where the patient was intubated—hospital intubations would be more secure than on-site intubations, where lack of optimal instrumentation, inadequate oropharyngolaryngeal suctioning and thereby inability to correctly visualize the glottis adds to to the injury list
- Details of securing the tube should be explored, as a wrongly secured tube in the posterior interarytenoid area increases the chances of a posterior glottic stenosis
- Level of consciousness and whether excessive movements due to inadequate sedation and ventilator movements are transmitted to the tube
- Route (orotracheal versus nasotracheal) of intubation
- Size of the tube and presence of a nasogastric tube.

Laryngeal Examination in Patients with Suspected Intubation Trauma

Extubated Symptomatic Patient

In an adult patient, awake dynamic airway examination is performed with a flexible fiberoptic nasolaryngoscope

to see the vocal cord mobility. Similar examination in children is performed under spontaneous respiration anesthesia with sevoflurane. All areas of the airway are examined systematically beginning with the nasal cavity, posterior choana, rhinopharynx, oropharynx, larynx, trachea, and bronchi. It must be pointed out that anesthetic drugs can modify the interpretation of dynamic airway functions, and hence the role of an experienced pediatric anesthetist and an optimal plane of anesthesia are very important. In a tracheostomized child, the cannula should be removed and the tracheostomy blocked temporarily to allow normal inspirium and expirium, thereby allowing precise identification of the airway obstruction.

Following dynamic examination, a direct laryngoscopy with 0° and angled optics should be performed for a complete evaluation of the endolaryngeal intubation injuries involving the supraglottis, glottis, and subglottis. During suspension microlaryngoscopy, examination with rigid 0° and 30° scopes is indispensable to identify injury at the posterior glottic level. A false vocal cord retractor is used to better expose the posterior glottis, which may show a cicatricial bridge between the two arytenoid cartilages. Direct palpation of the arytenoid cartilages may reveal fixation of the cricoarytenoid joints. The trachea, bronchi, and esophagus are carefully examined. It is not infrequent to see multisite airway narrowing, which eventually could affect patient treatment.

> **Note**
> Benjamin[2] advocates direct laryngoscopy in adult patients who had more than 7 days of intubation or in children 1 to 2 weeks after extubation that present with voice or respiratory symptoms and in infants after failed attempts at extubation.

Intubated Patient

Examination of the larynx is often challenging in an intubated patient. In patients who cannot be moved out of intensive care units, a bedside laryngoscopy with a McIntosh laryngosope and rigid 0° plus angled sinonasal endoscope is performed. In patients who are at high risk of developing a stenosis, the evaluation is made in the endoscopy suite aided by an anesthetist. During direct laryngoscopy, the ETT is removed, allowing complete examination of the glottis, the posterior glottis, and the subglottic region. The rest of the endoscopy protocol is similar to that described earlier for an extubated symptomatic patient. After visualizing the glottic injury, epinephrine-soaked cotton pledgets are used to decongest the laryngeal edema.

The patient is reintubated with an ETT that is one size smaller and an antibiotic–cortisone ointment plug is inserted into the glottis to calm the inflammatory process. Additional systemic corticosteroids and antibiotics are given (or continued). In children, if feasible, noninvasive ventilation methods like continuous positive airway pressure and bilevel positive airway pressure should be used as an alternative to continued endotracheal intubation. An intubated patient is under antibiotic cover and 24 hours before extubation, intravenous corticosteroid is administered to reduce the laryngeal edema and inflammation and aid the extubation. Epinephrine and steroid aerosols can be continued after extubation if needed.

> **Note**
>
> Patients brought to the endoscopy suite in an intubated state need to be evaluated during spontaneous respiration to rule out arytenoid fixation or other pre-existing extralaryngeal causes for airway obstruction, which could pose problems at extubation and after. This emphasizes the role of a previous detailed patient history.

- Supraglottis
  - Absent to minor lesions
  - Edematous protrusion of ventricular mucosa
  - Erythema or edematous swelling of the ventricular bands
- Glottis
  - Non-specific swelling in the Reinke space of the vocal cords
  - Pressure-induced ischemic necrosis
  - Ulcers at the medial aspect of the arytenoids with flanges of granulation tissue at vocal processes
  - Medial exposure of the cricoarytenoid joint
  - Posterior interarytenoid ulcer
- Subglottis
  - Nonspecific edematous swelling
  - Posterolateral cricoid ulcers
  - Concentric subglottis ulceration

Fig. 16.3 Acute postintubation injuries of the larynx.

Immediate/Acute Complications of Intubation

A myriad of nonspecific and unfortunate complications have been reported after attempted intubation of patients with difficult anatomy or performed by inexperienced clinicians. These include rare reports[7] of inadvertent esophageal intubation leading to swallowing of the ETT, laryngoscope bulb aspiration, and gastric perforation. More frequent complications include difficult intubation that may result in dental trauma, laceration to the mucosa of the oropharynx, hypopharynx, larynx, trachea, or esophagus, with the pyriform sinus being at the highest risk.[4] The endolarynx is especially vulnerable because of its delicate anatomy. Acute postintubation injuries are summarized in **Fig. 16.3** and illustrated in **Fig. 16.4**.

Dislocation of the Arytenoid Cartilage

Dislocation of the arytenoid cartilage is a rare acute complication of intubation. The most common symptom is hoarseness, followed by breathlessness, dysphagia and vocal fatigue. The diagnosis is usually made by detection of decreased vocal fold mobility and anterior tilting of the arytenoid at indirect or flexible laryngoscopy. The vocal-fold is lax with submucosal arytenoid hematoma and shortened compared with the opposite side. The most consistent finding is the two vocal folds showing an unequal level. Early repositioning of the arytenoid is best performed at the time of diagnosis because this improves

the likelihood of normal voice restoration. Prolonged dislocation may lead to cricoarytenoid joint ankylosis with complete joint fixation. However, there is no clear time period as to when this occurs and reductions as late as 1 year from the initial injury have shown dramatic improvement in voice quality.[1,8]

The arytenoid reduction procedure is performed under general anesthetic and suspension microlaryngoscopy. The dislocated arytenoid is repositioned posterolaterally and reaccommodated into the articular facet of the cricoid cartilage using a blunt-angled microlaryngoscopic instrument. It should be inserted into the Morgagni ventricle and pulled back until the arytenoid sits in its proper position. Sataloff et al[9] recommend local anesthesia and sedation because this allows assessment of the voice and vocal fold mobility intraoperatively. There are reports of patients with spontaneous reduction of the dislocation needing no further surgical intervention.[9] Bilateral ankylosed cricoarytenoid articular spaces together with a posterior glottic stenosis (PGS) present as *frozen larynx*, which is disastrous for the patient and a very difficult condition to treat.

Treatment of Acute Intubation Lesions

In clinical practice, two situations may occur: (1) swelling of the lax glotto–subglottic mucosa without ischemic necrosis, and (2) ulcers with fibrin and granulation tissue resulting from ischemic necrosis of the glottic and subglottic mucosa.

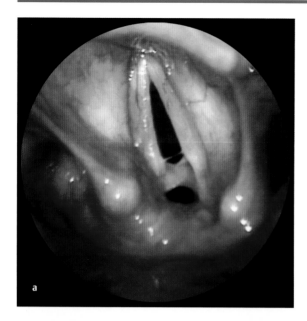

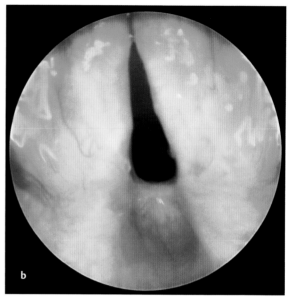

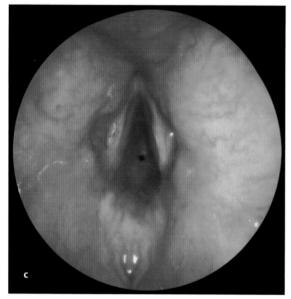

Fig. 16.4a–c Acute intubation lesions.

a Prominent edematous protrusion of ventricular mucosa.

b Ulcerated troughs with exuberant granulation tissue filling the posterior glottis.

c Annular interarytenoid ulceration with exposed cartilage, but no granulation tissue in an immunocompromised adolescent.

Treatment of Soft Tissue Stenosis without Mucosal Necrosis

Airway obstruction manifests itself within a few minutes of or up to a few hours after extubation. Premature babies are more prone than older children to develop this condition.[10] Treatment consists of:

- Topical decongestion with epinephrine pledgets
- Reintubation with an ETT that is one size smaller
- Application of an endolaryngeal plug of gentamycin–corticosteroid
- Ointment (Diprogenta [Merck, Sharpe and Dohme, worldwide])

- Systemic antibiotics, corticosteroids and antireflux treatment.

With the above conservative treatment, most patients can be extubated within 2 to 4 days.

Anterior Cricoid Split

This operation was introduced by Cotton and Seid in 1980[11] to avoid a tracheotomy in premature babies. It is indicated in the presence of adequate pulmonary reserve provided that no other upper or lower airway obstruction exists. Strict criteria for proper indications have been

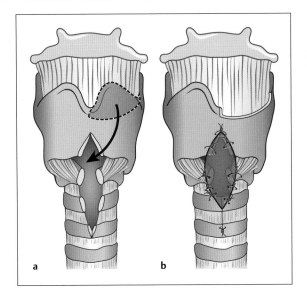

Fig. 16.5a,b Anterior cricoid split modified into an anterior laryngotracheal reconstruction.

a Anterior laryngotracheal incision. The cricoid ring springs partially open. Harvesting of the thyroid cartilage from the upper alar portion.
b Suturing the thyroid cartilage graft into position.

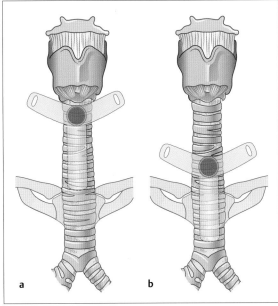

Fig. 16.6a,b Correct placement of tracheostomy with impending laryngotracheal stenosis.

a Tracheostoma situated immediately below the cricoid ring to maximally preserve normal trachea.
b Tracheostoma situated at the sixth to seventh or eighth tracheal rings to spare sufficient length of normal trachea between the stenosis and the tracheostomy.

established[12] and include: at least two extubation failures secondary to a subglottic laryngeal pathology, weight greater than 1500 g, off ventilator support for at least 10 days, supplemental oxygen requirement below 30%, noncongestive heart failure for at least 1 month, no acute respiratory tract infection, and no hypotensive medications for at least 10 days before the procedure.[13]

Anterior cricoid split is based on the principle that an anterior vertical midline transection of the cricoid ring allows the cartilage to *spring open.* This helps leakage of submucosal edema fluid through the wound. The surgery is illustrated in **Fig. 16.5**.

Tracheotomy in Impending Laryngotracheal Stenosis

After a complete airway examination, a rational decision is made regarding the safety of continued intubation or whether to proceed with tracheotomy. This decision, especially in children and infants can be very tricky and needs to be well discussed among the attending medical teams so as to avoid tracheotomy complications and sequelae. In infants, the time to perform the tracheotomy may be extended to several weeks and in neonates with good nursing, there is almost no length of intubation that is considered unsafe. The exact explanation for this is

unknown, but the immaturity and pliability of the laryngeal cartilages may play a significant role in reducing pressure necrosis of the mucosa.[2,7]

Contrary to the current rule stating that the tracheostomy site be placed at the second or third tracheal ring, in case the trachea needs to be maximally preserved in the event of a future airway reconstruction, the stoma must be placed either immediately below the cricoid ring or very low at the sixth, seventh, or eighth tracheal ring. In the first instance, a single-stage cricotracheal resection can be performed, without losing excessive normal trachea. In the second instance, good-quality vascularized tracheal rings are preserved between the anastomosis and the stoma, thereby preventing ischemic necrosis leading to anastomotic dehiscence. The stoma placement is illustrated in **Fig. 16.6**.

Sequelae of Prolonged Intubation

The presence of an ETT in the larynx for a long duration causes characteristic pathology (**Fig. 16.7**). In general, prolonged intubation would be more than 7 to 10 days in adults and 2 weeks in children.[4,7] The incidence of

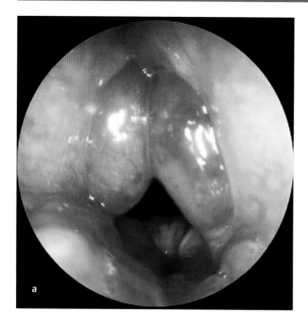

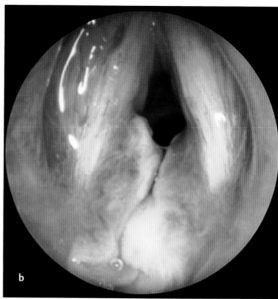

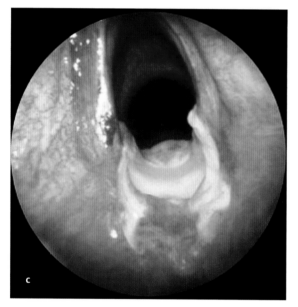

Fig. 16.7a–c Stenotic cicatricial sequelae due to prolonged endotracheal tube intubation.

a Posterior glottic stenosis without cricoarytenoid joint fixation.
b Posterior glottic stenosis with bilateral cricoarytenoid joint fixation.
c Cicatricial severe subglottic stenosis.

laryngeal complications after prolonged intubation is between 4 and 13%.[14] Benjamin[1] has described several stages of injury and the resultant chronic laryngeal changes that may be seen after prolonged intubation are discussed below.

Vocal Cord Edema

Edema is often marked in the mucosa of the laryngeal ventricle, causing a prolapse or protrusion of the mucosa into the laryngeal inlet persisting long after extubation as vocal cord edema and severe dysphonia.

Intubation Granuloma

Benjamin[1,2] describes "tongues of granulation" forming within 48 hours and extending from the vocal processes bilaterally anterior to the ETT. They may become large and prolapse into the glottis during extubation causing posterior airway obstruction with the need for immediate reintubation. In some instances, the granulation tissue resolves incompletely or matures into chronic laryngeal scarring. With incomplete healing and persistent perichondritis, an *intubation granuloma* may form. This is a localized, globular, yellow-red pedunculated rounded mass protruding from the site of ulceration, most commonly at the vocal process and medial surface of the arytenoid. Patients with intubation granuloma present weeks to months after extubation with voice changes, globus, or rarely airway obstructive symptoms. The treatment includes carbon dioxide laser excision under suspension microlaryngoscopy.

Cicatricial Furrows

Superficial cricoarytenoid ulceration is an early finding, occurring 4 to 6 hours after intubation (see **Fig. 16.2**). As the irritation from the endotracheal tube persists, the mucosal ulcerations deepen and are invaded by bacteria from the respiratory tract. At 48 hours, the inflammatory reaction extends into the perichondrium. Prolonged intubation results in progression of these changes. Deep ulcerations present as "ulcerated troughs", which can be seen only after removal of the endotracheal tube and appear as wide, deep erosions through the perichondrium and into the cartilage on the medial aspect of the arytenoid and cricoid cartilages. The cricoarytenoid joint is often exposed and may become inflamed leading to chronic fibrosis and ankylosis (**Fig. 16.7a**). Weeks to months after extubation, these ulcerated troughs heal and are noticed as "cicatricial furrows".

Interarytenoid Scarring and Posterior Glottic Stenosis (Fig. 16.7b)

Ulceration crossing the midline of the posterior glottis with no median residual strip of intact mucosa signifies a high risk for the formation of PGS upon scar maturation. In severe cases, this scarring matures into a thick fibrous band between the arytenoid cartilages. Abduction of the true vocal cords may be limited and be misdiagnosed as bilateral abductor paralysis, which is labeled as *pseudolaryngeal paralysis*. These patients usually have airway complaints ranging from dyspnea on exertion to near-complete obstruction. The voice is often near normal. Suspension microlaryngoscopic examination of the posterior glottis using 0° and 30° telescopes is of paramount importance. The transverse fibrotic scar appears as a firm, thick web in the posterior glottis between the arytenoid cartilages.

A palper is used to move the arytenoid in lateral and outward direction. In abductor palsy, this passive movement will not cause any movement of the opposite arytenoid. However, in PGS an outward movement of one arytenoid pulls the opposite arytenoid inward because of the transverse interarytenoid cicatricial bridge attaching both arytenoids. In the case of bilateral cricoarytenoid joint fixation, no arytenoid movement can be elicited. The cicatricial web may extend from the interarytenoid area into the glottis and the subglottis. Treatment of the

subglottic stenosis (SGS) is unlikely to be successful without addressing the posterior glottic scarring.

Subglottic Stenosis (Fig. 16.7c)

Prolonged intubation is the most common cause of SGS in both adults and children. Patients with abnormal cricoid cartilages and congenital SGS are more likely to have subglottic complications from intubation. Transglottic stenosis occurs when in addition to a glottic stenosis there is associated PGS and SGS. Such a severe grade of stenosis involves damage to intrinsic laryngeal muscles caused at the initial intubation injury or later by various surgical attempts during dilation, laser excision, or open procedures.

Vocal Cord Paralysis

True vocal cord paralysis may occur as a result of endotracheal intubation, though its occurrence has probably been largely overestimated. The paralysis is usually unilateral, but bilateral paralysis with airway obstruction has been reported.[14,15] Brandwein et al[16] examined the course of the anterior branch of the recurrent laryngeal nerve and discovered it to be vulnerable to compression between the inflated cuff of the ETT and the lateral projection of the abducted arytenoid and thyroid cartilages. It must be pointed out here that, cicatricial cricoarytenoid joint fixation is more frequent than actual vocal cord paralysis. Injury to the recurrent laryngeal nerve most commonly results in the cord lying in the paramedian position.

Ductal Retention Cysts

These may result from obstruction of the submucous glands by an indwelling ETT. They are most common in infants, occurring in the subglottis or undersurface of the vocal cords. Small cysts may be incidental findings, whereas larger cysts can cause airway obstruction and may need laser excision.

Surgical Treatment of Acquired Subglottic Stenosis

Laryngotracheoplasty and Laryngotracheal Reconstruction

The term laryngotracheoplasty describes a procedure aimed at enlarging the subglottic lumen by vertical incisions of the anterior and/or posterior cricoid ring and then splinting the two halves by a mold during the healing phase. In short, it implies an expansion procedure WITHOUT cartilage graft interposition. On the other hand, a laryngotracheal reconstruction (LTR) means an expansion procedure by cartilage grafts plus an indwelling laryngotracheal expander or mold. Also in an LTR, the cicatricial SGS is not resected so as to preserve residual mucosa in the stenotic tract, thereby facilitating the re-epithelialization process during the stenting and healing periods.

The LTR is less invasive than partial cricotracheal resection and is performed for grade II and less severe grade III SGS, especially in children. LTR can be performed as a single-stage or double-stage procedure. Costal cartilage is the best graft material, although conchal cartilage, nasal septum and the thyroid cartilage have been used with satisfactory results. Cartilage grafts can be used for anterior or posterior or both anterior and posterior airway expansion.

Surgical Steps of Laryngotracheal Reconstruction

- The operation starts with the neck stabilized in a hyperextended position. A collar incision is taken just above the superior edge of the tracheostoma. A subplatysmal flap is raised and the strap muscles are retracted in the midline to expose the larynx and the trachea.
- For SGS involving the glottis (PGS, vocal cord synechia, cricoarytenoid joint ankylosis) a full anterior midline laryngocricotracheal fissure is made taking great care while performing the midline thyrotomy to divide exactly at the anterior commissure and avoiding damage to the vocal cords. Upper one or two tracheal rings are divided without joining the incision distally into the tracheostoma. For isolated SGS without glottic involvement, an inferior midline thyrotomy in addition to a median cricotracheal fissure is performed, without incising the anterior commissure.
- A midline posterior cricoid split is performed cutting through the posterior cricoarytenoid muscle raphe, without damaging the retrocricoid mucosa. Cranially, the incision must extend into the interarytenoid muscle completely incising the posterior glottic fibrous band.
- Costal cartilage graft is harvested from the seventh or eighth rib preserving the anterior perichondrium. An anterior costal cartilage graft is sculpted with a sharp knife into a diamond shape and sutured into the anterior subglottic defect, with the perichondrium facing toward the airway (**Fig. 16.8b**). Slightly larger outer flanges measuring ~ 2 to 3 mm allow better fixing of the graft and avoid its medialization into the airway lumen. The thickness of the *spreader* graft should be equal to that of the expanded stenotic cricoid cartilage. 4–0/5–0 Vicryl is used to fix the graft on to the anterior thyrocricotracheal defect, making sure that there is a good mucosal approximation with the perichondrium (**Fig. 16.9**). A meticulous mucosa–perichondrium

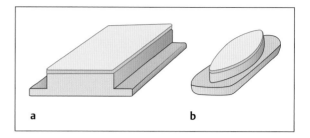

Fig. 16.8a,b Posterior and anterior costal cartilage grafts.

a The posterior cartilage graft is rectangular in shape with lateral flanges. The cartilage graft must be trimmed to an appropriate thickness (~ cricoid plate plus 1 or 2 mm).

b The anterior graft is diamond-shaped, preserving the superior, inferior, and lateral flanges of the cartilage.

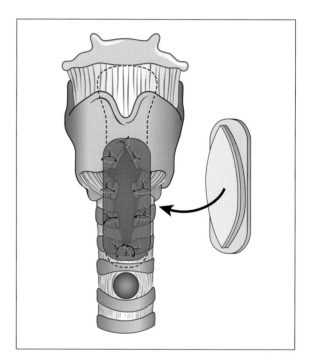

Fig. 16.9 Double-stage laryngotracheal reconstruction with anterior costal cartilage graft. The costal cartilage graft is sewn into position, with the perichondrium facing the lumen. Large flanges prevent prolapse of the costal cartilage graft into the airway. The reconstruction is stented by an LT-Mold (outline).

contact avoids postoperative exposure of the cartilage and granulation tissue formation.
- Costal cartilage graft is shaped as a rectangle when used for the posterior commissure expansion (**Fig. 16.8a**). Posterolateral flanges of the graft are sutured to the split posterior cricoid plate giving a snugly fitting interpositional reconstruction.
- In single-stage costal cartilage graft, a nasotracheal tube can be left in place for 5 to 7 days, which acts as a stent and avoids graft displacement.

- An LT-Mold stent is used in the double-stage procedure (**Fig. 16.9**) and the stent is fixed proximally (with thyroid cartilage) and distally (with trachea) using Prolene 3-0 stiches, which are removed endoscopically. Stenting is advocated for 3 to 12 weeks as required to allow optimal re-epithelialization.
- Fibrin glue is used all around the reconstruction to ensure an airtight closure. Thyroid isthmus and prelaryngeal muscles are resutured in the midline over the anterior graft, which is indispensible for the correct healing of cartilage grafts. The laryngofissure is closed using 3-0 Vicryl sutures, taking care to maintain a sharp anterior commissure and the neck is closed leaving in a Penrose drain. The procedure is performed under an antibiotic cover and antireflux treatment. There are no restrictions to the neck mobility as in a cricotracheal resection.

Postoperative Care

In single-stage LTR, the first endoscopic assessment is performed at 5 to 7 days. Early granulations are removed using biopsy forceps. Follow-up endoscopies are planned at 1 to 3 months. In double-stage LTR, the LT-Mold is removed endoscopically at 3 weeks to 3 months. Not earlier than 2 to 3 months, gentle dilation with Savary–Gilliard bougies may be required to open up and configurate the reconstructed airway. Complete mucosalization of the airway takes ~ 6 weeks to 3 months.

Complications during an LTR mainly include granulations and graft displacement. A free cartilage graft can become infected and may undergo necrosis, after which it is not rigid enough to keep the airway expanded. Fibrocicatricial healing in such cases can lead to severe laryngeal anatomy distortion and restenosis.

Cricotracheal Resection

Indications

Partial cricotracheal resection (PCTR) is the procedure of choice for the treatment of severe SGS (severe grade III and IV with > 70% luminal obstruction) of congenital or acquired origin. The surgery is performed as a single-stage operation (with concomitant resection of the tracheostoma during the surgery) when the stenosis is purely subglottic and the patient is otherwise healthy. In patients with multiple congenital anomalies, or impaired neurologic or cardiopulmonary function, a double-stage PCTR (with postoperative maintenance of the tracheostoma) is preferable.

If the SGS is combined with glottic involvement (PGS, cicatricial fusion of the vocal cords, anterior laryngeal web extending into the subglottis, or distortion of the laryngeal framework resulting from failed LTRs), PCTR

is supplemented with a posterior cricoid split and costal cartilage graft expansion that needs stenting and maintenance of the tracheostoma until a complete healing of the subglottic area is obtained. This procedure is called "extended PCTR" (E-PCTR).

Surgical Work-Up

When planning a CTR, a detailed dynamic airway examination is performed using a transnasal fibroscope to assess vocal cord mobility, malacic airway stenosis, or oropharyngeal (extralaryngeal) sites of obstruction. A rigid panendoscopy is performed at the same time observing the following.

- The location, extent, and degree of stenosis are assessed using telescopes (0°, 30°) and an intubation anesthetic laryngoscope.
- The exact location of the stenosis, with respect to the vocal folds, the tracheostoma (if existing) and the carina, is measured in millimeters and in number of residual normal tracheal rings above and below the tracheostoma.
- The endoscopy report should mention the presence of any localized tracheomalacia and a possible infection of the airway. A bacteriologic smear is routinely taken.
- Finally, in the presence of congenital SGS, a bronchoesophagoscopy is performed to rule out mediastinal malformations (e.g., tracheoesophageal fistula, tracheobronchial anomalies, extrinsic vascular compression of the airway).[17] If precise description and measurements of the stenosis are obtained from the endoscopy, then radiographs add little to the preoperative evaluation. When a malformation of the mediastinum is suspected, magnetic resonance imaging is the modality of choice.[18] Gastroesophageal reflux disease should be ruled out systematically and actively treated if present.[19]

Operative Technique

- The procedure is performed with the neck fully extended. Especially in small children, it is advisable to use magnifying glasses because of the small size of the structures being manipulated. It also aids in meticulous placement of the anastomotic sutures.
- A collar incision is usually made at the level of the second tracheal ring. In tracheotomized patients, a horizontal crescent-shape excision of the skin is made around the stoma.
- The subplatysmal skin flap is elevated, and the strap muscles are separated from the midline to provide exposure from the hyoid bone to the suprasternal notch. The isthmus of the thyroid gland is transected in the midline.
- The trachea is dissected anteriorly and laterally without identification of the recurrent laryngeal nerves by

staying in close contact with the underlying cartilaginous rings. The vascular supply coming laterally from the tracheoesophageal grooves should always be carefully preserved, especially in extensive mobilization of the distal trachea.

- At the level of the cricoid arch, the cricothyroid muscles are sharply dissected from the underlying cartilage until the cricothyroid joint is identified bilaterally.
- After having placed stay sutures to the distal normal tracheal wall, the inferior resection line is made first at the lower end of the stenosis or at the level of the tracheostoma if the latter is to be resected during the same surgical procedure.
- Unnecessary extensive separation of the trachea from the esophagus should be avoided to preserve vascularity of the posterior tracheal mucosa. The advancement of the distal tracheal stump upward is achieved by freeing the cartilaginous rings from the mediastinal structures only anteriorly and laterally. Because of its elasticity, the esophagus shortens spontaneously without anterior bulging.
- The superior incision is started at the inferior margin of the thyroid cartilage in front and is passed laterally just anterior to the cricothyroid joints, which results in the complete resection of the anterior cricoid arch while avoiding injury to the recurrent laryngeal nerves that run posteriorly to the joint. In the subglottis, the uppermost incision of the posterior mucosa is made just below the cricoarytenoid joints, and the submucosal fibrosis that constitutes the posterior aspect of the SGS is fully resected, so exposing the cricoid plate completely.
- In children and infants, the difference in diameter between the subglottic space and the tracheal stump is more pronounced than in adults, hence, the first normal tracheal ring used for the anastomosis must be adapted to the size of the subglottic lumen. Any attempt at reducing the caliber of the trachea should be avoided. Instead, one should enlarge the subglottic lumen as much as possible without compromising voice quality. This approach is best achieved by widening the cricoid plate posteriorly and laterally with a diamond bur and performing an inferior midline thyrotomy up to the level of the anterior commissure of the larynx without transecting it (**Fig. 16.10**). In this way, the subglottic lumen is enlarged considerably while the anterior commissure is kept intact, thus preserving a good voice. The triangular defect is filled in with a mucosa-lined cartilaginous wedge that is obtained from the first normal tracheal ring below the resected stricture. Inferior thyrotomy is not needed in adults. The denuded cricoid plate is covered with the membranous trachea after its upward mobilization.
- Depending on the patient's age, 3–0/4–0 Vicryl sutures are used for the thyrotracheal anastomosis. The first stitch is passed through the posterolateral

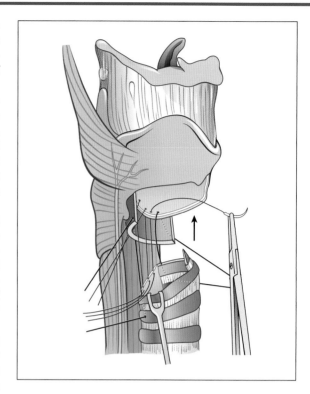

Fig. 16.10 Posterior cricotracheal anastomosis after partial cricotracheal resection. The posterolateral sutures (dark blue) are tied with the knots outside. Posterior sutures (light blue) are tied inside the lumen. Note the sharp dissection of the cricothyroid muscle, which is retracted laterally and thereby preserves the recurrent laryngeal nerve. Also seen is the inferior midline thyrotomy to enlarge the subglottic space.

aspect of the first normal tracheal ring and through the cricoid plate laterally (**Fig. 16.10**). It should emerge in a subperichondrial plane from the outer surface of the cricoid plate to avoid any damage to the recurrent laryngeal nerves. This stitch is important and should be placed as meticulously as possible to bring the mucosa of the subglottis in close contact with the mucosa of the trachea. Posterior anastomosis between the tracheal and posterior glottic mucosa is done using 4–0/5–0 Vicryl, either in a continuous running stitch or secured intermittently with the knots tied inside the lumen (**Fig. 16.11**). The anterior and lateral thyrotracheal anastomosis is completed by placing the sutures between the tracheal ring and the thyroid cartilage anteriorly, with the knots tied on the outside (**Fig. 16.12**). A tension-releasing suture is also placed between the third or fourth tracheal ring laterally and the inferior border of the cricoid plate.

Anastomotic Tension Release Procedures

Various techniques of tracheal and supralaryngeal release may be used to diminish the tension on the suture line,

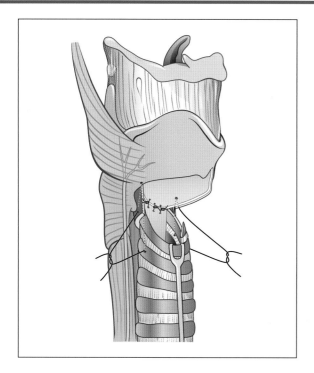

Fig. 16.11 Completion of the posterior cricotracheal anastomosis. Great care should be taken to achieve perfect mucosal approximation, the only guarantee for primary healing without scar tissue formation.

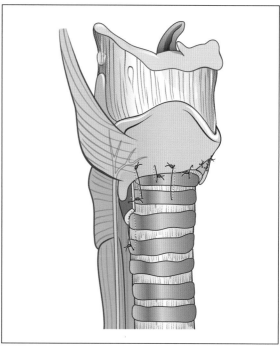

Fig. 16.12 Completion of thyrotracheal anastomosis. Note the alternate position of the stitches through the first and second tracheal rings so as to distribute the anastomotic tension onto different levels. An additional tension-releasing suture is placed between the posterolateral aspect of the cricoid plate and the trachea. Staying in the subperichondrial plane at the cricoid level is essential to avoid injury to the recurrent laryngeal nerves. The triangular wedge of pedicled trachea is trimmed to the size of the corresponding subcommissural defect to enlarge the subglottic space and sutured in place with two or three 5–0 Vicryl sutures.

depending on the length of the tracheal segment to be resected and on the individual anatomy. Usually, the advancement of the distal tracheal stump upward is much easier in children than in adults. If necessary, a laryngeal release suffices; hilar and pericardial mobilizations, sometimes used in adults, should remain as an exception in children.

At the end of the procedure, the neck is maintained in a flexed position. Sutures placed from the chin to the chest are never used to limit the extension of the neck during the postoperative period, although this measure has been recommended by certain authors.

Single-Stage Versus Double-Stage Partial Cricotracheal Resection

If a patient is fit for single-stage surgery, then two options usually exist, depending on the location of the tracheostoma. Either the stoma is close to the resection site and can be concomitantly excised during the primary procedure. Or, the stoma is away from the resection site with at

least three vascularized tracheal rings between the anastomosis and the stoma, in which case the distal stoma is maintained instead of risking a long resection and its attendant complications.

A single-stage PCTR (**Fig. 16.13**) with perioperative resection of the tracheostoma is chosen if no more than five tracheal rings must be resected with the SGS. The absence of a postoperative tracheostoma is favorable for healing of the anastomosis, and longer tracheal resections carry greater risk of anastomotic dehiscence.

Extended Partial Cricotracheal Resection

Partial cricotracheal resection with certain surgical modifications has proved to be efficient for treating combinations of SGS and glottic pathologies (PGS, cicatricial fusion of the vocal cords, anterior glottic web extending into the subglottis, combined supraglottic, glottic, and subglottic scarring, and distortion of the larynx after

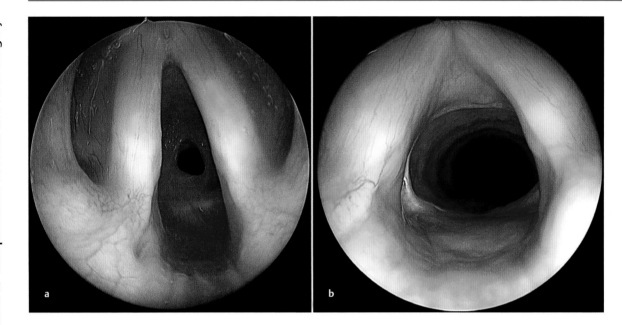

Fig. 16.13a,b Single-stage partial cricotracheal resection (PCTR) for isolated grade III subglottic stenosis.

a Preoperative view: the grade III subglottic stenosis is away from the normal vocal cords.

b Postoperative view: patent subglottic airway 2 years after single-stage PCTR. The anastomotic line is barely visible posterolaterally under the left vocal cord.

failed laryngotracheal reconstruction). To perform the E-PCTR, the surgical steps are identical to those in PCTR up to step 6 described earlier. The surgery is then modified as follows:

- A full anterior midline laryngocricofissure is made dividing exactly at the anterior commissure under direct vision. The anterior arch of the cricoid is cut open in the midline to expose the glotto–subglottic stenosis. The vocal cord adhesions are carefully excised preserving as many of the remaining vocal ligaments as possible, which are important for postoperative voice quality. The glotto–subglottic stenosis is excised along with the tracheostoma, if it is closer to the stenosis. As in PCTR, the resection margins rest anterior to the cricothyroid joint, thereby protecting the recurrent laryngeal nerves.

- The posterior cricoid plate is thinned down with a diamond bur and divided in the midline avoiding damage to the retrocricoid mucosa. The interarytenoid fibro-cicatricial posterior glottic stenosis is excised along with the transverse interarytenoid muscle preserving the posterior arytenoid mucosa.

- The posterior cricoid is sufficiently distracted and expanded with a costal cartilage graft harvested from the seventh or eighth rib. The graft must be flush with the cricoid plate, and the perichondrium facing the lumen (**Fig. 16.14**). Lateral cartilaginous extensions of the graft under the cricoid plate help to stabilize the graft, which is fixed in place with 4–0/5–0 Vicryl sutures.

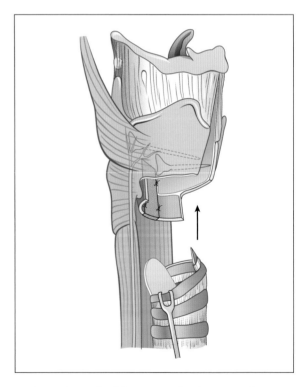

Fig. 16.14 Status after full anterior midline laryngocricofissure resection of the subglottic stenosis and posterior cricoid split with enlargement of the interarytenoid space with a posterior costal cartilage graft sutured into position with 4–0 Vicryl sutures.

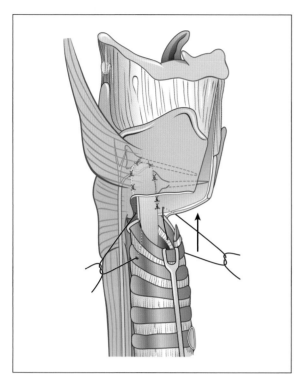

Fig. 16.15 Resurfacing of the cartilage graft and interarytenoid space. The pedicled flap of membranous trachea is sutured in a horseshoe fashion to the interarytenoid mucosa, so providing full cover of the posterior costal cartilage graft. Two posterolateral cricotracheal stitches are used as traction sutures to reduce tension on the posterior suture line.

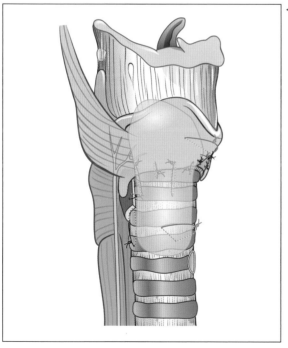

- As in PCTR, the trachea is mobilized cranially adding on a laryngeal drop procedure if needed. By resecting one or two additional rings of the tracheal stump distally, a pedicled flap of membranous trachea is created. A new tracheostomy is placed distally, leaving at least three vascularized tracheal rings caudal to the thyrotracheal anastomosis.
- The posterolateral anastomotic stitch is taken and the vascularized tracheal flap is sutured with the posterior commissure mucosa using 4–0/5–0 Vicryl (**Fig. 16.15**).
- The laryngofissure is closed over a stent, meticulously placing a 5–0 Vicryl suture exactly at the level of the vocal cords to restore a sharp anterior commissure (**Fig. 16.16**). At our institution, we use the laryngotracheal (Monnier) mold that conforms closest to the inner laryngeal contours, so restoring a normal laryngotracheal airway.[20] This prosthesis exists in ten different sizes (6 to 15 mm in diameter and a variety of lengths) for use in children and adults and can be placed intraoperatively and endoscopically. Newly designed metal guide templates help to choose the appropriate size of the LT-Mold. It is fixed to the thyroid cartilage and trachea by placing two 3–0 Prolene sutures passing transversally through the airway and stent with the knots tied on the outside.
- As in conventional PCTR, the lateral and anterior anastomoses are completed. Fibrin glue around the anastomosis allows an airtight closure. The thyroid isthmus and prelaryngeal muscles are resutured in the midline over the anastomosis and the neck incision is closed leaving a Penrose drain in place. A fully mucosalized

◁ **Fig. 16.16** Completion of thyrotracheal anastomosis with LT-Mold in situ. The lateral and anterior thyrotracheal stitches are placed alternately through the first and second rings on the tracheal side. Two transverse 3–0 Prolene stitches are used to fix the prosthesis in the supraglottis and at the upper tracheal level just above the tracheostoma. The anterior wedge of cartilage is trimmed to its final triangular shape and sutured into position using 5–0 Vicryl threads.

III B Surgery of the Larynx, Trachea, Hypopharynx, and Esophagus

Section III   Complications of Head and Neck Surgery

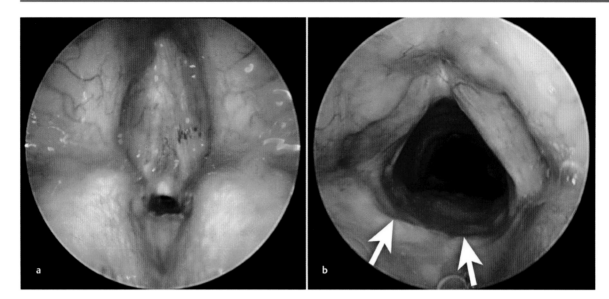

Fig. 16.17a,b Extended partial cricotracheal resection for glotto–subglottic stenosis with cicatricial fusion of the vocal cords.

a Preoperative view: acquired on congenital glotto–subglottic stenosis with fusion of the vocal cords and pinhole residual posterior opening.

b Postoperative view: patent glotto–subglottic airway, albeit with an overexpanded interarytenoid space. The posterior mucosal flap was sutured above the glottic level (white arrows).

glotto–tracheal anastomosis along with a posterior subglottic cartilage expansion is therefore obtained (**Fig. 16.17**).

E-PCTR in Cricoarytenoid Ankylosis

Cases with severe stenosis and fixation of the cricoarytenoid joints are extremely difficult to manage and often refractory to treatment. In our series of patients with fixed joints, recently, we have attempted to open the cricoarytenoid joint intentionally during open surgery and actively mobilize the joint space. We have been encouraged with satisfactory results. Every attempt must be made to restore mobility in these fixed cricoarytenoid joints and we stand to lose nothing by surgically opening these complex articular spaces.

If a *double-stage PCTR* is performed with stenting, no clinical information on subglottic airway patency is available, because the patient breathes through the tracheostoma. A control endoscopy at the third postoperative week is mandatory to assess the quality of healing at the site of the anastomosis.

Postoperative Care in PCTR and E-PCTR

After surgery, nontracheotomized pediatric patients stay under close supervision in the intensive care unit until extubation is achieved. All adult patients are extubated on-table immediately after the surgery, and shifted to intensive care units. The patient is kept in a neck flexed position avoiding any undue anastomotic tension. Children are sedated or paralyzed for a short duration, if needed. Broad-spectrum antibiotics and antireflux medications are given to all patients for a minimum of 10 days or until a mucosalized anastomosis is obtained. Systemic corticosteroids are started only on the day before extubation and continued for the following days, if necessary. A first control endoscopy is performed at 7 to 10 days postoperatively. In children, if there is only mild to moderate edema of the vocal folds and subglottis, then the child is tentatively extubated. In the case of significant edema, the child is reintubated with a one-size-smaller tube, and a plug of corticosteroid–gentamycin ointment is applied to the endolarynx. The next tentative extubation is planned for 2 days later. Additional endoscopic controls are routinely performed at 3 weeks and 3 months. The final result may then be optimized at 3 months by gentle bougienage with Savary–Gilliard dilators.

In E-PCTR and double-stage PCTR, the tracheostoma is left in place until complete healing of the subglottic anastomosis is obtained. Depending on the complexity of the reconstruction after an E-PCTR, stenting is maintained for 3 to 6 months or even longer, and then the LT-Mold is removed endoscopically. The tracheostomy is closed surgically once the patient has resumed oral feeds without bronchoaspiration, tolerates decannulation procedures (cannule capping trials or down-sizing) with adequate oxygen saturation and the airway is of optimal size and well mucosalized.

Conclusions

A physician asked to evaluate a patient for intubation injury should have a clear idea of the type of injury that may be encountered, as well as a thorough knowledge of ideal methods for its prevention and reconstruction. In many cases, the injury will resolve without sequelae, whereas in others the injury may lead to laryngotracheal stenosis. Frequently, the process can be corrected with good results at the acute or subacute stages if proper treatment is instituted at the right time.

A surgeon facing the problem of a patient with cicatricial SGS currently has a wide range of surgical options. The procedure must be tailored to the anatomy of the stenosis. Both LTR and CTR have achieved high decannulation rates, although no published data compare different surgical techniques in matched patients. CTR is the preferred option for grade IV and severe grade III stenoses that are clear of the vocal cords. LTR as a less extensive procedure and is preferred for some grade II and less severe grade III stenoses. Stenosis close to the vocal cords remains a challenge and can be treated by E-PCTR. Fixed cricoarytenoid joints are very complex situations. In our early series of patients, opening of the joint space and its active mobilization have been very encouraging but the sine qua non condition is to resurface the cricoarytenoid joint with a pedicled flap of the membranous trachea. We plan to open all ankylosed joints in the future as we stand to lose nothing. To achieve full mobility in these joints is a matter of further research.

References

1. Benjamin B. Prolonged intubation injuries of the larynx: endoscopic diagnosis, classification, and treatment. Ann Otol Rhinol Laryngol Suppl 1993;160:1–15
2. Benjamin B. Laryngeal trauma from intubation: endoscopic evaluation and classification. In: Cummings CW, et al, eds. Otolaryngology-Head & Neck Surgery. 3rd ed. St. Louis: Mosby, 1998:2013–2035
3. Donnelly WH. Histopathology of endotracheal intubation. An autopsy study of 99 cases. Arch Pathol 1969;88(5):511–520
4. Gaynor EB, Greenberg SB. Untoward sequelae of prolonged intubation. Laryngoscope 1985;95(12):1461–1467
5. Monnier P. Pediatric Airway Surgery: Management of Laryngotracheal Stenosis in Infants and Children. New York: Springer, 2011;Part I: 2 (pp 7–30), part III: 14 (pp 183–198)
6. Weiss M, Dullenkopf A, Fischer JE, Keller C, Gerber AC; European Paediatric Endotracheal Intubation Study Group. Prospective randomized controlled multi-centre trial of cuffed or uncuffed endotracheal tubes in small children. Br J Anaesth 2009;103(6):867–873
7. Keane WM, Denneny JC, Rowe LD, Atkins JP Jr. Complications of intubation. Ann Otol Rhinol Laryngol 1982;91(6 Pt 1):584–587
8. Weissler MC. Tracheotomy and intubation. In: Bailey BJ, ed. Head & Neck Surgery—Otolaryngology. 2nd ed. Philadelphia: Lippincott-Raven, 1998;803–818
9. Sataloff RT, Bough ID Jr, Spiegel JR. Arytenoid dislocation: diagnosis and treatment. Laryngoscope 1994;104(11 Pt 1):1353–1361
10. Pereira KD, Smith SL, Henry M. Failed extubation in the neonatal intensive care unit. Int J Pediatr Otorhinolaryngol 2007;71(11):1763–1766
11. Cotton RT, Seid AB. Management of the extubation problem in the premature child. Anterior cricoid split as an alternative to tracheotomy. Ann Otol Rhinol Laryngol 1980;89(6 Pt 1):508–511
12. Silver FM, Myer CM III, Cotton RT. Anterior cricoid split. Update 1991. Am J Otolaryngol 1991;12(6):343–346
13. Walner DL, Cotton RT. Acquired anomalies of the larynx and trachea. In: Cotton RT, Myer III, CM (Eds) Practical Pediatric Otolaryngology, Philadelphia/New York: Lippincott-Raven; 1999:524
14. Santos PM, Afrassiabi A, Weymuller EA Jr. Risk factors associated with prolonged intubation and laryngeal injury. Otolaryngol Head Neck Surg 1994;111(4):453–459
15. Volpi D, Lin PT, Kuriloff DB, Kimmelman CP. Risk factors for intubation injury of the larynx. Ann Otol Rhinol Laryngol 1987;96(6):684–686
16. Brandwein M, Abramson AL, Shikowitz MJ. Bilateral vocal cord paralysis following endotracheal intubation. Arch Otolaryngol Head Neck Surg 1986;112(8):877–882
17. Monnier P. Airway stenting with the LT-Mold: experience in 30 pediatric cases. Int J Pediatr Otorhinolaryngol 2007;71(9):1351–1359
18. Maddaus MA, Toth JL, Gullane PJ, Pearson FG. Subglottic tracheal resection and synchronous laryngeal reconstruction. J Thorac Cardiovasc Surg 1992;104(5):1443–1450
19. Jaquet Y, Lang F, Pilloud R, Savary M, Monnier P. Partial cricotracheal resection for pediatric subglottic stenosis: long-term outcome in 57 patients. J Thorac Cardiovasc Surg 2005;130(3):726–732
20. Alvarez-Neri H, Penchyna-Grub J, Porras-Hernandez JD, Blanco-Rodriguez G, Gonzalez R, Rutter MJ. Primary cricotracheal resection with thyrotracheal anastomosis for the treatment of severe subglottic stenosis in children and adolescents. Ann Otol Rhinol Laryngol 2005;114(1 Pt 1):2–6

17 Percutaneous Endoscopic Gastrostomy Complications

L. Samarà Piñol, J. Llach, M. Caballero

Enteral nutrition (EN) is defined as the administration of nutrients through the digestive tract. There are many options for digestive tract EN: oral, nasoenteric tubes, and enterostomies. For short-term (< 6 weeks) EN, nasogastric or nasoenteric tubes are the best choice. However, in long-term (> 6 weeks) EN, enterostomies are indicated, involving percutaneous endoscopic gastrostomy (PEG) or jejunostomy, fluoroscopic, image-guided gastrostomy, and surgical or laparoscopic gastrostomy.

The modality of choice for long-term enteral nutrition access is PEG, which was first described in 1980 by Gauderer and by Ponsky.[1,2] Although a PEG is generally safe and requires minimally invasive surgery (**Fig. 17.1**), it is associated with many potential complications related to both its insertion and the prolonged stay of a foreign body in the abdominal wall.

There are some absolute contraindications to PEG placement, which include pharyngeal or esophageal obstructions, coagulopathy, sepsis, and any other general contraindications to endoscopy. Obese patients, pregnancy, previous abdominal surgery, ascites, hepatosplenomegaly, and portal hypertension are relative contraindications.[3]

In this chapter, we summarize the most common PEG procedure-related (**Fig. 17.2**) and post-procedure-related (**Fig. 17.3**) complications.

Perforation

Perforation during upper endoscopy procedures, as an inadvertent puncture of the pharynx, esophagus, stomach, small bowel, colon, liver, or spleen, has an incidence rate of 0.008 to 0.04%.[4,5] Anatomic anomalies such as the finding of a transverse colon over the anterior gastric wall and those produced by radiotherapy, or previous surgery, contribute to the perforation in up to 50% of patients.[3] Patients typically present with tachycardia, fever, odynodysphagia, respiratory distress, or sepsis. Early (> 24 h) recognition is vital and its diagnosis is based on radiographic study. If diagnosed, broad-spectrum antibiotics, tube thoracostomy and a wide surgical procedure must be performed. In selected hemodynamically stable patients with small perforations, nonoperative management may be appropriate.

Pneumoperitoneum

Pneumoperitoneum is seen in up to 56% of patients after PEG placement procedures,[6] but is usually of no clinical importance[7] and conservative management is required. If a patient with pneumoperitoneum shows signs of sepsis or peritonitis, then imaging studies and appropriate treatment are mandatory.

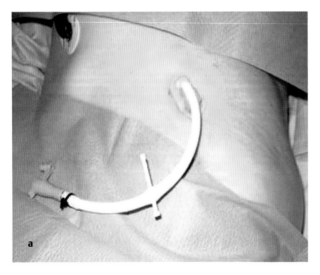
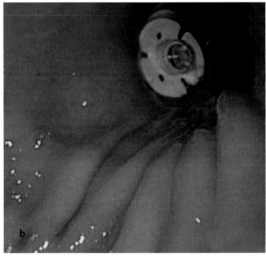

Fig. 17.1a,b Normal gastronomy placement.

a Normal external bolster.

b Normal internal bolster.

- Perforation
  - Early recognition
  - Consider any anatomy alteration secondary to previous surgery
- Pneumoperitoneum
  - Benign pneumoperitoneum is common after percutaneous endoscopic gastrostomy (PEG) tube insertion, it is usually self-limiting
  - Clinically concerning only when intra-abdominal air is increasing
- Peritonitis
  - Treat early with broad-spectrum antibiotics and surgical repair
- Bleeding
  - Correct coagulopathy and risk factors
  - Consider any anatomical alteration secondary to previous surgery
- Gastrocolocutaneous fistula
  - Late recognition
  - Diarrhea or feculent vomiting after the original PEG removal
- Ileus
  - Wait > 6 hours before beginning feeding post-PEG placement
  - If gastric distension occurs, uncap the PEG tube for easy decompression
- Aspiration
  - Avoid over-sedation and minimize air insufflation. Perform procedure efficiently

Fig. 17.2. Procedure-related complications.

- Percutaneous endoscopic gastrostomy (PEG) site infection
  - Prophylactic antibiotics and maintain proper tension between internal and external bolsters
  - For excessive granulation tissue (**Fig. 17.4**) topical silver nitrate may be beneficial
- Necrotizing fasciitis
  - Requires surgical debridement, broad-spectrum antibiotics and extensive patient support
- PEG site leakage/irritation
  - Prevent infection and excessive side torsion on the PEG tube
  - Correction of comorbidities
- Gastric ulceration (**Fig. 17.6a**)
  - Acid suppression and avoid lateral traction on the tube
- Buried bumper syndrome (**Fig. 17.6b**)
  - Avoid excessive tension between internal and external bolsters
  - Account for nutritional weight gain
- Inadvertent removal
  - Replace the PEG tube or place a nasogastric tube and broad-spectrum antibiotics. New PEG days later
- Clogged PEG tube
  - Flush water trough the PEG tube

Fig. 17.3. Post-procedure complications.

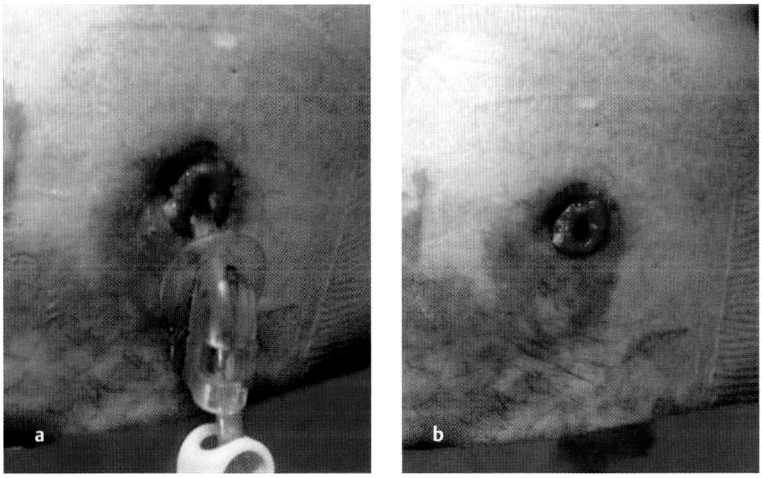

Fig. 17.4 Granulation tissue at the gastrostomy site.

a Granulation tissue around the external bolster.
b Granulation tissue with the external bolster removed.

Peritonitis

Peritonitis is a PEG complication that often carries a high mortality rate, and can be caused by removal or displacement of the tube before tract maturation, leakage from the PEG puncture site in the stomach or perforation of another visceral organ. It is manifested in post-PEG patients as abdominal pain, fever, leukocytosis, and ileus, and can result in significant morbidity if not identified and treated early with broad-spectrum antibiotics and surgical repair.[3]

Hemorrhage

Hemorrhage (**Fig. 17.5**) is an uncommon complication of PEG procedures (0.02 to 0.06% cases).[4,5] Risk factors include anticoagulation, antiplatelet therapy, portal hypertension (varices), and the presence of an anatomical anomaly. It may be caused by puncture of gastric wall vessels, gastric pressure ulcers, esophagitis, gastric wall erosion, liver or spleen laceration, and peptic ulcer disease. Management depends on the site of the bleeding and on the severity of the hemorrhage.

Cutaneous bleeding from the skin incision is common and usually self-limited. If not, tightening the external bolster (for not more than 48 hours) could stop the bleeding.

Fistulas

Gastrocolocutaneous fistula and fistulous tracts are a rare complication and happen when the PEG tube is placed

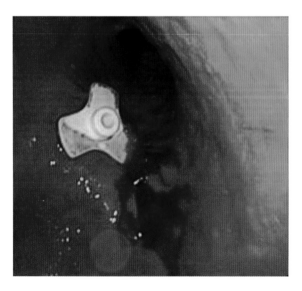

Fig. 17.5 Internal bleeding.

directly through the bowel or colon into the stomach. Normally discovered months after the PEG placement, when diarrhea or feculent vomiting appears after the original PEG tube is removed or manipulated. Removal of the tube is indicated with spontaneous closure of the track and a second gastrostomy can be performed.[8] If peritonitis is suspected, surgery may be required.

Ileus and Gastroparesis

Tube feeds may be safely initiated 3 hours after PEG placement and occasionally, postprocedural gastroparesis occurs.[3] In 1 to 2% of cases, prolonged ileus may follow PEG procedure, and should be managed conservatively.[9]

Aspiration

Aspiration can occur during the upper endoscopy (0.02 to 0.06% cases),[4,5] or after the PEG placement procedure. It can result in pneumonitis or pneumonia. This complication can be minimized by avoiding oversedation, optimizing gastric air insufflations by thoroughly aspirating gastric contents before and after the procedure, and performing the procedure efficiently.[3]

Wound Infection

Wound infection is the most common complication of PEG placement, occurring in up to 18% of patients who did not receive perioperative antibiotics. Antibiotic prophylaxis reduces the infection rate to ~ 3%.[3] Obesity, diabetes mellitus, malnutrition, and corticosteroid use represent patient-related factors. Small skin incisions and excessive traction on the PEG tube also increase infection risk. If diagnosed early, then an oral broad-spectrum antibiotic for 5 to 7 days may be all that is required for a PEG site infection.

Necrotizing Fasciitis

Necrotizing fasciitis is a very rare complication but a potentially life-threatening one. Patients with diabetes mellitus, chronic renal failure, malnutrition, poor immune system, or alcoholism appear to be at enhanced risk.[9] An overnight PEG tube tract wound can predispose the development of necrotizing fasciitis. Its prevention is imperative and treatment requires wide surgical debridement, planned operative reassessment, broad-spectrum antibiotics, and extensive patient support. Its mortality is still greater than 50% despite comprehensive management.[10]

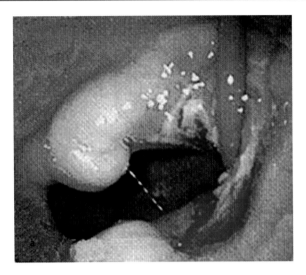
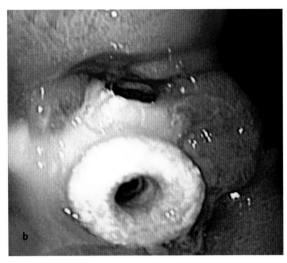

Fig. 17.6a,b Post-procedure complications.

a Gastric ulceration and hemorrrhage.

b Buried bumper syndrome.

Peristomal Leakage

Peristomal leakage appears early after PEG placement and is quite common (1 to 2%).[11] Treatment should include correction of comorbidities such as malnutrition and elevated glycemia, loosening of the external bolster, and local measures to address skin breakdown (such as skin protectants containing zinc oxide). If leakage persists, the PEG tube can be removed for several days and the tract allowed to partially close. Exchanging for a larger catheter only enlarges the stoma.

Buried Bumper Syndrome

Buried bumper syndrome (**Fig. 17.6**) is defined as migration of the PEG tube into the gastric wall because of a tight apposition of the external bolster.[12] The syndrome usually becomes apparent months to years after PEG placement as abdominal pain, difficulty with feeding or leakage around the tube, and an immobile catheter.[13] Risk factors include excessive tension between the internal and external bolsters, malnutrition, and poor wound healing. It may be confirmed endoscopically or radiographically and the treatment is removal of the tube, even if the patient is asymptomatic.

PEG Complications

Inadvertent PEG tube removal occurs in 1.6 to 4.4% of patients.[3] If recognized early, the PEG tube can be replaced. If recognition is delayed, a nasogastric tube should be placed, broad-spectrum antibiotics should be started and a new PEG should be placed within 7 to 10 days.[9]

Clogged PEG tube and tube dysfunction occurs in 45% of patients. Usually it is the result of medications or enteral formula clog. Prevention is critical, so we advocate flushing the PEG tube with water (30 to 60 mL) every 4 hours.[3]

Tumor implantation at the PEG site should be suspected in patients with head and neck cancer who develop unexplained skin changes at the PEG site.[3,9]

References

1. Gauderer MWL, Ponsky JL, Izant RJ Jr. Gastrostomy without laparotomy: a percutaneous endoscopic technique. J Pediatr Surg 1980;15(6):872–875
2. Ponsky JL, Gauderer MWL. Percutaneous endoscopic gastrostomy: a nonoperative technique for feeding gastrostomy. Gastrointest Endosc 1981;27(1):9–11
3. Schrag SP, Sharma R, Jaik NP, et al. Complications related to percutaneous endoscopic gastrostomy (PEG) tubes. A comprehensive clinical review. J Gastrointestin Liver Dis 2007;16(4):407–418
4. Kahn K. Indications for selected medical and surgical procedures – a literature review and rating of appropriateness. Diagnostic upper gastrointestinal endoscopy. Santa Monica, CA: The Rand Corporation, 1986
5. Froehlich F, Gonvers JJ, Vader JP, Dubois RW, Burnand B. Appropriateness of gastrointestinal endoscopy: risk of complications. Endoscopy 1999;31(8):684–686
6. Wiesen AJ, Sideridis K, Fernandes A, et al. True incidence and clinical significance of pneumoperitoneum after PEG placement: a prospective study. Gastrointest Endosc 2006;64(6):886–889
7. Wojtowycz MM, Arata JA Jr, Micklos TJ, Miller FJ Jr. CT findings after uncomplicated percutaneous gastrostomy. AJR Am J Roentgenol 1988;151(2):307–309

8. Schapiro GD, Edmundowicz SA. Complications of percutaneous endoscopic gastrostomy. Gastrointest Endosc Clin N Am 1996;6(2):409–422

9. Lynch C, Fang J. Prevention and management of complications of PEG tubes. Pract Gastroenterol 2004; (Nov):66–76

10. MacLean AA, Miller G, Bamboat ZM, Hiotis K. Abdominal wall necrotizing fasciitis from dislodged percutaneous endoscopic gastrostomy tubes: a case series. Am Surg 2004;70(9):827–831

11. Lin HS, Ibrahim HZ, Kheng JW, Fee WE, Terris DJ. Percutaneous endoscopic gastrostomy: strategies for prevention and management of complications. Laryngoscope 2001;111(10):1847–1852

12. Safadi BY, Marks JM, Ponsky JL. Percutaneous endoscopic gastrostomy. Gastrointest Endosc Clin N Am 1998;8(3):551–568

13. Horbach T, Teske V, Hohenberger W, Siassi M. Endoscopic therapy of the buried bumper syndrome: a clinical algorithm. Surg Endosc 2007;21(8):1359–1362

18 Complications of Tracheotomy

K. M. Kost

Introduction

Tracheotomy has a long and colorful history. The first reference to the procedure can be found in the sacred book of Hindu medicine, the *Rig Veda*, dated to ~ 2000 BC. Alexander the Great is reported to have performed a tracheotomy in the fourth century BC when he "punctured the trachea of a soldier with the point of his sword after he saw a man choking from a bone lodged in his throat".[1] For centuries, however, it would remain a marginal procedure, referred to as "the scandal of surgery" because of the associated high morbidity and mortality. The work of Armand Trousseau in 1834 and later Chevalier Jackson in 1909 demonstrated that by attention to technical detail and attentive postoperative care, the mortality of the procedure could be reduced to less than 2%. Jackson emphasized the importance of a long incision, avoidance of the cricoid cartilage, routine division of the thyroid isthmus, slow and careful surgery, use of a proper cannula, and meticulous postoperative care.

Chevalier Jackson's description of the "standard open tracheotomy", continues to be the standard against which all others are compared. This procedure can be performed in the operating room, at the bedside in the intensive care unit (ICU), or as an emergency on the ward as required. The most significant modification to tracheotomy was the introduction of an endoscopic percutaneous technique designed specifically for use at the bedside in intubated adult ICU patients.

Indications for Tracheotomy

The primary objective of a tracheotomy is to secure an artificial airway. Over the years, the indications for tracheotomy have continued to change in parallel with the evolution of medicine. Current major indications for tracheotomy include:

- Relief of upper airway obstruction (both acute and chronic)
- Providing a means for assisted mechanical ventilation
- Facilitating tracheobronchial toilet.

Currently over half of modern-day tracheotomies are performed on critically ill patients requiring prolonged mechanical ventilation.[2]

Tracheotomy Techniques

The standard open surgical tracheotomy is usually performed in the controlled setting of the operating room. Guiding surgical principles involve the following: (1) placement of the incision one to two fingerbreadths below the cricoid; (2) displacing or ligating the anterior jugular veins, as required; (3) displacing or dividing the thyroid isthmus to provide access to the anterior tracheal wall; (4) entering the trachea between the second and third, or third and fourth, tracheal rings; (5) placement of tracheal retention sutures to facilitate reinsertion of the tracheostomy tube in case of early dislodgement; and (6) meticulous postoperative wound care and suctioning. Although the technique is usually performed in the operating room, it may also be performed at the bedside in intubated ICU patients, or as an emergency life-saving procedure just about anywhere in the clinical setting.

Critically ill intubated ICU patients represent a special subset of the population by virtue of their multisystem disease and the complexity of the care they require. Tracheotomy is a frequently performed procedure in these patients, and, not surprisingly, is associated with a higher risk.[2] As such, special consideration is required in terms of indications, technique, and care. Moving these critically ill patients with their monitors requires additional personnel and carries several different risks, including accidental extubation and vital sign changes requiring pharmacologic intervention.[3,4] These factors served as the impetus for the development of a simple, yet safe bedside technique.

Seldinger's description[5] in 1953 of catheter replacement of the needle in percutaneous arteriography over a guidewire served as a basis for the development of a bedside percutaneous dilatational tracheotomy (PDT) technique. The "blind aspect" of the procedure was subsequently addressed by the addition of endoscopic guidance, first reported in 1990 in 61 patients by Marelli et al.[6] The technique is based on progressive dilatation of an initial tracheal puncture. Kost's series of 500 cases published in 2005,[7] demonstrated that, with bronchoscopic visualization and attention to technical detail, endoscopic PDT is a safe, cost-effective alternative to surgical tracheotomy in the operating theater for adult, intubated ICU patients.

Preventing Complications

> **Note**
>
> The vast majority of complications are preventable through:
> - Careful preoperative planning
> - Attention to technical detail during the procedure
> - Meticulous postoperative care.

Preoperative Planning

Traditionally, tracheotomy has been performed in the operating room, which is fully equipped with adequate lighting, suction, and assistance. Patients with an unprotected airway as well as those from the emergency room are best transferred to the controlled, monitored setting of the operating room whenever possible. Adult, intubated patients from the ICU may undergo tracheotomy (open or percutaneous) safely either at the bedside[8-10] or in the operating room[11,12] with comparable complication rates.

It is imperative to examine the patient preoperatively paying particular attention to the neck to anticipate and plan for special situations. The presence of a midline neck mass or high innominate artery may require modification of the level of incision or entry into the trachea, or both. Patients who have undergone previous surgery or radiotherapy to the neck are likely to have scarred, fibrotic, indurated tissue, which precludes the ability to identify any landmarks. In these cases, slow, careful, midline dissection prevents injury to adjacent structures such as the carotid artery and allows identification of the airway. Patients with severe cervical osteoarthritis, kyphoscoliosis, or other conditions, in whom the neck cannot be hyperextended; present a formidable surgical challenge.

It must be stressed that PDT is suitable only in adult intubated patients. This patient population accounts for almost two-thirds of all tracheotomies performed today.

Anatomical and medical suitability for PDT must be determined preoperatively by examining the patient with the neck extended.[7,13] Absolute contraindications to PDT include:
- The inability to palpate the cricoid cartilage above the sternal notch
- The presence of a midline neck mass or large thyroid gland
- A high innominate artery
- Patients with an unprotected airway, or patients with acute airway compromise
- Children, because of the different airway anatomy as well as the technical difficulties of maintaining adequate ventilation with a bronchoscope within a small endotracheal tube[13]

- Patients requiring a positive end-expiratory pressure ≥ 15 cmH$_2$O as they are at high risk for complications such as subcutaneous emphysema and pneumothorax.

Patients with the above conditions should undergo standard surgical tracheotomy (ST) in the operating room. Patients having had a previous tracheotomy may undergo PDT safely if they have no other contraindications.[7] Obese patients may also undergo PDT provided a proximally extended tracheostomy tube is used to reduce the risk of accidental decannulation.

Whether an ST or an endoscopic PDT is performed, every effort should be made to optimize the patient's comorbidities before surgery. Preoperative testing is minimal and includes a recent chest radiograph as well as serum determination of hemoglobin, prothrombin time, partial thromboplastin time, International Normalized Ratio, and platelets. Coagulopathies should be corrected to an International Normalized Ratio < 1.5, with > 50,000 functioning platelets. The use of aspirin or other nonsteroidal anti-inflammatory medications, and clopidogrel bisulfate (Plavix, Bristol-Myers Squibb Co., New York, NY, USA) should be discontinued for 7 days preoperatively, if at all possible. Aspirin and clopidogrel bisulfate are commonly used together in patients who have had cardiac stent placement, strokes or myocardial infarctions. Patients taking both drugs have a higher incidence of perioperative bleeding and at least one of these agents should be stopped before tracheotomy. Patients on warfarin should stop the drug 5 days before surgery or should receive infusions of fresh-frozen plasma or intravenous or oral vitamin K for rapid reversal of anticoagulation. A cross-match should be obtained if the hemoglobin is < 100 g/dL.

The anesthesia team plays an important role during the procedure: monitoring the airway and vital signs, and keeping the patient stable. Patients suffering from chronic respiratory insufficiency and high CO$_2$ levels may lose their respiratory drive or even develop pulmonary edema following establishment of an airway with tracheotomy. Support in the form of assisted ventilation and appropriate pharmacologic intervention is usually sufficient, although cardiopulmonary resuscitation may be necessary in severe cases.

The choice of tracheostomy tube is important. The purpose of a tracheostomy tube is to:
- Provide an airway
- Allow for mechanical positive-pressure ventilation
- Reduce the risk of aspiration
- Facilitate suctioning the tracheobronchial tree.[14]

Cuffed tubes should have a low-pressure, high-volume cuff to reduce the possibility of tracheal stenosis. Tubes with an inner cannula are preferable because the inner cannula can be quickly removed in the event of a mucus plug, leaving the open outer cannula in situ and the airway protected.

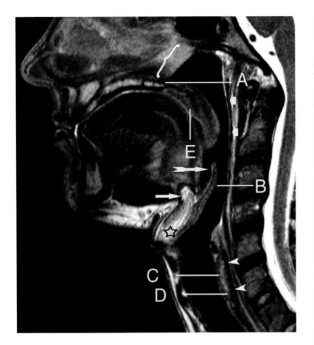

Fig. 18.1 Sectional anatomy of the pharynx and larynx. A = boundary plane between the nasopharynx and oropharynx at the level of the superior border of the soft palate. B = boundary plane between the oropharynx and hypopharynx at the level of the hyoid bone. C = boundary plane between the supraglottis and glottis through the apices of the laryngeal ventricles (not shown). D = boundary plane between the glottis and subglottis. E = boundary plane between the oral cavity and oropharynx at the level of the soft palate, vallate papillae (not shown), and palatine tonsils (not shown). Curly bracket = the posterior choanae form the boundary zone between the nasopharynx and nasal cavity. Short fat arrows = prevertebral fascia; tailed arrow = epiglottis; straight arrow = hyoid bone; open asterisk = pre-epiglottic space; arrowheads = postcricoid hypopharynx. (From Saleh A, Mathys C, Mödder U. Staging of head and neck cancer with imaging procedures (Part I: T staging). Radiologie up2date 2007;7(4):275–300).

Obese patients with thick pretracheal soft tissues are likely to require extended-length tubes to decrease the risk of accidental decannulation or tube displacement.[7] It has been shown that pretracheal soft tissue thickness can be reliably predicted within 4 mm in obese patients as a function of neck and arm circumference.[15] It can be seen that a patient with a neck circumference of 55 cm and an arm circumference of 50 cm would have a pretracheal soft tissue thickness of 3 cm. A proximally extended tracheostomy tube would be required in this patient because "standard" tubes have a much shorter proximal length (**Fig. 18.1**). It should be noted that tracheostomy tubes with either proximal or distal extensions are available. Tubes with adjustable flanges and those made of softer, thermolabile materials for anatomically difficult necks or tracheas are also available. Choosing the correct tracheostomy tube preoperatively is helpful in decreasing postoperative complications such as accidental decannulation,

skin maceration/infection, granulation tissue, and tracheitis, all of which may be related to ill-fitting tubes.

Patients with altered anatomy require special consideration. Patients with a history of radiotherapy with or without chemotherapy for head and neck malignancies often have stiff, indurated soft tissue and limited neck extension. Landmarks are predictably difficult to palpate or not palpable at all. Patients with kyphoscoliosis may also have poorly identifiable landmarks. These situations may present formidable surgical challenges. Preoperative localization of the airway with ultrasound is sometimes helpful. In all cases, careful midline dissection, frequent palpation of the laryngotracheal framework during the procedure, and identification of the airway with a needle, are all measures that help to reduce the probability of injury to adjacent structures and postoperative complications.

> **Note**
>
> For tracheotomies performed in the ICU, a fully equipped intubation cart should be readily available in the event of accidental extubation during the procedure.

As with all other minimally invasive techniques, there is a learning curve for endoscopic PDT. Familiarity with open surgical tracheotomy does not confer expertise in PDT and appropriate training should be obtained before using the technique. Careful selection of patients with anatomically favorable necks for the first 30 to 40 patients allows the surgeon to gain experience and reduce the likelihood of complications.

Attention to Technical Detail

For both ST and PDT, careful attention to technical details will help to minimize the risk of complications. Guiding surgical principles involve the following:

- Placement of the incision one to two fingerbreadths below the cricoid
- Displacing or ligating the anterior jugular veins, as required
- Displacing or dividing the thyroid isthmus to provide access to the anterior tracheal wall
- Entering the trachea between the second and third, or third and fourth tracheal rings
- Placement of tracheal retention sutures to facilitate reinsertion of the tracheostomy tube in case of early dislodgement
- Meticulous postoperative wound care and suctioning.

Technical details that are particular to endoscopic percutaneous tracheotomy include the following:

- The cricoid cartilage should be identified. Inability to palpate this important landmark constitutes an absolute contraindication to percutaneous tracheotomy.

- The procedure should only be performed under continuous endoscopic visualization. Complication rates increased two-fold when bronchoscopy is not used.[7] The bronchoscope ensures proper placement of the initial tracheal puncture, and allows visualization of the posterior tracheal wall.
- Force should never be used during dilatation or tracheostomy tube insertion. Resistance almost always indicates a problem, which must be identified and corrected before proceeding.
- Because of the tight tract, tracheostomy tube changes should be avoided for the first 5 to 7 days postoperatively. Accidental decannulation during this time should be addressed by reintubating the patient. Attempts to reinsert the tracheostomy tube are likely to result in creation of a false passage.
- In obese patients, a proximally extended tracheostomy tube should be placed.

Postoperative Care

Postoperative care of the tracheostomy site is facilitated if there is the opportunity for preoperative teaching. Knowing what to expect helps both children and adults adjust to this new way of breathing. Evidence indicates that patients undergoing tracheotomy experience a reduced quality of life.[16] Appropriate teaching, family counseling and highly skilled nursing care are all key factors in reducing anxiety and ensuring a smooth postoperative course. A multidisciplinary tracheotomy team involving a physician, nurse, respiratory therapist, and speech-language pathologist is ideal in coordinating and delivering the complex care that tracheotomy patients require.[17] The team assists with wound care, tracheostomy tube changes, deglutition, communication, decannulation, and teaching of the patient and caregivers. The presence of a multidisciplinary tracheotomy team produces measurable results in terms of decreased postoperative morbidity: the frequency of tube obstruction decreases, the use of speaking valves increases, and patients are decannulated more rapidly.[18]

In the initial postoperative period, patients are positioned with the head of the bed elevated 30° to 45° to maximize the ease of coughing and deep breathing, to facilitate suctioning, and to minimize discomfort. Vital signs require frequent monitoring because changes in blood pressure, respiratory rate, or pulse rate may indicate a new or ongoing respiratory problem, or that the tube may be plugged or have come out of the trachea. Agitation, anxiety, and restlessness may all indicate hypoxia and should not be dismissed or treated with anxiolytics.

Tracheal suctioning plays a key role in maintaining pulmonary toilet and patency of the tracheostomy tube. Initially, this should be done as aseptically as possible and

may be necessary as often as three or four times daily. Patients on mechanical ventilation are at risk for hypoxia and cardiac arrhythmias during suctioning because oxygen-rich air is suctioned and catheters may be too large. This can be prevented by ventilating the patient on 100% oxygen for at least five breaths before and after suctioning, and limiting suctioning to ≤ 12 seconds with a small catheter. As an alternative to this open technique, a closed, multiple-use suction catheter contained within a sheath may be used.[19] Similarly, to avoid mucus plugging of the tube, the inner cannula must be removed frequently for cleaning. Currently, inner cannulas are either disposable or reusable.

Humidification is extremely important in facilitating mucociliary transport of secretions and preventing serious complications such as crusting, accumulation of secretions, and eventual obstruction of the airway. Humidification is usually performed by a tracheal mask. T-tubes are best avoided because of the torque exerted on the tube, which traumatizes the tissue every time the patient moves.

The importance of meticulous local wound care cannot be overemphasized. The tracheostomy site should be cleaned as often as necessary (three or four times daily) with normal saline or hydrogen peroxide to prevent skin breakdown and infection. The neck tapes holding the tracheostomy tube in place should be changed, as necessary, when soiled. The skin under the tracheostomy neck plate should be kept dry with a thin nonadherent dressing such as Telfa (Covidien, Mansfield, MA, USA) to prevent skin maceration.

Following open surgical tracheotomy, it takes at least 48 to 72 hours for a tract to form, and therefore tracheostomy tube changes should be avoided during this period. Accidental decannulation in the early postoperative period can be very dangerous (even with stay sutures) because of the almost immediate soft tissue collapse, which greatly increases the possibility of tube misplacement in a false passage when reinsertion is attempted. In these cases, reintubation is the safest option. Tracheostomy tube change in the early postoperative period should be avoided unless there is a compelling reason, such as cuff failure, to do so. Should such a situation arise, skill and preparation are necessary for safe tube replacement. These requirements include:

- Optimal patient positioning
- Assistance
- Adequate light
- Tracheal hook
- Suction
- Two tracheostomy tubes: ideal and smaller size
- Tracheostomy tube exchanger.

The use of a tracheostomy tube exchanger may be a very helpful adjunct for early tracheostomy tube changes. The exchanger is a long semiflexible tube with a central lumen through which ventilation is possible. The exchanger is inserted into the tracheostomy tube, which is then removed and replaced with the new tube. The exchanger "guides" the new tracheostomy tube into the trachea. If for any reason the new tracheostomy tube is difficult to replace, ventilation may be temporarily continued through the exchanger.

The PDT technique is primarily dilatational with minimal tissue dissection resulting in a tight tract and a very snug fit of the tracheostomy tube. The technique does not allow for easy placement of traction sutures at the level of the trachea. Because of these factors, the patient should be reintubated orally in the event of accidental decannulation within the first 5 to 7 days of the procedure while the tract is still relatively immature. Attempts at forcefully replacing the tracheostomy tube in an emergent situation could result in bleeding, the creation of a false passage, pneumomediastinum, hypoxia, and even death.

Patients who do not require a cuffed tube may benefit from a Passy–Muir or speaking valve in the postoperative period. This one-way valve allows inspiration through the tracheostomy tube and closes on expiration, deflecting air through the vocal folds and permitting phonation. It has also been noted that these valves improve swallowing mechanics by restoring subglottic pressure, thereby facilitating deglutition. Contraindications for use of a speaking valve include: cuffed tracheostomy tube, upper airway obstruction, bilateral vocal fold paralysis, severe tracheal stenosis, copious inspissated secretions, and cognitive dysfunction.

Decannulation in adults can be safely accomplished by following a few simple steps. Indirect or flexible endoscopy should be used in both children and adults to ensure that the upper airway is adequate and the larynx is competent. Granulomas projecting into the stoma should be removed. The tube may then be downsized and plugged during waking hours. The period of plugging allows for adequate evaluation of airway adequacy. It also affords time for laryngeal adductor reflexes to be activated. The patient must be instructed to remove the plug in the event of dyspnea or shortness of breath. If the plug is not tolerated further, the nature of the obstruction must be investigated before further attempts at decannulation. If the patient tolerates the plug for 24 hours, then the cannula can be removed and the stoma can be covered with a light dressing and occlusive tape, which is changed as necessary. In the vast majority of cases, the stoma will close by secondary intention within a few days. The resultant scar from a transverse incision is cosmetically superior to that from a vertical incision.

General Considerations

Potential intraoperative and postoperative complications for ST and PDT are similar. Notable differences in terms of frequency will be discussed below. Interpreting the available data for both techniques can be difficult for several reasons.

- Uneven reporting of complications. Examples include desaturation, subcutaneous emphysema and infection, which frequently go unmentioned.
- Uneven threshold for reporting of complications. In some series even minor bleeding is reported whereas in others it is only mentioned if the loss is in excess of a "significant" amount (e.g., 200 mL). As there is no standard definition of "significant" amount, the quantity varies from one paper to another.
- Inhomogeneity of techniques, patient subsets and surgeons are observed in many studies.[20,21] Fundamentally different PDT techniques are frequently considered together and compared with ST, with misleading results.[20,21]

The patient subsets for PDT and ST are different and yet results from both groups are often compared. Patients undergoing PDT are relatively homogeneous and consist only of adult intubated ICU patients, identified as having a higher risk of complications. Most patients undergoing ST are neither intubated nor from the ICU. In the majority of reported PDT studies, the procedure is performed by nonsurgeons, whereas in virtually all ST studies the procedure is performed by surgeons. This fact can also bias results. These three factors, uneven reporting of complications, uneven threshold for reporting complications, and inhomogeneity of techniques, are all reflected in the widely varying incidences of complications reported in various studies. Finally, in many reports, including meta-analyses, several or all of these inhomogeneities coexist, which further complicates data analysis and interpretation.

With the above information in mind, some general statements can be made. Complication rates for endoscopic PDT in the literature vary widely from as low as 4%[22] to as high as 61%,[23] with an average of ~ 9%.[7] This compares favorably with that of ICU patients undergoing open surgical tracheotomy in the operating room, where complication rates of 14 to 66% have been reported,[7] or at the bedside where complication rates of 4 to 41% have been cited.[7] Procedure-related mortality is very low for both PDT (0.5%) and ST (< 2%). Comparative data on individual complications (e.g., bleeding, infection) for surgical and percutaneous tracheotomies vary widely from very low to very high, but overall PDT compares favorably with ST.

Although the use of continuous endoscopic visualization has been debated in the literature, the available data indicate that the complication rate of 16.8% without bronchoscopy is significantly higher than the complication rate of 8.3% in PDT with bronchoscopy ($p < 0.0001$). Particularly noteworthy is the reduced incidence of accidental extubation, false passage, pneumothorax, pneumomediastinum, and technical difficulties in the endoscopic PDT group. Arguments that bronchoscopy adds time, cost, and an increased complexity to the procedure and incurs risks such as difficulty in maintaining adequate ventilation, CO_2 retention, and elevated intracranial pressures are both unsupported and weak in comparison to the demonstrated benefits of bronchoscopy, which is crucial to the safety of the procedure and in reducing complications.[7,13]

Obese patients undergoing tracheotomy deserve special mention. Obese patients with a body mass index ≥ 30 are at higher risk for complications. This risk is further increased in obese patients who are "more ill" as assessed by the American Society of Anesthesia classification. The most common complication in this group is accidental decannulation owing to the thickness of the subcutaneous tissues. Use of a proximally extended cannula largely circumvents this problem. There are no data available on the risk of complications in obese patients undergoing open surgical tracheotomy, and therefore there is no evidence that the risk for this subset of patients is reduced in ST.[7] Early mortality in morbidly obese patients undergoing ST may be higher than in nonobese patients.[24] There are no data on early mortality in obese patients undergoing PDT.

Most descriptions of open surgical tracheotomy describe the placement of tracheal stay sutures as an added measure of safety. In the event of accidental decannulation in the early postoperative period, pulling on the stay sutures purportedly facilitates reinsertion of the tracheostomy tube. Although this makes intuitive sense, the real value of such sutures is unknown because, to the best of this author's knowledge, there are no data to support the use of such sutures. Furthermore, reinsertion of tracheostomy tubes into a false passage has been described even in the presence of tracheal sutures.[7,25] Similarly, the practice of routinely obtaining postoperative chest radiographs is described in almost all descriptions of tracheotomy, irrespective of technique. Again, to the best of this author's knowledge there are no data to support whether this practice is helpful or cost-effective in routine uncomplicated tracheotomies.

As with other minimally invasive endoscopic procedures, there is a learning curve for endoscopic PDT, and several studies have demonstrated a higher likelihood of complications in the first 20 or 30 patients.[7,26] Consequently, proper training in the procedure and careful selection of patients with anatomically favorable necks is advisable before proceeding to patients with thick or less favorable necks.[7] A "learning curve" of sorts has also occurred temporally over decades in the case of open surgical tracheotomy. Since Jackson's time, morbidity and mortality rates associated with ST have continued to decline.[27–29] In one study, tracheotomies performed before 1985 were associated with a much higher morbidity and mortality rate compared with those performed between 1985 and 1996.[20]

Complications

Complications of tracheotomy may be divided into intraoperative, immediate postoperative, and late postoperative complications. As stated previously, most complications can be prevented or minimized by optimizing preoperative planning, selecting the appropriate procedure, attention to technical detail, and meticulous postoperative care. However, when complications do occur, most will be noted in the postoperative period. For admitted patients or airway emergencies, the surgery is best done in the controlled setting of the operating room if possible. For those patients in respiratory distress, the airway should be secured whenever possible by insertion of an endotracheal tube before proceeding to the operating room. For adult intubated ICU patients, the procedure may also be safely performed one of two ways: (1) open at the bedside with adequate instruments, light, suction, and assistance, or (2) using an endoscopic percutaneous approach, which obviates the need for suction, cautery, and special lighting.

Intraoperative Complications

Desaturation

The real risk of this complication is unknown because it is infrequently reported in both the "open" and "percutaneous" tracheotomy literature. Brief episodes of mild oxygen desaturation may occur at the time of tracheostomy tube insertion, particularly in patients with compromised pulmonary function requiring high fraction of inspired oxygen concentrations.[7] The risk of such an occurrence may be minimized by thorough pre/intraoperative suctioning of secretions and by ventilating all patients on 100% oxygen for the duration of the procedure.

Hemorrhage

The reported incidence of bleeding varies widely in the literature from 0 to 37% for ST compared with 1 to 19% for PDT. Overall, the incidence of bleeding complications in larger series is lower in PDT compared with ST. This can be explained by the blunt nature of the technique as well as the tamponade effect of the tracheostomy tube against the tight tract which is created.[7,13]

Hemorrhage may be related to the patient ingesting anticoagulants, aspirin, or other nonsteroidal anti-inflammatory agents. These may contribute to excessive bleeding during the procedure and in the immediate postoperative period. The presence of coagulation disorders, such as hemophilia, leukemia, and liver disease, may also contribute to excessive bleeding. Every effort should be made to correct these problems preoperatively except in an emergency situation, in which case correction may be undertaken during the procedure and the surgeon must be meticulous with hemostasis.

Bleeding during tracheotomy may be minimized by careful attention to detail. When using local anesthesia, the procedure should not be begun until adequate vasoconstriction has been achieved. In open surgical tracheotomy, bleeding is usually minimized by staying in the midline with the dissection, being cautious to dissect layer by layer, and maintaining adequate light and assistance with retraction of the soft tissues. This is particularly important in the pediatric age group, where the great vessels are vulnerable because of their proximity to the surgical site. Bleeding from transection of the anterior jugular vein, or the thyroid isthmus, are possible and should be dealt with appropriately by identifying, and ligating or cauterizing the offending vessel. Careful preoperative examination allows identification of a high innominate artery and makes injury preventable. In the unlikely event of injury to the innominate artery, repair requires the expertise of a vascular surgeon. Introduction of the tracheal cannula may cause a paroxysm of coughing, and bleeding may occur at that time. Retraction, suction, and lighting will facilitate identification and ligation of the involved vessel. Tight packing should be avoided because extravasation of air through the packing during severe coughing may predispose to subcutaneous emphysema.

Occasionally, in endoscopic PDT, there is bleeding from a thyroid vein at the time of initial tracheal puncture. This can be addressed by removing the needle, applying pressure for 5 minutes and creating a new puncture. Alternatively, the procedure may be continued at the original puncture site, because the bleeding will stop with the tamponade effect of the tracheostomy tube. Minor oozing from wound edges can be controlled with simple pressure. Occasionally, a small amount of hemostatic packing may be helpful. Although there are isolated reports of life-threatening hemorrhage for both open and percutaneous techniques, this rare complication usually results from an unanticipated anatomical anomaly, from violating a major vessel, or, later, from erosion into the innominate artery.

Intraoperative Tracheoesophageal Fistula

Intraoperative tracheoesophageal fistula is unusual, but has been reported when the tracheal wall has been injured inadvertently, usually during an "urgent" open tracheotomy with overpenetration of the trachea itself. If this is recognized at the time, it may be necessary to open the neck once the airway has been established and individually close the wounds in the trachea and the esophagus.

In endoscopic PDT, occasional overzealous initial needle insertion may puncture the posterior wall, but this is clinically insignificant and is easily corrected by simply withdrawing the needle to the appropriate position. Serious posterior wall injury can be avoided by attention to technical detail (proper positioning of the guidewire, guiding catheter, and dilator) and, most importantly, constant endoscopic visualization of the posterior wall during the procedure.[7]

Pneumothorax

In ST, pneumothorax is most likely to occur in a patient suffering from air hunger. It may also be a result of direct puncturing of the pleura by the surgeon. This latter situation is most common in children, in whom the apex of the lung protrudes into the lower neck and is more vulnerable to injury. Pneumothorax may also occur when the tracheostomy tube is inserted between the anterior wall of the trachea and the soft tissues of the anterior mediastinum, creating a "false passage". This condition is much less likely to occur if the cannula is inserted with adequate exposure, retraction, and the use of traction sutures.

In the PDT technique, this potentially fatal complication can be almost completely avoided by continuous bronchoscopic visualization at every step of the procedure.[7] Excessive force should never be used during dilatation or tracheostomy tube insertion, and always indicates a technical problem.

Pneumomediastinum

Pneumomediastinum occurs more commonly in children and is usually noted on routine postoperative chest radiographs. Predisposing factors include excessive dissection of the paratracheal soft tissues, breathing against an obstructed airway, and excessive coughing that forces air from the open tracheostomy into the deeper planes of the neck. Patients with pneumomediastinum are generally asymptomatic, and no therapy is required. In PDT, this complication is rare with the use of continuous endoscopy.

Cardiopulmonary arrest may occur in patients who have had chronic air hunger and elevated CO_2 levels. Sudden relief of chronic upper airway obstruction may also result in congestive heart failure and pulmonary edema. This occurs from extravasation of fluid into alveoli from the sudden reduction of obstruction-induced positive end-expiratory pressure. This possibility should be considered with anesthesia in the event that cardiopulmonary resuscitation is necessary.

Fire

Fire during tracheotomy is a rare but catastrophic event. External burns may result from the use of electrocautery shortly after prepping the skin with alcohol-containing solutions. This is of particular concern in hirsute patients, in whom body hair interferes with the drying of the solution. Therefore, every effort should be made to ensure that the operative field is completely dry before electrocautery use, or the solutions should be avoided when possible.

Fire may also occur when using electrocautery in the presence of high concentrations of oxygen, whether delivered by mask (as in local procedures), or via the endotracheal tube under general anesthesia. Oxygen concentrations should be kept at a minimum safe concentration for the patient, and cautery should never be used to enter the airway. In the unfortunate instance of an airway fire, the immediate response includes turning off the oxygen, changing the endotracheal tube, and the use of water in the field, followed by bronchoscopy to assess the extent of injury. Medical treatment consists of antibiotics, steroids, and observation in the ICU. The best treatment consists of instituting all measures necessary to prevent such events.

The risk of fire in PDT is virtually nonexistent because cautery is not used.

Technical Misadventures

Technical misadventures are more likely to occur in endoscopic PDT. Loss of the puncture site and accidental removal of the J-wire are two of the possible technical mishaps. In these instances, the procedure must be continued from the previous step or started anew as dictated by the circumstances. Occasionally, dilatation may be difficult because resistance is encountered. If this is the case, the size of the incision and soft tissue "tunnel" should be verified. As a rule, the surgeon's index finger should fit comfortably in the incision and soft tissue tunnel. If not, additional spreading of the soft tissue should correct the problem. If the initial needle insertion is through a tracheal ring, dilatation will be difficult and the needle should be repositioned between rings. If the tracheostomy tube is difficult to insert, the tract should be "re-dilated". The use of excessive force, during any step of the procedure, always indicates a problem and should never be used because it is likely to lead to complications and damage of the instruments. Technical problems may prolong the procedure but rarely directly impact patient safety or outcome.[7]

Immediate Postoperative Complications

Tube Obstruction

Tube obstruction, a potentially fatal complication, may be caused by thick mucus or blood clots. This problem is largely preventable with attentive nursing care, proper humidification, and frequent suctioning. Routine use of a tracheostomy tube with an inner cannula allows regular inspection, cleansing, and suctioning. If for some reason the obstructed tube cannot be cleared, it should be removed and replaced.

Displaced Tracheostomy Tube

Displacement of the tracheostomy tube may occur at any time and is potentially fatal. This complication is most dangerous in the immediate postoperative period before a tract has formed in the soft tissues around the tracheostomy tube. Obese patients are particularly vulnerable to tube displacement because of the inadequate length of standard tracheostomy tubes. Insertion of an extended length tracheostomy tube at the time of surgery largely prevents this problem. Other patient factors that may predispose to displacement of the tube include excessive coughing, and agitation. Additional factors include incorrect placement of the opening into the trachea, creating a false passage, loosening of the neck tapes, poorly tied tracheotomy tapes, failure to suture the neck plate to the skin and use of bulky dressings.

Displacement of the tracheostomy tube should be suspected when a patient with a fresh tracheotomy develops respiratory distress or is suddenly able to speak. Tube displacement may be managed in one of two ways for open surgical tracheotomies. (1) Reinserting the tracheostomy tube. Pulling on previously placed traction sutures may be helpful. This effectively retracts the skin and may help bring the stoma into the wound. A tracheal hook, if available, may further improve visualization of the tracheal opening. The tracheostomy tube is then inserted and adequate ventilation is verified. (2) If reinserting the tube fails, is deemed too difficult, or if a patient is known to have difficult anatomy, it may be best to secure the airway by reintubating the patient and later identifying and opening the tracheostomy tract. The tight tract created with an endoscopic PDT technique essentially precludes safely reinserting a displaced tracheostomy tube within the first 5 to 7 days. In these cases, the patient should be reintubated, and the tracheostomy tube should be reinserted once the airway is protected.

Postoperative Hemorrhage

Postoperative bleeding may occur when the vasoconstriction from the epinephrine wears off or if vessels that were injured during surgery were not ligated and or cauterized. Treatment requires identification and ligation of vessels. For "oozing", use of a hemostatic packing such as Surgicel (Ethicon Inc., Somerville, NJ, USA) may be helpful. Coagulopathies should be identified and corrected. If there is significant bleeding, and visualization at the bedside is difficult, the patient should be returned to the operating room, the wound explored, and hemostasis secured.

Wound Infection

Overall, the incidence of wound infection in endoscopic PDT is lower than in ST. This is likely because of the very small wound and minimal soft tissue dissection, which effectively reduces the surface area available for bacterial growth.

The tracheal wound is colonized within 24 to 48 hours by many species of organisms, including *Pseudomonas* spp. and *Escherichia coli*, as well as gram-positive cocci.[30,31] It is not possible to prevent colonization. Tracheostomy tubes are also colonized by bacteria such as *Staphylococcus epidermidis*, which are embedded in biofilm. The longer the tube is in place, the heavier the load of biofilm. This biofilm functions as a "coat of armour" of sorts, effectively protecting bacteria from local and systemic antibiotics. A true infection of the tracheal stoma is uncommon. Antibiotics simply select for colonization by a resistant organism and should not be used. Regular tracheostomy tube changes every 2 weeks for patients in hospital, may decrease the incidence of granulation tissue and biofilm formation.[30]

The fundamental principles of tracheotomy wound care consist of meticulous hygiene with suctioning, cleansing, dressing and tie changes, and tube changes when necessary to remove crusts and necrotic debris, thereby reducing bacterial load. Traction sutures should be removed when the tract has formed (3 to 4 days). True infection with surrounding cellulitis is unusual and should be treated with organism-specific antibiotics as well as aggressive local wound care with debridement.

Tracheobronchitis may be a result of underlying disease or aspiration, or both. Treatment is with suctioning, vigorous pulmonary exercise (blow bottles, cupping and clapping, ambulation), and judicious administration of antibiotics.

Rarely, necrotizing stomal infections may occur, with substantial loss of soft tissue down to and including the tracheal wall. Further progression of the process may result in carotid artery exposure, with its attendant risks. Management includes aggressive wound debridement and cleaning with antiseptic dressings as well as culture-guided antibiotics. Rarely, local flaps may be necessary to provide soft tissue coverage to vital structures.

Subcutaneous Emphysema

Air may be forced into the subcutaneous tissues during or shortly after tracheotomy. Factors predisposing to this complication include excessive coughing, use of an uncuffed tracheostomy tube, tight suturing of the wound around the tracheostomy tube, and packing of the wound. Emphysema is usually mild and may be diagnosed by palpating crepitus in the tissues of the neck, chest, or face. Subcutaneous emphysema is generally prevented by using a cuffed tracheostomy tube and not packing the wound. If the condition is severe, the wound should be opened and any packing removed. Otherwise, no treatment is necessary because the air is slowly absorbed from the tissues.

Subcutaneous emphysema in association with PDT is rarely reported and probably occurs in patients requiring a positive end-expiratory pressure > 10 to 15 cmH$_2$O. For this reason, such patients should undergo ST.

Late Postoperative Complications

Granulation Tissue

Granulation tissue is considered to be a late complication or sequela of tracheotomy, variably reported as occurring in 3 to 80% of cases.[30] It is commonly seen in children, especially those in whom a fenestrated tube has been used. The clinical importance of granulation tissue lies in its ability to bleed, complicate tracheostomy tube changes, delay attempts at decannulation, and completely obstruct the tracheostomy tube with potentially catastrophic results. Factors thought to favor formation of granulation tissue include bacterial infection, gastroesophageal reflux, suture material, and powder from surgical gloves. Although several topical treatments such as steroid creams, antibiotic ointments, and silver nitrate have been suggested, larger amounts of granulation tissue, particularly when obstructive, may require surgical excision, with or without the use of the laser.

The prolonged presence of the same tracheostomy tube, which is a foreign body, elicits an inflammatory tissue response favoring the growth of granulation tissue, increased secretions, and bacterial colonization with biofilm production.[16] Regular tube changes on a schedule of every 2 to 3 weeks have been shown to dramatically reduce the incidence of this problem.[30]

Tracheoesophageal Fistula

Late tracheoesophageal fistula is rare and may result from an overinflated or improperly fitted cuff. A malpositioned tracheostomy tube pushed to the posterior wall of the trachea against an indwelling nasogastric tube may also result in the formation of a fistula. Penetration of the posterior tracheal wall during surgery, along with local infection may cause a tracheoesophageal fistula. Treatment consists of open repair with individual closure of the tracheal and esophageal defects, and interposition of soft tissue, such as muscle, in the defect. Although the passage of food through the tracheostomy may be an indication of a tracheoesophageal fistula, it is more often a manifestation of aspiration. This can be confirmed with a modified barium swallow.

Tracheoinnominate Artery Rupture

Rupture of the innominate artery usually occurs within the first 3 weeks after tracheotomy and may be fatal. This complication may occur in patients of any age and may be related to several factors:

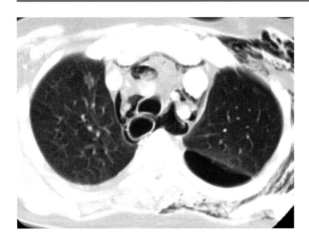

Fig. 18.2 Iatrogenic pneumomediastinum caused by injury to the left main bronchus during difficult intubation. (From van der Molen A, Prokop M, Galanski M, Schaefer-Prokop C. Ganzkörper-Computertomographie (RRR). 2nd ed. Stuttgart: Thieme; 2006.)

- Placing the tracheostoma too low, below the third tracheal ring where the inferior concave surface of the cannula may erode the artery (**Fig. 18.2**)
- Aberrant or abnormally high innominate artery
- Use of an excessively long or curved tube, with erosion of the tip through the trachea and into the vessel wall (**Fig. 18.3**)
- Prolonged pressure on the tracheal wall by an inflated cuff
- Tracheal infection.[32,33]

Rupture of the innominate artery is usually heralded by a "sentinel bleed", which may stop and be followed a few days later by a catastrophic hemorrhage. The patient coughs up bright-red blood from the tracheostomy tube. If this sign is recognized, the cuff of the tracheostomy tube should immediately be overinflated and suprasternal pressure applied in an attempt to control the hemorrhage. If the inflated tracheostomy cuff does not prevent

blood from entering the lungs, it can be changed for an endotracheal tube, which can be advanced to the desired level, and the cuff inflated to control bleeding and prevent aspiration of blood. These maneuvers generally control or reduce the bleeding at least temporarily. The patient should be cross-matched and transported to the operating room immediately, keeping continuous pressure between the anterior trachea and sternum. Sternotomy and ligation of the innominate artery is a lifesaving maneuver.

Tracheal Stenosis and Tracheomalacia

Tracheal stenosis and tracheomalacia are late complications. Steps toward decreasing the occurrence of these sequelae include:
- Proper placement of the tracheostomy tube between the first and third tracheal rings
- Use of the smallest possible tube size
- Minimizing cuff inflation pressures (< 25 mmHg)
- Minimizing cuff inflation times.

Tracheocutaneous Fistula

Tracheocutaneous fistula is a persistent opening between the trachea and skin following decannulation. It occurs when there is inward growth of the skin to meet the trachea. It is more likely to occur in longstanding tracheotomies. Another less frequent cause is partial upper airway obstruction, in which case the fistula compensates for the compromised airway. This can be easily verified with an endoscopic examination before undertaking any repair of the fistula.

A persistent tracheocutaneous fistula results in the following problems: difficulty speaking or coughing without digital occlusion of the fistula; moist, macerated skin from mucus; and social embarrassment. Although the simplest repair consists of excising the skin within the fistula and allowing the wound to close by secondary intention, a depressed scar is likely to result. A better method entails

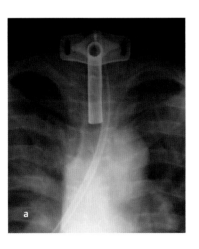
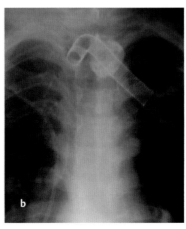

Fig. 18.3a,b Tracheostomy tube.

a Correct placement.

b Intratracheal segment of the tracheostomy tube is too short. The tip of the tube impinges against the lateral tracheal wall, with associated risk of pressure necrosis and perforation of the tracheal wall. (From Schaefer-Prokop C. Critical Care Radiology. Stuttgart: Thieme; 2011.)

removing a small ellipse of skin that includes the fistula. The skin is then dissected off the scar and widely undermined laterally. The strap muscles, which are scarred, are released from the trachea and reapproximated in the midline with absorbable sutures. This maneuver fills in the depressed area and separates the skin from the trachea. The skin is then closed and a light pressure dressing is applied to prevent air from escaping from the wound. Patients should be instructed to apply pressure to the area if they need to cough. The procedure requires general anesthesia in children but can be performed under local anesthesia in the outpatient setting in adults.

Depressed Scar

A depressed scar is visible when the skin is adherent to the underlying trachea. Such scars are unsightly and draw attention because the skin moves with the trachea every time the patient swallows. They can be repaired under local anesthesia by excising the involved skin, widely undermining the edges of skin, freeing and reapproximating the intervening layer of scarred strap muscles, and closing the skin without tension.

Summary

Complications related to tracheotomy are largely preventable. Careful preoperative planning allows for the anticipation and advance problem-solving of potential difficulties. Appropriate patient selection for an open versus percutaneous technique and attention to technical detail help to ensure an uncomplicated intraoperative course. Meticulous postoperative care with the help of a multidisciplinary tracheotomy care team reduce the incidence of postprocedure morbidity.

References

1. Frost EA. Tracing the tracheostomy. Ann Otol Rhinol Laryngol 1976;85(5 Pt.1):618–624
2. Zeitouni AG, Kost KM. Tracheostomy: a retrospective review of 281 cases. J Otolaryngol 1994;23(1):61–66
3. Warren J, Fromm RE Jr, Orr RA, Rotello LC, Horst HM; American College of Critical Care Medicine. Guidelines for the inter- and intrahospital transport of critically ill patients. Crit Care Med 2004;32(1):256–262
4. Shirley PJ, Bion JF. Intra-hospital transport of critically ill patients: minimising risk. Intensive Care Med 2004;30(8):1508–1510
5. Seldinger SI. Catheter replacement of the needle in percutaneous arteriography; a new technique. Acta Radiol 1953;39(5):368–376
6. Marelli D, Paul A, Manolidis S, et al. Endoscopic guided percutaneous tracheostomy: early results of a consecutive trial. J Trauma 1990;30(4):433–435
7. Kost KM. Endoscopic percutaneous dilatational tracheotomy: a prospective evaluation of 500 consecutive cases. Laryngoscope 2005;115(10 Pt 2):1–30
8. Futran ND, Dutcher PO, Roberts JK. The safety and efficacy of bedside tracheotomy. Otolaryngol Head Neck Surg 1993;109(4):707–711
9. Wease GL, Frikker M, Villalba M, Glover J. Bedside tracheostomy in the intensive care unit. Arch Surg 1996;131(5):552–554, discussion 554–555
10. Upadhyay A, Maurer J, Turner J, Tiszenkel H, Rosengart T. Elective bedside tracheostomy in the intensive care unit. J Am Coll Surg 1996;183(1):51–55
11. Stauffer JL, Olson DE, Petty TL. Complications and consequences of endotracheal intubation and tracheotomy. A prospective study of 150 critically ill adult patients. Am J Med 1981;70(1):65–76
12. Dayal VS, el Masri W. Tracheostomy in intensive care setting. Laryngoscope 1986;96(1):58–60
13. Kost KM. Percutaneous tracheostomy: comparison of Ciaglia and Griggs techniques. Crit Care 2000; 4(3):143–146
14. Hunsaker DH. Anesthesia for microlaryngeal surgery: the case for subglottic jet ventilation. Laryngoscope 1994; 104(8 Pt 2, Suppl 65)1–30
15. Szeto C, Kost K, Hanley JA, Roy A, Christou N. A simple method to predict pretracheal tissue thickness to prevent accidental decannulation in the obese. Otolaryngol Head Neck Surg 2010;143(2):223–229
16. Hashmi NK, Ransom E, Nardone H, Redding N, Mirza N. Quality of life and self-image in patients undergoing tracheostomy. Laryngoscope 2010;120(Suppl 4):S196
17. Kost KM. Tracheostomy in the intensive care unit setting. In: Myers EN JJ, editor. Tracheotomy: Airway Management, Communication, and Swallowing. San Diego: Plural Publishing; 2008:83–116
18. de Mestral C, Iqbal S, Fong N, et al. Impact of a specialized multidisciplinary tracheostomy team on tracheostomy care in critically ill patients. Can J Surg 2011;54(3):167–172
19. Deppe SA, Kelly JW, Thoi LL, et al. Incidence of colonization, nosocomial pneumonia, and mortality in critically ill patients using a Trach Care closed-suction system versus an open-suction system: prospective, randomized study. Crit Care Med 1990;18(12):1389–1393
20. Dulguerov P, Gysin C, Perneger TV, Chevrolet JC. Percutaneous or surgical tracheostomy: a meta-analysis. Crit Care Med 1999;27(8):1617–1625
21. Oliver ER, Gist A, Gillespie MB. Percutaneous versus surgical tracheotomy: an updated meta-analysis. Laryngoscope 2007;117(9):1570–1575
22. Barba CA. Percutaneous dilatational tracheostomy has been advocated by many to be the procedure of choice for a patient requiring a tracheostomy. J Trauma 1997;42(4):756–758
23. Graham JS, Mulloy RH, Sutherland FR, Rose S. Percutaneous versus open tracheostomy: a retrospective cohort outcome study. J Trauma 1996;41(2):245–248, discussion 248–250
24. Darrat I, Yaremchuk K. Early mortality rate of morbidly obese patients after tracheotomy. Laryngoscope 2008;118(12):2125–2128
25. Cheng E, Fee WE Jr. Dilatational versus standard tracheostomy: a meta-analysis. Ann Otol Rhinol Laryngol 2000;109(9):803–807
26. Massick DD, Yao S, Powell DM, et al. Bedside tracheostomy in the intensive care unit: a prospective randomized trial comparing open surgical tracheostomy with endoscopically guided percutaneous dilational tracheotomy. Laryngoscope 2001;111(3):494–500
27. Pemberton LB. A comprehensive view of tracheostomy. Am Surg 1972;38(5):251–256
28. Salmon LF. Tracheostomy. Proc R Soc Med 1975;68(6): 347–356

29. Goldenberg D, Golz A, Netzer A, Joachims HZ. Tracheotomy: changing indications and a review of 1,130 cases. J Otolaryngol 2002;31(4):211–215

30. Yaremchuk K. Regular tracheostomy tube changes to prevent formation of granulation tissue. Laryngoscope 2003;113(1):1–10

31. Sottile FD, Marrie TJ, Prough DS, et al. Nosocomial pulmonary infection: possible etiologic significance of bacterial adhesion to endotracheal tubes. Crit Care Med 1986;14(4):265–270

32. Ozlugedik S, Ozcan M, Unal A, Yalcin F, Tezer MS. Surgical importance of highly located innominate artery in neck surgery. Am J Otolaryngol 2005;26(5):330–332

33. Allan JS, Wright CD. Tracheoinnominate fistula: diagnosis and management. Chest Surg Clin N Am 2003; 13(2):331–341

19 Complications in Transoral Laser Microsurgery of Malignant Tumors of the Larynx and Hypopharynx

M. Bernal-Sprekelsen, I. Vilaseca, J.-L. Blanch

Introduction

Complications may arise during and after surgery and can be divided into minor and major complications:

- Minor complications are those that can be treated medically without sequelae for the patients or that can be dealt with using a "wait-and-see" policy.
- Major complications are those needing a blood transfusion, or either a revision surgery, or treatment in an intensive care unit or both.

In this chapter, potential complications and their rates will be analyzed; prognostic factors and tips and tricks to prevent and to manage complications will be addressed.

> **Note**
>
> Complications may reduce the quality of life because of the need for a temporary or even permanent tracheostomy or gastrostomy.

Risk Factors and Incidence

Transoral laser microsurgery has become the standard procedure for the resection of malignant tumors of the larynx and hypopharynx. Recent reports show good results also for advanced tumors.[1,2] Although in experienced hands the laser approach seems to be a safe procedure,[3–6] this is mainly because most studies deal with small glottic tumors. Large tumors and those located in the hypopharynx or the supraglottic region are usually well vascularized presenting a potentially high risk of postoperative bleeding. Also, the extension of the resection may jeopardize deglutition from microaspirations to aspiration pneumonia.

> **The following factors are significantly related to the complication rate**
>
> - The site of the primary, the extension of the resection, and the level of experience of the surgeon have a significant influence on the complication rate.[5,7]
> - pT: early tumors (pT1–pT2) versus large (pT3–pT4): $p > 0.014$
> - Surgical experience: $p > 0.010$

Our experience on over 900 consecutively treated patients with primary curative intention by means of transoral laser resection, could rule out the following potential factors: gender, arterial hypertension, diabetes mellitus, and tumor exposure, which therefore have no significant influence on the incidence of postoperative complications.

Table 19.1 reflects the incidence of severe complications for microsurgical transoral laser resections.

Intraoperative Complications

Most intraoperative complications refer to anesthesic problems related to the use of the CO_2 laser and include accidental burning, ignition of the upper airways, ocular lesions, mucosal edema, and obstruction of the airway. Most of them were already described during the initial period of laser use, between the 1970s and 1990s,[8–11] which led to protocols of general recommendations to avoid them.[12,13]

Nowadays, little or no anesthesiologic complications are to be expected if the recommendations in the use of the carbonic laser are strictly followed. Hence, Steiner and Ambrosch[14] report a 0% rate of anesthesiologic

Table 19.1 Relevant (severe) complications depending on tumor location and T classification

Location / T-classification	T1	T2	T3	T4	Total
Supraglottis (n = 255)	0 / 50	7 / 84 (8.3%)	16 / 105 (15.2%)	3 / 16 (18.8%)	26 (10.2%)
Glottis (n = 597)	1 / 339 (0.3%)	8 / 182 (4.4%)	5 / 69 (7.2%)	0 / 7	14 (2.3%)
Hypopharynx (n = 55)	2 / 11 (18.2%)	4 / 29 (13.8%)	3 / 14 (21.4%)	0 / 1	9 (16.4%)
Total (n = 907)	3 / 400 (0.7%)	19 / 295 (9.7%)	24 / 188 (12.7%)	3 / 24 (12.5%)	49 (5.4%)

complications in a large series of 704 patients with malignant tumors of the larynx and hypopharynx. We observed the ignition of steristrips, used to fix both tubes employed during jet ventilation, which was resolved without any major complication.[15]

Postoperative Complications

Following the literature, the rate of postoperative complications after transoral laser surgery is lower than after conventional external partial surgery.[16–20] Nevertheless, the fact that after larger transoral resections patients are kept without a tracheostomy, leaves them in a potentially risky situation if a complication arises. Therefore, some authors recommend keeping patients intubated overnight who have undergone an extensive resection particularly of the supraglottic region[18,21] or in patients of advanced aged. Others advocate temporary (preventive) tracheostomy after large resections.

Postoperative Hemorrhage

This is probably the most feared complication after transoral resections, with a calculated mortality rate of 0 to 0.3%.[14,19,22] The reported incidence is ~ 5% by Hinni et al,[1] 6% by Rudert et al.[23] and 7% by Ambrosch and Steiner.[24] In a recent review on 1,528 cases, Ellies and Steiner[25] had 72 patients (4.7%) with postoperative bleeding. In seven of these the external carotid artery needed to be ligated. In our series of 905 patients, 33 patients (3.6%) had postoperative bleeding as a major complication, two of them died as a consequence, one at postoperative day 7 (in hospital), the other at postoperative day 10 (at home).

> **Note**
> The incidence of postoperative hemorrhage is directly related to the extension of the resection and the tumor location.[9,22]

Glottic tumors rarely bleed, even after larger resections, whereas the risk increases considerably in supraglottic and hypopharyngeal tumors, even when the local extension is small.[18,26,27] In our experience postoperative bleeding tends to occur during the first 48 hours after surgery or is delayed until around 7 to 10 days later. To reduce the risk of early bleeding some authors advocate leaving patients intubated for 24 to 48 hours after extended resections.[18,21] Delayed hemorrhages may be associated with severe sequelae or even death.[1,7,19,22]

When a simultaneous neck dissection is planned in extended tumor resections, the ligation of laryngeal or hypopharyngeal vessels can be performed in the neck.

For the resection of larynx tumors there are two areas with a higher tendency to bleed: the posterior and lateral, just in front of the arytenoid; and the superior and

lateral to the thyroid cartilage. In supraglottic tumors, the laryngopharyngeal plicae contain the major vessels and in tumors of the hypopharynx, the lateral wall is at risk.

Management of postoperative hemorrhage depends on the amount of bleeding and its potential tendency to be self-limiting, but it sometimes includes the need for general anesthesia to cope with the vessel. Most bleeding can be resolved by identifying the vessel and applying electrocautery or clipping (vascular) forceps.[14,18,23,24,28] However, it may become difficult to identify an intermittently oozing vessel in the middle of a large operated surface with extensive fibrin exudation. Exceptionally, ligation of the external carotid artery may be indicated[14] or a supraselective embolization of the involved vessel.[7] The latter was needed in just one of our patients.

> **Note**
> The best treatment for postoperative bleeding is its prevention. Larger vessels should be dissected or identified during surgery and double-clipped (**Figs. 19.1, 19.2, 19.3, 19.4**). Coagulation alone may not be sufficient.

Dyspnea

After primary laser resections, dyspnea is rarely to be expected and can be medically treated, the need for a tracheotomy being extremely rare.[7,14,29] In our series, we found nine patients (1%) with temporary dyspnea.

In isolated cases or in patients previously treated with radiotherapy, the simple manipulation of the upper airway may result in edema or stenosis compromising the upper airway.[17,18] Also, edema after radiotherapy or chemoradiotherapy may induce edema formation requiring transoral laser resections to ensure the patency of the upper airways. Stenosis producing dyspnea may

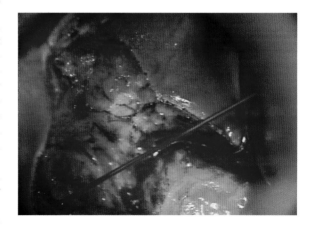

Fig. 19.1 Arterial bleeding from the aryteno-apiglottic fold toward the lateral wall of the hypopharynx.

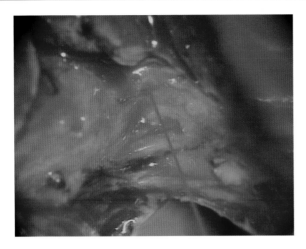

Fig. 19.2 Arterial bleeding from the anterior wall of the pyriform sinus.

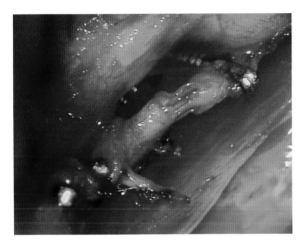

Fig. 19.3 Clipping of a vessel in the left parapharyngeal space.

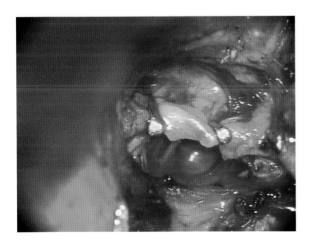

Fig. 19.4 Clipping of a vessel in the pyriform sinus.

occur after extensive or repeated resections, particularly involving the thyroid cartilage or the posterior commissure (**Fig. 19.5**). The treatment in these patients is surgical and will depend on the extension and location of the stenosis.

Cervical Emphysema

This is a rare complication that may occur after resection even of small tumors located in the anterior commissure of the larynx and the subglottis.[7,14,27] In particular, it may occur in cases where the cricothyroid membrane was opened and, at the same time, the glottic level remains competent. Under these circumstances an increased subglottic pressure, such as may happen at the moment of extubation or after coughing, may produce leakage and dissection of the subcutaneous spaces.

Minor emphysemas do resolve spontaneously or can be managed with a conservative treatment including the external application of a dressing or asking the patients themselves to apply external compression while coughing.

In one patient (with a T3 glottic tumor), we found an extended emphysema that extended to the neck and the mediastinum, needing a tracheotomy and intubation for some days (**Figs. 19.6 and 19.7**).

> **Note**
>
> In large tumor resections even with extended exposure of the thyrohyoid or the cricothyroid membrane, emphysemas are rarely seen, because the resections usually include parts of the glottis, which leaves the glottis incompetent and prevents the increase in subglottic pressure.

Local Infection

Only around 1% of patients suffer from an infection of the operated region after transoral laser resections.[19] The presence of fibrin exudations, even extensive ones, should not be confused with an infection (**Figs. 19.8 and 19.9**). Isolated cases of delayed abscess formation have been described after resection of pharyngolaryngeal tumors needing debridement.[14,25,27]

The most common form of infection is perichondritis of the thyroid cartilage, with or without cartilage sequestration, in patients in whom the cartilage has been exposed and denuded extensively. These cases present as multiple granulation tissue formation, erythema of the skin, locally painful, and oral malodor. Patients who have received previous radiotherapy may have an increased tendency to acquire an infection. Medical treatment with conventional antibiotics may prevent a true chondritis. Long-term granulation tissue formation, refractory to antibiotic treatment, may indicate the presence of

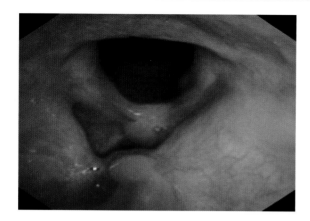

Fig. 19.5 Partial synechia of the anterior commissure after transoral tumor resection.

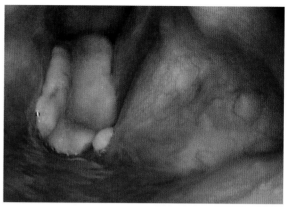

Fig. 19.8 Fibrin exudation after transoral laser microsurgery of the anterior commissure. It is recommended to remove it to avoid extensive synechiae. Application of mitomycin C may be helpful in reducing fibrin formation and prevention of synechiae.

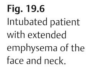

focal   cartilage

Fig. 19.6
Intubated patient with extended emphysema of the face and neck.

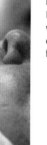

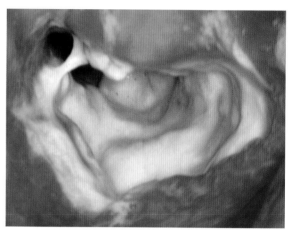

Fig. 19.9 Infectious fibrin exudation over the whole resection area requiring antibiotic treatment.

necrosis needing surgical revision with resection of the sequester (**Fig. 19.10**).

Pneumonia

The presence of symptoms related to microaspiration, such as occasional cough, can be considered normal after transoral tumor resections. In some patients, however, aspiration can lead to pneumonia, be it in the immediate postoperative period or delayed, requiring a more aggressive treatment or preventive management.

In our series, we found 89 patients (9.8%) with temporary microaspiration and 10 (1.1%) with severe aspiration pneumonia, most of them after supraglottic resections. Ellies and Steiner[25] found only five (0.3%) pneumonias and six (0.4%) patients with temporary aspiration. Because of aspiration, in a series of 507 patients with T2 to T4 tumors, 15 (2.9%) temporary and four (0.8%)

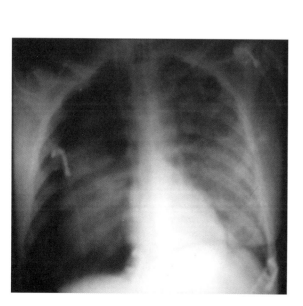

Fig. 19.7 X-ray of the same patient shown in **Fig. 19.6** displaying drainage for severe emphysema of the mediastinum and pleura.

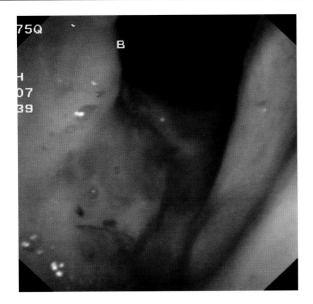

Fig. 19.10 Bed of granulation tissue formation after cordectomy type III to V of the right vocal cord with mucopurulent exudation indicating perichondritis. Antibiotic treatment is indicated.

definitive gastrostomies were needed, and one definitive tracheotomy.[16,25,30]

Microaspiration during hospital stay can be identified through repeated elevations of the body temperature. Most aspiration pneumonia was delayed until after hospital discharge, more rarely it occurred in the immediate postoperative period.[31]

The combination of piperazillin–tazobactam covers most microorganisms during hospital treatment of an aspiration pneumonia.[32] Persisting problems with the deglutition or a delayed rehabilitation of swallowing is directly related to the extension of the resection and the tumor location, sometimes needing a temporary or definitive gastrostomy or even tracheotomy. Conversion into a total laryngectomy for functional reasons is rare.[16,32] We needed to perform this in one patient with severe recurrent aspirations.

> **Note**
> - If problems in deglutition can be anticipated, it is easier to place a nasogastric feeding tube while the patient is under general anesthesia and remove it when swallowing proves to be safe.
> - Rehabilitation of deglutition is key to avoid (micro) aspirations and should be started as early as possible to improve function, particularly after resection of tumors of the supraglottis and the hypopharynx.

Tracheotomies

The need for a tracheotomy cannot necessarily be seen as a complication of transoral laser microsurgery itself, as many patients undergoing transoral laser microsurgery needed to have their airways secured either because of asphyxia, or immediately before surgery, because intubation was not feasible.

Prophylactic tracheotomies are not performed regularly, not even after extended (T3 to T4) resections. Hence, the majority of the tracheotomies in our series were temporary (45/905; 5%) and only a few were definitive ($n = 15$; 1.6%), leaving 850 cases without any type of tracheotomy.

> **Note**
> The level of expertise in transoral laser microsurgery has a direct, statistically significant influence on the rate of complications ($p < 0.01$), particularly in locations with a high complication rate, such as the supraglottis and the hypopharynx.[7]

General Recommendations

Considering that postoperative bleeding and aspiration are the two most frequent complications, the following recommendations can be made:

- *Improve hemostasis* Use all technical methods available: clips, vascular forceps, and monopolar coagulation, tumor reduction in continuous scanner mode (more hemostatic than superpulse), ligation of vessels during simultaneous neck dissection. For larger (supraglottic or hypopharyngeal vessels) clip the vessel adequately: two clips are preferable to coagulation. Cautery alone may be insufficient.
- *Improve patient selection* Select those cases in which good rehabilitation of swallowing can be anticipated, either because of the extension of the resection or because of the physical conditions of the patients. Contrary to other partial external laryngectomies, age of the patient is not a formal contraindication for transoral laser microsurgery.
- *Simultaneous neck dissection* has not proven to be a risk factor for dyspnea, in our hands, moreover, the neck approach can secure hemostasis by the ligation of laryngeal vessels; for these reasons, we have abandoned delayed neck dissections.

> **Note**
> Leave extended tumors (such as large T2 to T3 or very selected T4) to surgeons with more experience.

References

1. Hinni ML, Salassa JR, Grant DG, et al. Transoral laser microsurgery for advanced laryngeal cancer. Arch Otolaryngol Head Neck Surg 2007;133(12):1198–1204
2. Vilaseca I, Blanch JL, Bernal-Sprekelsen M, Moragas M. CO2 laser surgery: a larynx preservation alternative for selected hypopharyngeal carcinomas. Head Neck 2004;26(11):953–959
3. Steiner W, Ambrosch P. Endoscopic Laser Surgery of the Upper Aerodigestive Tract. Stuttgart: Georg Thieme Verlag. 2000; 147 p
4. Rudert HH, Werner JA. Endoscopic resections of glottic and supraglottic carcinomas with the CO2 laser. Eur Arch Otorhinolaryngol 1995;252(3):146–148
5. Peretti G, Nicolai P, Redaelli De Zinis LO, et al. Endoscopic CO2 laser excision for Tis, T1, and T2 glottic carcinomas: cure rate and prognostic factors. Otolaryngol Head Neck Surg 2000;123(1 Pt 1):124–131
6. Peretti G, Piazza C, Cocco D, et al. Transoral CO2 laser treatment for T(is)–T(3) glottic cancer: the University of Brescia experience on 595 patients. Head Neck 2010;32(8):977–983
7. Vilaseca-González I, Bernal-Sprekelsen M, Blanch-Alejandro JL, Moragas-Lluis M. Complications in transoral CO2 laser surgery for carcinoma of the larynx and hypopharynx. Head Neck 2003;25(5):382–388
8. Ossoff RH, Hotaling AJ, Karlan MS, Sisson GA. CO2 laser in otolaryngology-head and neck surgery: a retrospective analysis of complications. Laryngoscope 1983;93(10):1287–1289
9. Fried MP. Complications of CO2 laser surgery of the larynx. Laryngoscope 1983;93(3):275–278
10. Meyers A. Complications of CO2 laser surgery of the larynx. Ann Otol Rhinol Laryngol 1981;90(2 Pt 1):132–134
11. Padfield A, Stamp JM. Anaesthesia for laser surgery. Eur J Anaesthesiol 1992;9(5):353–366
12. Ossoff RH, Karlan MS. Safe instrumentation in laser surgery. Otolaryngol Head Neck Surg 1984;92(6):644–648
13. Ossoff RH. Laser safety in otolaryngology—head and neck surgery: anesthetic and educational considerations for laryngeal surgery. Laryngoscope 1989; 99(8 Pt 2, Suppl 48)1–26
14. Steiner W, Ambrosch P. Complications. In: Endoscopic Laser Surgery of the Upper Aerodigestive Tract. Stuttgart: Georg Thieme Verlag. 2000; 112–113
15. Santos P, Ayuso A, Luis M, Martínez G, Sala X. Airway ignition during CO2 laser laryngeal surgery and high frequency jet ventilation. Eur J Anaesthesiol 2000;17(3):204–207
16. Steiner W, Ambrosch P. Advantages of transoral laser microsurgery over standard therapy. In: Endoscopic Laser Surgery of the Upper Aerodigestive Tract. Stuttgart: Georg Thieme Verlag. 2000; 44–45
17. Zeitels SM, Koufman JA, Davis RK, Vaughan CW. Endoscopic treatment of supraglottic and hypopharynx cancer. Laryngoscope 1994;104(1 Pt 1):71–78
18. Ambrosch P, Kron M, Steiner W. Carbon dioxide laser microsurgery for early supraglottic carcinoma. Ann Otol Rhinol Laryngol 1998;107(8):680–688
19. Oliva Domínguez M, Bartual Magro J, Roquette Gaona J, Bartual Pastor J. Results of supraglottic laryngeal cancer treatment with endoscopic surgery using CO2 laser. [Article in Spanish] Acta Otorrinolaringol Esp 2003;54(8):569–574
20. Peretti G, Piazza C, Cattaneo A, De Benedetto L, Martin E, Nicolai P. Comparison of functional outcomes after endoscopic versus open-neck supraglottic laryngectomies. Ann Otol Rhinol Laryngol 2006;115(11):827–832
21. Rudert H. Laser surgery for carcinomas of the larynx and hypopharynx. In: Naumann HH, ed. Head and Neck Surgery. Volume 3: Neck. Panje WR and Herberhold C, eds. Stuttgart: George Thieme Verlag. 1998; 355–370
22. Kremer B, Schlöndorff G. Late lethal secondary hemorrhage after laser supraglottic laryngectomy. Arch Otolaryngol Head Neck Surg 2001;127(2):203–205
23. Rudert HH, Werner JA, Höft S, Transoral carbon dioxide laser resection of supraglottic carcinoma. Ann Otol Rhinol Laryngol 1999;108(9):819–827
24. Ambrosch P, Steiner W. Komplikationen nach transoraler Lasermikrochirurgie von Mundhöhlen-, Rachen- und Kehlkopfkarzinomen. Otorrhinolaryngol Nova 1995; 5:268–274
25. Ellies M, Steiner W. Peri- and postoperative complications after laser surgery of tumors of the upper aerodigestive tract. Am J Otolaryngol 2007;28(3):168–172
26. Motta G, Esposito E, Testa D, Iovine R, Motta S. CO2 laser treatment of supraglottic cancer. Head Neck 2004; 26(5):442–446
27. Moreau PR. Treatment of laryngeal carcinomas by laser endoscopic microsurgery. Laryngoscope 2000;110(6):1000–1006
28. Rudert HH, Werner JA, Höft S. Transoral carbon dioxide laser resection of supraglottic carcinoma. Ann Otol Rhinol Laryngol 1999;108(9):819–827
29. Eckel HE, Schneider C, Jungehülsing M, Damm M, Schröder U, Vössing M. Potential role of transoral laser surgery for larynx carcinoma. Lasers Surg Med 1998;23(2):79–86
30. Bernal-Sprekelsen M, Vilaseca-González I, Blanch-Alejandro JL. Predictive values for aspiration after endoscopic laser resections of malignant tumors of the hypopharynx and larynx. Head Neck 2004;26(2):103–110
31. Rudert HH, Werner JA. Endoscopic resections of glottic and supraglottic carcinomas with the CO2 laser. Eur Arch Otorhinolaryngol 1995;252(3):146–148
32. Mensa J, Gatell JM, Jiménez de Anta MT, Prats G, Domínguez Gil A. Guía de terapéutica antimicrobiana. Barcelona: Ed.Masson. 2003

20   Complications after Total Laryngectomy, Pharyngolaryngectomy, and Conservative Laryngeal Surgery

J. Herranz González, J. Gavilán

Introduction

Some complications are unpredictable, some are unpreventable and some are incurable. They may be further aggravated by a failure in conscientious reporting. There is a natural disposition to avoid emotional confrontation with all types of disappointment and emphasize the positive aspect of these encounters. This should never supersede the necessity of the open and frank study of all complications so that their full impact is comprehended on the personal and scientific levels. This scholarly and humanizing experience will make medicine a noble profession.

John J .Conley

According to the National Comprehensive Cancer Network Practice Guide in Oncology v.2.2010, "in tumors of the larynx, the decision to perform either total laryngectomy or conservation laryngeal surgery (i.e., laser resection, hemilaryngectomy, supraglottic laryngectomy, etc.) will be decided by the surgeon but should adhere to the principle of complete tumor extirpation with curative intent".[1] There are multiple treatments and different options and consequences, and the most appropriate one should be the decision of a multidisciplinary team, considering patient preferences, tumor characteristics, experience and facilities available.[2-4]

Surgery for laryngeal or hypopharyngeal carcinomas can be indicated either as initial treatment or as a salvage procedure. When properly indicated and performed, surgery achieves 90% local control.[2,5,6] Total laryngectomy is mostly employed for recurrent disease after failure of previous treatment, although it is a good option for advanced tumors that are not suitable for organ preservation because of oncologic criteria, patient status, or health system resources.[7] Conservative laryngeal surgery, when properly indicated, avoids the permanent undesirable sequelae of total laryngectomy, namely permanent tracheostoma and alaryngeal speech, allowing the patient to swallow without aspiration.[4-7] Salvage surgery after failure of radiotherapy or chemoradiotherapy increases the risk of short-term and long-term complications,[8] and reduces the chances for partial surgery options.[9-12]

Complications after surgery of the laryngopharynx result in prolonged hospitalization, increased morbidity related to local infections, tissue necrosis and vascular rupture, resource utilization, and patient anxiety. Rehabilitation and additional postoperative treatments may be delayed beyond the recommended time.

The incidence of complications ranges from 7% to 41%, with pharyngocutaneous fistula being the most frequent.[13,14] After partial surgery, every effort is made to avoid aspiration, so the selection procedure should include a thorough investigation of the patient's capacity to tolerate pulmonary complications.[5-8]

A major challenge for the surgeon is the identification of patients and surgical scenarios with a higher risk of complications, and attempting to prevent their occurrence while favoring early detection of symptoms.

Total Laryngectomy and Pharyngolaryngectomy

Total laryngectomy is a dreadful intervention in which the surgeon admits late diagnosis and the inability for conservative surgery, but it should not be avoided at all costs because life is more important than voice;[15] a lung-powered voice can also be achieved through a tracheo-esophageal fistula. A good quality of life can be maintained after total laryngectomy.[16] Although conservation surgery is possible after radiotherapy failure, only around 30% of patients are suitable.[17]

Prophylactic Antibiotics

According to the National Clinic Guide for surgical prophylaxis from the Scottish Intercollegiate Guidelines Network, for head and neck surgery (contaminated/clean-contaminated), there is consistent evidence that a single dose of an antibiotic with a half-life long enough to achieve activity throughout the operation is adequate.[18] There is evidence from several studies of antibiotic prophylaxis during surgery that dosages with longer duration have no increased benefit over a short course. A single standard therapeutic dose of antibiotic is sufficient for prophylaxis under most circumstances. Intravenous prophylactic antibiotics should be given up to 30 minutes before incision.

> **Note**
>
> Local policy makers have the experience and information required to make recommendations about specific drug regimens based on an assessment of evidence, local information about resistance and drug costs. Narrow-spectrum, less expensive antibiotics should be the first choice for prophylaxis.

Surgery

The best way to avoid complications after total laryngectomy is through careful and meticulous technique, with minimum mucosal damage and accomplishing a watertight pharyngeal mucosa closure without tension. If possible, tracheotomy should be avoided before definitive surgery because of the higher incidence of local infection; the tissue around a previous tracheotomy should be removed.

Approach

All efforts should be made to avoid entering the larynx close to the tumor, keeping in mind the spatial needs for safe margins. For intralaryngeal tumors the approach can be made through the vallecula, removing the tumor under direct vision. If the tumor invades the upper part of the epiglottis, the vallecula or base of the tongue, the approach is made from behind the arytenoids, in an upward direction.

During endoscopic evaluation of the patient, tumor extension to the pyriform fossa mucosa should be recorded. If no infiltration is found, the mucosa is detached from the internal side of the thyroid cartilage, preserving as much mucosa as possible. This will help during pharyngotomy closure, avoiding both tension and stenosis.

Pharyngeal Mucosal Closure

Pharyngeal mucosal closure can be done in two different ways, through either the usual т-shaped closure or the tobacco-pouch technique. The former is made using a Connell suture pattern, but trying not to enter the mucosa of the pharyngeal wall. A 2–0 Vicryl suture is used. The suture goes from the outside toward the pharyngotomy border without entering the mucosa, ~ 0.5 cm. At the opposite side, the sutures enter the pharyngeal wall close to the pharyngotomy border and exit, without entering

the mucosa, after 0.5 cm. Independent stitches are made from the inferior border of the pharynx toward the tongue base. It is important to make sure that the suture inverts the mucosal edges into the pharynx. This makes the vertical part of the т. For the horizontal arms of the т, a similar technique is used crossing from the upper pharyngeal mucosa to the tongue base until the midline is reached. Care must be taken to avoid damage to the hypoglossal nerve and the lingual artery during this maneuver. A second layer can be made with the inferior constrictor muscles, to reinforce pharyngeal closure, although this may increase hypopharyngeal tension, making esophageal speech acquisition more difficult.

The tobacco pouch, described in 1945 by García-Hormaeche, is possible when sufficient pharyngeal mucosa is preserved for direct closure.[19] Two parallel continuous suture lines are placed around the hypopharyngeal opening. The first one is placed 2 or 3 mm from the mucosal edge, without entering the mucosa, inserting the needle every 6 to 8 mm. By gently pulling from both ends of the sutures, the mucosal edges are approximated and turned inward, creating a safe primary closure. The second line starts at the tongue base and is placed 5 mm lateral and parallel to the first one. The aim of the second stitch is to relieve tension from the first and to retract the suture below the tongue base.

When there is insufficient hypopharyngeal mucosa for direct closure, an apron platysma myocutaneous flap is a fast and reliable reconstruction method with no additional morbidity.[20] Reconstruction begins by suturing the base of the tongue to the superior base of the apron platysma flap. The lateral and inferior edges are sutured to the inner surface of the apron flap.

A Montgomery salivary bypass tube (Boston Medical Co., Boston, MA, USA) may be used to buttress the closure, especially in cases of closure with free flaps or in patients with a high risk of pharyngocutaneous fistula. Sectioning both sternal insertions of the sternocleidomastoid muscle results in a more superficial and accessible stoma, facilitating cleaning maneuvers and occlusion in patients with a tracheoesophageal shunt for voice rehabilitation.

Creating a half-moon section in the superior skin flap at the midline results in a circular-shaped stoma, reducing the chances of stomal stenosis. Tracheal opening should avoid cutting the cartilage itself, by making an incision between two tracheal rings. Cartilage exposure and infection should be avoided by using vertical mattress stitches in the skin covering the tracheal stump.

We usually place a Jackson–Pratt drain adjacent to the pharyngotomy closure and keep it in place until swallowing is recovered. This drain helps in early identification of saliva leak, reduces patient discomfort, and simplifies postsurgical care.[21]

> **Note**
> - The main advantage of the tobacco pouch is that it allows oral feeding with a soft diet by the 3rd postoperative day.
> - With an apron platysma myocutaneous flap, the anterior wall of the neopharynx allows a wide food passage in spite of the small amount of remaining pharyngeal mucosa.
> - A stable, adequate-sized, accessible stoma significantly improves the quality of life of the laryngectomized patient.
> - A half-moon section in the superior skin flap at the midline should reduce the chances of tracheostoma stenosis.

Postoperative Care

Drains

Neck drains are removed once output is less than 20 mL in 24 hours, usually around the third postoperative day.

Skin Flap

The neck aspect should be checked often in the first 48 hours, mainly in patients with cough or nausea in the early postoperative period, to identify hematoma formation. Hematoma may be hidden behind a bulky neck dressing and a nonfunctional drain. An empty drain does not rule out hematoma formation.

A pressure dressing prevents fluid collection, but should be loose enough to avoid venous or arterial interference. To check adequate pressure, a finger should easily be placed underneath the dressing. Slight elevation (30 to 45°) of the patient's head should be maintained to avoid postoperative edema. Pressure dressings are removed 24 hours after drains are taken out.

> **Note**
> Fever, foul odor or a suture line that is inflamed, ischemic, or under tension should be investigated for abscess or hematoma formation.

Tracheotomy

A cuffed, high-volume, low-pressure laryngectomy tube is placed for the first 24 hours to prevent aspiration in case of acute hemorrhage. It is important to check cuff pressure to avoid necrosis of tracheal wall mucosa and secondary stenosis. A cuffed tube is replaced by a silicon non-cuffed tube after 24 or 48 hours, or the cuff can be deflated in patients at low-risk of aspiration. Airway humidity can be achieved by using moisture and heat exchangers.[22,23]

The tracheostomy should be carefully cleaned, avoiding tracheal and tube crusting, and it is important to keep the airway clear. Coughing and deep breathing should be encouraged to clear secretions and expand the lungs. In case of ineffective cough or thick secretions, aspiration should be performed every 2 to 3 hours. Saline irrigation of the trachea, 2 to 3 mL, will render secretions more easily removable.

X-ray Control

Regular chest X-ray is not necessary unless pulmonary symptoms are present: pulmonary auscultation is sufficient.

Blood Test

Blood test for hemoglobin, protein, leukocytes, and renal function should be performed 12 hours after surgery and on the 4th postoperative day. Thyroid hormones should be checked in previously radiated patients.

Enteral Feeding

Before enteral feeding is started, the tube position should be checked. Diet selection depends on the proteic and caloric requirements of the patient, and should be controlled by a nutritionist.

Oral Feeding

Instruct the patient to avoid swallowing saliva during the first operative days. Average time to initiate oral feeding ranges between 7 and 10 days,[23] unless signs that indicate a fistula are present (odor, fever, skin erythema, saliva in suction drain). Although this is common practice, some authors believe that the time of oral feeding has little to do with fistula formation, with the nasogastric tube exerting a more traumatic effect than oral feeding.[24]

Emotional Support

In the postoperative period the patient and family face the real sequelae of the operation, and such a new unknown and stressful situation may induce depression. Psychologic and emotional support should be given to the patient to encourage active participation in the rehabilitation process. Family instruction about the basic needs of patient care will make it easier for them to understand the patient's needs and how to provide assistance.

Wound Care

There are multiple factors that may affect wound healing:
- General factors:
  - Nutrition. Nutritional status may interfere with adequate oxygen transport and tissue perfusion.

Low hemoglobin, protein deficiency, and dehydration reduce wound healing.

- Co-morbidity. Diabetes, tobacco, and obesity all delay healing.
- Drugs. Steroids and nonsteroidal anti-inflammatory drugs reduce fibroblast proliferation and decrease collagen synthesis.
- Local factors:
  - Ischemia. Poor tissue perfusion reduces the inflammatory response, an essential part of wound healing. Previous radiotherapy, diabetes, hematoma, infection, or peripheral vascular disease may be responsible for ischemia.
  - Foreign bodies, hematoma, necrosis, and suture all prolong the inflammatory process and increase the risk of infection.
  - Infection. Reduces local tissue oxygenation and has a collagenolytic effect.
  - Pressure. Pressure dressing is a potential risk of local ischemia, and should be carefully checked, mainly in chronic infections.

Note

- Preoperative and postoperative patient evaluation should identify all potential risk factors for adequate wound healing by optimizing nutritional (protein, calories), biochemical (hormones, glucose levels, ions, renal function), and physical (pulmonary, cardiac, hepatic, hematologic) status.
- Wound signs like odor, warmth, swelling, and pain should warn of complications.
- Every effort should be made to eliminate necrotic tissue and infection by debridement, and to promote wound healing by regular cleaning with hydrogen peroxide or antibiotic solutions.
- Iodoform gauze may be used to pack the wound and promote granulation tissue and healing by secondary intention.

Complications after Total Laryngectomy and Pharyngolaryngectomy

Hematoma/Seroma

Vacuum drains should be checked in the immediate postoperative period. The most frequent area of vacuum failure is the stoma–skin suture, which may be easily corrected if identified. Sudden bulging of the skin flap in the early postoperative period should act as a warning of hematoma or seroma formation. It is usually soft and cystic, and involves oozing under the flap and suction drain obstruction. Exploration and drainage under sterile

conditions is mandatory. A Penrose drain and pressure dressings are used to avoid recurrence. If active bleeding is found, the patient must be taken to the operating room to identify and control bleeding points.

Note
Pressure dressing is not recommended if active bleeding is found because blood cloths can be disseminated around the surgical field, increasing the risk of infection.

Airway Obstruction

Blood aspirated during surgery and drying of the normal mucus may produce crusting and mucus plugs that obstruct the trachea. The patient has noisy breathing, dyspnea, and weak airflow through the stoma. When suspected, the tracheostomy tube should be removed and checked for obstruction at the tube lumen and trachea. In case of dyspnea due to tracheal crusting, avoid removal with forceps. The patient should be asked to slowly take a deep breath while the trachea is irrigated with 2 to 3 mL of saline, and to force exhalation so that the tracheal plug can be removed. This should be done repeatedly until the plug is removed. Adequate humidification of inhaled air will decrease tracheal crusting.[22,23]

Pharyngocutaneous Fistula

Incidence and Risk Factors

Pharyngocutaneous fistula is the most frequently reported complication after total laryngectomy, with rates ranging from 2 to 65%.[14] Many factors are reported to predispose to this complication, including preoperative radiotherapy, preoperative tracheotomy, concurrent radical neck dissection, postoperative hemoglobin level, technique of pharyngeal closure, antibiotic prophylaxis, positive margins, tobacco use, comorbidity, and poor nutritional status.[13,24–30] In a meta-analysis of 26 published studies, a hemoglobin level lower than 125 g/dL, previous tracheotomy, preoperative radiotherapy, and concurrent neck dissection are associated with an increased risk of pharyngocutaneous fistula.[30] Fistulas after radiotherapy were larger and took longer to heal,[28] and a significant number of patients required surgery for closure.[29] However, the significance of these risk factors has been questioned because of the small sample size, selection criteria, and event definition.[13,14]

Signs and Symptoms

Pharyngocutaneous fistulas usually occur 4 to 10 days postoperatively, in primary cases, and up to 4 to 6 weeks

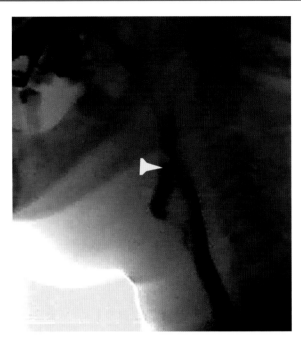

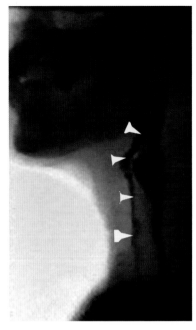

Fig. 20.2 White arrows show the course of a salivary fistula from the tongue base to the tracheostoma area, parallel to the esophageal lumen.

Fig. 20.1
Videofluoroscopic examination showing a short-course salivary fistula in the tongue-base area (arrow).

later in salvage surgery after chemoradiotherapy. Saliva can leak through the pharyngotomy closure line, accumulating in subcutaneous spaces. This situation precedes abscess formation, tissue necrosis, and sepsis. Symptoms include foul odor, fever, leukocytosis, skin erythema and edema, and purulent secretion around the tracheostoma. Purulent material can be found in the suction drain and the drain may lose vacuum because of air and saliva entering the subcutaneous space during swallowing.

Videofluoroscopic imaging or a methylene blue swallowing test are useful to confirm diagnosis and locate the fistula (**Figs. 20.1 and 20.2**). Early identification is important to reduce morbidity (risk of sepsis and infection with major vessel rupture), allowing more conservative management. When a fistula occurs, saliva and pus create an abscess underneath the skin flap that will make a tract to outflow through the skin incision, in the most recumbent area, usually the tracheostoma–skin suture line.

Treatment

Treatment is directed to reduce infection, necrosis, large vessel rupture, and a sizable fistulous tract. If the fistula is adjacent to a working suction drain, and no signs of local infection are visible, the drain should be kept in place. This will evacuate pus and saliva, keeping the skin flap seated next to the underlying bed.[2] If an abscess is detected, or if the drain is absent or not working properly, the abscess should be opened, drained, and medialized with insertion of a Penrose drain, because the entire

surgical field may become infected. Fistula location and course should be evaluated by asking the patient to swallow while pressing with a finger over the potential location, most frequently in the tongue-base area. A skin incision is made over the potential fistula location to reduce the length of the fistula track and avoid saliva reaching the large vessels and tracheostoma.

Most fistulas in uncomplicated cases will heal spontaneously. Conservative treatment with control of infection by cleaning the wound twice a day, cleaning the fistula with iodoform gauze, and applying a pressure dressing to avoid dead spaces, is satisfactory in most cases. Even in large fistulas, once infection and necrosis are controlled, fistula reduction and closure by secondary intention is frequent. If infection or tissue necrosis appear, then skin slough and fistula exteriorization are frequent, with greater risk after radiotherapy or chemoradiotherapy (**Figs. 20.3, 20.4, 20.5, 20.6**). Surgery is necessary to close large and sometimes refractory fistulas by using local, regional, or free vascularized tissue once infection is fully controlled (**Fig. 20.7a–d**).

For patients at high risk because of general or comorbidity factors, or those receiving salvage surgery after chemoradiotherapy, debridement and wide opening, with exteriorization of the fistula, is mandatory, with special attention to avoid infection of large vessels. If granulation tissue appears, then evolution is positive and skin graft or regional flaps can be used. A pectoralis major muscle flap is a good option to bring well-vascularized nonirradiated tissue to the neck, reinforcing pharyngeal

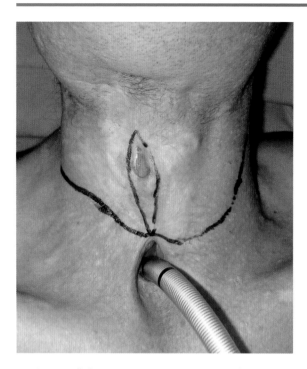

Fig. 20.3 Small pharyngostoma opening superior to the tracheostoma.

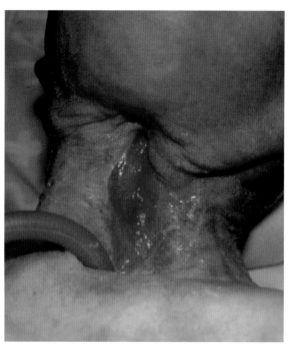

Fig. 20.5 Pharyngostoma with complete necrosis of the pharyngeal mucosa and neck skin from the tongue base to the esophagus entrance.

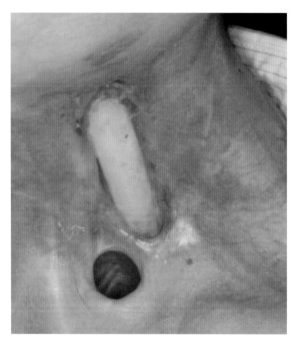

Fig. 20.4 Large pharyngostoma with skin slough. A salivary tube is placed to avoid saliva exit to the neck.

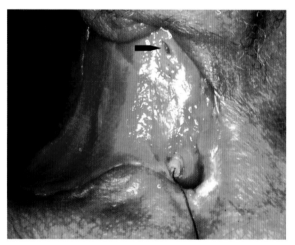

Fig. 20.6 Large skin necrosis after neck infection due to a pharyngocutaneous fistula at the tongue base (black arrow).

Tracheostomal Stenosis

Stomal stenosis is a late complication after total laryngectomy, with an incidence that varies between 4 and 42%.[35] A higher incidence has been associated with female sex and stoma infection, whereas other factors such as fistula, neck dissection, previous radiotherapy, primary tracheoesophageal puncture, or myocutaneous use have not been

closure. Free vascularized tissue reinforcement (jejunum, thigh or radial forearm flap) has also been used to reduce major complications.[31–34]

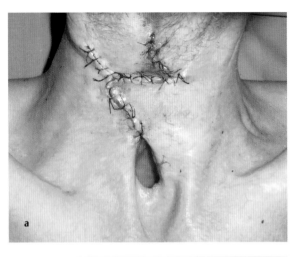

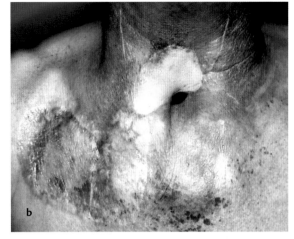

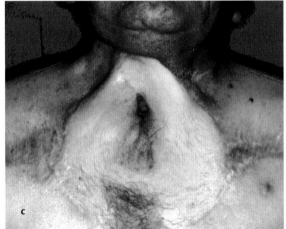

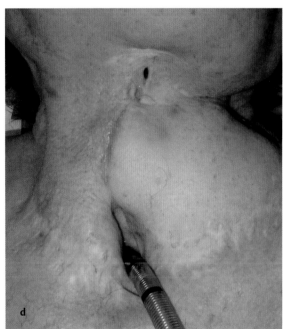

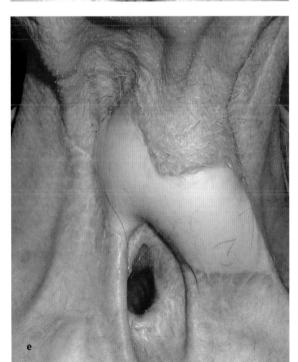

Fig. 20.7a–e Different surgical techniques for salivary fistula closure.

a Local z-plasty.
b Unilateral Bakamjian flap.
c Bilateral Bakamjian flap.
d Pectoralis major myocutaneous flap.
e Radial fasciocutaneous free flap.

confirmed.[35,36] Stomal recurrence should always be ruled out as an underlying cause (**Fig. 20.8**).

To avoid tracheostomal stenosis, careful surgical technique is mandatory at the time of laryngectomy, especially in patients at higher risk (irradiated, female, previous tracheostoma, poor nutritional status). To prevent stomal stenosis, the trachea is cut horizontally between two tracheal rings until the point where the cartilage meets the membranous posterior portion of the trachea, making an upper flap with the membranous mucosa to increase the tracheostoma size without cutting or exposing cartilage.[37]

Different techniques have been described to treat stomal stenosis, all with the basic idea of removing the circumferential scar and introducing new tissue from the surrounding area to prevent a new circular scar.

Pharyngeal Stenosis

Pharyngeal stenosis is infrequent, and is mostly related to pharyngeal closure that is too tight because of extensive removal of mucosa without reconstruction. As is the case in tracheostomal stenosis, tumor recurrence should always be ruled out and excluded once dysphagia is present in a laryngectomized patient several months after laryngectomy. Videofluoroscopic examination is useful to identify the stenosis and evaluate the peristaltic movements of the pharyngoesophageal muscles (**Fig. 20.9**). Dilatation is usually effective to obtain an adequate lumen for nutrition. In more severe cases that are not resolved by dilatation, augmentation of the free flaps may be necessary.

Conservative Laryngeal Surgery

The maintenance of nonaided respiratory, swallowing, and phonatory functions is the objective of conservative laryngeal surgery. Complications after both horizontal supraglottic laryngectomy and supracricoid partial laryngectomies, are mainly related to the ability of the patient to swallow without aspiration and to breathe without an open tracheostoma. Both procedures heavily modify the airway protective function of the larynx, increasing the risk of aspiration pneumonia and atelectasis.

Contraindications and Limitations

For this reason, severe irreversible pulmonary conditions, chronic and ineffective cough, and severe pulmonary restrictions, like the inability to climb two flights of stairs without shortness of breath, are contraindications for conservative surgery. Age should also be considered based on general health and pulmonary status.

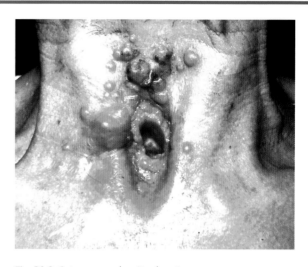

Fig. 20.8 Cutaneous and peritracheostoma recurrence.

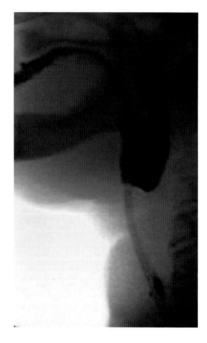

Fig. 20.9 Videofluoroscopic examination showing pharyngeal stenosis at the tongue-base area.

Most patients with laryngeal or hypopharyngeal cancer are heavy smokers and have chronic bronchitis, a condition than can sometimes be improved before surgery. Accurate clinical evaluation is important in the selection procedure. General conditions like diabetes, arteritis, and gastroesophageal reflux should be considered and actively treated before surgery.

Supraglottic Horizontal Laryngectomy

The rate of complications relates to the extent of the operation, with a rate of permanent aspiration between 1.5 and 21%, and between 0 and 50% for nondecannulated patients.[38] Following our selection criteria,[39] in 51% of our patients the feeding tube was removed by day 20 after surgery. No patient had aspiration pneumonia, and 0.9% underwent a total laryngectomy because of permanent aspiration 3 months after surgery. Decannulation was possible in 94.5% of patients.[40] Sevilla et al reported a 9% incidence of total laryngectomy due to intractable aspiration, and a 15% incidence of permanent tracheostomy due to laryngeal stenosis or edema.[41] They found significant association between the decannulation rate and primary tumor stage, and an age over 65 years. Bron et al report 98.5% larynx preservation, with 100% decannulation and no total laryngectomy needed for intractable aspiration.[42] On the other hand, removing one arytenoid, the pyriform sinus, one hypoglossal nerve, or a large portion of tongue base is associated with a higher incidence of aspiration and delayed rehabilitation.[40–43] The effects on swallowing of superior laryngeal nerve preservation, cricopharyngeal myotomy, and hyoid bone preservations are yet to be demonstrated.[44,45]

Airway obstruction of the laryngeal remnant may be the result of either fibrosis and glottic stenosis (**Fig. 20.10**) or an arytenoid mucosa edema acting as a valve during inspiration (**Fig. 20.11**). To avoid glottic stenosis, all the supraglottic tissue should be removed close to the upper surface of the true vocal cord and anterior face of the arytenoids (**Fig. 20.12a,b**). We avoid mucosal flaps to cover the arytenoid to reduce the risk of mucosal edema.

Postoperative Management

Swallowing rehabilitation is essential. Patients are instructed to flex their head anteriorly to touch the sternum with the chin. By doing this, the laryngeal remnant gets closer to the tongue base, closing the laryngeal inlet and avoiding aspiration (**Fig. 20.12c, d**).

Postoperative radiotherapy increases mucosal edema of the irradiated area. Careful evaluation of the indications for postoperative radiotherapy should be made because local control is very high after horizontal laryngectomy.[40,41,46–48] Postoperative radiation to the laryngeal remnant because of positive margins should be avoided by careful intraoperative margin histologic examination, changing to a total or near total laryngectomy if clean margins are not obtained. Relying on radiotherapy for incomplete tumor removal violates the first principle of oncologic surgery, which is complete tumor removal with curative intent.[1]

Supraglottic laryngectomy demands more effort and courage from the patient. It takes time, and the patient must learn how to avoid aspiration and clear the larynx after swallowing. The best way to avoid pulmonary problems and major complications is by never performing a supraglottic horizontal laryngectomy in a patient who is not likely to overcome pulmonary complications. In the early postoperative period, a cuffed tracheostomy

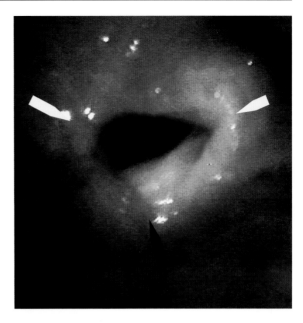

Fig. 20.10 Stenosis after a supraglottic horizontal laryngectomy, due to fibrosis between arytenoids (white arrows) and tongue base (black arrow).

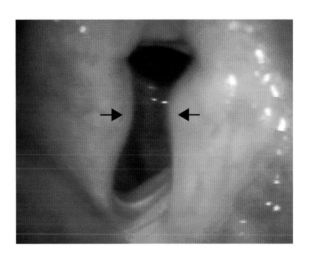

Fig. 20.11 Arytenoid edema over both arytenoids (black arrows).

tube is maintained for 2 or 3 days and then replaced by a fenestrated uncuffed tube. The patient is encouraged to cork the tube and breath through the nose. By day 5 or 6, swallowing rehabilitation is initiated with semisolid food (banana, yogurt, puddings). Careful pulmonary function control is undertaken to avoid pneumonia secondary to chronic aspiration.

The tracheostomy tube is removed as soon as the patient is able to breathe with the tube corked for 48 hours, and endoscopic examination shows patent glottic passage. If postoperative radiotherapy is necessary, the tracheostomy tube is maintained until treatment is completed to avoid having to reopen the tracheostomy

Section III Complications of Head and Neck Surgery

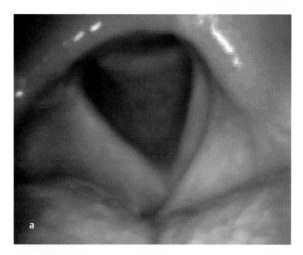

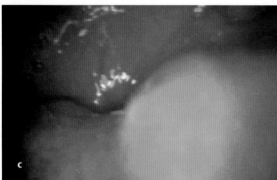

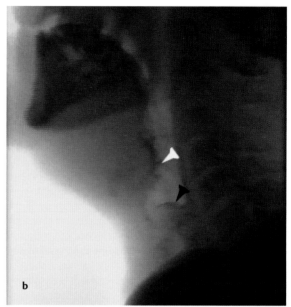

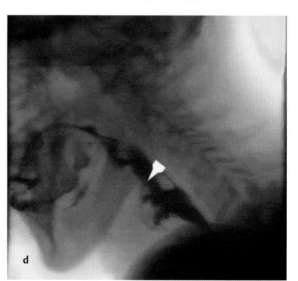

Fig. 20.12 **(a)** Vocal cords and tongue base after horizontal supraglottic laryngectomy. **(b)** Fluoroscopic view shows the tongue base (white arrow) away from the arytenoids (black arrow). **(c)** Once the head is flexed over, the tongue base covers the larynx entrance. **(d)** Fluoroscopic view shows tongue base and arytenoids in contact (white arrow), avoiding aspiration.

because of airway obstruction secondary to arytenoid mucosal edema.

Supracricoid Partial Laryngectomy

Indications

Indications for supracricoid partial laryngectomy (SCPL) are selected cases of supraglottic and transglottic carcinomas.[5]

There are a few key surgical tips to avoid postoperative complications after SCPL.[5,49]

- Elevate the superior platysma flap 2 cm above the hyoid bone
- Incise the infrahyoid muscles at the superior border of the thyroid cartilage
- Vallecula mucosa should be resected and not used in closure
- Blunt finger dissection along the anterior wall of the cervicomediastinal trachea

- Preserve at least one intact mobile cricoarytenoid unit
- Spare the main trunk of both superior laryngeal nerves
- If one arytenoid is removed, preserve the posterior mucosa
- Do not preserve the posterior third of the false and true cord in the noninvolved side
- Suture the arytenoid anteriorly to the cricoid
- Reposition the pyriform sinus
- If hypertonia is found, cricopharyngeal myotomy should be performed.

Contraindications

The main contraindication for supracricoid laryngectomy with cricohyoidoepiglottopexy or with cricohyoidopexy is preoperative evidence of severe respiratory impairment.

Patients with pulmonary disease do not have sufficient pulmonary reserve to tolerate the increased aspiration that occurs in the immediate postoperative period.[49]

Complications

Aspiration pneumonia is the most common complication after SCPL. Joo et al[50] reported a 32.4% rate of postoperative complications, with significant correlation with age, chronic lung disease, and smoking. Benito et al[51] reported, in a series of 457 patients, normal swallowing in 58.9% of patients, finding a correlation of aspiration with increased age, cricohyoidopexy, not repositioning the pyriform sinus, and removal of one arytenoid. Management of aspiration required permanent gastrostomy in 0.6%, and completion total laryngectomy in 1.5% of patients, with no death related to aspiration complications. At Johns Hopkins, 1 of 24 patients underwent a completion total laryngectomy, and 95.8% achieved successful tracheostomy tube decannulation.[52] Laccourreye et al[53] reported no mortality in 69 patients over 65 years of age, with early medical complications in 10.1% and early surgical complications in 13.1%. Tracheal tube removal was achieved in 97.2% of patients, and 52.1% achieved normal swallowing in the first postoperative month. Aspiration pneumonia developed in 21.7%, and by the end of the first year the incidence of completion total laryngectomy and permanent gastrostomy was 1.4%. In a series of 240 patients, in which the resection included the pyriform sinus mucosa, 87.4% reported normal or satisfactory deglutition, with a recovery period that may take up to 1 year.[54] They reported a rate of 1.25% for deaths related to aspiration pneumonia, and 4.5% for completion laryngectomy for bronchopneumonia-related aspiration.

Conservative Surgery as a Salvage Procedure

Conservative laryngeal surgery as a salvage procedure is an option in very selected cases. Patients with tumors that extend beyond their original site are not candidates for these salvage procedures.[55] SCPL as a salvage procedure is related to a higher incidence of complications caused by mucosa edema and reduced capacity for healing,[56] although this finding is not reported in all series.[57,58] Ganly et al[59] reported an increased incidence of complications, with pharyngocutaneous fistula being the most frequent postoperative complication. Pellini et al,[60] in a multi-institutional study on SCPL as salvage surgery, reported satisfactory functional recovery, decannulation, and satisfactory swallowing in 97.4% of patients, with an incidence of 27% for early complications, and 17.9% for late complications. The small number of patients included in most series, and the variety of tumor locations, techniques reported, and expertise, require a careful interpretation of the causes and incidence of complications.

Conclusions

An important part of the treatment of complications after laryngeal surgery is their prevention and anticipation. The surgeon must be aware of the surgical indications based on patient health condition, tumor extension, and possible sequelae, selecting the proper surgical technique. It is always easier to prevent complications than to treat them.

Conservative laryngeal surgery encompasses sound oncologic techniques, with very acceptable functional results, but potential complications related to swallowing demand careful patient selection. Postoperative swallowing rehabilitation is important to obtain good functional results. Postoperative radiotherapy of the laryngeal remnant should be individualized, and avoided if not indicated, to reduce mucosal edema that may affect decannulation. Tissue management, mainly in patients with recurrence after chemoradiotherapy or radiotherapy, should be delicate, avoiding tension and ischemia. Free flaps or myocutaneous flaps should be considered when large defects demand vascularized tissue for reconstruction or protection of large vessels. In the early postoperative period, the surgeon must be aware of symptoms and local signs that act as warnings of the presence of a complication or a potential complication to reduce morbidity by prompt and adequate management.

References

1. National Comprehensive Cancer Network. Clinical Practice Guidelines in Oncology. Head and Neck Cancer v.2.2010. Available at: www.nccn.org
2. Lefebvre JL. Surgery for laryngeal SCC in the era of organ preservation. Clin Exp Otorhinolaryngol 2009; 2(4):159–163
3. DeSanto LW. T3 glottic cancer: Options and consequences of the options. Laryngoscope 1984;94:1311–1315
4. Ferlito A, Silver CE, Howard DJ, Laccourreye O, Rinaldo A, Owen R. The role of partial laryngectomy resection in current management of laryngeal cancer: a collective review. Acta Otolaryngol 2000; 120:456–465
5. Brasnu DF. Supracricoid partial laryngectomy with cricohyoidopexy in the management of laryngeal carcinoma. World J Surg 2003;27:817–823
6. Herranz J. Supraglottic laryngectomy: functional and oncologic results. Ann Otol Rhinol Laryngol 1996;105:18–22
7. Silver CE, Beitler JJ, Shaha AR, Rinaldo A, Ferlito A. Current trends in initial management of laryngeal cancer: the declining use of open surgery. Eur Arch Otorhinolaryngol 2009;266:1333–1352
8. Ganly I, Patel S, Matsuo J, Bhuvanesh S, Kraus D, Boyle J, et al. Postoperative complications of salvage total laryngectomy. Cancer 2005;103:2073–2081
9. Ganly I, Patel S, Matsuo J, Bhuvanesh S, Kraus D, Boyle J, et al. Results of surgical salvage after failure of definitive radiation therapy for early-stage squamous cell carcinoma of the glottic larynx. Arch Otolaryngol Head Neck Surg 2006; 132:59–66
10. Gleich LL, Ryzenman J, Gluckman JL, Wilson KM, Barret WL, Redmond KP. Recurrent advanced (T3 or T4) head and

neck squamous cell carcinoma. Is salvage possible? Arch Otolaryngol Head Neck Surg 2004.130:35–38

11. Goodwin WJ. Salvage surgery for patients with recurrent cell carcinoma of the upper aerodigestive tract: When do the ends justify the means? Laryngoscope 2000;110 (Suppl. 93):1–18

12. Leon X, Quer M, Orus C, López M, Gras R, Vega M. Results of salvage surgery for local or regional recurrences after larynx preservation with induction chemotherapy and radiotherapy. Head Neck 2001;23:520–523

13. Schwartz SR, Yueh B, Maynard C, Daley J, Henderson W, Khuri S. Predictors of wound complications after laryngectomy: A study of over 2000 patients. Otolaryngol Hean Neck Surg 2004;131:61–68

14. Paydarfar JA, Birkmeyer NJ. Complications in head and neck surgery. A meta-analysis of postlaryngectomy pharyngocutaneous fistula. Arch Otolaryngo Head Neck Surg 2006;132:67–72

15. DeSanto LW, Pearson BW. Initial treatment of laryngeal cancer. Principles of selection. Minnesota Medicine 1981;64:691–698

16. Woodward TD, Oplatek A, Petruzzelli GJ. Life after total laryngectomy: a measure of long-term survival, function and quality of life. Arch Otolarynglo Head Neck Surg 2007;133:526–532

17. Holsinger FC, Funk E, Roberts DB, Díaz EM. Conservation laryngeal surgery versus total laryngectomy for radiation failure in laryngeal cancer. Head Neck 2006;28:779–784

18. Antibiotic prophylaxis in surgery. A national clinical guideline. Scottish Intercollegiate Guidelines Network (July 2008). Avalilable at: www.sign.ac.uk/pdf/sign104.pdf

19. García-Hormaeche D. Avance sobre un Nuevo procedimiento de técnica quirúrgica para realizar las laringuectomía sub totales y totales. Rev Esp Am Laringol Otol Rinol 1945;3:99–120

20. Gavilán C, Cerdeira MA, Gavilán J. Pharyngeal closure following total laryngectomy: the "tobacco pouch" technique. Oper Tech Otolaryngol Head Neck Surg 1993;4:292–302

21. Bastian RW, Park AH. Suction drain management of salivary fistulas. Laryngoscope 1995;105:1337–1341

22. Hilgers FJ, Aaronson NK, Ackerstaff AH, Schouwenburg RF, Zandwijk NV. The influence of a heat and moisture exchanger (HME) on the respiratory symptoms after total laryngectomy. Clin Otolaryngol 1991;16:152–156

23. Ackerstaff AH, Hilgers FJ, Aaronson NK, De Boers MF, Meeuwis; CAKnegt PPM, et al. Heat and moisture exchanger as a treatment option in the post-operative rehabilitation of laryngectomized patients. Clin Otolaryngol 1995; 20:504–509

24. Seven H, Calis AB, Turgut S. A randomized controlled trial of early oral feeding in laryngectomized patients. Laryngoscope 2003;113: 1076–1079

25. Violaris N, Bridger M. Prophylactic antibiotics and post laryn-gectomy pharyngo-cutaneous fistulae. J Laryngol Otol 1990; 104:225–228

26. van Bokhorst-de van der Schueren MA, van Leeuwen PA, Sauerwein HP, et al. Assessment of malnutrition parameters in head and neck cancer and their relation to postoperative complications. Head Neck 1997;19:419–25

27. Herranz J, Sarandeses A, Fernández MF, Barro CV, Vidal JM, Gavilan J. Complications after Total Laryngectomy in Nonradiated Laryngeal and Hypopharyngeal Carcinomas. Otolaryngol Head Neck Surg 2000; 122:892–898

28. Pinar E, Oncel S, Calli C, Guclu E, Tatar B. Pharyngocutaneous fistula alter total laryngectomy: enphasis on lymph node metastases as a new predisposing factor. Otolaryngol Head Neck Surg 2008;37:312–318

29. Virtaniemi JA, Kumpulainen EJ, Hirvikoski PP, Johansson RT, Kosma VM. The incidence and etiology of postlaryngectomy fistulae. Head Neck 2001,23:29–33

30. Paydafar JA, Birkmeyer NJ. Complications in head and neck surgery: a meta-analysis of postlaryngectomy pharyngocutaneous fistula. Arch Otolaryngol Head and Neck Surg 2006;132:67–72

31. Cavalot AL, Gervasio CF, Nazionale G, Alvera R, Bussi M, Staffieri A, et al. Pharyngocutaneous fistula as a complication of total laryngectomy: Review of the literature and analysis of case records. Otolaryngol Head Neck Surg 2000; 123:587–592

32. Fung K, Teknos TN, Vanderberg CD, Lyden TH, Bradford CR, Hogikyan ND, et al. Prevention of wound complications following salvage laryngectomy using free vascularized tissue. Head Neck 2007;28:425–430

33. Dubsky PC, Stift A, Rath T, Kornfehl J. Salvage surgery for recurrent carcinoma of the hypopharynx and reconstruction usin jejunal free tissue transfer and pectoralis major muscle pedicled flap. Arch Otolaryngol Head Neck Surg 2007;133:551–555

34. Withrow KP, Rosenthal EL, Gourin CG, Peters GE, Magnuson JS, Terris DJ, et al. Free tissue transfer to manage salvage laryngectomy defects after organ preservation failure. Laryngoscope 2007;117:781–784

35. Wax MK, Touma J, Ramadan HH. Tracheostoma stensosis after laryngectomy: incidence and predisposing factors. Otolaryngol Head Neck Surg 1995;1113:242–247

36. Capper R, Bradley PJ. Etiology and management of tracheostoma stenosis. Current Opinion Otolaryngol Head Neck Surg 2002;10:123–128

37. Tucker HM. Total laryngectomy: Technique. Operative Tech Otolaryngol Head Neck Surg 1990;1:42–44

38. Herranz González-Botas J, Gavilán J, Gavilán C (1999). Cirugía de los tumors supraglóticos. En: Tratado de Otorrinolaringología y cirugía de cabeza y cuello. Madrid: Proyectos Médicos SL, 1999; pp. 3040–3057

39. Herranz J, Martínez Vidal J, Gavilán J. Horizontal supraglottic laryngectomty: modifications to Alonso´s technique. Opererative Tech Otolaryngo Head Neck Surg 1993;4:252–257

40. Herranz-González J, Gavilán J, Martínez Vidal J, Gavilán C. Supraglottic laryngectomy: Functional and oncologic results. Ann Otol Rhinol Laryngol 1996;18–22

41. Sevilla MA, Rodrigo JP, Llorente JL, Cabanillas R, López F, Suárez C. Supraglottic laryngectomy: analysis of 267 cases. Eur Arch Otorhinolaryngol 2008;265:11–16

42. Bron LP, Soldati D, Monod ML, Mégevand C, Brossard E, Monnier P, et al. Horizontal partial laryngectomy for supraglottic squamous cell carcinoma. Eur Arch Otorhinolaryngol 2005;262:302–306

43. Prades JM, Simon PG, Timoshenko AP, Dumollard JM, Schmitt T, Martin C. Extended and standard supraglottic laryngectomies: a review of 110 cases. Eur Arch Otorhinolaryngol 2005; 262:947–952

44. Hirano M, Kurita S, Tateishi M, Matsuoka H. Deglutition following supraglottic horizontal laryngectomy. Ann Otol Rhinol Laryngol 1987;96:7–11

45. Flores TC, Wood BG, Levine HL, Koegel L Jr, Tucker HM. Factors in successful deglutition following supraglottic laryngectomy surgery. Ann Otol Rhinol Laryngo 1982;91:579–583

46. Bocca E, Pignataro O, Oldini C, Sambataro G, Cappa C. Extended supraglottic laryngectomy. Review of 84 cases. Ann Otol Rhinol Laryngol 1987; 96:384–386

47. Ferlito A, Shaha AR, Gavila J, Buckley JG, Rinaldo A, Herranz J, et al. Is radiotherapy recommended after supraglottic laryngectomy? Acta Otolaryngol 2001; 121:877–880

48. Sessions DG, J Lenox, Spector DJ. Supraglottic laryngeal cancer: analysis of treatment results. Laryngoscope 2005;115:1402–1410

49. Lai SY, Weistein GS (October 2001). Conservation laryngeal surgery, supracricoid laryngectomy. Available at: http://emedicine.medscape.com/article/851248-overview

50. Joo YH, Sun DI, Cho JH, Cho KJ, Kim MS. Factors that predict postoperative pulmonary complications after supracricoid partial laryngectomy. Arch Otolaryngol Head Neck Surg 2009; 135:1154–1157

51. Benito J, Holsinger BJ, Perez-Martin A, García D, Weinstein GS, Laccourreye O. Aspiration after supracricoid partial laryngectomy: Incidence, risk factors, management, and outcomes. Head Neck 2011;33(5):679–685

52. Ferrag TY, Koch WM, Cummings CW, Abou-Jaoude PM, Califano JA, Flint PW. Supracricoid laryngectomy outcomes: The Johns Hopkins experience. Laryngoscope 2007; 117:129–132

53. Laccourreye O. Brasnu D, Périé S, Muscatello L, Ménard M, Weinstein G. Supracricoid partial laryngectomy in the elderly: Mortality, complications, and functional outcome. Laryngoscope 1998; 108:237–242

54. Laccourreye H, Sr Guily JL, Brasnu D, Fabre A, Menard M. Supracricoid hemilaryngopharyngectomy. Analysis of 240 cases. Ann Otol Rhinol Laryngol 1987; 96:217–221

55. Shah JP, Loree TR, Kowalski L. Conservation surgery for radiation failure carcinoma of the glottic larynx. Head Neck 1990;12:326–331

56. Laccourreye O, Weinstein G, Naudo P, Cauchois R, Laccourreye H, Brasnu D. Supracricoid partial laryngectomy after failed laryngeal radiation therapy. Laryngoscope 1996;106:495–498

57. Spriano G, Pellini r, Tomano G, Muscatello L, Roselli R. Supracricoid partial laryngectomy as salvage surgery after radiation failure. Head Neck 2002;24:759–765

58. Luna-Ortiz K, Pasche PO, Tamez-Velarde M, Villavicencio-Valencia V (2009). Supracricoid partial laryngectomy with cricohyoidoepiglottopexy in patients with radiation therapy failure. Available at: www.wjso.com/content/7/1/101

59. Ganly I, Patel SG, Matsuo J, Singh B, Kreaus D, Boyle J, et al. Analysis of postoperative complications of open partial laryngectomy. Head Neck 2009;31:338–345

60. Pellini R, Pichi B, Ruscito P, Ceroni AR, Caliceti U, Rizzotto G, et al. Supracricoid partial laryngectomy after radiation failure: a multi-institutional series. Head Neck 2008;28:372–379

III B Surgery of the Larynx, Trachea, Hypopharynx, and Esophagus

21 Cricotracheal Resection and Anastomosis

G. Peretti, C. Piazza

Tracheal resection and anastomosis (TRA) and its different cranial extensions involving the cricoid cartilage (cricotracheal resection and anastomosis, CTRA) are one-stage procedures aimed at complete, circumferential removal of a stenotic tract of the upper airway with consequent terminoterminal anastomosis of the upper and lower segments to re-establish a patent air passage. First described as surgical treatments of posttraumatic, postintubation, and posttracheotomy benign laryngotracheal stenoses, these procedures have been subsequently applied even to the management of primary tumors of the cricotracheal junction or neoplasms of the thyroid gland infiltrating the airway.

Even though this surgery must be specifically tailored to each clinical condition and scenario, from a didactic point of view it can be useful to distinguish at least three essential types of procedure that we usually classify as follows:

- Type A (removal of tracheal rings only, with subsequent cricotracheal anastomosis if resection starts from the first tracheal ring or tracheotracheal anastomosis if the resection involves more distal portions of the trachea, preserving the first tracheal rings) (**Fig. 21.1**)

- Type B (removal of the first tracheal rings in association with the anterior arch of the cricoid cartilage with subsequent thyrocricotracheal anastomosis) (**Fig. 21.2**)

- Type C (removal of the anterior cricoid arch and part of the cricoid plate, potentially up to the cricoarytenoid joints, with subsequent thyrocricotracheal anastomosis) (**Fig. 21.3**).

Generally speaking, the technical difficulty encountered going from Type A to Type C procedures increases, as well as the prevalence of postoperative complications and the risk of failure in terms of patent airway. Overall success rate (usually defined as a patent airway without respiratory distress during daily life) for TRA and CTRA has been reported to range between 86 and 100%.[1–11] Mortality rate (mainly due to cardiovascular and respiratory distress and major anastomotic dehiscence) is reported in the range from 0 to 3%.[4,8,12–14]

In this chapter, we will discuss in detail specific strategies to minimize the occurrence of complications in this kind of demanding surgery.

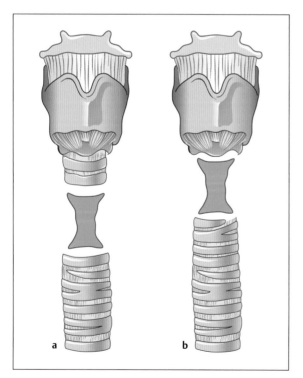

Fig. 21.1 Diagram of Type A resection (with tracheotracheal or cricotracheal anastomosis).

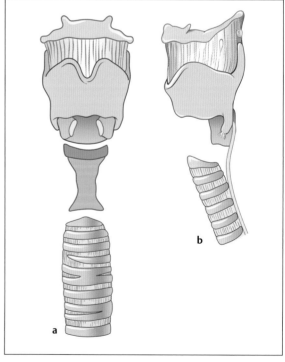

Fig. 21.2 Diagram of Type B resection (with anterior thyrocricotracheal anastomosis posteriorly reaching the inferior border of the preserved cricoid plate).

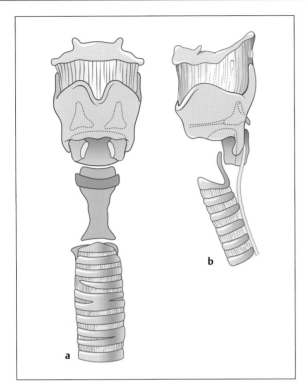

Fig. 21.3 Diagram of Type C resection (with anterior thyrocricotracheal anastomosis posteriorly reaching the level of the cricoarytenoid joints after partial removal of the inner portion of the cricoid plate).

Recurrent Laryngeal Nerve Lesion

Recurrent laryngeal nerve (RLN) lesion, either temporary or permanent, unilateral or bilateral, during TRA or CTRA is reported in a range from 0 to 12%.[2,4,5,8,9,13–15] Identification of the RLN during this type of procedure is not systematically performed, except when the airway resection follows thyroidectomy performed for thyroid cancer infiltrating the cricotracheal junction, in which case the RLNs have usually already been identified during thyroidectomy. To prevent any RLN lesion during TRA and CTRA performed for benign stenoses, surgical dissection of the trachea and cricoid should always be conducted in a subperichondral plane, leaving laterally any scar tissue in which the nerves could be embedded. Particular attention must be paid when isolating the stenotic part of the airway, where the tracheal deformation can cause alteration to the normal course of the RLN. At the level of the cricoid, surgical dissection is performed safely if maintained in between the cricothyroid joints and inside the posterior aspect of the perichondrium of the cricoid plate.

The use of gauze soaked in warm water and epinephrine may be of help in minimizing the use of bipolar forceps for small vessels, especially in heavily inflamed surgical fields. Ligatures and clips are also useful. Monopolar cautery should be avoided whenever in close proximity to the RLNs, whereas cautious bipolar use should be associated with simultaneous saline irrigation of the surgical field to reduce the risk of thermal damage to the nerves.

Extubation, either in the operating room immediately after surgery or during the following day(s) in the intensive care unit, is performed under endoscopic control by a flexible fiberscope with a suction channel through the nose. If bilateral RLN palsy is diagnosed, immediate reintubation and tracheotomy, performed at least two or three tracheal rings below the anastomotic line, are required. Subsequently, in case of failure to recover the function of at least one RLN, an elective posterior cordotomy by CO_2 laser can be considered as an option. In the case of postoperative unilateral RLN palsy, serious airway problems are usually not observed, unless this lesion is associated with an anterior arytenoid subluxation or laryngeal edema (e.g., in the case of extensive neck dissection for neoplastic disease involving the cricotracheal junction). Aerosol of racemic epinephrine, elevation of the head of the bed, absolute voice rest, and a judicious use of intravenous corticosteroids usually help in reducing laryngeal edema in the first 2 to 3 days after surgery. Speech therapy to optimize the phonatory compensation usually starts not earlier than 1 month after surgery, unless concomitant swallowing problems are observed. In the case of incomplete glottic closure in spite of intense speech therapy, delayed vocal fold augmentation phonosurgical procedures will be proposed to the patient.

An expected sequela of CTRA involving the cricoid arch or cricoid plate is a certain degree of vocal fold detensioning as the result of the removal of part of the cricoid cartilage and cricothyroid muscles. This condition is usually associated with persistent mild dysphonia with limitations in pitch and intensity modulation of the voice (**Fig. 21.4**).

Postoperative Bleeding

Both TRA and CTRA present a risk of postoperative bleeding similar to other head and neck surgical procedures but the delicate situation of the airway in these patients (usually without postoperative tracheotomy) requires an urgent revision of the surgical field within a few hours to avoid laryngeal edema and respiratory distress. The source of bleeding is usually located at the thyroid gland level where the use of bipolar cautery is reduced as much as possible to avoid the risk of causing thermal damage to the RLNs. Moreover, in the case of TRA or CTRA for neoplastic disease, the surgical field can be extended to the entire thyroid and lateral cervical regions, resulting in the presence of other potential sources of postoperative bleeding.

III B Surgery of the Larynx, Trachea, Hypopharynx, and Esophagus

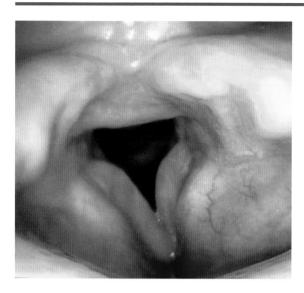

Fig. 21.4 Postoperative laryngoscopy in a patient treated by Type B cricotracheal resection and anastomosis. Vocal cord mobility was bilaterally preserved but postoperative persistent mild dysphonia was present because of vocal fold de-tension after cricoid arch and cricothyroid muscle removal.

Compressive dressings at the end of the procedure are generally less effective than after other major head and neck operations, because of the need to avoid airway discomfort and because of the position of the patient, with the head flexed on the thorax by chin to chest sutures. The absence of any protective tracheotomy after TRA and CTRA also means an increased risk of coughing in the postoperative period. The repeated Valsalva maneuvers may be the cause of hypertensive episodes predisposing to postoperative bleeding. The vacuum drainage that is usually inserted in the surgical field may also lose its effectiveness if the anastomosis is not perfectly sealed, especially during coughing.

For all these reasons, medical and nursing monitoring of wound drainage in such patients should be particularly close in the first 24 to 48 hours. An unrecognized postoperative hemorrhage, although minor, can quickly lead to respiratory distress as the result of pharyngolaryngeal edema or oozing of blood from the anterior cervical compartment through the anastomosis into the airway. As soon as the complication is diagnosed, the patient should be reintubated under endoscopic guidance, extending the head as little as possible to avoid anastomotic rupture. The hematoma is then drained through a redo-cervicotomy approach and hemostasis is performed with scrupulous care not to damage the RLNs. A small tracheotomy, performed at least two or three rings below the anastomotic line, is recommended to prevent any airway compromise from the the laryngopharyngeal edema that is usually associated with further revision maneuvers.

Another event that may lead to important, often fatal, bleeding after TRA or CTRA is the erosion of the innominate trunk by an extremely low anastomosis at the cervicomediastinal junction. Fortunately, this is an extremely rare complication (ranging between 0.3 and 0.7% for postintubation and inflammatory stenoses and between 1.2 and 4.3% for neoplastic ones), in which a dominant role is played by the greater extent of airway resection, removal of paratracheal metastatic lymph nodes, especially when associated with total thyroidectomy, and previous radiotherapy. Other predisposing factors can be a high position in the neck of the innominate trunk, as occurs in young, thin, and female patients, or the low location of the trachea itself, as observed in the elderly. This type of hemorrhage virtually disappeared after the abandonment of the Neville silicone prosthesis, used in the 1960s and 1970s for tracheal reconstruction after resection of more than 5 cm of airway length (with a reported incidence of tracheoesophageal innominate fistula around 57%).[12,16,17]

The safest and easiest way to prevent such a catastrophic event is to insert soft tissues (e.g., thymus, thyroid, or muscle flaps) between the anastomosis and these large vessels. The appearance of the fistula, resulting in a high risk of rupture of the artery, is usually anticipated by late hemoptysis (around the 6th to 10th postoperative day). Its emergent treatment, whenever feasible, is based on the immediate reopening of the cervicotomy with inspection of the vessel and subsequent vascular repair or ligation.

Anastomotic Dehiscence

Anastomotic dehiscence is a potentially life-threatening complication that, in its complete form, certainly represents one possible cause of CTRA or TRA failure, requiring a redo-anastomosis in healthy tissue (when feasible), or placement of a tracheotomy or a Montgomery's T-tube prosthesis. Its reported incidence in the literature ranges between 4 and 14%.[4,7–11,14,18]

Several preoperative, intraoperative, and postoperative measures can be taken to reduce its incidence, at least in its most dramatic form. First, use of corticosteroids, both systemically or through inhalation, should be restricted as much as possible in the preoperative and postoperative periods, for their well-known action in considerably slowing down the healing process of the anastomotic site. Moreover, elective TRA and CTRA should always be performed under optimal airway conditions, i.e., after adequate antibiotic and anti-inflammatory therapy, to obtain a stable, mature, and well-defined cicatricial stenosis, without granulation tissue and local infection.

During surgery, every attempt should be made to preserve as much as possible the cricotracheal blood supply coming from the thyroid gland (which is usually divided on the midline through an isthmotomy and separated from the underlying airway to expose the stenotic site), from the cervicomediastinal tissues adjacent to the trachea, and from the esophagus itself (from which the residual trachea should never be separated for more than 1 cm). At the end of airway resection, before the anastomotis, proximal and distal "stay sutures" should be placed at the two airway stumps to manually simulate their approximation and appreciate their degree of tension. If this shows excessive tension while maintaining a flexed position of the patient's head of ~ 30°, release maneuvers are mandatory. The most frequently used technique is represented by blunt finger dissection of the cervicomediastinal soft tissues from the anterolateral walls of the lower trachea up to the innominate trunk (**Fig. 21.5**). Laryngeal release maneuvers should be strictly reserved for selected cases with an airway resection longer than 4 to 5 cm or shorter resections but a rigid airway (as observed in elderly patients). Several techniques have been described to lower the larynx to reduce the gap between it and the trachea. Basically, these comprise sectioning the muscles above or below the hyoid bone, including sometimes the lower pharyngeal constrictor muscles and the thyrohyoid ligaments.[19,20] We usually prefer the infrahyoid laryngeal release for its easier performance through a standard collar incision, for reduced risk of bleeding and lesions to the hypoglossal nerves, and apparently decreased incidence of postoperative long-lasting dysphagia. As a matter of fact, laryngeal release maneuvers are certainly effective in lowering the proximal stump of the airway (by ~ 1.5 cm) and reducing the anastomotic tension, but they can be a source of swallowing problems, especially in elderly patients or in those with pre-existing central neurologic problems, sometimes lasting for months.[21]

After the anastomosis has been accomplished, it should be covered by the thyroid isthmus and prelaryngeal muscles (if still present) or, if they had been removed as happens for thyroid cancers infiltrating the airway, with pedicled locoregional muscle flaps (sternocleidomastoid or pectoralis major). Sealing the anastomotic line with an outer layer of fibrin glue can prevent the formation of small dehiscences between anastomotic stitches during coughing, particularly after complex thyrocricotracheal anastomosis. In these circumstances, subcutaneous cervical emphysema (usually moderate and self-limiting) can be prevented by compressive dressings of the neck.

The patient's head is usually kept flexed at ~ 30°, after surgery up to the 8th postoperative day, with two heavy chin-to-chest stitches ("guardian sutures"), to prevent dangerous tension on the anastomotic site during the healing process (**Fig. 21.6**). Muscle relaxants may be added to help the patient to tolerate such an uncomfortable and forced postoperative position in the first days after surgery. A devastating, although very rare (five reported cases only in the literature), intraoperative complication of excessive forward flexion of the head during the anastomosis is immediate tetraplegic spinal cord ischemia. To prevent this, the surgeon should always be

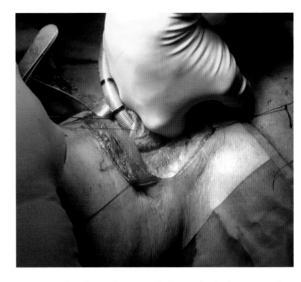

Fig. 21.5 Blunt finger dissection during tracheal release up to the innominate trunk before accomplishment of the anastomosis.

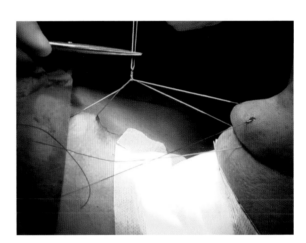

Fig. 21.6 Heavy chin-to-chest "guardian sutures" with the head flexed at ~ 30° at the end of surgical procedure.

able to interpose an inch between the chin and chest of the patient after positioning of the "guardian sutures".[22] Additional attention must be paid preoperatively and intraoperatively to this detail, in every instance when the spine may be affected by arthritic disease processes, or in the presence of a history of craniovertebral trauma.

The first sign of an impending partial or complete anastomotic dehiscence is usually represented by persistent cough (with or without cervical emphysema) and onset of stridor (typically around the 3rd to 8th postoperative day). Careful flexible endoscopy should allow evaluation of abundant anastomotic fibrin, fresh granulomas, small bleeds, and inflamed and edematous laryngotracheal mucosa (**Fig. 21.7**). In severe cases, anastomotic stitches may be partially or frankly torn and intraluminally exposed. More rarely, a complete gap between

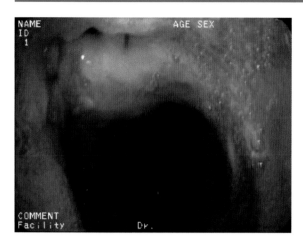

Fig. 21.7 Posterior complete anastomotic dehiscence in a patient treated by Type A resection with tracheotracheal anastomosis after failure of radiotherapy.

the two airway stumps is clearly visible. Management of such a condition is almost invariably surgical and, if feasible, should include removal of one or two more tracheal rings with accomplishment of a redo-airway anastomosis within healthy tissues. When this option is not realistic, tracheotomy should be performed through the dehiscence, or below it, and the airway should be stented with a T-tube. In case of minor dehiscence, which usually evolves to restenosis of the anastomotic line, a viable alternative is represented by the endoscopic placement of a silicone Dumon prosthesis (Novatech, La Ciotat, France) to be left in place for at least 6 months (**Fig. 21.8**).

Anastomotic Granuloma

Postoperative granuloma formation at the level of the anastomotic line is one of the most frequently encountered complications. In the past, it was much more common due to the use of nonabsorbable stitches (such as those in Tevdek, Dacron, Mersilene, Prolene, and Nylon). Since the introduction of Vicryl (polyglactin 910), a braided synthetic medium- to long-lasting absorbable thread, the incidence of this problem has greatly decreased, from 23.6% in the first series to 1.6% in the most recent studies.[22,23] Prevention of granuloma formation is essentially based on the accurate and, whenever possible, submucosal placement of the anastomotic stitches. Inflamed mucosa, bare cartilages, and suboptimal closure of the anastomosis are all factors potentially associated with redundant granuloma formation.

The postoperative appearance of small granulomas at the anastomotic level (usually 1 to 2 weeks after surgery) is still observable in the most complex CTRAs, in which the three-dimensional alignment of the laryngeal and tracheal stumps can be technically demanding (**Fig. 21.9**).

When solitary and limited in their volume, anastomotic granulomas are usually asymptomatic and should be conservatively treated with anti-inflammatory drugs. Corticosteroids are suggested only 2 to 3 weeks after surgery because of their well-known tendency to cause anastomotic dehiscence. In the case of persistence, endoscopic removal, and subsequent mitomycin C application, can represent an alternative approach. Rarely, after CTRA performed for neoplastic diseases, a differential diagnosis

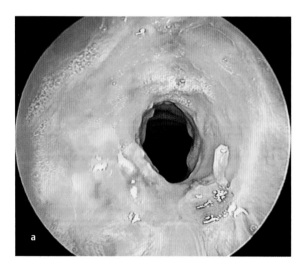

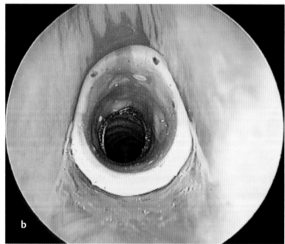

Fig. 21.8a,b Anastomotic dehiscence and restenosis.

a Partial anastomotic dehiscence and restenosis in a patient treated by Type B resection 10 days before.

b After endoscopic removal of stitches and granuloma under general anesthesia, stenosis was dilated and a Dumon prosthesis was inserted. The endotracheal stent was left for 1 year and subsequently removed with good functional outcomes (no dyspnea during daily life).

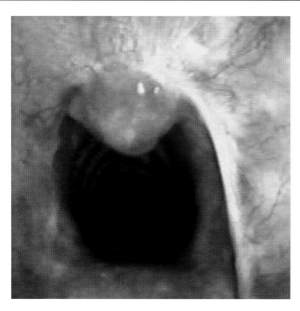

Fig. 21.9 Anterior granuloma formation in a patient treated by Type B resection 2 months before, at the beginning of our series, before the introduction of Vicryl stitches. Endoscopic removal under local anesthesia was successful and granuloma did not recur.

issue with possible tumor recurrence can be raised and solved by histopathologic evaluation of the removed tissue.

Diffuse granuloma formation along the entire anastomotic line and cervical scar can also rarely occur as an allergic reaction to Vicryl or any other suture. In such a case, a gradual endoluminal extrusion of the stitches is seen within a month from surgery, and can be associated with the same phenomenon at the level of the cervicotomy. Stridor can be present and, according to the type of complication, anti-inflammatory and antibiotic therapy can be associated with the endoscopic removal of the extruded stitches.

Comorbidities Potentially Causing Complications

Any respiratory pathologic condition (e.g., chronic obstructive or restrictive pulmonary disease) should be carefully evaluated, even though lung function tests in these patients are usually unreliable because of the presence of the airway stenosis itself. Bronchoscopy and chest computed tomography in selected cases may be of great help. Postoperative intensive care support by a staff specifically committed to the treatment of these patients can be of invaluable help, as well as the early start of an aggressive program of respiratory physiotherapy.

Any motor deficit (posttraumatic paraparesis or tetraparesis associated with diaphragmatic or accessory respiratory muscle deficits, or forced bed rest with ambulation

problems for orthopedic trauma), must also be taken into account. After major head trauma, a predisposition to seizure disorders is also frequently present, especially in the postoperative period, because of the added surgical stress. Any cognitive impairment should be carefully evaluated to ensure full patient compliance during the first days after surgery. In all subjects with a history of craniovertebral trauma, the cervical spine should be preoperatively checked by dynamic flexion–extension radiographs to rule out any instability of the vertebral bodies, which may be potentially increased during and after surgery by the forced flexion of the head.

Particular attention should be devoted to the evaluation of possible swallowing problems, potentially masked in patients with tracheotomy and a complete laryngotracheal stenosis. Fiberoptic evaluation of swallowing with methylene blue and, in doubtful cases, videofluoroscopy may reveal the presence of subclinical aspiration.

Hypertension and coagulation should be carefully controlled to reduce the risk of postoperative bleeding. Diabetes, as in any kind of surgical procedure, predisposes to slow wound healing with possible superinfection (especially by *Staphylococcus aureus*). Gastroesophageal reflux must be prevented by means of high-dose proton-pump inhibitors even in asymptomatic patients.

References

1. Grillo HC, Mathisen DJ, Wain JC. Laryngotracheal resection and reconstruction for subglottic stenosis. Ann Thorac Surg 1992;53(1):54–63
2. Laccourreye O, Brasnu D, Seckin S, Hans S, Biacabe B, Laccourreye H. Cricotracheal anastomosis for assisted ventilation-induced stenosis. Arch Otolaryngol Head Neck Surg 1997;123(10):1074–1077
3. Peña J, Cicero R, Marín J, Ramírez M, Cruz S, Navarro F. Laryngotracheal reconstruction in subglottic stenosis: an ancient problem still present. Otolaryngol Head Neck Surg 2001;125(4):397–400
4. Macchiarini P, Verhoye JP, Chapelier A, Fadel E, Dartevelle P. Partial cricoidectomy with primary thyrotracheal anastomosis for postintubation subglottic stenosis. J Thorac Cardiovasc Surg 2001;121(1):68–76
5. Rea F, Callegaro D, Loy M, et al. Benign tracheal and laryngotracheal stenosis: surgical treatment and results. Eur J Cardiothorac Surg 2002;22(3):352–356
6. Ashiku SK, Kuzucu A, Grillo HC, et al. Idiopathic laryngotracheal stenosis: effective definitive treatment with laryngotracheal resection. J Thorac Cardiovasc Surg 2004;127(1):99–107
7. Ciccone AM, De Giacomo T, Venuta F, et al. Operative and non-operative treatment of benign subglottic laryngotracheal stenosis. Eur J Cardiothorac Surg 2004;26(4):818–822
8. George M, Lang F, Pasche P, Monnier P. Surgical management of laryngotracheal stenosis in adults. Eur Arch Otorhinolaryngol 2005;262(8):609–615
9. Primov-Fever A, Talmi YP, Yellin A, Wolf M. Cricotracheal resection for airway reconstruction: The Sheba Medical Center experience. Isr Med Assoc J 2006;8(8):543–547
10. Amorós JM, Ramos R, Villalonga R, Morera R, Ferrer G, Díaz P. Tracheal and cricotracheal resection for laryngotracheal

stenosis: experience in 54 consecutive cases. Eur J Cardiothorac Surg 2006;29(1):35–39

11. Marulli G, Rizzardi G, Bortolotti L, et al. Single-staged laryngotracheal resection and reconstruction for benign strictures in adults. Interact Cardiovasc Thorac Surg 2008;7(2):227–230, discussion 230

12. Grillo HC, Zannini P, Michelassi F. Complications of tracheal reconstruction. Incidence, treatment, and prevention. J Thorac Cardiovasc Surg 1986;91(3):322–328

13. Donahue DM, Grillo HC, Wain JC, Wright CD, Mathisen DJ. Reoperative tracheal resection and reconstruction for unsuccessful repair of postintubation stenosis. J Thorac Cardiovasc Surg 1997;114(6):934–938, discussion 938–939

14. Krajc T, Janik M, Benej R, et al. Urgent segmental resection as the primary strategy in management of benign tracheal stenosis. A single center experience in 164 consecutive cases. Interact Cardiovasc Thorac Surg 2009;9(6):983–989

15. Mansour KA, Lee RB, Miller JI Jr. Tracheal resections: lessons learned. Ann Thorac Surg 1994;57(5):1120–1124, discussion 1124–1125

16. Deslauriers J, Ginsberg RJ, Nelems JM, Pearson FG. Innominate artery rupture. A major complication of tracheal surgery. Ann Thorac Surg 1975;20(6):671–677

17. Couraud L, Bruneteau A, Martigne C, Meriot S. Prevention and treatment of complications and sequelae of tracheal resection anastomosis. Int Surg 1982;67(3):235–239

18. Wright CD, Grillo HC, Wain JC, et al. Anastomotic complications after tracheal resection: prognostic factors and management. J Thorac Cardiovasc Surg 2004;128(5):731–739

19. Dedo HH, Fishman NH. Laryngeal release and sleeve resection for tracheal stenosis. Ann Otol Rhinol Laryngol 1969;78(2):285–296

20. Biller HF, Munier MA. Combined infrahyoid and inferior constrictor muscle release for tension-free anastomosis during primary tracheal repair. Otolaryngol Head Neck Surg 1992;107(3):430–433

21. Grillo HC, Mathisen DJ. Primary tracheal tumors: treatment and results. Ann Thorac Surg 1990;49(1):69–77

22. Grillo HC. Complications of tracheal reconstruction. In: Grillo HC, ed. Surgery of the Trachea and Bronchi. Hamilton, London: BC Decker Inc. 2004

23. Grillo HC, Donahue DM, Mathisen DJ, Wain JC, Wright CD. Postintubation tracheal stenosis. Treatment and results. J Thorac Cardiovasc Surg 1995;109(3):486–492, discussion 492–493

22 Complications of Surgery of the Salivary Glands and Sialoendoscopy

H. Iro, J. Zenk

Introduction

Surgery of the major salivary glands (parotid gland, submandibular gland, and sublingual gland) is often challenging despite the standardization of surgical procedures in recent years and the aids now available to surgeons. Avoiding complications requires more than surgical skill and adequate surgical instruments: the surgeon must also be familiar with the complex anatomy of the facialis nerve and other adjacent vascular and neural structures. The more tissue structures and anatomy have been altered by inflammation, tumors, previous surgeries and radiation treatments, the more important these aspects become. Potential complications and their treatment as well as measures to prevent and avoid complications during surgery of the major salivary glands are the subject of the present chapter.

Diagnostics

Clinical Examination

In addition to an exhaustive anamnesis of the nature and duration of individual symptoms, a complete clinical examination of the patient by an Ear, Nose and Throat specialist is an absolute necessity. It is important to palpate the gland and neck to obtain a characterization of the localization, dimension, mobility, and pressure sensitivity of any masses. The main purpose of gland massage is to facilitate the evaluation of the saliva secreted through the ostia. Preoperative clinical assessment of facialis nerve function is made according to the criteria formulated by House and Brackmann.[1]

Imaging

The method of choice for imaging the anatomy and pathology of the major salivary glands in both the preoperative and postoperative periods is ultrasonography. It is noninvasive, economical, and involves no exposure to radiation or contrast agents. With this method, the localization and number of stones are just as easy to determine as those of tumors and other pathologic changes.[2] For some time, sialoendoscopy of the Stenson and Wharton ducts has, in the case of unclear swellings, closed a diagnostic gap in the differentiation of stones, duct strictures, and inflammatory changes in the deferent ducts.[3,4]

What, in our view, would be supplemental imaging with magnetic resonance imaging or computed tomography is used, for example, for tumors in the deep lobe of the parotid gland or infiltrative tumor growth into adjacent tissues (bone, base of skull). Positron emission tomography is indicated when searching for distant metastases of undifferentiated carcinomas or in the detection of recurrence.[5]

> **Note**
>
> Ultrasonography is the method of choice for preoperative and postoperative evaluation of anatomy and pathology of the major salivary gland.

Fine Needle Aspiration Cytology, Core Needle Biopsy, and Intraoperative Frozen Sections

The assessment of the significance of fine-needle aspiration cytology (FNAC) in the diagnosis of salivary gland lesions is varied. Factors favoring FNAC include the virtual absence of complications (hemorrhaging, infections) and easier planning of surgical procedures. Bleeding can usually be staunched by simple compression. Antibiotics effective against staphylococci and streptococci are indicated if infections occur. However, good results are obtained with FNAC alone when the procedure is performed by the pathologist.

On the other hand, there is a criticism that FNAC allows insufficient differentiation of tumor types, and therefore has little influence on therapeutic planning. The sensitivity and specificity of the method have been assessed by various studies to be between 55 and 98%.[6] Ultimately, surgery is indicated in the majority of patients even with negative FNAC. In the case of a suspected malignancy, intraoperative frozen section diagnostics should also be used for further clarification, even if this method may deviate considerably from the reference standard of histology.[7] For example, if a decision concerning resection of the facialis nerve is involved and the frozen section diagnosis is unclear, then waiting for definitive histology and a two-session procedure is indicated.

> **Note**
> - FNAC is indicated in patients with high levels of surgical and anesthesiologic risk or who reject surgery for other reasons, to rule out a malignancy.
> - A core-needle biopsy represents an exceptional measure that is appropriate in certain situations and should be avoided with salivary gland tumors because of the risk of tumor cell spillage.

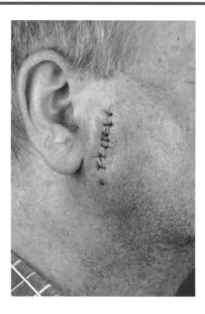

Fig. 22.1
Inadequate biopsy in a pleomorphic adenoma with the risk of tumor spillage. The skin around the biopsy has to be removed during definitive surgery.

Intraoperative Aids

Facialis Monitoring and Facialis Stimulation

Intraoperative neuromonitoring of the facialis nerve makes it easier to identify the nerve and facilitates continuous monitoring of neural function.[8,9] Whereas intraoperative monitoring of the facialis nerve is considered useful in difficult cases, such as revision surgeries, the necessity of neuromonitoring in routine parotid surgery is still controversial.[10,11]

Arguments frequently heard against the routine use of neuromonitoring include, besides the additional time required, a false sense of security leading to hasty and less careful work. Most studies have not, however, described any false-negative responses.[9] However, there could be legal consequences if monitoring is not performed.[10] In our experience, the small amount of additional time required can be compensated for by briefer surgery times.[9] Nerve monitoring, when properly performed, does not cause complications, so there would seem to be no solid arguments against its use, although it cannot of course replace the anatomical knowledge and experience of the surgeon.

> **Note**
> Monitoring of the facialis nerve in extracapsular dissections is a conditio sine qua non (see below).

Use of Microscope or Loupes

Depending on the intraoperative situation, preparation of the facialis nerve and its branches can be performed either with the naked eye or with the help of optical aids such as loupes or a microscope. Dogmatic statements on this would be out of place here. Such aids are normally useful and indicated for revision procedures and reconstructive surgery.

Surgery of the Parotid and Submandibular Glands

In the majority of cases, benign and malignant glandular tumors represent indications for open surgical procedures on the parotid or submandibular glands. Justifications for surgical procedures may also include unclarified systemic diseases (e.g., Sjögren syndrome or sarcoidosis), or inflammatory changes such as sialolithiasis or chronic recurrent sialadenitis.

Techniques

The following parotid gland procedures can be differentiated according to their level of invasiveness.

Specimen Biopsies

Biopsies can be taken with a relatively low level of risk, for example, from the pretragal region of the parotid tissue. Indications for this would normally be the clarification of inflammatory salivary gland diseases or suspected lymphoma. Inadequate specimen biopsies from tumors such as pleomorphic adenoma should be avoided because of the risk of tumor cell spillage (**Fig. 22.1**).

Enucleation

In the historical sense, enucleation is the surgical opening of the tumor capsule followed by intracapsular tumor reduction. The technique is used today, for example, in neurosurgical intervention on brain tumors. It can be considered obsolete for parotid tumors.

Extracapsular Dissection

This technique describes the extirpation of a tumor from outside the capsule in healthy tissue, ideally together with a surrounding layer of healthy parotid tissue. Extracapsular dissection is often incorrectly called enucleation, an error that must be avoided. In contrast to partial parotidectomy, the main trunk of the facialis nerve is not exposed.[12]

Partial Parotidectomy

Following exposure of the main trunk of the facialis nerve, only part of the parotid gland is removed along with the tumor and surrounding glandular tissue. Most of the gland remains in situ.

Lateral or Superficial Parotidectomy

Following exposure of the main trunk of the facialis nerve and its peripheral branches, the entire lateral segment of the gland is removed.

Total Parotidectomy

This term refers to the complete removal of the gland with exposure of the facial nerve and its branches. The synonymous term "near total parotidectomy", which frequently corresponds to the intraoperative finding, reflects the fact that some glandular lobes are usually left in situ.

Radical Parotidectomy

In the case of malignancies that infiltrate the facialis nerve over a wide area, this term refers to resection of parts or the entirety of the facial nerve, usually accompanied by reconstructive measures. In addition to direct neural suture, nerve grafts and other techniques of static or dynamic rehabilitation of the paralyzed face are used.[13,14] Dynamic rehabilitation is performed, for instance, with the help of the temporal or masseter muscles.[15] Static rehabilitation is done by harnessing, in which the fascia lata and contemporaneous tarsorraphy or tarsal tongue plasty is used and a gold or platinum weight is implanted in the upper lid.[16]

Submandibulectomy

The submandibular gland is usually extirpated through a horizontal skin incision parallel to the mandibula. The glandular parenchyma (including the uncinatus process) is completely removed along with parts of the main deferent duct. Partial resections are not performed because of the risk of salivary fistula.

Normal Postoperative Course

> **Note**
> - There is normally no pronounced swelling or pain in the wound area. If this should occur, then the possibility of a complication must be considered and investigated accordingly.
> - Bandage changes and wound control procedures, as well as clinical functional tests of the facialis nerve, should be performed at regular intervals.

Wound Drainage

At the end of the intervention, subtle hemostasis and insertion of a drainage tube help to prevent the development of postoperative hematomas and seromas. Views differ on the use of Redon drains in parotid surgery. Due to possible direct contact with the facialis nerve, we prefer a rubber drain to a Redon drain in parotid gland procedures. In extirpations of the submandibular gland, we also use a standard size Redon (10 Fr) drain under suction until the 2nd postoperative day. Removal of the drain depends on how much material is still being drained off in each individual case (< 20 mL/day).

The volume of postoperative wound secretion correlates with the histology of the tumor (malignant > benign) and is independent of the age and sex of the patient, intraoperative blood loss and the presence of hypertension.[17] A drain is not required in minor procedures such as a specimen biopsy or circumscribed extracapsular dissection.

Wound Management

Wound bandaging types and techniques are often the subject of discussions on how to achieve normal wound healing. Clinical practice undoubtedly favors the use of tight compression bandages to prevent the development of hematomas, seromas, sialoceles, and salivary fistulas, especially if no drains have been used or the wound areas are large (**Fig. 22.2a, b**). Jianjun et al[18] emphasize the importance of compression bandages in their publication, in which they proposed a special setup (similar to headphones) for the reduction of postoperative fistulas and wound healing disturbances: such a setup was employed with a high level of success in a controlled study.

There are, however, exceptional cases in which the administration of perioperative antibiotic prophylaxis is expedient (known cardiac defect, immunosuppression, inflammatory changes in the salivary gland, procedure lasting > 4 hours), but it should not be practiced routinely.[19]

The removal of dermal sutures can be performed safely from the 7th postsurgical day onward.

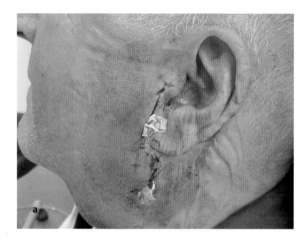

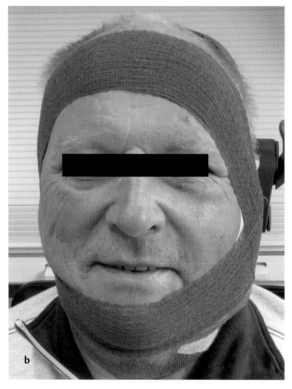

Fig. 22.2a,b Postoperative hematoma.

a Drainage of a postoperative hematoma with placing of rubber drains.

b After removal and drainage of the hematoma, a compression bandage is useful to inhibit bleeding and swelling.

Typical Postoperative Complications

Typical complications of salivary gland surgery include defective wound healing, wound infections including otitis externa, dehiscences and hypertrophic scars, seromas, hematomas, sialoceles, salivary fistulas, anesthesias and paresthesias around the dermal incision or the area supplied by the great auricular nerve, temporary and permanent facialis pareses and, in the later course, Frey syndrome or gustatory sweating.[20]

Hematomas and Impaired Wound Healing

Immediate postoperative impaired wound healing is frequently associated with the development of hematomas, seromas, and sialoceles, and for this reason these phenomena are discussed together here. In addition to specific patient characteristics (status of blood coagulation, vascular status, immune status), factors contributing to the occurrence of these problems also include the wound surface size and the extent of the procedure. Subtle hemostasis with bipolar coagulation and the interruption of flow in larger veins (retromandibular vein) or arteries (maxillary artery) can contribute to the prevention of major postoperative hemorrhaging. The frequency of postoperative hematomas is around 3 to 7%. The most frequent causes are insufficient intraoperative hemostasis and sudden increases in venous or arterial blood pressure.[21,22]

> **Note**
>
> Coagulation inhibitors (phenprocoumon, clopidogrel, acetylsalicylic acid) should be discontinued at least 1 week before the procedure. If anticoagulation cannot be discontinued, a switch to low-molecular-weight heparin or full heparinization is recommended.

The first sign of a complication is usually painful swelling around the wound. If such a swelling develops rapidly after a total parotidectomy, acute postoperative hemorrhage with hematoma is the first possibility that comes to mind. This is usually characterized by a livid skin color, but sometimes by swelling alone (**Fig. 22.3a, b**)

Depending on the extent of hemorrhaging or the hematoma, emergency measures are required because of the loss of blood or secondary swelling of the soft tissues of the neck: the cutaneous and subcutaneous sutures must be opened wide and the hematoma must be removed either by suction or digitally, while at the same time sparing the facialis nerve. In case of severe bleeding in the deep soft tissues of the neck, the respiratory passages must be protected. If the hemorrhaging does not cease under compression, surgical revision is indicated (**Fig. 22.4**). Otherwise, flushing of the wound area, placement of a rubber drainage tube, and application of a compression bandage will suffice.

If the swelling does not develop until days 3 to 5 after surgery, following removal of the drain, and if the salivary gland parenchyma has been retained, sialoceles, or even seromas, have probably formed and saliva is being retained in the wound. In cases of extensive findings with pronounced pain, reopening of the wound

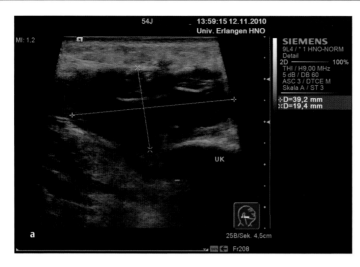

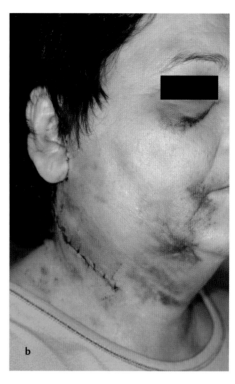

Fig. 22.3a,b Hematoma in a 54-year-old woman.

a Postoperative ultrasound image of a right parotid gland. Extensive partially organized hematoma (+...+ 4 × 2 cm) after total parotidectomy in a patient on anticoagulative agents.

b Clinical view 1 week after removal of the hematoma. Blue and yellow areas are still visible as a sign of resorption of the bleeding. Notice that there is also a diffuse hematoma at the location where facialis nerve monitoring was performed (lateral mouth and eye).

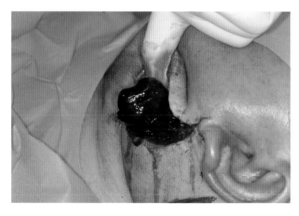

Fig. 22.4 Surgical removal of a large hematoma after partial parotidectomy. The use of bare fingers may prohibit facialis nerve damage in the beginning.

and removal of the secretion with the insertion of another wound drain is recommended. In the case of hematomas, seromas, or sialoceles, the administration of an antibiotic is warranted to avoid the development of secondary infections. Flushing with antiseptic solutions and physiologic saline solutions is then indicated. In less severe cases, sonography can be used to assess their dimensions, after which a decision can be made on whether to puncture and use a compression bandage or whether to puncture only. Whichever is chosen, these patients require further monitoring until the findings have resolved.

If pronounced reddening has developed in the postoperative course as a sign of a phlegmon, an antibiotic is indicated. Abscesses must be punctured or split. The normal cutaneous germs as well as *Staphylococcus aureus* should be taken into account as the most frequent causes of postoperative wound infections. The antibiotics that would be indicated in these cases are amoxicillin with a β-lactamase inhibitor, a second-generation cephalosporin or, in the case of a penicillin allergy, clindamycin. In individual cases, antibiosis should be performed in keeping with the results of a smear test. In addition to antibiotic treatment, we also consider opening and drainage to be necessary in the case of abscesses.

Necrosis of the skin flap is a rare postparotidectomy complication.[21] The necrosis usually develops inframastoidally at the caudal end of the flap (**Fig. 22.5**). In particular, if extensive cutaneous flaps are prepared for cosmetic improvement, as in a facelift, the risk of necrosis is increased. In addition to cautious intraoperative handling of the skin flap (drying, pressure), the main causal factors of such a complication may primarily include nicotine abuse, diabetes mellitus, or previous radiotherapy.[23,24] Therapy comprises the removal of the necroses and secondary wound closure after healing.

Sialoceles, Seromas, and Salivary Fistulas

Sialoceles may occur following surgery of the salivary glands and are also observed as a consequence of penetrative injuries of the salivary gland (**Fig. 22.6a, b**). A

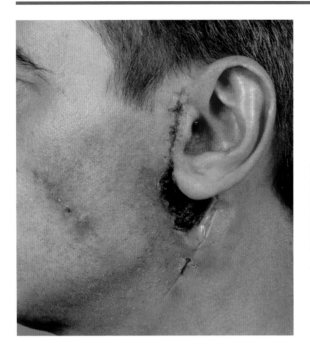

Fig. 22.5 Necrosis of the skin flap after parotidectomy.

sialocele is defined as an accumulation of saliva, either in a deferent duct (also called a retention cyst) or after trauma or other injury to the glandular parenchyma, in such cases often defined by an inflammatory reaction, such as in a pseudocyst. The incidence is described as 5 to 10% following partial or lateral parotidectomy.[22,25] A seroma shows a similar clinical picture, but is characterized by a lower concentration of amylase. This is of no practical consequence, however.

The therapeutic options described in the literature are in most cases anecdotal.[26] The descriptions include repeated punctures with aspiration and the application of suitable compression bandages. Restitutio ad integrum follows in most cases after 4 to 6 weeks. If the sialocele is allowed to drain to the outside by opening the wound area, a salivary fistula may form, which usually closes within 6 weeks at the latest.[27] Antibiotic treatment that also considers the possibility that a staphylococcus could be the pathogen can be administered, if the tissue shows corresponding inflammatory changes.

> **Note**
>
> In the rare cases of persistent sialoceles, oral anticholinergics (ipatropium bromide) or dermal anticholinergic applications (transdermal scopolamine) can be used.

The relevant contraindications and potential systemic adverse effects are to be taken into account below. Nowadays, a neurectomy of the chorda tympani is certainly contraindicated. Successful treatments with botulinum toxin have also been described recently.[28] A study by Witt[26] confirmed that sialoceles occur with significantly greater frequency following partial resections of the parotid gland than after total parotidectomy. Regardless of whether the sialocele was punctured, healing without further complications was observed in all cases within 4 weeks. The author concluded that it is permissible to wait at least 4 weeks following surgery to carry out ultrasonographic evaluation before considering any further therapeutic alternatives.

Considering the development of postoperative wound healing defects, including salivary fistulae, our investigation (n = 452), which covers all parotid gland surgeries, revealed an incidence level of 9% (**Fig. 22.7**). The lowest level of occurrence was after partial parotidectomy.

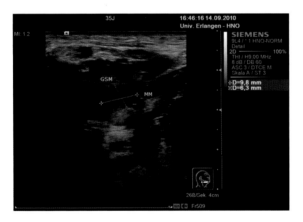

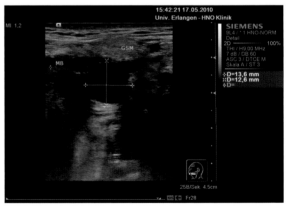

Fig. 22.6a,b Sialocele of the submandibular gland.

a Ultrasound image (longitudinal plane) of a sialocele of the right submandibular gland after sialendoscopy and a duct slitting procedure for stone removal. MM, mylohyoid muscle; GSM, submandibular gland; +...+, sialocele.

b Ultrasound image of a sialocele of the left submandibular gland after transoral stone removal (longitudinal plane). GSM, submandibular gland; MB, floor of the mouth; +...+, sialocele.

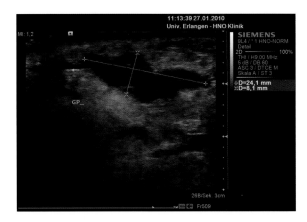

Fig. 22.7 Ultrasound image (horizontal plane, GP: parotid gland) of a salivary fistula and sialocele of the right parotid gland after removing a mass near the masseter muscle. Stensens duct (arrow) was opened during surgery.

Salivary flow ceased an average of 2.3 weeks after total parotidectomy, 4.6 weeks after lateral parotidectomy and 4 weeks after partial parotidectomy. All fistulae had healed within 11 weeks.[12,20] Jianjun et al described covering the defect with a flap taken locally from the parotid fascia, which significantly reduces the frequency of salivary fistula.[29] Application of a compression bandage is a further measure that reportedly reduces the frequency of occurrence.[18] Similar to that of sialoceles, therapy of salivary fistulas involves the administration of anticholinergic agents (see p. 235). According to our own experience and the literature, local injection of tetracyclines can accelerate the healing process.[30–32] The local inflammatory reaction results in a closure of the fistula. Botulinum toxin can also be used successfully to inhibit salivary gland secretions.[33] If the fistula persists, the application of botulinum toxin can be supplemented by a circumscribed surgical revision with freshening of the wound margins and, if necessary, the insertion of a TachoSil patch (Takeda Pharmaceuticals, Zurich, Switzerland) (a sponge containing the active substances human fibrinogen and thrombin as well as horse albumin and collagen).

Before considering major surgical revision with removal of the residual salivary gland and the attendant risk of injury to the facialis nerve, it is now possible to consider local irradiation of the residual salivary gland tissue with up to 30 Gy[34] (**Fig. 22.8a–d**). The last resort would then be surgical removal of the residual gland.

Sensory Defects in the Area of the Cutaneous Incision or in the Supply Area of the Great Auricular Nerve

Whereas temporary haptic disturbances in the area of the cutaneous incision are unavoidable, attempts should always be made to preserve the great auricular nerve.

The smaller the parotid gland procedure, the greater the chances of achieving this will be. The literature reports the occurrence of sensory defects and dysesthesias after parotidectomy in 57% of patients.

The symptoms abate to normal in somewhat more than half of these cases.[35,36] Nitzan et al[32] published average scores of moderate intensity for this parameter, which were, however, not of significant importance in overall quality of life. Problems arise in connection with the wearing of earrings, the use of telephone receivers, shaving and combing the hair. Colella et al[37] report that sensory defects in the supply area of the great auricular nerve usually cause only minor discomfort and are not considered to be genuine complications by patients. Qualitative and quantitative tests reveal an increase in surface sensitivity in 80% of cases with only moderate dysfunction in the remaining 20%.[38] On the other hand, postoperative evaluation has shown that both visual analog scores for quality of life and sensory deficits were significantly better in patients in which the great auricular nerve was preserved.[39]

In cases in which ulcerations occur following damage to the great auricular nerve, a primary psychiatric ailment (psychoses, personality disorders) of an autoaggressive nature must always be considered. After sacrificing the great auricular nerve, a neuroma may develop as a very rare complication. Operative resection is required in these cases to define histology and to differentiate from tumor recurrence (**Fig. 22.9a, b**).

Facial Nerve Injuries and Pareses

Temporary Facial Nerve Paresis

The incidence of temporary or early postoperative facial nerve paresis is reported in the literature in 18 to 65% of cases with an incidence of permanent paresis in 0 to 19%. It is associated with significant morbidity, disturbed daily activity and impaired cosmetic appearance.[8,21,40–42] Temporary facial nerve paresis was observed in our patient cohort after total parotidectomy in 38% of cases, after lateral parotidectomy in 26% and after partial parotidectomy in 5.9% of cases[20] (**Fig. 22.10a, b**). In cases of extracapsular dissection, the frequency is below 5%.[12] No studies have been published on the efficacy of postoperative cortisone in cases of pronounced postoperative paresis.

Permanent Facialis Nerve Paresis

Depending on the surgical method (partial, lateral, or total parotidectomy), permanent facialis nerve pareses occurred in our patients in 0 to 3.1% of cases with no significant differences.[20] The literature also reports frequencies of 6% and 10%.[43–45] The prognosis and course of a postoperative paresis can be estimated by electromyographic examinations, which do not show significant results until

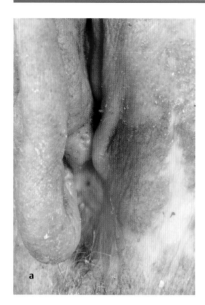

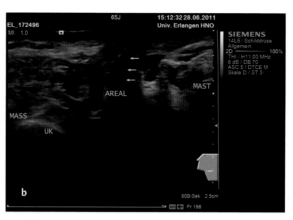

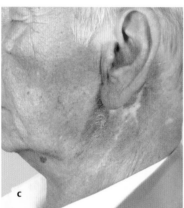

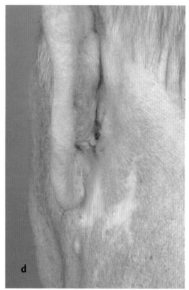

Fig. 22.8a–d Ongoing salivary fistulas after partial parotidectomy in a 65-year-old patient. There were 10 attempts in another hospital and two surgical attempts including botox and tetracycline in our own institution to close the fistula. Because of the risk to the facialis nerve in case of removal of the remaining parenchyma of the parotid gland, the patient underwent local radiotherapy (30 Gy).

a Clinical view.

b Salivary fistulae before radiotherapy seen by ultrasound (arrows) in a horizontal plane. MASS, masseter muscle; MAST, mastoid bone; UK, mandibula; AREAL, area of the fistula reaching down to the facial nerve trunk.

c Salivary fistulae directly after radiotherapy. The skin is burned within the region of radiation.

d Image 3 months after radiotherapy showing the absence of visible fistula.

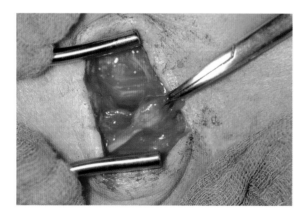

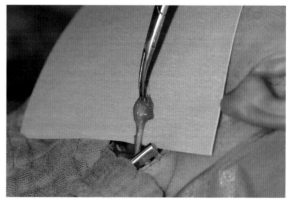

Fig. 22.9 Neuroma of the great auricular nerve several years after parotidectomy and sacrificing the nerve.

a Neurinoma within the clamp localized on the sternocleidomastoid muscle together with the proximal part of the greater auricular nerve.

b Neurinoma at the end of the greater auricular nerve prior to extirpation.

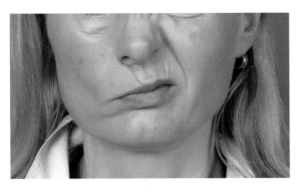

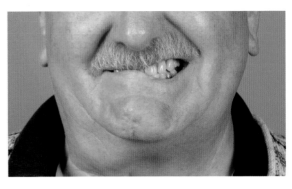

Fig. 22.10a,b Facial nerve paresis.

a Permanent facial nerve paresis (House V) 6 months after radical parotidectomy in the case of a malignant tumor of the right parotid gland. No reinnervation is yet visible after nerve grafting with the great auricular nerve.

b Transient facial nerve paresis (House III) after partial parotidectomy.

days 10 to 12 after the occurrence of the damage. In pronounced facial nerve pareses (House Index V and VI), it is particularly important to prevent damage to the cornea if lid closure is dysfunctional. In addition to eye ointments (e.g., retinol palmitate [vitamin A], thiamine chloride–HCl [vitamin B₁], calcium pantothenate), a watch-glass bandage is recommended during the night.

Definitive surgical treatment in the sense of a static or dynamic rehabilitation cannot be recommended until after at least 1 year because the nerve can continue to regenerate during this period. If the nerve is definitely not expected to recover until such a lengthy period has passed, a gold weight or platinum chain can be implanted until normal function is restored. This procedure can be reversed at any time.[46] It appears highly questionable whether manual physiotherapy, electrostimulation, biofeedback methods, or active exercise therapy will improve prognosis and the healing rate of facialis nerve pareses. Regarding Bell palsy, Teixeira et al[47] performed a systematic literature search, wherein these measures were not seen to have any significant efficacy. Other authors are of the opinion that physiotherapeutic measures can be used in the conservative treatment of peripheral facial nerve paresis and have a positive effect on the healing phase. The domain of physiotherapeutic measures is the treatment of medium-grade acute lesions and chronic partial lesions of the facialis nerve. In high-grade lesions, therapy concentrates more on functional improvement achieved by compensatory movements.[48] Synkinesis of the facial musculature during the healing phases can be treated effectively with injections of botulinum toxin.[49]

Frey Syndrome

Frey syndrome or gustatory sweating is reported to have an incidence of 2 to 80% depending on which method is applied in the investigation. Treatment is necessary in 10 to 15% of cases.[21,50] According to Nitzan et al,[32] 57% of all patients complain of this symptom following parotid surgery, albeit without any influence on the quality of life. The literature is concerned mainly with the avoidance of this complication. The interposition of fat transplants, fasciae, muscle, superficial musculoaponeurotic system [SMAS], or allogeneic material between the wound area and the subcutaneous tissue has been shown, more or less, to be questionable with variable long-term success.[51–53]

The decisive factor in avoiding the development of Frey syndrome is the extent of the surgical procedure. The lowest incidence in our patients was observed after partial surgical parotidectomy, and a significant positive correlation was found between the extent of the removed tissue and the incidence of Frey syndrome. Patient scores reflected the clinical results and correlated significantly with the extent of gland tissue removed. These findings are reflected in the literature.[20] If the gustatory sweating is very disturbing and cannot be influenced by local ointment or deodorant stick applications,[54,55] intracutaneous injection of botulinum toxin is currently the therapy of choice.

Affected skin areas are rendered visible by the Minor test and divided into areas of 1 cm² each. Then, 2.5 units botulinum toxin A are injected into each of these areas. Symptoms are suppressed for 6 to 9 months, after which the treatment must be repeated[49] (**Fig. 22.11a–c**). Alternatively, the efficacy of 1 to 2% glycopyrrolate (an anticholinergic) was also confirmed in an older double-blind study.[54] The effects lasted for several days after local application of ointment or cream.

Tumor Recurrence

Recurrence in malignant salivary gland tumors, and especially benign pleomorphic adenomas, can be considered a late complication (**Fig. 22.12a, b**). This particularly

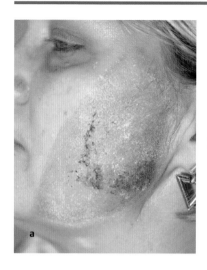

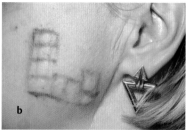

Fig. 22.11a–c Minor test.

a Frey syndrome after total parotidectomy. Minor test shows the skin regions (blue) of sweating.

b Skin marking and botox application in the areas of positive Minor test.

c Minor test 4 weeks after botox treatment. No visible gustatory sweating is present.

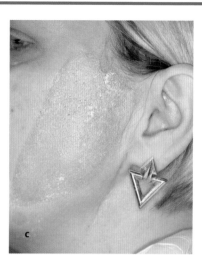

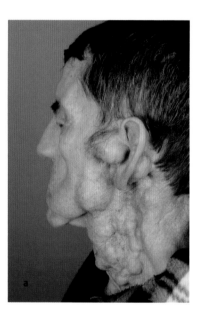

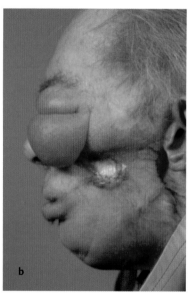

Fig. 22.12a,b Recurrences.

a Multiple recurrences of a benign pleomorphic adenoma in a 60-year-old male patient from Romania. He was operated on 30 years ago in his home country and again several years later. The facial nerve was already paretic. Though a benign disease, in this case radical surgery with removal of skin and tissue, together with a lateral thigh flap, had to be performed. Postoperative radiotherapy would have been useful in such a case.

b Recurrence of an undifferentiated salivary gland carcinoma after radical parotidectomy and chemoradiotherapy. A large edema of the orbit and free bone is visible. In this case, there was a clear indication for palliative therapy.

applies to advanced-stage and undifferentiated tumors. Therefore, postoperative monitoring of salivary gland malignancies for 10 years or longer is always obligatory.[56]

The situation is different for benign tumors, especially in the case of pleomorphic adenomas. The responsibility for recurrences has been repeatedly placed on inadequate resection (bare area) or tumor cell entrainment when tumors are opened during surgery.[57] The extent of primary tumor resection is a further factor currently being discussed in the literature.

The main argument against techniques of circumscribed partial resection, such as extracapsular dissection and partial parotidectomy, is the supposed increased risk of recurrence postulated to occur with these procedures. In this context, a clear distinction must be made between

the modern technique of extracapsular dissection and the historical technique of enucleation, which has recurrence rates of 20 to 40%. Several studies have shown that the recurrence rate of pleomorphic adenomas is no higher with extracapsular dissection than with superficial or total parotidectomy.[45,56,58,59] For example, after a mean follow-up period of 12.5 years, McGurk et al[60] found a recurrence rate of 2% with both extracapsular dissection ($n = 380$) and superficial parotidectomy ($n = 95$). Rehberg et al[45] reported recurrence rates of 2.3% after extracapsular dissection, 0% after superficial parotidectomy, and 15.4% after total parotidectomy. The recurrence rate reported with extracapsular dissection is therefore similar to that reported with superficial and total parotidectomy, namely 0 to 5%.[21,44,58,60]

The theoretical argument is that recurrence increases, in particular, in cases of pleomorphic adenomas, in cases of incomplete tumor capsules, and in the presence of pseudopodia or satellite nodules pushing through the capsule. Consequently, it would seem axiomatic that the risk of tumor recurrence is greater if dissection is performed on or close to the tumor in contrast to en bloc removal in superficial parotidectomy. Several studies have challenged the theory that an incomplete capsule is the main source of recurrence. Donovan and Conley[57] found that in 60% of supposedly en bloc resections performed as part of superficial parotidectomy, the tumor capsule was partially exposed when the facial nerve was dissected off its surface. Moreover, in 21% of cases, the tumor extended to the edge of the histologic specimen, whereas in a further 40% of cases, only an extremely narrow resection margin was present. Despite this, no increase in recurrence rate was demonstrated.

To define risk factors for recurrence, Ghosh et al[61] analyzed a series of 83 pleomorphic adenomas by re-evaluating the histologic slides. After a mean follow-up of 12.5 years, they found a recurrence rate of 17.6% in cases where tumor cells were present at the margin, but only 1.8% if they were found within 1 mm of, but not directly at, the margin. They therefore concluded that a layer of connective tissue consisting of a mere one or two cell rows is sufficient to prevent recurrence.

In a retrospective analysis of histologic specimens published in 2002, Witt[62] found that both extracapsular dissection and superficial and total parotidectomy almost always resulted in focal capsular exposure and that the recurrence rate did not differ between the various techniques.

Treatment of recurrence comprises an attempt to remove the often multilocal tumors entirely. As a final consequence, this may also frequently involve resection of the facial nerve. Radiotherapy can prevent a further recurrence in cases of microscopic residual tumors.[63]

Cosmetic Considerations and Quality of Life

Cosmetic results after parotid gland resection are discussed in the recent literature.[60,62,64] Nitzan et al[32] reported that, when asked in a questionnaire, 70% of patients stated that they felt disturbed by a change in their appearance after superficial or total parotidectomy, 60% because of scarring and 58% because of a local depression. However, a significant impact of these parameters on the overall quality of life could not be detected. Marshall et al[50] reported that 26.9% of patients recognized an altered shape of the skin soon after the operation, but only 3.1% reported long-term problems. Impaired cosmetic appearance after conventional parotid gland surgery was also described by physicians who were asked to judge patients using a visual analog scale from 0 to 10.[64]

The literature demonstrates that there is a need for therapy, and numerous modifications of the surgical technique designed to improve cosmetic results have been described. Particularly, the amount of gland tissue removed seems to be associated with depression of the facial contour. Roh et al[58] reported that patient scores regarding scar and cosmetic appearance were significantly better after performing partial compared with superficial or total parotidectomy. In our study, comparing total, superficial, and partial parotidectomy, nearly 80% of patients were not fully satisfied with the cosmetic result, but the mean scores were not severe. It is noteworthy that no significant correlation was determined between perception of cosmetic appearance and incidence of facial nerve paresis. The mean score value regarding their perceived general condition indicates no significant impact of any parotid surgery on this parameter.[20] This was in agreement with other previous studies, which failed to show any significant impact of parotidectomy on quality of life or global health status.[32,65,66] However, if only those patients who sustained complications were considered, the scores showed significant positive correlations with the scores of facial nerve paresis, Frey syndrome, sensory deficit of the auricle, and cosmetic appearance ($p = 0.01$ for each). This significant correlation points to a potential impact and need for prophylaxis or therapy.

The main factor for the avoidance of tissue deficit is to strive for the greatest possible circumscription of the procedure. For extensive defects, free fat transplants, pedicled rotation plasty of the sternocleidomastoid muscle, fillers such as Alloderm (LifeCell, Bridgewater, NJ, USA) or even free microvascular muscle flaps have been described.[67-69] To further hide the barely noticeable scars, the cutaneous incision can be made behind the tragus as in a facelift, then continued in the retroauricular direction up to the hairline.

Complications Following Submandibulectomy

Apart from problems such as scar formation, disturbances of skin sensation, and injury to the lingual nerve, McGurk et al[70] have published an update of the literature (16 series) concerning nerve morbidity and other possible complications in submandibular sialoadenectomy. The incidence of non-neural complications in 1,798 patients was as follows: hemorrhage 0 to 14%, fistula 0 to 4%, postoperative infection 0 to 14%, altered skin sensations 0 to 16%, and problems with scar formation 0 to 16%, transient and permanent palsy of the mandibular branch of the facial nerve was seen in 9.6% and 3.3% of patients, respectively. Regarding the effects on the lingual and hypoglossal nerves, transient palsies were encountered in 1.9% and 0.5% of patients, respectively, and permanent problems were found in 1.6% and 1.4% of patients, respectively.

Moreover, unilateral excision of the submandibular gland also leads to a significant reduction of the non-stimulated flow of saliva, which may have an important impact on oral hygiene, risk of caries, and development of xerostomia.[71]

For the avoidance of, as well as the treatment of, complications, the same conditions as for parotid gland surgery essentially apply. In this connection, it must also be mentioned that the most effective prevention of complications is to avoid the removal of the gland and the application and indication of gland-preserving methods. Iro et al[72] demonstrated, for example, that, only 3% of the glands need to be removed in the case of obstructive sialadenitis.

Sialendoscopy and Transoral Surgery

Sialendoscopy

Sialendoscopy is a minimally invasive method for the direct diagnosis of the pathologies of the duct system by direct visual inspection (diagnostic endoscopy) or the treatment of these pathologies (interventional endoscopy). The interventions include, apart from basket extraction or stone fragmentation, the widening and opening of duct stenoses. The procedures are accompanied in each case by retrograde irrigation with Ringer or physiologic saline solution, which can always cause post-interventional swelling and pain or even purulent sialadenitis.[3,4,73] The extent of the swelling correlates with the duration of the procedure. Other minor surgical measures in connection with sialoendoscopy include papillotomy with distal duct slitting of the Wharton duct and so-called minipapillotomy of Stenson duct. Extensive slitting of Stenson duct with marsupialization or duct reinsertion should be avoided as much as possible and are more of the nature of an last resort because of the high risk of duct stenosis[3] (**Fig. 22.13a, b**).

> **Note**
> Occasionally, manipulations at the duct ostium may result in painful swelling persisting for several days.

The follow-up after diagnostic endoscopy with no abnormalities includes gland massage by both the patient and physician. It is better to massage the gland vigorously three or four times a day than to do it gently once an hour. The important thing is to press first on the glandular parenchyma and then exert pressure with the hand moving outward toward the distal duct ostium. This must, without fail, be demonstrated repeatedly to the patient.

As a result of the risk of a bacterial sialadenitis following retrograde irrigation, each patient receives perioperative antibiotic prophylaxis, which is extended for 3 to 5 days depending on the duration of the procedure and symptoms immediately following surgery. The antibiotics of choice are: amoxicillin/sulbactam, amoxicillin/clavulanic acid, second-generation cephalosporin, roxythromycin, or clindamycin. Postoperative administration of nonsteroidal anti-inflammatory agents (e.g., naproxen 250 mg) allows, on the one hand, for adequate gland massage to be performed, and on the other, also reduces swelling. In the case of pronounced pain, medical therapy must be changed, e.g., to oral metamizole or intravenous paracetamol etc.

Management is the same for interventional endoscopy and diagnostic endoscopy. However, we recommend intravenous administration of the antibiotic and inpatient monitoring for 1 or 2 days after procedures that last more than 45 minutes. A single dose of 250 mg prednisolone is very effective in cases of highly pronounced postoperative glandular swelling.

If a minipapillotomy or distal duct slitting has been performed, stenosis prophylaxis is very important. If no secretion emerges by postoperative gland massage, the ostium should be carefully dilated, if necessary under local anesthesia and microscope control. We use a conical dilator, which is also used in tear duct surgery, to dilate the lacrimal puncta.

It is important to mention that, if the duct restenoses and the wound area shows clear signs of inflammation, immediate reopening of the duct is not necessary as a matter of principle. On the contrary, it is much more helpful to allow the local swelling and inflammation to heal first if the patient can tolerate the symptoms. After an interval of 4 to 6 weeks, it is much easier to carry out renewed surgical measures or a repeated endoscopy.

Chronic recurrent sialadenitis, in both adults and children, represents a special case regarding follow-up. After interventional endoscopy with intraoperative cortisone irrigation, the intraductal application of prednisolone (50 mg in adults) is recommended for 6 to 8 weeks. Following surface anesthesia with, for example, xylocaine spray, and dilatation of the ostium of the deferent duct, it is usually easy to introduce a 22-G venous indwelling needle into the duct. The medication is then introduced into the duct under relatively high pressure. The patient must then fast for 1 hour and not massage the gland, to allow the cortisone to act locally for as long as possible. Depending on the level of cooperation, the same procedure is, with exception, possible in children who are more than 5 to 7 years of age.

Repeated duct endoscopy is part of the follow-up in cases of persisting symptoms.

Transoral Surgery of the Salivary Glands

Transoral surgery of the salivary glands includes intervention on the deferent ducts of the submandibular,

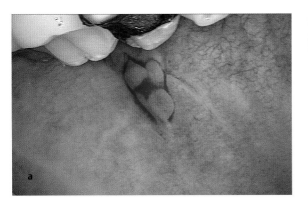

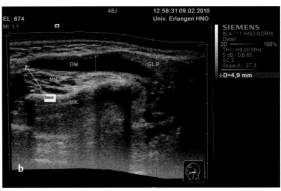

Fig. 22.13a,b Stensen duct.

a Stenosis and granulation tissue at the orifice of Stensen duct of the left side after the attempt at transoral stone removal in another institution. The stone was removed, although severe and painful stenosis developed weeks after the surgery.

b Horizontal plane of the ultrasound image showing a dilated Stensen duct (+...+ 4.9 mm, DW) proximal to the stenosis of the duct (arrow) on its course over the masseter muscle. Reopening of the duct was not possible, and parotidectomy was performed. MM, masseter muscle; UK, mandible; GLP, parotid gland.

sublingual, and parotid glands. In addition, tumors of the minor salivary glands, a ranula and the sublingual gland can be completely removed transorally. Transoral removal of the submandibular gland has also been described, but has not been established to date.[23]

Healing of the oral mucosa usually progresses well, so that even after extensive surgery, oral nutrition can initially be reinstated very quickly with liquids or pureed food. Patients undergoing extended duct slitting into the glandular hilus of the submandibular gland can usually begin with the re-establishment of a normal diet on the evening of the procedure.

Follow-up must focus on proper wound healing, prevention of infections and duct stenoses as well as on the recognition of complications (lesions of the lingual nerve [< 1%] or ranula after duct slitting [< 1%]).

Based on 1,000 transoral surgeries, the following measures have proved useful:[71,72]

- Use of absorbable suture material (Vicryl P3 4–0) avoids suture removal, which can be unpleasant.
- In the case of potentially inflammatory changes in the salivary glands, perioperative antibiotic prophylaxis is administered and can be extended according to the intraoperative findings.
- For the prophylaxis of postoperative edema and swelling, and therefore painful symptoms, a single perioperative dose of 250 mg prednisolone is particularly advisable for extensive surgical procedures. Caution is advised for patients with diabetes, gastric or duodenal ulcers, and glaucoma. In these cases, appropriate measures, such as monitoring blood glucose, administration of proton-pump inhibitors, or ophthalmologic monitoring are recommended.
- Antiseptic mouthwashes, such as Meridol (chlorhexidine-bis (D-gluconate) or Salviathymol (sage oil,

eucalyptus oil, peppermint oil, cinnamon oil, clove oil, fennel oil, anise oil, laevomenthol, thymol) are used to promote wound healing and cleaning, and can be applied hourly beginning immediately after surgery.

- In cases of severe postoperative pain and pain during glutition, pain relievers must be administered intravenously (e.g., paracetamol). In our experience, the administration of metamizole has proven useful. The administration of analgesics should be performed at regular intervals during the first days, and not just as required, because this facilitates food intake and therapeutic measures such as gland massage.

Typical Postoperative Complications

Rare postoperative bleeding can usually be stopped under local anesthesia with bipolar forceps or by compression with swabs. The avoidance of duct stenoses, especially in cases of extensive duct slitting, is achieved by checking the neo-ostium, which is located in the hilus of the gland, daily for the first 3 days, i.e., anterocaudal of the tonsillar region of the floor of the mouth. By medializing the tongue with the tongue depressor and exerting pressure on the affected gland, the expulsion and condition of saliva can be assessed. Dilatation may become necessary. Obstruction of the gland, impaired wound healing, swelling and the entire course of wound healing can be assessed with the aid of ultrasonography, but this is rarely performed after these interventions (less than 5%).

Marsupialization of a ranula due to reunification of the superficial mucosal layers may result in recurrence (**Fig. 22.14**). Attaching swabs with sutures has been recommended in the literature as a prophylactic measure.[74]

However, if a recurrence should still develop, the method of choice is complete removal of the sublingual gland with preservation of the submandibular duct and lingual nerve.

Postoperative disturbances in the supply area of the lingual nerve are usually caused by a stretching or pinching of the nerve. Total recovery usually occurs within 9 to 12 months. If the nerve itself, or part of it, is severed during intraoperative manipulation, neural suture should be attempted. Restoration of function is reported in ~ 90% of cases after 1 year.[75] The possibility of such an option should be discussed preoperatively with the patient. Overall, the likelihood of permanent nerve injury is significantly less than 1%.[71]

Extracorporeal Shock Wave Lithotripsy

During extracorporeal shock wave lithotripsy, shock waves are focused on a sialolith under ultrasound guidance. The stone is broken apart, ideally into fragment sizes of < 1.5 mm.

Although adverse effects are not generally observed, patients should be informed of the following major theoretical risks of the use of shock waves in the head-and-neck region:

- Bleeding, petechia
- Infection, formation of abscesses (< 5%)
- Subsequent gland removal (< 5%)
- Hearing impairment, tinnitus (< 0.1%)
- Potential tooth damage and eye injuries (in the case of improper use) (not seen reported).

Absolute contraindications are coagulation disorders and acute inflammation of the gland.[71]

Before shock wave treatment, as well as 1 hour and 1 day after lithotripsy, B-scan ultrasonography of the diseased gland is routinely performed. At the same time, a pure tone audiogram is performed in all patients before and 24 hours after treatment, to detect any potential treatment-related hearing loss.[71,76] Before treatment, oral analgesics may only be administered to patients who are very sensitive to pain. The treatment is performed under general anesthesia in children under 10 years of age.[76]

Before localization of the calculus in the instrument focus, cotton for hearing protection is inserted in the outer ear canal to protect the inner ear from acoustic trauma that could be caused by the loud pop resulting from shock wave generation.

After the equipment settings are established with the aid of sonography, shock wave application begins at

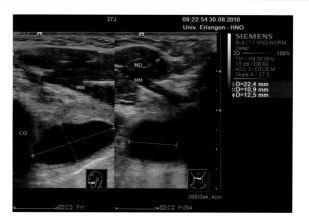

Fig. 22.14 Longitudinal and horizontal ultrasound image of a recurrent ranula (+...+) which developed after transoral surgery for a salivary stone and recurred even after marsupialization within the left sublingual gland. In this case, removal of the sublingual gland was indicated. CO, oral cavity very anteriorly near the chin; MM, mylohyoid muscle; MD, digastric muscle.

low intensity. With continuous ultrasound guidance and increasing intensity, treatment is continued up to the maximum shock wave count (3,000 to 5,000).

> **Note**
> Treatment is stopped prematurely if the sonographer can no longer locate the stone because it has been completely fragmented, or if a lack of cooperation on the part of the patient renders further treatment impossible.

Once a sialolith has been fragmented by the applied shock waves, the fragments are flushed out through the natural deferent duct of the gland. This process can be supported by so-called auxiliary measures performed by both the patient and the treating physician.

Sialagogues and gland massage ensure a continuous flow of saliva. In addition, the elimination of concrements is facilitated by a dilatation of the natural ostium, which is the narrowest part of the deferent duct system. If individual fragments are palpable or sonographically visible in the distal duct system near the ostium, extraction is attempted using a Dormia basket, guided either endoscopically or sonographically.

All patients receive oral doses of a prophylactic antibiotic (e.g., roxythromycin) and an anti-inflammatory agent (e.g., naproxen) administered on the day of treatment and continued for the first 2 days posttreatment.

Two or four months after this initial treatment, if symptoms still persist and/or residual concrements are still sonographically detectable, a second or third therapy session is held.

References

1. House JW, Brackmann DE. Facial nerve grading system. Otolaryngol Head Neck Surg 1985;93(2):146–147
2. Zenk J, Iro H, Klintworth N, Lell M. Diagnostic imaging in sialadenitis. Oral Maxillofac Surg Clin North Am 2009;21(3):275–292
3. Zenk J, Koch M, Bozzato A, Iro H. Sialoscopy—initial experiences with a new endoscope. Br J Oral Maxillofac Surg 2004;42(4):293–298
4. Koch M, Zenk J, Bozzato A, Bumm K, Iro H. Sialoscopy in cases of unclear swelling of the major salivary glands. Otolaryngol Head Neck Surg 2005;133(6):863–868
5. Cermik TF, Mavi A, Acikgoz G, Houseni M, Dadparvar S, Alavi A. FDG PET in detecting primary and recurrent malignant salivary gland tumors. Clin Nucl Med 2007;32(4):286–291
6. Salgarelli AC, Capparè P, Bellini P, Collini M. Usefulness of fine-needle aspiration in parotid diagnostics. Oral Maxillofac Surg 2009;13(4):185–190
7. Zbären P, Nuyens M, Loosli H, Stauffer E. Diagnostic accuracy of fine-needle aspiration cytology and frozen section in primary parotid carcinoma. Cancer 2004;100(9):1876–1883
8. Dulguerov P, Marchal F, Lehmann W. Postparotidectomy facial nerve paralysis: possible etiologic factors and results with routine facial nerve monitoring. Laryngoscope 1999;109(5):754–762
9. Wolf SR, Schneider W, Suchy B, Eichhorn B. Intraoperative facial nerve monitoring in parotid surgery. [Article in German] HNO 1995;43(5):294–298
10. Witt RL. Facial nerve monitoring in parotid surgery: the standard of care? Otolaryngol Head Neck Surg 1998;119(5):468–470
11. Olsen KD, Daube JR. Intraoperative monitoring of the facial nerve: an aid in the management of parotid gland recurrent pleomorphic adenomas. Laryngoscope 1994;104(2):229–232
12. Klintworth N, Zenk J, Koch M, Iro H. Postoperative complications after extracapsular dissection of benign parotid lesions with particular reference to facial nerve function. Laryngoscope 2010;120(3):484–490
13. Miehlke A. Die Chirurgie des Nervus facialis. Munich/Berlin: Urban & Schwarzenberg; 1960
14. Thumfart WF, et al. Operative Zugangswege in der HNO-Heilkunde. Stuttgart/New York: Thieme; 1998
15. Schauss F, Schick B, Draf W. Regional muscle flapplasty and adjuvant measures for rehabilitation of the paralyzed face. [Article in German] Laryngorhinootologie 1998;77(10):576–581
16. El Shazly M, Guindi S. Static management of lagophthalmos following facial nerve paralysis using standardized weights. Rev Laryngol Otol Rhinol (Bord) 2008;129(4-5):263–266
17. Mofle PJ, Urquhart AC. Superficial parotidectomy and postoperative drainage. Clin Med Res 2008;6(2):68–71
18. Jianjun Y, Haofu W, Yanxia C, et al. A device for applying postsurgical pressure to the lateral face. Oral Surg Oral Med Oral Pathol Oral Radiol Endod 1999;88(3):303–306
19. Wacha H, et al. Perioperative Antibiotika-Prophylaxe. Empfehlungen einer Expertenkommission der Paul-Ehrlich-Gesellschaft für Chemotherapie e.V. Chemother J 2010;19:70–84
20. Koch M, Zenk J, Iro H. Long-term results of morbidity after parotid gland surgery in benign disease. Laryngoscope 2010;120(4):724–730
21. Laccourreye H, Laccourreye O, Cauchois R, Jouffre V, Ménard M, Brasnu D. Total conservative parotidectomy for primary benign pleomorphic adenoma of the parotid gland: a 25-year experience with 229 patients. Laryngoscope 1994;104(12):1487–1494
22. Bova R, Saylor A, Coman WB. Parotidectomy: review of treatment and outcomes. ANZ J Surg 2004;74(7):563–568
23. Kauffman RM, Netterville JL, Burkey BB. Transoral excision of the submandibular gland: techniques and results of nine cases. Laryngoscope 2009;119(3):502–507
24. Rees TD, Liverett DM, Guy CL. The effect of cigarette smoking on skin-flap survival in the face lift patient. Plast Reconstr Surg 1984;73(6):911–915
25. Langdon JD. Complications of parotid gland surgery. J Maxillofac Surg 1984;12(5):225–229
26. Witt RL. The incidence and management of siaolocele after parotidectomy. Otolaryngol Head Neck Surg 2009;140(6):871–874
27. Chow TL, Kwok SP. Use of botulinum toxin type A in a case of persistent parotid sialocele. Hong Kong Med J 2003;9(4):293–294
28. Vargas H, Galati LT, Parnes SM. A pilot study evaluating the treatment of postparotidectomy sialoceles with botulinum toxin type A. Arch Otolaryngol Head Neck Surg 2000;126(3):421–424
29. Jianjun Y, Tong T, Wenzhu S, et al. Use of a parotid fascia flap to prevent postoperative fistula. Oral Surg Oral Med Oral Pathol Oral Radiol Endod 1999;87(6):673–675
30. Nixon PP, Ward SE. Tetracycline sclerotherapy for the treatment of recurrent pooling of plasma in the submandibular tissue space: case report. Br J Oral Maxillofac Surg 1999;37(2):137–138
31. Metson R, Alessi D, Calcaterra TC. Tetracycline sclerotherapy for chylous fistula following neck dissection. Arch Otolaryngol Head Neck Surg 1986;112(6):651–653
32. Nitzan D, Kronenberg J, Horowitz Z, et al. Quality of life following parotidectomy for malignant and benign disease. Plast Reconstr Surg 2004;114(5):1060–1067
33. Ellies M, Gottstein U, Rohrbach-Volland S, Arglebe C, Laskawi R. Reduction of salivary flow with botulinum toxin: extended report on 33 patients with drooling, salivary fistulas, and sialadenitis. Laryngoscope 2004;114(10):1856–1860
34. Christiansen H, Wolff HA, Knauth J, et al. Radiotherapy: an option for refractory salivary fistulas. [Article in German] HNO 2009;57(12):1325–1328
35. Schultz JD, Dodson TB, Meyer RA. Donor site morbidity of greater auricular nerve graft harvesting. J Oral Maxillofac Surg 1992;50(8):803–805
36. Patel N, Har-El G, Rosenfeld R. Quality of life after great auricular nerve sacrifice during parotidectomy. Arch Otolaryngol Head Neck Surg 2001;127(7):884–888
37. Colella G, Rauso R, Tartaro G, Biondi P. Skin injury and great auricular nerve sacrifice after parotidectomy. J Craniofac Surg 2009;20(4):1078–1081
38. Biglioli F, D'Orto O, Bozzetti A, Brusati R. Function of the great auricular nerve following surgery for benign parotid disorders. J Craniomaxillofac Surg 2002;30(5):308–317
39. Yokoshima K, Nakamizo M, Ozu C, et al. Significance of preserving the posterior branch of the great auricular nerve in parotidectomy. J Nippon Med Sch 2004;71(5):323–327
40. Witt RL. Facial nerve function after partial superficial parotidectomy: An 11-year review (1987–1997). Otolaryngol Head Neck Surg 1999;121(3):210–213
41. Gaillard C, Périé S, Susini B, St Guily JL. Facial nerve dysfunction after parotidectomy: the role of local factors. Laryngoscope 2005;115(2):287–291
42. Guntinas-Lichius O, Gabriel B, Klussmann JP. Risk of facial palsy and severe Frey's syndrome after conservative parotidectomy for benign disease: analysis of 610 operations. Acta Otolaryngol 2006;126(10):1104–1109

43. McGurk M, Renehan A, Gleave EN, Hancock BD. Clinical significance of the tumour capsule in the treatment of parotid pleomorphic adenomas. Br J Surg 1996;83(12):1747–1749
44. Guntinas-Lichius O, Kick C, Klussmann JP, Jungehuelsing M, Stennert E. Pleomorphic adenoma of the parotid gland: a 13-year experience of consequent management by lateral or total parotidectomy. Eur Arch Otorhinolaryngol 2004;261(3):143–146
45. Rehberg E, Schroeder HG, Kleinsasser O. Surgery in benign parotid tumors: individually adapted or standardized radical interventions?. [Article in German] Laryngorhinootologie 1998;77(5):283–288
46. Silver AL, Lindsay RW, Cheney ML, Hadlock TA. Thin-profile platinum eyelid weighting: a superior option in the paralyzed eye. Plast Reconstr Surg 2009;123(6):1697–1703
47. Teixeira LJ, Soares BG, Vieira VP, Prado GF. Physical therapy for Bell's palsy (idiopathic facial paralysis). Cochrane Database Syst Rev 2008; (3):CD006283
48. Paternostro-Sluga T, Herceg M, Frey M. Conservative treatment and rehabilitation in peripheral facial palsy. [Article in German] Handchir Mikrochir Plast Chir 2010;42(2):109–114
49. Laskawi R. The use of botulinum toxin in head and face medicine: an interdisciplinary field. Head Face Med 2008;4:5
50. Marshall AH, Quraishi SM, Bradley PJ. Patients' perspectives on the short- and long-term outcomes following surgery for benign parotid neoplasms. J Laryngol Otol 2003;117(8):624–629
51. Kim JT, Naidu S, Kim YH. The buccal fat: a convenient and effective autologous option to prevent Frey syndrome and for facial contouring following parotidectomy. Plast Reconstr Surg 2010;125(6):1706–1709
52. Ye WM, Zhu HG, Zheng JW, et al. Use of allogenic acellular dermal matrix in prevention of Frey's syndrome after parotidectomy. Br J Oral Maxillofac Surg 2008;46(8):649–652
53. Dulguerov P, Quinodoz D, Cosendai G, Piletta P, Marchal F, Lehmann W. Prevention of Frey syndrome during parotidectomy. Arch Otolaryngol Head Neck Surg 1999;125(8):833–839
54. Hays LL, Novack AJ, Worsham JC. The Frey syndrome: a simple, effective treatment. Otolaryngol Head Neck Surg 1982;90(4):419–425
55. Boles R. Parotid neoplasms: surgical treatment and complications. Otolaryngol Clin North Am 1977;10(2):413–420
56. Spiro RH. Salivary neoplasms: overview of a 35-year experience with 2,807 patients. Head Neck Surg 1986;8(3):177–184
57. Donovan DT, Conley JJ. Capsular significance in parotid tumor surgery: reality and myths of lateral lobectomy. Laryngoscope 1984;94(3):324–329
58. Roh JL, Kim HS, Park CI. Randomized clinical trial comparing partial parotidectomy versus superficial or total parotidectomy. Br J Surg 2007;94(9):1081–1087
59. Smith SL, Komisar A. Limited parotidectomy: the role of extracapsular dissection in parotid gland neoplasms. Laryngoscope 2007;117(7):1163–1167
60. McGurk M, Thomas BL, Renehan AG. Extracapsular dissection for clinically benign parotid lumps: reduced morbidity without oncological compromise. Br J Cancer 2003;89(9):1610–1613
61. Ghosh S, Panarese A, Bull PD, Lee JA. Marginally excised parotid pleomorphic salivary adenomas: risk factors for recurrence and management. A 12.5-year mean follow-up study of histologically marginal excisions. Clin Otolaryngol Allied Sci 2003;28(3):262–266
62. Witt RL. Minimally invasive surgery for parotid pleomorphic adenoma. Ear Nose Throat J 2005;84(5):308, 310–311
63. Samson MJ, Metson R, Wang CC, Montgomery WW. Preservation of the facial nerve in the management of recurrent pleomorphic adenoma. Laryngoscope 1991;101(10):1060–1062
64. Fee WE Jr, Tran LE. Functional outcome after total parotidectomy reconstruction. Laryngoscope 2004;114(2):223–226
65. Beutner D, Wittekindt C, Dinh S, Huttenbrink KB, Guntinas-Lichius O. Impact of lateral parotidectomy for benign tumors on quality of life. Acta Otolaryngol 2006;126(10):1091–1095
66. Kahn JB, Gliklich RE, Boyev KP, Stewart MG, Metson RB, McKenna MJ. Validation of a patient-graded instrument for facial nerve paralysis: the FaCE scale. Laryngoscope 2001;111(3):387–398
67. Walter C. The free dermis fat transplantation as adjunct in the surgery of the parotid gland (author's transl). [Article in German] Laryngol Rhinol Otol (Stuttg) 1975;54(5):435–440
68. Nosan DK, Ochi JW, Davidson TM. Preservation of facial contour during parotidectomy. Otolaryngol Head Neck Surg 1991;104(3):293–298
69. Baker DC, Shaw WW, Conley J. Reconstruction of radical parotidectomy defects. Am J Surg 1979;138(4):550–554
70. McGurk M, Makdissi J, Brown JE. Intra-oral removal of stones from the hilum of the submandibular gland: report of technique and morbidity. Int J Oral Maxillofac Surg 2004;33(7):683–686
71. Zenk J, Gottwald F, Bozzato A, Iro H. Submandibular sialoliths. Stone removal with organ preservation. [Article in German] HNO 2005;53(3):243–249
72. Iro H, Zenk J, Escudier MP, et al. Outcome of minimally invasive management of salivary calculi in 4,691 patients. Laryngoscope 2009;119(2):263–268
73. Koch M, Zenk J, Iro H. Diagnostic and interventional sialoscopy in obstructive diseases of the salivary glands. [Article in German] HNO 2008;56(2):139–144
74. McGurk M. Management of the ranula. J Oral Maxillofac Surg 2007;65(1):115–116
75. Bagheri SC, Meyer RA, Khan HA, Kuhmichel A, Steed MB. Retrospective review of microsurgical repair of 222 lingual nerve injuries. J Oral Maxillofac Surg 2010;68(4):715–723
76. Iro H, Schneider HT, Födra C, et al. Shockwave lithotripsy of salivary duct stones. Lancet 1992;339(8805):1333–1336

23 Minimally Invasive Approach to the Thyroid and Parathyroid Glands

P. Miccoli, G. Materazzi

Introduction

In 1996, Gagner[1] described endoscopic subtotal parathyroidectomy for secondary hyperparathyroidism, which represented the first application of a minimally invasive technique to the field of endocrine neck surgery. Since then, several minimally invasive approaches to the thyroid gland[2-7] have been described, all aiming to improve cosmetic outcome, reduce postoperative pain and improve postoperative recovery, either by performing the incision in an area that is not visible such as the axilla or around the nipple, or by minimizing hyperextension of the neck to reduce the length of the scar in the neck. **Table 23.1** summarizes the different mini-invasive approaches.

The development of these new techniques also added new types of complications to those already typical of traditional thyroid and parathyroid surgery. Subcutaneous emphysema was described first by Gottlieb et al[8] after endoscopic parathyroidectomy,[1] although this complication, also associated with hypercarbia and tachycardia, is possible during any endoscopic neck procedure in which the operative space is maintained by gas insufflation. In fact, the neck cannot be considered a predetermined cavity because it is not circumscribed by a continuous serosal layer such as the pleura or the peritoneum, which avoids massive passage of carbon dioxide from the cavity to the bloodstream. Some authors with extensive experience with the procedure suggest that lowering the carbon dioxide pressure to 4 mmHg can help to avoid subcutaneous emphysema.[9,10]

The gasless anterior neck skin-lifting method described by Shimizu and Tanaka[11] and based on the Nagai method for the abdomen,[12] in which the edges of the chest wall wound and the lateral neck wound are pulled by sutured threads to create the working space, can potentially create a new complication, namely the rupture of the skin through excessive traction.

In this chapter, we will discuss complications following a minimally invasive approach to the neck, both for thyroid and parathyroid glands, with particular focus on minimally invasive video-assisted thyroidectomy (MIVAT) and parathyroidectomy (MIVAP).

Video-assisted Thyroidectomy and Parathyroidectomy

These two techniques were first described in 1997 in Pisa, and, after more than 10 years, have gained acceptance worldwide as the preferred mini-invasive techniques for the surgical treatment of thyroid and parathyroid diseases, not only because they have similar results to traditional techniques concerning safety and curative results, but also because of improvements in postoperative course and cosmetic outcome.

Technique

Briefly, both techniques are characterized by a single central cervical incision, 1.5 cm in length, at the same level as Kocher's incision. Operative space is maintained by small retractors without gas insufflation. The operation is performed mostly endoscopically under magnified vision with a 30° 5-mm endoscope (**Fig. 23.1**). The dissection of the thyrotracheal groove is completed by using small (2 mm in diameter) instruments: atraumatic spatulas in different shapes, spatula-shaped sucker, ear-nose-throat forceps and scissors (**Fig. 23.2**). Coagulation and sectioning of principal vessels can be performed with any energy device (ultrasonic, high frequency, etc.) or by vascular clips and cauterization.

Indications

> **Note**
>
> Up to 15% of thyroid diseases with surgical indications can be treated by MIVAT, and ~ 80% of patients affected by primary hyperparathyroidism can be treated by MIVAP.

Table 23.1 Endoscopic minimally invasive thyroidectomy: different approaches

Cervical access	Breast access	Axillary access
Miccoli (video-assisted) central	Ohgami (endoscopic)	Ikeda (endoscopic)
Gagner (endoscopic)		
Shimizu (video-assisted) skin lifting method		

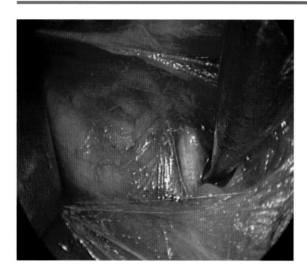

Fig. 23.1 Endoscopic vision during minimally invasive video-assisted thyroidectomy: the inferior laryngeal nerve is easily identified.

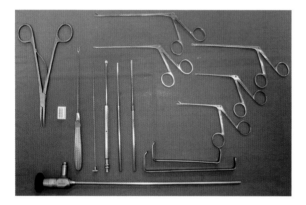

Fig. 23.2 Instruments for minimally invasive video-assisted thyroidectomy.

Exclusion criteria for these two techniques are: active thyroiditis, parathyroid adenomas > 4 cm, parathyroid carcinoma, goiter > 25 mL in total thyroid volume, thyroid carcinomas > 2 cm or synchronous metastases at the central or lateral compartments. Therefore, careful selection of patients is the only guarantee of a low incidence of complications and good outcome. An important limit is, at present, the volume of both the nodule and the gland. The parathyroid adenoma, as well as the thyroid nodule, has to be removed without disrupting their capsule because of the necessity for accurate histologic evaluation and to avoid cellular spread. Other limits of these techniques are the presence of adhesions that can make dissection difficult: this can happen in revision surgery, and also in thyroiditis unveiled both by increased thyroid antibodies and ultrasound aspects.

Complications

Injuries to the Inferior Laryngeal Nerve and External Branch of the Superior Laryngeal Nerve

During thyroidectomy and parathyroidectomy both the inferior laryngeal nerve (ILN) and the external branch of the superior laryngeal nerve (EBSLN) can be transiently or definitively injured. Nerve injury can be temporary (resolution within 6 months to 1 year) or definitive, monolateral or bilateral. The causes most frequently responsible for nerve damage are accidental sectioning of the nerve, perineural edema consequent to manipulation, stretching, and heating.

The EBSLN innervates the cricothyroid muscle, which is responsible for vocal fold tension and pitch modulation. The nerve is jeopardized during sectioning of the upper pedicle because of the variability of its course. The incidence of this complication is underestimated because symptoms are moderate and objective demonstration of damage is difficult. During MIVAT, endoscope magnification provides an optimal view of the EBSLN, which is far better than in an open field (**Fig. 23.3**).

The rate of injury to the ILN is highly variable depending on the characteristics of disease, type of procedure, and surgeon's experience. The rate of definitive palsy is around 1%, but ranges from 0.5 to 14% in the literature.[13-18] In our MIVAT series, the rate of injury to the ILN (both temporary and definitive) did not differ from literature reports. Complications included transient monolateral ILN palsy in 2.4% of cases, definitive monolateral palsy in 1.1%, and bilateral transient palsy in 0.3% of cases (**Table 23.2**). In addition, the ILN can be easily identified during MIVAT thanks to the magnification provided by the endoscope.

An excellent anatomical landmark when searching for the ILN is the posterior lobe of the thyroid because it generally lies over the nerve. In conventional surgery, the ILN is generally prepared where it emerges from the thoracic outlet, but this area can be difficult to visualize with the endoscope; the middle part of the thyroid gland is clearly visible and optimal nerve dissection can be performed.

Some concerns should be expressed about stretching the parenchyma and the ILN during the extraction phase. At the beginning of our experience, we recorded some transient nerve palsies that were probably a result of this maneuver. Since then, complete dissection of the nerve during the endoscopic phase and placing lower traction on the lobe during extraction have avoided this type of complication.

In addition, the incorrect use of the new harmonic scalpel can jeopardize the nerve. The surgeon should always remember to keep the inactive blade of the

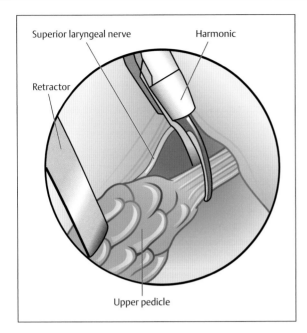

Superior laryngeal nerve

Harmonic

Retractor

Upper pedicle

Fig. 23.3 During the upper pole section, the surgeon should always keep the inactive blade of the instrument oriented to avoid jeopardizing the external branch of the superior laryngeal nerve, which always lies posterior to it.

instrument oriented during artery sectioning to avoid jeopardizing the nerve, which always lies posterior to it and is very sensitive to heat transmission (**Fig. 23.3**). Safety of the harmonic scalpel, with low thermal injury or energy diffusion, has been demonstrated by other authors.[19-24] However, we think that a minimal distance should be maintained between the inactive blade and the nerve, and small clips should be used when dealing with

Table 23.2 Minimally invasive video-assisted thyroidectomy: complications

Complication	Incidence
Transient monolateral recurrent nerve palsy	2.4%
Transient bilateral recurrent nerve palsy	0.3%
Definitive monolateral recurrent nerve palsy	1.1%
Transient hypoparathyroidism[a]	5.1%
Definitive hypoparathyroidism[a]	0.4%
Postoperative bleeding	0.3%
Wound infection	0.2%

[a] Hypoparathyroidism and recurrent nerve bilateral palsy rate is calculated on total thyroidectomies.

small vessels crossing the nerve near its entrance into the larynx.

During MIVAT and MIVAP, intraoperative nerve monitoring can also be used. In fact, nerve and laryngeal palpation or the use of magnifying glasses during MIVAT and MIVAP are not feasible given the small cervical incision. Some authors demonstrated that intraoperative nerve monitoring is feasible, easy, safe, and effective during MIVAT.[25-28] Terris et al[25] demonstrated that intraoperative nerve monitoring serves as an adjunct to visual identification of nerves in different minimal access thyroid procedures performed through incisions < 6 cm in length, both endoscopic, nonendoscopic, and reoperative cases. Dionigi et al[26] proposed a standardized intraoperative nerve monitoring technique with vagal stimulation during MIVAT. Regarding voice and swallowing changes in the absence of laryngeal nerve injury, MIVAT seems to have significant advantages compared with conventional thyroidectomy. Lombardi et al,[29] in a recently published study, found that even if voice and swallowing changes were reported in both groups of patients (MIVAT and conventional thyroidectomy), their comparison demonstrated that MIVAT had significant advantages. Indeed, patients in the MIVAT group had significantly lower postoperative scores at each time-point and showed a trend toward more rapid return to the preoperative condition. A similar trend was also observed for swallowing impairment. Patients who underwent MIVAT reported significantly lower scores at 1 week and 1 month after surgery. In conclusion, the study found that voice and swallowing changes are significantly less important and show a tendency to recover more rapidly in patients who undergo MIVAT.

This important finding likely has multiple causes. First, the reduction in surgical trauma of thyroidectomy seems to determine a better outcome. Nonetheless, the less extensive and finer dissection of the thyroid bed, which characterizes MIVAT, could be responsible for a reduced risk of lesion to the perivisceral neural plexus, formed by small branches connecting the recurrent laryngeal nerve, EBSLN and the sympathetic chain, which is considered to be involved in the pathogenesis of postthyroidectomy aerodigestive symptoms by some authors.[30,31] Finally, a functional component related to the reduced local neck pain, and consequently reduced psychologic reaction to postoperative stress, should be taken into account.[32]

Bleeding

> **Note**
>
> Bleeding is considered the most life-threatening neck complication.

Postoperative bleeding can be defined as early (within 10 hours) or delayed (after 10 hours). The former are often massive and require immediate reintervention for compressive hematoma, whereas delayed bleeding does not usually cause airway obstruction and is treated conservatively.

Intraoperative bleeding during either MIVAP or MIVAT can be controlled and resolved endoscopically with a hemostatic energy device or vascular clips. It is obvious that, as with any endoscopic procedure, it may be difficult to control high-flow bleeding because of the narrow space in which the surgeon is operating.

In our series, we have never experienced an intraoperative or postoperative hemorrhage after MIVAP, although there have been cases of intraoperative and postoperative bleeding after MIVAT. In most cases of intraoperative bleeding, we were able to control the vessel, but when required, a conversion to traditional cervicotomy was performed. This occurred in 0.08% of cases (two conversions in 2,383 cases for upper pedicle intraoperative bleeding). Postoperative bleeding after MIVAT occurred in nine patients (0.3%). In all patients, reoperation was required and traditional cervicotomy was the preferred option to re-explore the neck.

After MIVAT and MIVAP, no suction drainage is left in the neck. The wound is closed using glue, so the operative space must be completely dry at the end of the procedure. A partial advantage is the fact that MIVAT is performed only on small glands (maximum thyroid volume 25 mL), so additional risks from large vessels, highly vascularized glands, or large dissections are absent. Furthermore, energy devices (ultrasonic, radiofrequency scissors) assure good and usually definitive hemostasis.

Hypoparathyroidism

Hypoparathyroidism can be transitory (resolution within 6 months to 1 year) or definitive. It is considered to be the most frequent complication following total thyroidectomy. Transitory hypocalcemia is reported to be present in 0.5 to 16% of cases, and definitive hypocalcemia ranges from 0.5 to 12%.[13–18] In our MIVAT series, 5.1% of patients undergoing total thyroidectomy exhibited transient hypocalcemia, but only five complained of permanent hypocalcemia that necessitated substitutive therapy, so reducing the rate of permanent hypoparathyroidism to 0.4%. Parathyroid glands are generally visualized easily thanks to endoscope magnification, and their manipulation with spatulas is easier than in open surgery.

The incidence of transient and permanent hypoparathyroidism in our series is comparable to that described in the literature for traditional thyroidectomy. During the minimally invasive approach, we observed less trauma to parathyroid glands, confirmed by the healthy appearance of most glands at the end of the procedure and by the low rate of transient hypoparathyroidism. This can

probably be explained both by technically correct dissection (vascular supply is preserved by selective ligature of the branches of the inferior thyroid artery), and by the low lateral spread of energy produced by the harmonic scalpel.[33,34]

Wound Morbidity

The incidence of wound morbidity after thyroidectomy is 2 to 7%.[35–43] Wound complications after MIVAT or MIVAP are similar to those after traditional cervicotomy and are represented by seroma, hematoma, infection, cheloids, and adhesions. It is well accepted that video-assisted neck surgery is less traumatic than open surgery because the wound is minimal (1.5 to 2 cm) and tissue manipulation and dissection are reduced.[44,45] Literature reports confirm better cosmetic outcomes when comparing MIVAT with traditional thyroid surgery,[46,47] but paradoxically the small access through which instruments are introduced, stretching of wound edges by retractors and the use of energy (heating) devices, can be additional risks for unsightly scars after MIVAT and MIVAP.

We suggest covering the skin with a sterile film (Tegaderm; 3M, St. Paul, MN, USA) and using electrocautery with its blade protected by a thin film of sterile drape, leaving just the tip able to coagulate, to avoid damage to the skin or the superficial planes. At the end of the procedure wound edges are reapproximated by a few subcutaneous stitches and glue to avoid any external suture.

Only one study comparing wound outcome after MIVAT with traditional cervicotomy was published recently.[48] The author compared two groups of 56 patients undergoing thyroidectomy with a mean follow-up of 9 ± 2 months and found a significant difference in favor of MIVAT. In fact, in the control group, there were two seroma, one hematoma, three wound infections, and two cheloids, whereas only one cheloid was noted in the MIVAT group.

A minor proinflammatory response, fewer immunosuppressive effects and shorter hospitalization probably contribute to the lower rate of wound morbidity.

References

1. Gagner M. Endoscopic subtotal parathyroidectomy in patients with primary hyperparathyroidism. Br J Surg 1996;83(6):875
2. Hüscher CS, Chiodini S, Napolitano C, Recher A. Endoscopic right thyroid lobectomy. Surg Endosc 1997;11(8):877
3. Miccoli P, Berti P, Conte M, Bendinelli C, Marcocci C. Minimally invasive surgery for thyroid small nodules: preliminary report. J Endocrinol Invest 1999;22(11):849–851
4. Ohgami M, Ishii S, Arisawa Y, et al. Scarless endoscopic thyroidectomy: breast approach for better cosmesis. Surg Laparosc Endosc Percutan Tech 2000;10(1):1–4

5. Ikeda Y, Takami H, Sasaki Y, Kan S, Niimi M. Endoscopic neck surgery by the axillary approach. J Am Coll Surg 2000;191(3):336–340

6. Shimizu K, Akira S, Jasmi AY, et al. Video-assisted neck surgery: endoscopic resection of thyroid tumors with a very minimal neck wound. J Am Coll Surg 1999;188(6):697–703

7. Gagner M, Inabnet WB III. Endoscopic thyroidectomy for solitary thyroid nodules. Thyroid 2001;11(2):161–163

8. Gottlieb A, Sprung J, Zheng XM, Gagner M. Massive subcutaneous emphysema and severe hypercarbia in a patient during endoscopic transcervical parathyroidectomy using carbon dioxide insufflation. Anesth Analg 1997;84(5):1154–1156

9. Ochiai R, Takeda J, Noguchi J, Ohgami M, Ishii S. Subcutaneous carbon dioxide insufflation does not cause hypercarbia during endoscopic thyroidectomy. Anesth Analg 2000;90(3):760–762

10. Yeung GH. Endoscopic surgery of the neck: a new frontier. Surg Laparosc Endosc 1998;8(3):227–232

11. Shimizu K, Tanaka S. Asian perspective on endoscopic thyroidectomy—a review of 193 cases. Asian J Surg 2003;26(2):92–100

12. Ohki J, Nagai H, Hyodo M, Nagashima T. Hand-assisted laparoscopic distal gastrectomy with abdominal wall-lift method. Surg Endosc 1999;13(11):1148–1150

13. Bergamaschi R, Becouarn G, Ronceray J, Arnaud JP. Morbidity of thyroid surgery. Am J Surg 1998;176(1):71–75

14. Rosato L, Avenia N, Bernante P, et al. Complications of thyroid surgery: analysis of a multicentric study on 14,934 patients operated on in Italy over 5 years. World J Surg 2004;28(3):271–276

15. Gonçalves Filho J, Kowalski LP. Surgical complications after thyroid surgery performed in a cancer hospital. Otolaryngol Head Neck Surg 2005;132(3):490–494

16. Zambudio AR, Rodríguez J, Riquelme J, Soria T, Canteras M, Parrilla P. Prospective study of postoperative complications after total thyroidectomy for multinodular goiters by surgeons with experience in endocrine surgery. Ann Surg 2004;240(1):18–25

17. Shen WT, Kebebew E, Duh QY, Clark OH. Predictors of airway complications after thyroidectomy for substernal goiter. Arch Surg 2004;139(6):656–659, discussion 659–660

18. Fewins J, Simpson CB, Miller FR. Complications of thyroid and parathyroid surgery. Otolaryngol Clin North Am 2003;36(1):189–206, x

19. Ortega J, Sala C, Flor B, Lledo S. Efficacy and cost-effectiveness of the UltraCision harmonic scalpel in thyroid surgery: an analysis of 200 cases in a randomized trial. J Laparoendosc Adv Surg Tech A 2004;14(1):9–12

20. Cordón C, Fajardo R, Ramírez J, Herrera MF. A randomized, prospective, parallel group study comparing the Harmonic Scalpel to electrocautery in thyroidectomy. Surgery 2005;137(3):337–341

21. Gao L, Xie L, Li H, et al. Using ultrasonically activated scalpels as major instrument for vessel dividing and bleeding control in minimally invasive video-assisted thyroidectomy. [Article in Chinese] Zhonghua Wai Ke Za Zhi 2003;41(10):733–737

22. Shemen L. Thyroidectomy using the harmonic scalpel: analysis of 105 consecutive cases. Otolaryngol Head Neck Surg 2002;127(4):284–288

23. Miccoli P, Berti P, Raffaelli M, Materazzi G, Conte M, Galleri D. Impact of harmonic scalpel on operative time during video-assisted thyroidectomy. Surg Endosc 2002;16(4):663–666

24. Siperstein AE, Berber E, Morkoyun E. The use of the harmonic scalpel vs conventional knot tying for vessel ligation in thyroid surgery. Arch Surg 2002;137(2):137–142

25. Terris DJ, Anderson SK, Watts TL, Chin E. Laryngeal nerve monitoring and minimally invasive thyroid surgery: complementary technologies. Arch Otolaryngol Head Neck Surg 2007;133(12):1254–1257

26. Dionigi G, Boni L, Rovera F, Bacuzzi A, Dionigi R. Neuromonitoring and video-assisted thyroidectomy: a prospective, randomized case–control evaluation. Surg Endosc 2009;23(5):996–1003

27. Witzel K, Benhidjeb T. Monitoring of the recurrent laryngeal nerve in totally endoscopic thyroid surgery. Eur Surg Res 2009;43(2):72–76

28. Inabnet WB, Murry T, Dhiman S, Aviv J, Lifante JC. Neuromonitoring of the external branch of the superior laryngeal nerve during minimally invasive thyroid surgery under local anesthesia: a prospective study of 10 patients. Laryngoscope 2009;119(3):597–601

29. Lombardi CP, Raffaelli M, De Crea C, et al. Long-term outcome of functional post-thyroidectomy voice and swallowing symptoms. Surgery 2009;146(6):1174–1181

30. Pereira JA, Girvent M, Sancho JJ, Parada C, Sitges-Serra A. Prevalence of long-term upper aerodigestive symptoms after uncomplicated bilateral thyroidectomy. Surgery 2003;133(3):318–322

31. Lombardi CP, Raffaelli M, D'Alatri L, et al. Voice and swallowing changes after thyroidectomy in patients without inferior laryngeal nerve injuries. Surgery 2006;140(6):1026–1032, discussion 1032–1034

32. Lombardi CP, Raffaelli M, Princi P, et al. Safety of video-assisted thyroidectomy versus conventional surgery. Head Neck 2005;27(1):58–64

33. Miccoli P, Berti P, Dionigi G, D'Agostino J, Orlandini C, Donatini G. Randomized controlled trial of harmonic scalpel use during thyroidectomy. Arch Otolaryngol Head Neck Surg 2006;132(10):1069–1073

34. Meurisse M, Defechereux T, Maweja S, Degauque C, Vandelaer M, Hamoir E. Evaluation of the Ultracision ultrasonic dissector in thyroid surgery. Prospective randomized study. [Article in French] Ann Chir 2000;125(5):468–472

35. Bergamaschi R, Becouarn G, Ronceray J, Arnaud JP. Morbidity of thyroid surgery. Am J Surg 1998;176(1):71–75

36. Max MH, Scherm M, Bland KI. Early and late complications after thyroid operations. South Med J 1983;76(8):977–980

37. Flynn MB, Lyons KJ, Tarter JW, Ragsdale TL. Local complications after surgical resection for thyroid carcinoma. Am J Surg 1994;168(5):404–407

38. Johnson JT, Wagner RL. Infection following uncontaminated head and neck surgery. Arch Otolaryngol Head Neck Surg 1987;113(4):368–369

39. Brown BM, Johnson JT, Wagner RL. Etiologic factors in head and neck wound infections. Laryngoscope 1987;97(5):587–590

40. Tabet JC, Johnson JT. Wound infection in head and neck surgery: prophylaxis, etiology and management. J Otolaryngol 1990;19(3):197–200

41. Dionigi G, Rovera F, Boni L, Castano P, Dionigi R. Surgical site infections after thyroidectomy. Surg Infect (Larchmt) 2006;7(Suppl 2):S117–S120

42. Dionigi G, Rovera F, Boni L, Dionigi R. Surveillance of surgical site infections after thyroidectomy in a one-day surgery setting. Int J Surg 2008;6(Suppl 1):S13–S15

43. Bergenfelz A, Jansson S, Kristoffersson A, et al. Complications to thyroid surgery: results as reported in a database from a multicenter audit comprising 3,660 patients. Langenbecks Arch Surg 2008;393(5):667–673

44. Wichmann MW, Hüttl TP, Winter H, et al. Immunological effects of laparoscopic vs open colorectal surgery: a prospective clinical study. Arch Surg 2005;140(7):692–697

45. Dionigi R, Dominioni L, Benevento A, et al. Effects of surgical trauma of laparoscopic vs. open cholecystectomy. Hepatogastroenterology 1994;41(5):471–476

46. Dionigi G. Evidence-based review series on endoscopic thyroidectomy: real progress and future trends. World J Surg 2009;33(2):365–366

47. Duh QY. Presidential Address: Minimally invasive endocrine surgery—standard of treatment or hype? Surgery 2003;134(6):849–857

48. Dionigi G, Boni L, Rovera F, Rausei S, Dionigi R. Wound morbidity in mini-invasive thyroidectomy. Surg Endosc 2011;25(1):62–67

24 Open Neck Thyroid and Parathyroid Surgery

J. P. O'Neill, A. R. Shaha

Introduction

The great Greek physicians Hippocrates and Galen defined disease as a natural process and based treatment on observation and experience. Hippocrates is credited with naming cancer as *karkinoma* (carcinoma) because a tumor looked like a "crab" with its blood vessels extending from a hard, solid body like legs. The pain of cancer was also likened to the pinch of a crab. Galen used *oncos* to describe all tumors, the root for the modern word oncology. These visionary scientists believed that a tumor may arise from too much blood in the veins, or a flux of black bile mixed with blood producing a scirrhus, a tumor that could transmute into cancer. Cancers were identified, with warnings against treatment of the more severe forms. This approach set the template for Islamic medicine, which rapidly spread throughout the Arab Empire. Rhazes, the great Persian physician, warned that surgery generally made matters worse unless the tumor was completely removed and the incision was cauterized, while Paré confessed that he had never seen cancer cured by the knife. We have come a long way in terms of surgical oncology and tumor ablation but complications and morbidity are daily consequences of surgical adventure and ingenuity.

The American Cancer Society estimated that 46,670 new cases of thyroid cancer would be diagnosed in 2010 (American Cancer Society 2010). Surgical ablation is the main treatment of thyroid tumors within the thyroid bed and surrounding central and lateral lymphatic drainage basins. Thyroid tumors represent a fascinating group of heterogeneous neoplasms. Thyroid cancer is broadly divided into differentiated and undifferentiated cancers. Papillary and follicular carcinoma (well-differentiated thyroid carcinomas) arise from the follicular epithelium and are the most common thyroid malignancies. Thyroid differentiated cancers are followed by medullary thyroid carcinoma, anaplastic thyroid carcinoma and thyroid lymphoma (according to traditional teaching). A rare form of thyroid cancer would be metastases from breast or colon disease.

The male to female ratio is ~ 2.5 : 1, but this may be a conservative estimate. Presentation is largely during the fourth to fifth decades of life with a median age at presentation of 47 years. A thyroid nodule is the usual presenting feature of a thyroid neoplasm, with 275,000 new nodules detected annually in the United States.[1] An increasing number of incidental thyroid nodules are being identified through the use of ultrasonography by primary-care physicians. In general, the majority of patients with well-differentiated thyroid carcinoma have a favorable long-term prognosis with 10-year survival exceeding 90%. Several prognostic factors have been identified to segregate patients with well-differentiated thyroid carcinoma into a large group with a low risk of mortality and a small group with a high risk of mortality. At Memorial Sloan Kettering Cancer Center we stratify thyroid cancers as low, intermediate, or high risk using GAMES criteria: key prognostic factors include Grade, Age > 45 years old, Metastases, Extrathyroidal extension, and Size > 4 cm.[2] Almost 80% of patients fit into the low-risk category, with an overall mortality rate of 1 to 2%. About 20% of patients fit into the high-risk category with a mortality rate of nearly 50%. Thyroid cancer is controversial, because differentiated thyroid malignancies are implicated in the carcinogenesis of the most aggressive human tumor, anaplastic thyroid cancer.

Historically, thyroid surgery, for both benign and malignant disease, was a feared procedure with high mortality rates related to vascular and septic insults. The term "thyroid" (Latin: "shield-shaped") is attributed to Bartholemeus Eustacius of Rome while Thomas Wharton of London named it "glandular thyroidoeis" in his *Adenographia* in 1656. In the late eighteenth century, Frederick Ruysch of Leyden suggested that the gland had a secretory role whereas Caleb Hillier Parry of Bath described thyroid function as a vascular reservoir preventing "brain engorgement". In more recent times, the Nobel Prize winner Theodor Kocher was appointed to the Chair of Surgery in Bern in 1872 and began his landmark surgery with the use of antiseptic techniques, arterial ligation, and precise dissection within the capsule. His progressive understanding of the dangers of capsular trauma rendered the operation less morbid and increasingly oncologic. He initially recorded mortality rates of 13 of 101 procedures, but Kocher also collected data on a further 268 operations performed since 1877, finding that mortality for nonmalignant goiter had fallen to 12% and for malignant goiter to 57%. As more patients survived the surgery, greater insights into the postoperative sequelae were experienced, including recurrent laryngeal nerve injury, myxedema, and tetany. These were identified as serious postoperative complications, encouraging a more cautious resection and a more precise technique by extracapsular dissection. By the time Kocher was awarded the Nobel Prize, with dedicated surgical appraisal and modification, the mortality for a thyroidectomy for simple goiter, in his hands had fallen to less than 1%.[3]

The parathyroid glands were first discovered in the Indian Rhinoceros by Richard Owen in 1850. It took a further 30 years before Ivar Viktor Sandström (1852–1889), a Swedish medical student, in 1880 identified these organs in humans. It was the last major organ to be recognized in humans.[4]

Anatomy

Thyroid Gland

Vascularity

The thyroid is a highly vascular gland located anteriorly in the lower neck, extending from the fifth cervical vertebra down to the first thoracic vertebra. The gland is formed by two elongated lateral lobes with superior and inferior poles connected by a median isthmus (with an average height of 12 to 15 mm) overlying the second to fourth tracheal rings. Each lobe is 50 to 60 mm long, with the superior poles diverging laterally at the level of the oblique lines on the laminae of the thyroid cartilage. Thyroid weight varies but averages 25 to 30 g in adults. A conical pyramidal lobe often ascends from the isthmus or the adjacent part of either lobe (more often the left) toward the hyoid bone. The vascularity stems from the superior thyroid artery, which is the first branch of the external carotid artery, the inferior thyroid artery originating from the thyrocervical trunk and occasionally a thyroid ima vessel originating from the aortic arch or brachiocephalic artery. Detailed understanding of the surgical anatomy including anomalous anatomy is necessary for low surgical morbidity.

Lymphatic Drainage

Lymphatic drainage of the thyroid gland is extensive and flows multidirectionally. The lymphatics are key to thyroid surgery and have obvious implications for oncologic surgery. Four principal lymphatic collecting trunks drain the thyroid. The inferomedial channels drain into the pretracheal and paratracheal lymph nodes (most common route of metastasis). The superomedial channels terminate in the prelaryngeal node ("Delphian node"). The superolateral channels drain into the nodes of the upper internal jugular vein and finally the inferolateral channels extend into the supraclavicular and jugulo-subclavian nodes.

Rouvière described a lymphatic vessel that occurred in one-fifth of the cadaver dissection specimens. This vessel (the posterosuperior collecting trunk) drains the upper pole of the thyroid into the retropharyngeal lymphatic system. Several authors state that the retropharyngeal space communicates with the parapharyngeal space through a dehiscence of the fascia of the superior constrictor muscle. This dehiscence allows metastatic disease to involve the parapharyngeal space.

Parathyroid Glands (Fig 24.1)

The parathyroid glands are four or more small glands located on the posterior surface of the thyroid gland. The parathyroid glands usually weigh between 25 and 40 mg in humans. Occasionally, some individuals may have six parathyroid glands. The parathyroid glands are quite easily recognizable histopathologically from the thyroid, as they have densely packed cells, in contrast with the follicular structure of the thyroid. However, in surgery, they are harder to differentiate from the thyroid or fat and may be devascularized, especially during a central neck dissection for disseminated thyroid cancer.

Recurrent Laryngeal Nerve

The recurrent laryngeal nerve (RLN) innervates the intrinsic laryngeal musculature and supplies sensory innervation to the glottis. The embryology of this nerve begins in its relation to the sixth branchial arch and is associated with the sixth arch arteries. The ventral aspects of the sixth arch arteries become the pulmonary arteries. The dorsal aspects of the sixth arch arteries disappear, allowing the RLN to ascend to the larynx. The fifth arch arteries regress early in development so the RLN is hooked by the

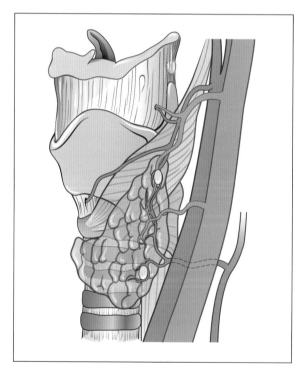

Fig. 24.1 The parathyroid glands receive their blood supply from branches of the inferior thyroid artery and, less frequently, from the superior thyroid artery.

fourth arch vessels. The fourth arches on the right and left sides become the subclavian artery and the aortic arch.

Axons of the recurrent laryngeal nerve are grouped within the vagus nerve. As this nerve travels through the skull base via the jugular foramen it lies anterior to the jugular vein. The left vagus nerve follows the carotid artery into the mediastinum crossing the aortic arch anteriorly. The left RLN loops under the aorta medially and ascends the tracheoesophageal groove and is approximately 12 cm from the aorta to the cricothyroid joint. Multiple studies have attempted to document the relationship of the inferior thyroid artery to the RLN.[5] The inferior thyroid artery lies anterior to the left RLN in 50 to 55% of patients. The nerve lies anterior to the artery in 11 to 12% of patients. In all remaining patients the nerve rests between the distal arteriolar branches.

The right RLN is a shorter nerve at 5 to 6 cm from the subclavian to the cricothyroid joint. As the right vagus nerve courses along the cowmmon carotid artery, at the division of the innominate artery the right RLN loops around the subclavian artery and travels along the right superior lobe pleura. It enters the tracheoesophageal groove more laterally than the left side behind the common carotid artery. In less than 1% of patients the nerve branches directly from the right vagus at the level of the thyroid gland and is always associated with an anomalous retroesophageal location of the right subclavian artery. The variability of this vessel and its position relative to the RLN make it a poor surgical landmark; however, ligation of the artery should not be performed until the RLN has been correctly identified. At the inferior constrictor muscle the nerve passes deep, posterior to the cricothyroid joint. It is within the larynx where the nerve splits into sensory and motor components. Extralaryngeal division of the RLN is well described and estimated at 35 to 80% of dissections.[6] The consistent theme on reports of the course of this nerve is the variability of its anatomical path. Traditional techniques advocate identification of the mid to inferior segment close to the inferior thyroid artery; however, many surgeons search for the distal segment just below Berry's ligament. This has the advantage of preventing disruption of the blood supply to the inferior parathyroid gland. The only disadvantage of identification of the nerve at the distal segment is the presence of a large tubercle of Zuckerkandl. This tubercle can be classified as grade I, II, and III and can be found in up to 80% of patients undergoing thyroidectomy. Grade I < 0.5 cm, grade II 0.5 to 1.0 cm and grade III > 1 cm. In an otherwise small goiter, a grade III tubercle may be associated with significant compressive symptoms.

The anomalous position of a nonrecurrent laryngeal nerve predisposes the nerve to injury during thyroid surgery and compression by a thyroid mass. A nonrecurrent nerve arises when the fourth arch on the right side disappears and the right subclavian artery arises from the dorsal part of the aortic arch. The right RLN now does not have a recurrent route and directly joins the larynx. There are no convincing reports of a left sided nonrecurrent nerve. Nonrecurrent RLNs are rare but an awareness of their existence and correct surgical technique will prevent the surgeon from iatrogenic trauma if one is encountered.

Thyroid Surgery

Thyroidectomy is not an infrequent operation. In the modern era surgical specialization and correct oncologic management demand a more sophisticated approach to thyroid and parathyroid surgery. Anything less may contribute to early tumor recurrence, incorrect therapeutic approach to lateral neck disease, or unnecessary postoperative sequelae. There are definitive data to suggest that low operative volume is associated with a higher incidence of complications. This is true for both surgical trainees and established surgeons.[7] Surgical volume also influences the failure pattern after parathyroidectomy for hyperparathyroidism.[8] From a technical point of view, the experienced thyroid surgeon is well versed in the normal and aberrant anatomy of the thyroid gland and the necessary maneuvers required preventing complications. More importantly, the surgeon is equipped to identify and deal with unexpected pathology that may require additional procedures such as jugular vein resection, central compartment nodal dissection, or selective lateral compartment nodal dissection. As a tertiary referral center, we often deal with patients who have had suboptimal thyroid surgery, and with issues in reoperative thyroid surgery. Hence, we have made a conscious attempt to reduce the need for secondary thyroid surgery. Shaha[9] reported less than 3% incidence of completion thyroidectomy, suggesting that the best and most appropriate treatment decisions are made during the first surgical procedure. This was achieved through careful preoperative and intraoperative assessment of the primary pathology and correct surgical management during the first procedure.

Superior Laryngeal Nerve (Figs. 24.2, 24.3, 24.4)

Injury to the external branch of the superior laryngeal nerve (SLN) is often underestimated, and there are no objective measurements in place to confirm it. Patients usually complain of voice fatigue, inability to shout, scream, or sing. This can be a significant morbidity to professionals, such as singers, whose voice is the basis of their careers. Injury rates have been reported to range from 1 to 5%, but the actual figure is likely to be higher as confirmation of SLN injury may be difficult. Patients at risk include those with high-riding thyroid glands, with a nodule at the upper pole, or large goiters. Direct visualization of the nerve is possible in more than 60%

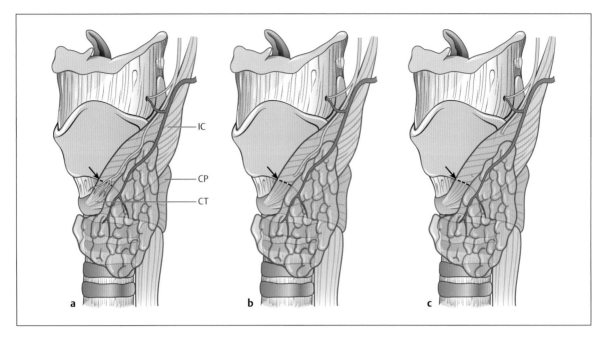

Fig. 24.2a–c Variations in the anatomic relationship of the main trunk of the external branch of the superior laryngeal nerve to the inferior constrictor (IC) muscle and superior thyroid pedicle.

a The external branch of the superior laryngeal nerve descends superficial to the inferior constructor (IC) muscle along the superior thyroid vessels so that it is visible in its entire course before innervating the cricothyroid (CT) muscle.

b The external branch of the superior laryngeal nerve pierces the inferior constructor (IC) muscle ~ 1 cm above the cricothyroid membrane (red arrow) so that only its upper portion is at risk for injury.

c The external branch of the superior laryngeal nerve runs deep to the inferior constructor (IC) muscle and, therefore, is protected from unintended injury during dissection in the vicinity of the superior thyroid pole. The cricopharyngeus muscle is marked CP.

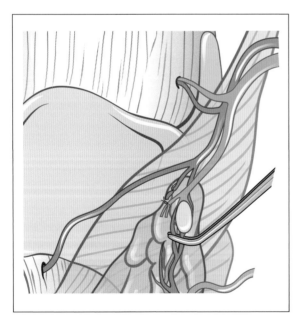

Fig. 24.3 The technique of individual vessel ligation allows the surgeon to delineate the thyroid parenchymal tissue at the superior pole from its surrounding structures, minimizing risk for injury to the external branch of the superior laryngeal nerve.

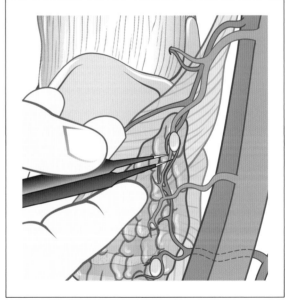

Fig. 24.4 As the superior pole tissue drops down away from the external branch of the superior laryngeal nerve, the remaining small blood vessels, especially those in the vicinity of the superior parathyroid gland, can be cauterized safely with fine-tipped bipolar electrocautery.

of cases. This, however, places the nerve at unwanted increased risk of injury. When dissecting the prelaryngeal and pretracheal fascia, care should be taken not to injure the cricothyroid muscle, which may be adherent to the thyroid gland.

An improved technique of SLN protection involves downward and lateral traction of the superior pole, which exposes the Joll triangle, the anatomical space between the superior thyroid vessels, superior pole of the thyroid, and cricothyroid muscle. The superior thyroid vessels are then ligated and divided close to the upper pole. This maneuver is effective in preventing SLN injuries in most situations.

Recurrent Laryngeal Nerve (Figs. 24.5 and 24.6)

A rich heritage of scientific investigation and research has considered the complexity of vocal cord function, laryngoscopic presentation, and surgical rehabilitation. In 1855, Garcia, an opera teacher, first described mirror laryngoscopy which, despite flexible endoscopy, remains an excellent, fast, and safe investigation, especially in the preoperative thyroid setting for evaluation of symmetrical vocal cord mobility or evaluation of tongue-base tumors. From this technique came direct laryngoscopy and laryngotracheal intubation.

Injury to the RLN can be caused by a variety of insults. The best way to avoid morbidity is routine identification of the nerve. Vocal fold paresis or paralysis may have a devastating impact on the patient's life especially in an unanticipated situation. Furthermore, hoarseness is likely to become a more disabling condition as voice recognition becomes central to forms of technology and replaces manual information entry such as typing and keyboarding.

What is crucial to RLN injury is that the extent of the injury is not necessarily apparent at the time of surgery. This also corresponds to the fact that RLN dysfunction may be present in the preoperative condition without obvious clinical indication. Therefore, in the interest of best practice the surgeon must protect the patient's interests and his own.

Neural disruption may be mediated by iatrogenic means, thermal damage, sharp dissection, stretching, retraction and compression, neurotoxic pharmaceutics and endocrine alteration at the time of operating, existing pathologic process, and neoplastic changes exerting pressure on the laryngeal nerves or strap muscles in thyroid surgery and inducing paresis or paralysis on the vocal fold. Despite no apparent surgical insult, up to 2% of patients may have an RLN vocal cord paralysis without any recognized intraoperative event. Up to 50% of patients with paralysis of their vocal cord may be asymptomatic.[10,11] Given its length, the left RLN is more frequently involved and therefore may encounter a greater number of pathologies and surgical interventions. Multiple series within the literature still hold surgery accountable for more RLN injury than tumor. One study estimates that in 75% of their 325 patients, the RLN paralysis was secondary to surgical intervention.[12] Thyroid surgery, above all interventions, remains the most common surgical procedure associated with iatrogenic RLN paralysis. Estimation

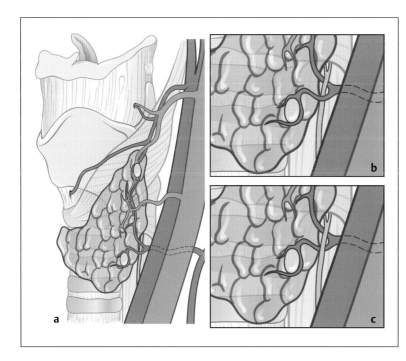

Fig. 24.5 Variations in the relationship of the recurrent laryngeal nerve (RLN) to the inferior thyroid artery and its branches. Most commonly, the RLN courses deep to the inferior thyroid artery and its branches (a), but it may lie between the branches (b) or anterior (c) to the artery.

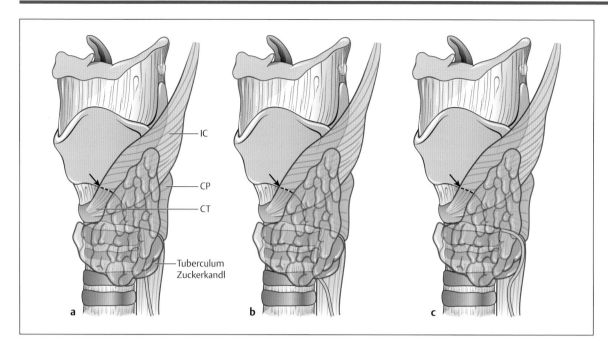

Fig. 24.6a–c Variations in anatomic relationships of the recurrent laryngeal nerve (RLN) to the Zuckerkandl tubercle. The RLN generally courses deep to the Zuckerkandl tubercle and superficial to the lateral border of the trachea **(a)** but it may run medial to it **(b)**. Nodular enlargement of thyroid tissue in the location of the tubercle **(c)** may displace the RLN laterally around it, placing the nerve at risk for injury if this variation is not recognized. IC, inferior constrictor muscle; CP, cricopharyngeus muscle; CT, cricothyroid muscle.

of nerve damage varies and has been reported as 0.2%,[13] 6.6%,[14] and 13.2%[15] of patients.

All endocrine surgeons should be competent at vocal cord evaluation. The American Association of Endocrine Surgeons has embraced this idea and is now developing courses in basic laryngeal fiberoptic evaluation. This can be interpreted as a clear change in policy ideology as their 2002 guidelines fail to even mention preoperative endoscopic evaluation.

Flexible endoscopy is a fast, cost-effective, safe and high yielding procedure that works in the interests of best practice. In protecting the patient, you are also protecting the surgeon. Preoperative visualization aids counseling the patient, outlines the operative degree of dissection and compartmental clearance strategy, and minimizes the medicolegal ramifications of iatrogenic injury. This is standard procedure in leading oncology institutions internationally.[11]

Operative Assessment

Recurrent laryngeal nerve monitoring is controversial. Many conventionally trained surgeons believe that visual identification and meticulous dissection obviate the necessity of RLN monitoring. Increasingly surgeons in training are accustomed to nerve monitoring and, provided an attitude of dependence is not fostered, this can be a helpful adjunct.

Conventional RLN monitoring techniques consist of electrode placement at the cricoarytenoid muscle either by direct needle placement, endoscopic hook, or a special endotracheal tube and a stimulator electrode in contact with the nerve. Monitoring does not significantly change the occurrence of transient recurrent laryngeal nerve paralysis; however, it has been reported to reduce the incidence of permanent paralysis and is a safe and easy to use surgical tool. Neuromonitoring has also been advocated to reduce the risk of vocal cord palsy and to predict postoperative vocal cord function. It must be acknowledged, however, that the literature has recently reflected reports of an overall statistical dissatisfaction with this method. Intraoperative neuromonitoring during thyroid surgery is not necessary for all thyroid surgical cases. We believe that it is of benefit in high-risk patient populations. A recent assessment of 1000 nerves at risk found that RLN monitoring during thyroid surgery conferred no benefit compared with routine RLN identification. They did however report that within their high-risk patients undergoing secondary thyroidectomy, a positive trend emerged in the reduction of overall, transient, and permanent postoperative RLN palsy rates from 19%, 14.2%, and 4.8% to 7.8%, 5.2%, and 2.6%.[16,17]

Intraoperative determination of RLN function may also be evaluated using a nerve stimulator and palpating for a contraction of the posterior cricoarytenoid muscle while the stimulus is applied. Postoperative assessment of RLN integrity is then determined by direct or indirect laryngoscopy to visualize vocal fold mobility. This technique reports a sensitivity of 75% and specificity of 92.2%.[18] In the postoperative course, RLN and vocal cord mobility can be inspected by a variety of means including nerve stimulation, cricothyroid palpation, or the use of bronchoscopic equipment for direct visualization (employment of the Hopkins II rod or flexible laryngoscopy).

Previous thyroid surgery, external beam radiation or radioiodine therapy can increase the risk of accidental RLN disruption. In these cases, it may be prudent for the surgeon to use a nerve monitoring device such as the NIM Response 2.0 Nerve Integrity Monitoring system, which we commonly use in difficult scenarios. This is an electromyographic system that uses a specialized endotracheal tube with electrodes that monitor activated laryngeal musculature secondary to a stimulus, which can be unwanted pressure, thermal activation from electrocautery, or deliberate stimulation using a special probe/wand. While some studies have shown an advantage in using this system, others have suggested that nerve monitoring adds no further advantage to careful identification and meticulous dissection of the nerve. We feel that the greatest benefit in nerve monitoring is in situations where we anticipate extensive disease and a hostile neck secondary to scarring from previous procedures. Hence we limit our use of the nerve monitoring system to cases where we anticipate technical difficulties.

Managing nerve injury is usually disappointing. If a transected nerve is identified intraoperatively, every effort should be made to repair this either directly by suturing the perineural layer using fine nonabsorbable sutures (7–0 or 8–0 Prolene) or a cable graft using an adjacent nerve (ansa cervicalis or branches of the cervical plexus). Permanent paralysis may require medialization procedures such as cord injection (using collagen, fat, or hydroxyapatite) or a type 1 thyroplasty using a Gore-Tex implant. Patients at risk for bilateral nerve injuries require careful extubation and fiberoptic examination of their vocal cords before transfer out of the operating room. If both cords are paralyzed, the patient may require a tracheotomy.

Complications (Fig. 24.7)

Bleeding and Wound Hematoma

Hematoma after thyroid surgery is reported at 1%.[19] Postoperative bleeding often warrants rapid intervention to prevent airway issues and hypoxia. The major issues are evacuating the hematoma and securing the airway, and there may be a need to achieve this at the bedside. If the wound needs to be opened, it is important for the physician (often a junior resident) to open both superficial and

- Bleeding and hematoma
- Nerve injuries
  - Recurrent laryngeal nerve
  - Superior laryngeal nerve
  - Cervical sympathetic trunk (Horner syndrome)
- Parathyroid injury and hypoparathyroidism
  - Temporary
  - Permanent
- Airway problems
  - Tracheal injury
  - Tracheomalacia
  - Laryngeal edema
- Wound issues
  - Seroma
  - Infections
- Scar issues
  - Hypertrophic scar
  - Keloids
- Chyle leak
- Hypothyroidism
- Recurrent hyperthyroidism
- Recurrent malignant disease
  - Thyroid bed
  - Nodal

Fig. 24.7 Complications of thyroid surgery.

deep layers to relieve the pressure effect of the hematoma. Intubation is usually still possible despite the laryngeal edema, but may have to be presumptive: the vocal cords are usually not seen and the tube may have to be guided just behind the epiglottis. Fiberoptic laryngoscopy and intubation may be considered in select circumstances. In these cases, an experienced Head and Neck Surgeon may be required to perform a fiberoptic nasoendoscopy and intubation. Rarely, an emergency tracheotomy may be required, but this can be easily achieved when the wound is opened, as the trachea would be completely exposed once the deep muscle layer is opened. Re-exploration often does not yield a specific bleeding source. After irrigation, it may be prudent to line the thyroid bed with one of many commercially available procoagulant materials and leave a drain before closure.

Airway obstruction does not occur secondary to tracheal compression, but as the result of a "central compartment pressure and congestion" that results in laryngeal edema. More than half of these cases occur within the first 6 hours after surgery; however, a further 25 to 40% can still occur between 6 and 24 hours postoperatively, which is why many surgeons remain reluctant to embrace the concept of "day case" ambulatory thyroid surgery.

- Extensive malignant primary disease
  - Concomitant Graves disease
  - Extensive nodal disease
  - Extrathyroidal extension
  - Substernal extension
- Extensive planned surgery
  - Paratracheal dissection
  - Neck dissection
  - Manubrium/sternal split
- Reoperative thyroid surgery
- Previous external beam radiation
- Previous radioactive iodine treatment
- Reoperation for hematoma
- Inexperienced surgeon

Fig. 24.8 Risk factors for increased complication rates.

Preoperative identification of at-risk patients is important to reduce the overall consequence of bleeding (**Fig. 24.8**). This includes identification of patients with bleeding diatheses or on antiplatelet or anticoagulant drugs. We have a general policy to stop the intake of antiplatelet agents (e.g., aspirin, clopidogrel, ticlopidine) at least 7 to 10 days before surgery. Patients with Graves disease are also at higher risk for postoperative bleeding. Lugol iodine may also be used before surgery to reduce the vascularity of the gland. Iodine reduces thyroid cellularity and vascularity and therefore is used in the preparation of patients for thyroidectomy. This effect transiently blocks thyroid hormone generation, with thyroid hormone synthesis recovering in a few days or weeks. It has been related to decreases in both angiogenic stimuli and blood flow in Graves disease. Decreased angiogenesis and blood flow results in a significantly decreased number of vessels. This has therefore been estimated to have a significant reduction in intraoperative blood loss.[20]

Meticulous hemostasis is mandatory during surgery. This can be achieved with the available armamentarium of existing devices available for hemostasis. Novel devices such as the "Harmonic scalpel" and "Ligasure" have been shown to be effective in ensuring hemostasis, without the need to leave foreign body material in the thyroid bed. However, simple ligation with silk or vicryl sutures is just as effective, particularly for all named vessels. Monopolar electrocautery should be used with caution to prevent thermal injury to the nerve; hence many prefer the use of bipolar diathermy for cautery and dissection. The harmonic scalpel is an excellent device for superior vascular pedicle ligation and division of the isthmus. It has also been shown to be effective in sealing lymphatic channels and reducing chyle leaks, especially when dealing with bulky nodal disease left in the level IV region.

We advocate a Valsalva maneuver up to 40 mmHg before closure. Most bleeding points will be evident with these simple steps. Several studies have also shown the value of commercially available agents (e.g., collagen, fibrin, cellulose) in reducing bleeding and serum collection. It is hence our practice to line the surgical bed with oxidized regenerated cellulose (Surgicel, Fibrillar; Ethicon Inc., Somerville, NJ, USA). Upon closure of the wound, the strap muscles should be loosely approximated with interrupted sutures, as opposed to water-tight continuous closure of this layer. This prevents the accumulation of blood in the deep compartment of the neck. The most common cause of postoperative bleeding is believed to be a sudden rise in pressure during extubation or coughing in the postoperative setting. Good communication with your anesthesiologist is essential. Some have advocated manual pressure on the neck with a sponge during extubation.

Routine drainage has been shown to have no benefit in most cases, and to have no advantage in early detection of postoperative bleeding. A meta-analysis of 11 randomized controlled trials showed that the only significant difference between drainage and no drainage was the length of hospital stay, which was expectedly prolonged in patients with drainage. The major indications for drainage include large and substernal goiters with a substantial dead space, extensive dissection, concomitant neck dissection, and considerable oozing of the thyroid bed. In these cases, a closed-suction drain is usually left in place for 24 to 48 hours. Drainage is also recommended in patients who have undergone re-exploration for postoperative bleeding.[21]

Parathyroid Injury

The mantra for any endocrine surgeon is that "total thyroidectomy is a parathyroid gland preserving procedure." Transient hypocalcemia is common after total thyroidectomy; postoperative rates have been reported at 20 to 40% for asymptomatic and 10% for symptomatic hypocalcemia. Permanent hypoparathyroidism is fortunately less common, with a reported incidence ranging from 2 to 5%, with rates below 2% in specialized high-volume units. Hypoparathyroidism can be predicted based on rapid parathyroid hormone analyses performed 6 hours after surgery. Patients with normal parathyroid hormone levels are unlikely to develop serious hypocalcemia, and patients with abnormal levels can be prophylactically treated with a combination of calcium and calcitriol (vitamin D) before discharge. Permanent hypoparathyroidism is a debilitating complication, which is difficult to manage and requires life-long calcium and vitamin D supplementation. Unintentional removal of the parathyroid gland has been reported in up to 15% of thyroidectomy specimens. The cause of hypofunctioning glands may also not be a result of direct injury.

High-risk patients are those with previous neck irradiation or radioiodine treatment, those who require additional procedures such as central compartment nodal clearance, extended resection for thyroid cancers, large multinodular or substernal goiters or significant inflammatory changes secondary to thyroiditis, and in patients undergoing reoperative or secondary thyroidectomies. Similarly, patients with Graves disease or primary hyperparathyroidism (undergoing a concomitant parathyroidectomy) will almost always develop postoperative hypocalcemia and should be prophylactically treated with vitamin D and calcium.

Technical considerations in parathyroid surgery include ligating branches of the inferior thyroid artery close to the thyroid gland and avoiding further shock to the parathyroid glands with excessive irrigation with cold saline. Be careful with suctioning the thyroid bed overenthusiastically and suctioning out the the parathyroid glands!

Examine the thyroid bed after the main dissection to confirm parathyroid viability. If the gland is congested, the capsule and hematoma may be incised to relieve the pressure. If there is any doubt about the viability of the gland, it should be removed, diced and autotransplanted in a suitable muscle pocket, such as the sternocleidomastoid muscle or trapezius. The failure rate is reported to be as high as 21 to 43%. Hence, we suggest autotransplantation only if there is any doubt about viability, inadvertent removal of a gland, or if there is heavy paratracheal nodal disease where it is safer to excise the gland and reimplant.

Despite these efforts, the cause of hypoparathyroidism may not be apparent in all cases. Several authors have suggested routine autotransplantation of at least one parathyroid gland as a means to prevent permanent hypoparathyroidism. Two studies have shown that this simple technique results in no permanent hypoparathyroidism, although the reported transient hypocalcemia rates were high. Postoperative recognition of hypoparathyroidism is advantageous because it allows early calcium replacement thereby offsetting the sequelae of hypocalcemia. Traditionally, calcium levels can be measured every 6 to 8 hours during the first 24 hours postoperatively, and treatment of patients who actually develop hypocalcemia can take place. Alternatively, trending of calcium levels at 6 and 23 hours can be used to predict patients who are likely to develop hypocalcemia, and they can be treated prophylactically. There has been much interest in the role of parathyroid hormone assay in predicting which patients are likely to require calcium supplementation, and most studies have shown that postoperative parathyroid hormone levels are a faster and more reliable predictor of hypocalcemia. Parathyroid hormone levels of less than 10 pg/mL at 4 to 6 hours after surgery are nearly 100% sensitive and specific in detecting hypocalcemia, and these patients should be started on prophylactic calcium replacement, comprising calcium and calcitriol. Conversely, parathyroid hormone levels of more than 30 pg/mL are an accurate predictor of normocalcemia. Asymptomatic patients should be treated with oral supplementation.

Uncommon Complications

Wound Infection

Thankfully, wound infections are rare in these surgeries because this is a clean, highly vascular case. Rates should typically be less than 0.5%. There is no correlation between infection rates and prophylactic antibiotic usage; hence we do not recommend routine use of antibiotics, except in uncommon circumstances dictated by patients' histories (e.g., immunodeficiency, valvular heart disease). We routinely insert a subcuticular suture (5–0 Monocryl) with a longitudinal sheet of steristrips. If there are any problems with the wound site, patients are encouraged to contact our support staff immediately.

Tracheal Injury

Tangential dissection of the thyroid off the tracheal cartilage/ligament of Berry makes tracheal damage or injury rare. Tracheal injuries tend to occur in the pediatric population, where the cartilage is soft. This can easily be repaired with interrupted absorbable sutures (such as Vicryl or Monocryl). It is important to remember to deflate the endotracheal tube cuff so that that the stitches do not puncture or stitch through the tube, making subsequent extubation a challenge. It is also useful to reapproximate the strap muscles over the repair site to bolster the repair. A nonsuction drain should then be employed to avoid surgical emphysema.

Tracheomalacia

True tracheomalacia is very rare but will often arise in surgeon–anesthetist conversations. It is an uncommon complication, and tends to occur consequent to pressure exerted by a longstanding, large goiter compressing the trachea. When suspected, the surgeon should palpate the trachea after the thyroid gland has been removed with the endotracheal cuff deflated. If the trachea is found to be soft, it may be safer to keep the patient intubated for 24 hours and allow scar tissue to form in the area, after which a trial extubation can be attempted.

Horner Syndrome—Injury to Sympathetic Trunk

Care must be taken when dissecting the carotid sheath from the prevertebral fascia, especially in the setting of neck dissections for significant nodal metastases. This is a largely avoidable sequela and surgical experience is required.

Summary

Prevention is the key to avoiding the morbidities of thyroid surgery. An intimate knowledge of thyroid gland anatomy and physiology is mandatory. There is no place in this day and age for the occasional thyroid surgeon especially considering the spectrum of heterogeneous neoplasms occurring in the thyroid. When complications do occur, anticipation and rapid treatment can prevent prolonged suffering for the patient and risks of litigation for the surgeon. There are unambiguous data that complication rates are significantly lower in high-volume centers and with experienced thyroid surgeons. Surgeons must be aware of their own limitations, audit their own complication rates at an individual or institutional level, maintain an insight in the literature, and keep patients fully informed of the optimal treatment strategies and potential morbid sequelae of thyroid and parathyroid disease.

References

1. Castro MR, Gharib H. Thyroid nodules and cancer. When to wait and watch, when to refer. Postgrad Med 2000;107(1): 113–116, 119–120, 123–124
2. Shaha A. Treatment of thyroid cancer based on risk groups. J Surg Oncol 2006;94(8):683–691
3. Giddings AE. The history of thyroidectomy. J R Soc Med 1998;91(Suppl 33):3–6
4. Eknoyan G. A history of the parathyroid glands. Am J Kidney Dis 1995;26(5):801–807
5. Moreau S, Goullet de Rugy M, Babin E, Salame E, Delmas P, Valdazo A. The recurrent laryngeal nerve: related vascular anatomy. Laryngoscope 1998;108(9):1351–1353
6. Miller FR. Surgical anatomy of the thyroid and parathyroid glands. Otolaryngol Clin North Am 2003;36(1):1–7, vii
7. Shaha A, Jaffe BM. Complications of thyroid surgery performed by residents. Surgery 1988;104(6):1109–1114
8. Chen H, Wang TS, Yen TW, et al. Operative failures after parathyroidectomy for hyperparathyroidism: the influence of surgical volume. Ann Surg 2010;252(4):691–695
9. Shaha AR. Revision thyroid surgery—technical considerations. Otolaryngol Clin North Am 2008;41(6):1169–1183
10. Shaha AR. Invited commentary: vocal cord evaluation in thyroid surgery. Surgery 2006;139(3):363–364
11. Randolph GW, Kamani D. The importance of preoperative laryngoscopy in patients undergoing thyroidectomy: voice, vocal cord function, and the preoperative detection of invasive thyroid malignancy. Surgery 2006;139(3):357–362
12. Laccourreye O, Papon JF, Kania R, Ménard M, Brasnu D, Hans S. Unilateral laryngeal paralyses: epidemiological data and therapeutic progress. [Article in French] Presse Med 2003;32(17):781–786
13. Kark AE, Kissin MW, Auerbach R, Meikle M. Voice changes after thyroidectomy: role of the external laryngeal nerve. Br Med J (Clin Res Ed) 1984;289(6456):1412–1415
14. Lo CY, Kwok KF, Yuen PW. A prospective evaluation of recurrent laryngeal nerve paralysis during thyroidectomy. Arch Surg 2000;135(2):204–207
15. Holt GR, McMurray GT, Joseph DJ. Recurrent laryngeal nerve injury following thyroid operations. Surg Gynecol Obstet 1977;144(4):567–570
16. Chan WF, Lang BH, Lo CY. The role of intraoperative neuromonitoring of recurrent laryngeal nerve during thyroidectomy: a comparative study on 1000 nerves at risk. Surgery 2006;140(6):866–872, discussion 872–873
17. Chan WF, Lo CY. Pitfalls of intraoperative neuromonitoring for predicting postoperative recurrent laryngeal nerve function during thyroidectomy. World J Surg 2006;30(5):806–812
18. Otto RA, Cochran CS. Sensitivity and specificity of intraoperative recurrent laryngeal nerve stimulation in predicting postoperative nerve paralysis. Ann Otol Rhinol Laryngol 2002;111(11):1005–1007
19. Bhattacharyya N, Fried MP. Assessment of the morbidity and complications of total thyroidectomy. Arch Otolaryngol Head Neck Surg 2002;128(4):389–392
20. Erbil Y, Ozluk Y, Giriş M, et al. Effect of Lugol solution on thyroid gland blood flow and microvessel density in the patients with Graves' disease. J Clin Endocrinol Metab 2007;92(6):2182–2189
21. Sanabria A, Carvalho AL, Silver CE, et al. Routine drainage after thyroid surgery—a meta-analysis. J Surg Oncol 2007;96(3):273–280

25 Neck Dissections

C. Piazza, F. Del Bon, P. Nicolai

Introduction

Neck dissections (NDs) include a wide spectrum of surgical procedures aimed at removal of different neck lymph nodes groups, distinguished in seven levels as proposed by the American Head and Neck Society and American Academy of Otolaryngology—Head and Neck Surgery.[1] According to the same classification and its subsequent proposal for revision,[1,2] ND can range from a very extensive and morbid procedure, such as extended radical neck dissection, passing through radical (RND) and modified radical (MRND) neck dissections, to less invasive ones such as selective or so-called superselective neck dissection (SND; aimed at targeted removal of two adjacent neck levels after nonsurgical organ preservation strategies).

Therefore, both the prevalence and severity of complications and sequelae of ND can vary greatly in relation to the type of procedure, and are diversely affected by several variables mainly in relation to their association with synchronous primary tumor removal, reconstructive surgical techniques adopted, and postradiotherapy (RT) or chemoradiotherapy (CRT) setting. Adverse events after ND may significantly impact the overall health and quality of life of head and neck cancer patients in both the short-term and long-term. Their anticipation in patient counseling, prevention, management, and evaluation play an essential role in such a demanding surgical intervention.

Complications Related to Skin Incisions

Different skin incisions for ND have been reported and may be chosen according to several criteria. The most important is certainly the potential need for associated tumor resection. In case of oral/oropharyngeal lesions, the incision should start from the mastoid process extending to the mid-third of the sternocleidomastoid (SCM) muscle, then reaching the midline of the submental level or chin (**Fig. 25.1**). In the event of bilateral NDs, this incision goes from one mastoid process to the contralateral one, passing through the cricothyroid membrane (**Fig. 25.2**). In case of parotid, auricular, or parapharyngeal lesions, a posterosuperior extension of the incision should be performed at the level of the preauricular or retroauricular region, while for thyroid, hypopharyngeal, or laryngeal primaries, a classic "apron" or "hemi-apron"

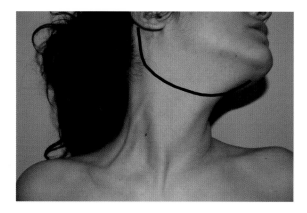

Fig. 25.1 Skin incision used in case of unilateral selective neck dissection (levels I–III).

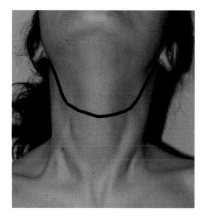

Fig. 25.2 Skin incision used for bilateral selective neck dissection (levels I–III).

flap is raised to include tracheotomy in the same incision as needed (**Fig. 25.3**).

As a general rule, removal of neck lymph nodes from levels I to IV and VB can be easily accomplished through a horizontal incision from the posterior midthird of the SCM muscle to the cricothyroid membrane, while dissection of level VA usually needs a more posterior and caudal extension of the incision reaching the level of the supraclavicular fossa. Dissection of level VI and VII must be usually addressed through a skin flap involving the jugular notch. A thorough dissection from levels I to VII can be accomplished by the MacFee incision (**Fig. 25.4**), which allows excellent cosmetic results at the price of a more tedious and time-consuming dissection. Apart from these variables, the general rules to be observed include performing horizontal more than vertical incisions for

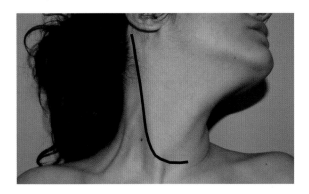

Fig. 25.3 "Hemi-apron" or "hockey stick" incision.

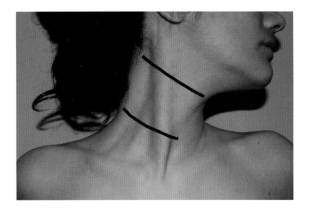

Fig. 25.4 MacFee incision.

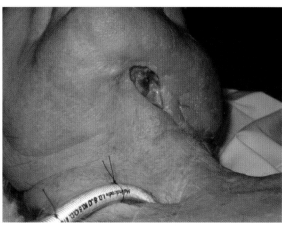

Fig. 25.5 Cutaneous dehiscence after surgery on a preirradiated neck. (Image courtesy of M. Bernal, MD.)

cosmetic reasons, and following whenever possible pre-existing skin creases.

Every neck scar or previous incision should be incorporated into the new one. When composite skin incisions are required, it is imperative to avoid acute angles at their intersection point. For this reason, we usually avoid skin incisions such as Martin double-Y, Schobinger, and H incisions. When this is not possible, the areas of potential skin devascularization and dehiscence should be placed away (usually posteriorly) from the major vessels. Every effort should be made to carefully plan such incisions, especially in patients with a previously irradiated neck because of their well-known higher propensity for cutaneous dehiscence and infection, with potential vascular exposure and blowout. Along the same lines, every care should be taken in patients with fragile tissues to protect the skin flaps during surgery, by gentle handling, applying moist gauzes or wet towels, and performing frequent saline irrigation, so avoiding intraoperative desiccation of the flap.

In spite of all these preventive measures, dehiscences at the level of the surgical wound may still occur (**Fig. 25.5**). A limited gap can be managed conservatively by aggressive and frequent medication to stimulate healing by secondary intention. In case of more extensive flap

necrosis with potential exposure of major blood vessels or associated local infection for fistula formation, regional pedicled or free flaps may be required. Hyperbaric oxygen therapy, especially in a previously irradiated and infected field, can play a role in this setting, both as an attempt to promote spontaneous healing, and in preparation of the following reconstructive procedure.[3,4]

Locoregional Infections

Wound infections are more frequently encountered when ND is performed in association with upper aerodigestive tract procedures followed by development of oral/oropharyngeal or pharyngocutaneous fistulas. Moreover, previous RT or CRT may increase their prevalence by several fold (**Figs. 25.6 and 25.7**). The most frequent cause of local infection after ND that is not associated with upper aerodigestive tract procedures is represented by formation of seroma or hematoma. This can be avoided by meticulous intraoperative hemostasis, placement of at least one suction drainage on each side of the neck, and control of its correct postoperative functioning. Frequently, poor functioning of suction drainage is related to inadequate suture around the tracheostomy site or along the incision itself. Early evaluation and solution of these problems are mandatory. When seroma or hematoma is suspected, it must be aggressively treated by drainage through a small opening of the previous suture or via a separate stab wound to prevent superinfection. If this develops, it is usually accompanied by sudden spiking fever, chills, malaise, increase in white cell count, odor, purulent discharge from the incision or from the drainage, edema and hyperemia of the skin flaps, and swelling at the level of the surgical field. Once infection is diagnosed, its management is based on broad-spectrum antibiotics, drainage of the wound, and, if wound breakdown occurs, covering of large vessels by a pedicled myofascial

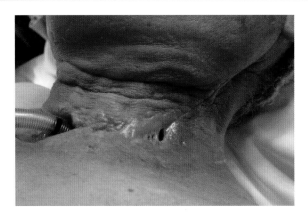

Fig. 25.6 Pharyngocutaneous fistula after surgery on an irradiated neck. (Image courtesy of M. Bernal, MD.)

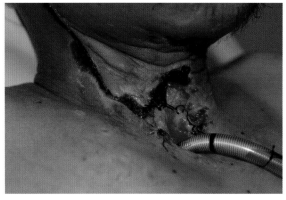

Fig. 25.7 Local wound infection with partial necrosis after surgery on an irradiated neck. (Image courtesy of M. Bernal, MD.)

pectoralis major flap to obliterate the dead space. This is strongly suggested, especially in association with RND or major pharyngocutaneous fistula. Every effort should also be directed to the correction of possible predisposing factors like malnutrition, electrolytic alterations, and diabetes.

Prevention of local infections with a liberal use of antibiotics is still debated. While antibiotic prophylaxis for isolated ND in nonirradiated patients is not considered beneficial by most authors, the evidence for antibiotic prophylaxis in ND associated with upper aerodigestive tract opening and for patients previously undergoing RT or CRT is less clear-cut. Different antibiotics have been reported (penicillins with or without sulbactam, cephalosporins, clindamycin, metronidazole), with various associations, dose, and time of administration that are largely dependent on personal preferences and specific institutional policies. Patients treated by salvage surgery on the larynx, hypopharynx, and oropharynx with concomitant ND after failure of nonsurgical organ preservation strategies certainly require a more cautious approach.[5,6]

Complications Related to Lymphatic Vessels

Prevalence of lesions of the thoracic duct (during left ND) and right lymphatic duct (an inconstant and smaller structure formed by the union of the right jugular, subclavian, and bronchomediastinal trunks entering the neck across the medial border of the anterior scalenus muscle and leading to the junction of the right subclavian and internal jugular vein [IJV]), during clearance of level IV, is reported in around 1.5% of MRND[7,8] and in 1 to 3% after RND.[9] However, this figure is probably an underestimate of the actual prevalence of chylous leaks (CL), accounting for only the most evident ones, being reported in up to 5.8% of cases.[10] Of these, only ~ 25% occur on the right side of the neck.[11]

Predisposing factors are previous RT, which renders identification of lymphatic vessels difficult and makes their walls more fragile during surgical dissection, and some anatomic variations such as a more cranial ending of the thoracic duct (reported as high as 5 cm above the clavicle) or multiple terminations. Presence of large metastatic lymph nodes also seems to be associated with hypertrophy of the lymphatic drainage system, with an increased number of collectors identified during dissection and a higher risk of intraoperative injury.

The best treatment of CL is prevention by careful and bloodless dissection at level IV.[9,12] In case of intraoperative injury of a lymphatic vessel, CL may be detected macroscopically as a milky, oily, partially transparent fluid. Not infrequently, it is possible to see the tear in the thoracic duct itself by using operating loops. Otherwise, to help in identifying the point of leak, the anesthesiologist may be asked to apply positive pressure ventilation, so raising central venous pressure.[10] Placing the patient in the Trendelenburg position may also be useful, in addition to moderate external pressure on the abdominal wall.

A CL can be treated by ligation and oversewing of the bed of the thoracic duct with nonabsorbable suture, being careful not to further damage the thin-walled duct.[10,13] In case of missed identification of the CL source, a tobacco pouch suture should be made in the possible area of origin. Various local and regional flaps have been described to primarily cover the CL site, ranging from the scalenus anterior muscle flap, which is not recommended because of the risk of damage of the brachial plexus, to the clavicular head of the SCM.[12,14] During all of these surgical maneuvers, significant effort should be made to preserve both phrenic and vagal nerves. Various aids have been proposed to increase the likelihood of CL closure, including the use of fibrin glue or sclerosing agents. The main advice is against neck closure and patient awakening if the leakage is not completely controlled. Dietary modifications such as a low-fat diet should be initiated the day after surgery and continued for at least 7 days if a CL has been intraoperatively detected. Medium-chain triglycerides are recommended[10,12,15] because they are absorbed directly into portal venous circulation, bypassing the lymphatic system.[9] If this dietary restriction is not successful, total parenteral nutrition is warranted.[10] It bypasses the normal breakdown of long-chain fatty acids in the small bowel, decreasing the amount of chyle production; but it requires central venous catheterization with possible complications. Suction drainage should be avoided whenever feasible on the CL neck side or removed as soon as possible.

Even after the best control of all visible leakage sites, patients with intraoperative CL still remain at high risk for postoperative leakage, which occurs in 25 to 75% of patients.[9] This may not appear until several days after surgery (generally on the third postoperative day). Postoperative CL is manifested by unexpectedly high drain outputs, or by the appearance of creamy, greasy, oily, yellow-white fluid in the drainage. Differential diagnosis includes saliva if the ND was performed in association with surgery of the upper aerodigestive tract or major salivary glands. Confirmation of CL can be obtained by the analysis of the drainage content searching for amylases (in case of saliva) or triglycerides (in case of CL).

Postoperative CL should be promptly and aggressively addressed. Left untreated, it may give rise to other complications such as an intense inflammatory reaction, wound infection, and dehiscence with possible exposure of major vessels. Moreover, a long-lasting high-output CL may result in electrolyte disturbance.[11] Conservative management is recommended in the case of CL less than 600 mL/day. It comprises bed rest in an anti-Trendelenburg position, removal of suction drainages allowing them to drain naturally, application of pressure dressing at the level of the supraclavicular region, and dietary management. This conservative management can be prolonged for many days, but in the case of planned postoperative RT, this approach is advisable for no more than 30 days.[10] Reoperation at the CL site may be troublesome, and finding the leakage site can be facilitated by feeding the patient with heavy cream a couple of hours before surgery.[9] After exploration of the surgical field, use of fibrin glue, mattress suture around the leakage site or even harvesting of myocutaneous pectoralis major or latissimus dorsi flaps can be useful in case of massive leakage or in patients with fragile tissue conditions (diabetes, post-RT scenario).

General consensus in the literature advocates prompt revision surgery in case of CL exceeding 600 mL/day (high-output CL) for 4 to 5 consecutive days. In these cases, a longer conservative approach is risky, and can lead to worsening of the patient's general condition, associated with excessive granulation and scar tissue formation, which makes revision surgery even more troublesome.

Some controversies exist about the use of sclerosing and bonding agents such as tetracyclines in the management of postoperative persistent CL after failure of medical or surgical treatment. Of special note are concerns about outcomes, which seem to be late and unpredictable. It is certain that they are associated with intense local fibrosis that renders subsequent surgical revision technically more challenging.

Chylothorax

Chylothorax is a rare event after ND: as for CL the most affected site is the left one. The site of injury of the thoracic duct is usually unclear, and it is not possible to exclude that chyle extravasation in the chest is the result of backpressure after ligation of the main duct in the neck. In such a situation, chyle may pass through the cervical fascia, reaching the mediastinum and thoracic cavity. Another possible mechanism explaining chylothorax when macroscopic tearing of the pleura is not visible is progressive pleural infiltration and soaking because of the prolonged stagnation of chyle in the supraclavicular fossa. Following this, unilateral chylothorax could spread bilaterally by the same mechanism. Massive pleural effusion may cause cardiorespiratory failure as a result of mechanical compression on the lung and major thoracic vessels.

Therapy encompasses dietary restrictions and medical precautions as mentioned above for CL. Puncture and drainage of subcutaneous collection can be associated with one or more thoracenteses or left thoracostomy drainage. Pleurodesis via talc introduced into the pleural space through a chest drain to obtain a scar reaction and subsequent pleural obliteration is an alternative approach. Surgical revision should be left as the last option. Prognosis of this rare complication, when promptly recognized, is good and without major respiratory complications.

Lymphocele

Described as a circumscribed collection of fluid without an endothelial lining, lymphocele may develop as a late complication of CL. It is an extremely rare condition, even though it can be accidentally encountered during postoperative magnetic resonance follow-up (**Fig. 25.8a, b**). First described by Chantarasak and Green in 1989[16] as the consequence of a low-output CL into the healing tissues, lymphocele formation may be the result of the presence of a wall of scar tissue preventing the CL from spreading along the fascial layers into the adjacent anatomic compartments. Differential diagnosis with hematoma, seroma, abscess, nodal persistence, or recurrence with cystic degeneration is of paramount importance. Lymphocele usually appears as a taut-elastic swelling, generally located in the supraclavicular region, mostly on the left, in patients with a history of intraoperative or postoperative CL. Neck ultrasound is useful in identifying its fluid content and defining relationships with the IJV and subclavian vein, SCM, and deep neck muscles.

Complications Related to Blood Vessels

Internal Jugular Vein Blowout

Calearo and Teatini[7] reported that the prevalence of IJV rupture was 0.8% after an MRND type III procedure. After unilateral RND, during contralateral ND this event can cause severe complications because of increased intracranial pressure. Intraoperative injury of the middle portion of the IJV can usually be controlled easily, while its tearing at the skull base or below the clavicle may be more troublesome, requiring, respectively, mastoidectomy with sigmoid sinus obliteration or clavicle disarticulation to properly control bleeding. Injury of the subclavian vein can also be associated with IJV damage, and its ligature may cause postoperative upper limb edema. Lesion of the IJV or a major collateral vessel may be complicated by fatal air embolism. To prevent this rare event, the patient should always be placed in a Trendelenburg position during the steps of ND in which the IJV is at risk.

Internal Jugular Vein Thrombosis

Even after SND, minor injuries to the IJV may occur causing its complete or partial thrombosis. Some factors responsible for this event are: complete mobilization of the vessel from the clavicle to the jugular foramen with its excessive handling and traction resulting in loss of vasa vasorum, inappropriate ligation of large side branches with formation of possible thrombogenic pockets, heat damage of the venous wall through an excessive use of monopolar cautery or bipolar forceps, and dehydration of the vessel wall, which is exposed to the air during long procedures. These technical factors are complemented by others, such as maintenance of inadequate intraoperative blood volume, reduction of blood flow, hypotension during surgery and in the immediate postoperative period, and a hypercoagulable state characteristic of some cancer patients because of an increase in factor VIII, the number of platelets, and their adhesiveness. Use of a bulky myocutaneous flap for reconstruction (causing compression of the IJV), salivary fistula, wound infection, and sepsis are other predisposing factors. The role of RT is still controversial. Diagnosis of IJV thrombosis may be easily made with high-resolution Doppler ultrasound, which allows a rapid, noninvasive, and accurate assessment of vein patency.[19–22] Computed tomography and magnetic resonance imaging are clearly more expensive, but can add information regarding anatomic structures surrounding the IJV.

Several studies have confirmed that IJV thrombosis may occur in up to 30% of patients within a week after MRND, with recanalization within 3 months between 60 and 80%, and vessel patency after surgery estimated to be around 95%.[21,23–30]

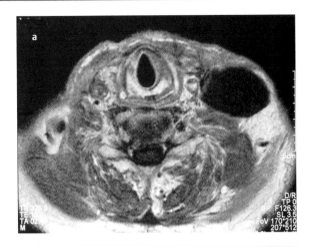

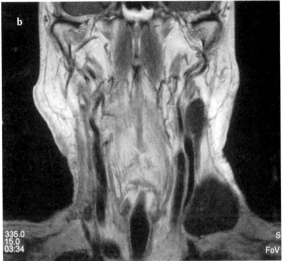

Fig. 25.8a,b Magnetic resonance contrast-enhanced T1 sequence on axial (**a**) and coronal (**b**) planes. Lymphocele appears homogeneously hypointense with no contrast enhancement. It is located at the confluence of the subclavian vein with the internal jugular vein, medially displaced, and posteriorly in contact with the anterior scalenus muscle.

Ultrasound-guided fine needle aspiration allows confirmation of the nature of the fluid, and temporary drainage of the fluid collection. Computed tomography and magnetic resonance imaging may be useful in the case of planned surgical revision.

The treatment modality of lymphocele is not standardized in the literature because of its rare occurrence. However, it can be treated either by a conservative medical approach (drainage, local washing of the cavity by iodine solution, injection of sclerosing chemical agents like OK-432,[17] application of compressive dressings in the supraclavicular region, and appropriate diet), or by surgical revision as described for CL.[16,18]

Complications Related to Venous Congestion

The main consequence of ND is the obvious alteration of head and neck lymphatic drainage, associated with venous congestion in case of IJV sacrifice, especially on the right side, where venous flow is usually dominant because of the larger dimensions of the transverse sinus, jugular foramen, and IJV.

Unilateral IJV ligation leads to a transitory three-fold increase of the intracranial pressure, whereas after bilateral IJV occlusion this value can even be five times higher than normal.[31] Prolonged intracranial pressure increase may reduce the reabsorption of cerebrospinal fluid through collapse of the dural venous sinuses, especially the superior sagittal one, with consequent cerebral edema.

Mortality after bilateral simultaneous RND ranges between 10 and 14%, but it decreases to 0 to 3% in staged interventions scheduled at least 1 month apart. However, even applying this precaution, the morbidity of bilateral RND remains high and includes facial and conjunctival edema and chemosis, papillary stasis, potential obstruction of the upper aerodigestive tract, headache, nausea, vomiting, amaurosis, stroke, and possible evolution to coma and death. Options to reduce morbidity include the reconstruction of one IJV using an autologous saphenous graft[32] or by a heterologous prosthesis made of various materials. The latter procedures are usually associated with poorer functional outcomes. However, the main issue concerning bilateral RND remains its oncologic indication, because of the overall dismal prognosis usually observed in these patients.

Visual Loss

Visual loss following head and neck surgery has been rarely reported,[33] but ischemic optic neuropathy is the most frequently reported cause of permanent visual loss. Deterioration of vision generally occurs immediately after surgery and progresses in 2 to 3 days. Risk factors include combinations of prolonged surgical times, hypotension, anemia due to blood loss, and prone positioning.[34] Balm et al[35] and Marks et al[36] reported six cases of complete blindness due to permanent intracranial hypertension after bilateral RND (performed simultaneously in four patients, delayed in two), while de Vries et al[37] reported nine cases of amaurosis and other visual disturbances associated with transient increases of intracranial pressure and papilledema after unilateral RND. In these cases, the sudden and sustained increase in intracranial pressure would act as a primary cause, leading to papilledema and difficulty of the ophthalmic veins to drain into the cavernous sinus. The increase in cerebrospinal fluid pressure at the level of the optic nerve sheath and compression by the adjacent ophthalmic veins may compromise arterial perfusion of the nerve itself.

Amaurosis

In case of persistent and worsening amaurosis, placement of a lumbar cerebrospinal fluid drain and assisted hyperventilation are warranted.[35] The need for urgent surgical decompression of the optic nerve has been exceptionally reported.[38] In the case of marked swelling of the face with exophthalmos and eyelid edema, a temporary tarsorrhaphy may be required to prevent corneal damage.

Syndrome of Inappropriate Antidiuretic Hormone Secretion

Some cases of syndrome of inappropriate antidiuretic hormone (ADH) secretion (SIADH or Schwartz–Bartter syndrome) after unilateral RND have been observed. In case of unilateral IJV ligation, anatomical abnormalities of the venous system may preclude the formation of an effective shunt to the contralateral IJV with overloading of the collateral vessels responsible for venous drainage (vertebral and paravertebral venous plexuses, occipital vein and other veins of the scalp, orbital and ophthalmic veins, pharyngoesophageal veins and pterygoid plexus).

SIADH is characterized by an increased ADH plasma concentration and consequent marked diuresis contraction, increase in urine-specific gravity, and hyponatremia. Beyond the possible paraneoplastic syndromes associated with malignant tumors of the head and neck leading to increased secretion of ADH, this clinical picture has been observed with several etiopathogenic conditions associated with increased intracranial pressure.[39] Therefore, it is conceivable that even in SIADH after bilateral or unilateral RND, the causal factor of autonomization of ADH secretion is attributable to an increase in intracranial pressure.

If not promptly recognized and properly treated, this syndrome involves worsening of the clinical picture with headache, lethargy, anorexia, convulsions, cardiac arrhythmias, and dangerous altered states of consciousness leading to coma. However, this is a complication that can be prevented by reducing intraoperative and postoperative fluid infusion in patients at increased risk.

Carotid Artery Lesions

Excessive manipulation of the carotid axis can lead to embolus detachment from atherosclerotic plaques and to cardiovascular changes as the result of stimulation of the carotid sinus. These can range from bradyarrhythmia with hypotension to ventricular fibrillation, especially in digitalized patients. Subadventitial infiltration of the carotid sinus with intravenous injection of 1% xylocaine or atropine is usually sufficient to control these adverse events. In case of failure in controlling bradyarrhythmia, further manipulations of the carotid sinus should be avoided.

Extremely rare, but potentially fatal, is the intraoperative rupture of the common or internal carotid artery, due to an unrecognized abnormal tortuosity of these vessels, typically seen in the elderly, with a convex posterolateral curvature at levels IIA and IIB.

Relatively more frequent is postoperative carotid blowout, a complication that can occur even some weeks after surgery, with a reported prevalence up to 3 to 4% in older studies and reduced to 0 to 1.2% in more recent ones. The most frequent site of carotid rupture is at the level of the common carotid artery, followed by the external and internal carotid arteries, in descending order of frequency. Wherever the source of bleeding is located, it remains a serious complication with a high mortality rate both in the case of planned surgery for impending risk of rupture, as well as in the setting of an emergency procedure. Morbidity, mostly related to cerebral ischemia, ranges from 19 to 60% and can occur either immediately after vessel ligation or within weeks.

The pathogenic mechanism of carotid rupture is linked to thrombosis of the adventitial vasa vasorum, resulting in fibrosis and weakening of the vessel wall. The main cause of this complication is excessive thinning of the adventitia as a consequence of an aggressive peeling of metastatic lymphadenopathies strictly adhering to the carotid axis. In this regard, Freeman et al[40] recommend resection and immediate reconstruction of the portion of the carotid artery involved with the tumor: such a procedure (complemented by intraoperative RT) would improve not only the possibility of local control of disease (67 versus 50%), but also survival (47 versus 36%) compared with traditional subadventitial peeling. This assumption holds true in the presence of disease infiltrating the carotid axis alone. Unfortunately, lymph nodes involving the carotid artery are usually found to extensively infiltrate the deep cervical fascia and muscles beyond any form of radical surgery. However, every planned carotid artery resection should be preceded by a preoperative balloon occlusion test, still considering that the morbidity of this intervention is not negligible,[41] and the predictive value of a negative test, especially if associated with hypotensive challenge, is high but not absolute.[42]

Other factors potentially leading to carotid blowout are RND, preoperative RT or CRT, cervical flap necrosis with wound dehiscence (especially if associated with local infection and salivary fistula), and tumor persistence or recurrence. In case of wound dehiscence and simple carotid artery exposure, covering it with a pectoralis major myocutaneous or myofascial pedicled flap can effectively prevent artery rupture. Carotid blowout can be heralded by small "sentinel" bleeds from brownish eschar formed at the level of the damaged area, sometimes in correspondence with pseudoaneurysmatic vessel dilation. These early signs should immediately prompt carotid ligation before the clinician is faced with a dramatic emergency.

An alternative option to control bleeding is the interventional neuroradiologic approach with carotid artery occlusion using an inflatable balloon.[43] Even endovascular embolization has been successfully employed as an alternative to surgical ligation.[44] This approach is feasible for prevention of acute bleeding, such as that occurring during vessel exposure through a dehiscent wound or after "sentinel" bleeding. The results of this technique are encouraging, even during complete carotid blowout. In fact, this technique seems better tolerated from a cardiovascular point of view than traditional surgery, because it involves less manipulation of the carotid sinus, it is possible to perform it with the patient under sedation, and it can precisely identify the source of bleeding. In a series of 15 patients, Citardi et al[43] reported a survival rate of 83%, without major neurologic complications, and a single case of ipsilateral Claude–Bernard–Horner syndrome. Acute carotid bleeding has also been successfully managed by placement of endovascular stents, even though long-term sequelae as a result of the presence of a foreign body in a potentially contaminated field make this solution questionable.[45]

Prevention of postoperative carotid artery rupture is best accomplished by covering the vascular axis by liberal use of a pedicled or free myofascial flap, so separating it from the upper aerodigestive tract in the presence of high-risk conditions for salivary fistula and wound dehiscence.

Complications of the Peripheral Nervous System

Marginal Branch of the VII Cranial Nerve

Cabra et al[8] reported that the prevalence of paralysis of the marginal branch of cranial nerve VII was 2.6% among patients undergoing MRND. Others reported a prevalence of temporary and permanent marginal branch palsy as high as 29% and 16%, respectively, after ND involving level I.[46] Because of its location and its small caliber, this nerve can be easily damaged, even without a real discontinuation, both during skin flap raising and submental (IA) and submandibular (IB) lymph nodes dissection. This risk is higher in the presence of metastatic lymphadenopathies adjacent to the anterior facial artery and vein (prefacial and postfacial submandibular lymph nodes), most frequently encountered in tumors of the nose, lips, cheek, and floor of mouth.

Marginal nerve palsy causes important aesthetic alterations, with asymmetric static and dynamic lower lip appearance, as well as functional limitations in chewing and swallowing, with possible oral incontinence and salivary drooling. Its prevention involves careful identification of the nerve before any dissection of the region, limiting to a minimum the use of electrostimulation (which can potentially leading to neuroapraxia), and asking the anesthesiologist to avoid using muscle relaxants during nerve isolation. The most useful landmark for its safe and quick identification is the angle of the mandible, posterior to the facial vessels and submandibular gland tail. The marginal nerve is almost always found at this level, closely adjacent to the fascia of the masseter muscle. From here, it arches down laterally to the facial artery and veins (where it is usually located ~ 1.5 cm lower than the mandibular body) and the submandibular gland, with a variable course depending on its branching pattern. The marginal branch may be confused with the cervical one, which serves the platysma and is usually located a few inches below the former. Between the two, an anastomosis can be present, and the cervical branch should be preserved whenever possible because of its contribution to lower lip movement through innervation of platismatic fibers with peroral insertion.

When level IA–IB dissection is not required, the marginal branch can be safely kept outside the surgical field by ligation and division of the anterior facial vein just below the submandibular gland and lifting up its stump (Hayes Martin's maneuver). This will also elevate the cervical skin flap and fascia, and with them, the marginal nerve wrapped in a protective sheath.

In case of marginal branch neurotmesis, its immediate neurorrhaphy with 9–0 or 10–0 monofilament nylon is warranted.

Cranial Nerve X

Lesions of this nerve can accidentally occur, especially during RND when dealing with IJV isolation and ligation. Neurorrhaphy, although immediate and accurate, is rarely successful because of the frequent occurrence of random reinnervation along the two stumps, resulting in dysfunctional synkynesia and/or dyskinesia (adductor fibers reinnervating abductor muscles and vice versa, so causing chaotic muscle activation with an outcome worse than the paralysis). Vagal palsy is commonly associated with moderate dyspnea, dysphonia, dysphagia, inefficient cough with possible aspiration pneumonia, and stypsis.

Cranial Nerve XI

The most relevant functional sequela of RND is undoubtedly impairment of shoulder function as the result of sectioning the spinal accessory nerve (SAN) and the ensuing denervation of the upper trapezius muscle. Nahum et al[47] first coined the term "shoulder syndrome" to describe a clinical picture consisting of pain (possibly radiating from

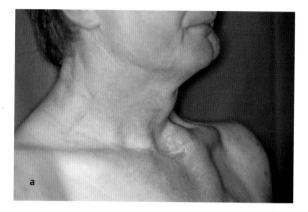

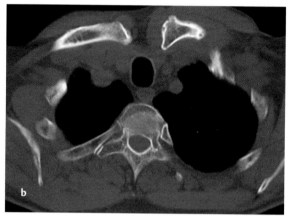

Fig. 25.9a,b Clinical picture **(a)** and computed tomography scan **(b)** of sternoclavicular joint hypertrophy after left radical neck dissection.

the neck to the face), limited abduction of the shoulder and upper limb, stiffness of the neck, full passive range of motion, and anatomic deformities such as scapular flaring, droop, and protraction. Pain is attributed to strain placed on supporting muscles, such as the rhomboids and levator scapulae, as a consequence of shoulder drooping. A frequent ancillary sign of shoulder syndrome is sternoclavicular joint hypertrophy caused by abnormal torque-like forces applied to the medial head of the clavicle, potentially complicated by stress fracture of the middle third of the clavicle[48] (**Fig. 25.9**). Shoulder syndrome-like symptoms may also originate from cervical plexus neuralgia, adhesive capsulitis of the scapulohumeral joint, with myofascial pain starting not only from the upper trapezius, but also from elevator scapulae and rhomboid muscles.[49]

The SAN is usually described purely as a motor nerve, providing innervation to the SCM and upper trapezius muscles. After loss of nerve function, paralysis of both muscles occurs: while loss of SCM activity is generally of secondary importance, upper trapezius denervation is mainly responsible for the complex clinical picture of shoulder syndrome. However, there is still considerable debate on the pattern of innervation of the upper trapezius. While some authors consider the SAN as the only motor nerve of this muscle,[50,51] others make it clear that this cranial nerve and the cervical plexus can provide independent motor contributions to the upper trapezius.[52,53] In particular, the anatomical studies by Kierner et al[54–56] have highlighted these relationships. Based on their observations, innervation of the upper trapezius would be ensured by a thin branch of the SAN, without any contribution from the cervical plexus. Indeed, no anastomosis was found between this branch and the component of the nerve that passes into the muscle or in a more distal anastomosis at the Erb's point. The only exception to this condition is in subjects (30%) in which the SAN does not pass through the SCM, but begins dorsally to the muscle. Moreover, one to three branches of the cervical plexus going to the middle and lower thirds of the trapezius (always running in the subfascial plain, at the level of the posterior triangle of the neck, but independently from the main trunk of the SAN and rarely intermingling with it) have been identified. It was finally pointed out that there is a wide range of variability in both the number and level (both intracranial and extracranial) of anastomotic connections between the SAN fibers and the C2, C3, and C4 roots. This fact could explain the various degrees of shoulder joint dysfunction observed in patients submitted to the same type of ND.

Surprisingly, even after RND, only 60 to 80% of patients present a complete shoulder syndrome picture, likely to be counterbalanced in its appearance by the action of accessory muscles. Even in patients in whom the SAN is anatomically preserved during ND, it is possible to find electromyographic and clinical signs of shoulder syndrome. These apparently contradictory results can be explained on the basis of the influence of various factors such as age, sex, dominant side, presence of concomitant neuropathy or myopathy, and need for complementary treatment, especially RT.[57] A review of the recent literature reported shoulder syndrome symptoms in 18 to 77% of patients undergoing MRND and in 29 to 39% of those treated by SND.[58] This can be explained on the basis of a sequence of iatrogenic "minor" insults (traction, skeletonization and devascularization resulting in segmental demyelination, neuroapraxia, and axonotmesis) to the SAN that, even though anatomically preserved, suffers during dissection of sublevels IIB and VA, together with the thin branches from the cervical plexus, and is potentially damaged during levels IV and V clearance.

Some precautions can be useful in reducing the damage to the cranial portion of the SAN during dissection of sublevel IIB. An interesting study by Rafferty et al[59] demonstrated the utility of using the sternomastoid branch of the occipital artery (or superior SCM muscle vascular pedicle) as an intraoperative landmark for reliable identification of the entry point of the SAN in the SCM itself. These vessels cross the SAN at a mean distance of 6.2 mm

(range 1 to 11) below the point where it enters the muscle. In a ventral to dorsal direction, surgeons always come across this vascular pedicle before encountering the nerve itself, located slightly deeper.

The accidental transection of the nerve during MRND or SND not entailing the sacrifice of the nerve for oncologic reasons has an incidence of 1.68% in a large European series.[60] An improvement of shoulder function in the postoperative period using immediate reconstruction by a microsurgical technique using a great auricular nerve cable graft has been described.[61] Other techniques include use of the sural, anterior branch of medial antebrachial cutaneous, or thoracodorsal nerve as interposition grafts. A major concern regards the increased cost in terms of donor-site morbidity of these surgical techniques. In fact, some patients do not benefit from this procedure because of neuroma formation and ingrowth of fibrous tissue blocking the axon sprouting from the proximal nerve stump, particularly when a long and nonvascularized graft is required and postoperative RT is needed. An alternative method to restore SAN conduction is the technique described by Guo et al[62] using the proximal portion of the SCM and the great auricular nerve as a composite myo-fascial-nervous pedicled flap. The major advantages of this approach are vascularization by the underlying fascia and muscle of the interposition graft, and its very limited donor site morbidity. A key aspect is to leave the SAN intact in the posterior triangle of the neck, whenever oncologically feasible. A large series of patients, however, still needs to be evaluated to assess the actual advantages of this method in restoring postoperative function after RND. If the repair of the nerve has not been performed at the time of its sectioning, it should still be accomplished by a secondary intervention after a maximum time of 20 months.[63]

Once shoulder syndrome has been properly diagnosed and quantified, it is necessary for the patient to undergo appropriate shoulder function rehabilitation. This ideally includes exercises that patients, adequately educated, should perform every day at home. The main goal is to start as early as possible to counteract the pathologic reduction in the range of shoulder mobility, before glenohumeral joint fibrosis, tightening of capsule and ligaments, and atrophy of the shoulder muscles develop. By prevention of restriction of shoulder passive mobility in the first few months after surgery, a more rapid recovery of the active motility will be obtained once the upper trapezius has recovered its full functionality. In particular, Salerno et al[64] have stressed the value of an early (within 15 to 30 days after surgery) and continuous rehabilitation program for a long period (up to 6 months). In their experience, this should include exercises such as passive forward elevation of the upper limb on the same plane as the scapula, passive forward elevation with joined hands and movements of elongation, shoulder rotation with elbow flexed and abducted to 90°, and internal rotation with the hand placed behind the back. By applying these exercises, the authors observed a significant gain of passive and active global mobility of the shoulder, improvement in the quality of life in terms of pain reduction, return to previous habits and recreational activities, and objective normalization of electromyography of the upper trapezius, supraspinatus, infraspinatus, and levator scapulae.

Cranial Nerve XII

Cabra et al,[8] in their series of MRNDs, found a prevalence of unilateral hypoglossal nerve lesion of 1.69%, whereas Calearo and Teatini[7] reported a prevalence of 0.4%. It is therefore a rare event, mostly related to the presence of extensive lymph node metastases at levels IB and IIA.

Cervical Sympathetic Chain

Cabra et al[8] reported cervical sympathetic chain injury in 0.78% of patients, which is comparable to the 0.8% cited by Calearo and Teatini.[7] Its clinical consequence is Claude–Bernard–Horner syndrome (including ptosis, miosis, enophthalmos, and head and neck anhidrosis, and is rarely associated with increased salivary viscosity, changes in cerebral blood flow, and blood pressure instability). The point of risk for such a nervous structure, especially during RND, is lymph node dissection in the parapharyngeal or retropharyngeal spaces. In some instances, the superior cervical sympathetic ganglia are barely distinguishable from small lymphadenopathies.

Cervical Roots, Brachial Plexus, and Phrenic Nerve

Sectioning of C2–C4 roots preserving only the phrenic nerve is a commonly performed surgical maneuver in both RND and MRND.[7] As a consequence, hypoesthesia or even complete anesthesia in an area that extends from the outer ear to the anterior chest below the clavicle is an expected sequela of this surgery. These sensory deficits can spontaneously recover, at least in part, in a few months, except for the earlobe. During elective dissections, preservation of C2 to C4 roots is possible, at the cost of an increase in surgical time.

Amputation neuroma is a rounded swelling, usually not larger than 2 cm, consisting of a hard, painful mass, associated with local paresthesia. It usually originates from the stump of sensory cutaneous nerves cut during surgery as a result of posttraumatic disorganized neural regeneration. It may be confused with local recurrence or lymph node metastasis, but usually its clinical picture is sufficient for correct differential diagnosis. Otherwise, fine needle aspiration cytology should help in resolving the clinical dilemma. By contrast, excisional biopsy is almost invariably followed by further neuroma formation at the new residual stump. Symptomatic therapy is performed by infiltration of local anesthetics (temporary effect) or ethanol (more lasting effect).

The possibility of injuring the nerve roots of the brachial plexus is extremely rare and limited to RND. Gacek[65] described four cases out of 350 NDs with a redundant course of the primary division of C5 (which provides the most cranial contribution to the brachial plexus), running in the supraclavicular adipose tissue. In such an aberrant position, this motor root can be confused with C4 sensory nerves running from medial to lateral in the neck. Therefore, in the case of uncertain dissection at level IV, VA, and VB, surgeons should always suspect the existence of an abnormal anatomic structure crossing this plain and are at risk if not properly identified. Consequence of lesion of a motor root of the brachial plexus is paralysis or paresis of the upper limb muscles.

The prevalence of phrenic nerve injury is significantly higher (around 10 to 11%) in series including only RND, compared with those that consider patients undergoing MRND, in which it ranges from 0 to 1%.[7] This complication is most often asymptomatic, although a wide range of signs and symptoms affecting the respiratory tract (cough, dyspnea, chest pain, subcyanosis, and lung base atelectasia), cardiovascular system (palpitations, tachycardia, and extrasystoles due to the mediastinal shift toward the unaffected side of the diaphragm), and gastrointestinal tract (abdominal pain, nausea, vomiting, and heartburn caused by malposition of the abdominal viscera for altered diaphragmatic motility) has been reported. Diagnosis of phrenic nerve palsy is based essentially on chest X-ray (hemidiaphragm elevation corresponding to the injured nerve) and radioscopic examination (immobility, hypomobility or paradoxical movement of a hemidiaphragm during inspiration, or in conditions with increased effort such as those produced during sniffing, and pendular swing of the mediastinum toward the healthy side).[66]

The phrenic nerve is rarely sacrificed for the sake of oncologic radicality. More frequently, it is damaged in the presence of fibrosis and post-RT edema, neoplastic infiltration of adjacent structures or major bleeding requiring vessel ligation or electrocautery in conditions of limited visibility. In case of unilateral PN injury, impairment of lung function with limitations in daily activities is rarely seen; even spirometric parameters are generally not significantly altered. However, this complication should always be feared in patients with heavily impaired pulmonary conditions. Bilateral phrenic nerve palsy can result in a fatal event or, in case of bilateral temporary neuroapraxia, may require prolonged mechanical ventilation.

Systemic Complications

According to Weber et al,[67] complications involving the lower respiratory tract are the most frequent source of systemic morbidity in head and neck cancer surgery. Especially after prolonged procedures, focal or diffuse lung atelectasias, usually resolving with an adequate respiratory physiotherapy, are frequently encountered on postoperative chest X-ray. This condition can evolve, in predisposed patients, to bacterial pneumonia (with *Staphylococcus aureus* as the causal agent in 62% of cases according to McCulloch et al[68]), possibly associated with pleuritis or pulmonary embolism (with a prevalence of 1.7% and 0.5%, respectively, according to Cabra et al[8]). Pneumothorax is less frequent, and is usually secondary to placement of a central venous catheter into the subclavian vein or to injury of the pleural dome during supraclavicular fossa dissection. This rarely causes symptoms, and is most frequently followed by spontaneous resolution when unilateral.

Concerning the digestive tract, postoperative gastrointestinal bleeding, acute pancreatitis, and stress ulcers have been observed with an incidence of 0.3%, 0.2%, and 0.2%, respectively, in the series of Cabra et al.[8]

The cardiovascular system may be affected by postoperative myocardial infarction. A more complex scenario is the QT prolongation syndrome, an abnormal electrocardiographic finding that some authors[69] have associated with sympathetic chain injury during right ND. An important and seemingly stable QT prolongation may lead to torsion of the tips and subsequent malignant arrhythmias such as ventricular fibrillation and cardiac arrest. On the other hand, as demonstrated in animal models, injury to the left cervical stellate ganglion can cause QT interval shortening. Others tend to minimize the importance of ND as a possible cause of ECG alterations and conclude that, in the absence of other concomitant risk factors such as congenital anomalies, metabolic disorders or pharmacologic effects, ND has the same low probability of causing malignant arrhythmias as any other surgical maneuver on the neck.[70]

Prevalence of perioperative cerebrovascular complications in head and neck surgery is around 4.8%, whereas it is reduced to 3.2% when considering only ND.[71] The etiology of this serious complication is undoubtedly multifactorial, including hyperextension and rotation of the head with compression of the C1 transverse process on the carotid artery contralateral to ND, with possible changes at the level of the intimal layer resulting in detachment of atheromatous emboli or thrombogenesis. According to Rechtweg et al,[72] the risk of perioperative stroke is 1% if the patient has one to three risk factors for cerebrovascular disease, reaching up to 20% in the presence of more than three factors. In the latter group of patients, these authors recommend careful evaluation of the vascular supra-aortic trunks and, in the presence of severe carotid stenosis, its surgical treatment before or even simultaneously to ND is warranted.

References

1. Robbins KT, Clayman G, Levine PA, et al. Neck dissection classification update: revisions proposed by the American Head and Neck Society and the American Academy of Otolaryngology-Head and Neck Surgery. Arch Otolaryngol Head Neck Surg 2002;128(7):751–758

2. Ferlito A, Robbins KT, Shah JP, et al. Proposal for a rational classification of neck dissections. Head Neck 2011;33(3):445–450

3. Grim PS, Gottlieb LJ, Boddie A, Batson E. Hyperbaric oxygen therapy. JAMA 1990;263(16):2216–2220

4. Neovius EB, Lind MG, Lind FG. Hyperbaric oxygen therapy for wound complications after surgery in the irradiated head and neck: a review of the literature and a report of 15 consecutive patients. Head Neck 1997;19(4):315–322

5. Simo R, French G. The use of prophylactic antibiotics in head and neck oncological surgery. Curr Opin Otolaryngol Head Neck Surg 2006;14(2):55–61

6. Pang L, Jeannon JP, Simo R. Minimizing complications in salvage head and neck oncological surgery following radiotherapy and chemo-radiotherapy. Curr Opin Otolaryngol Head Neck Surg 2011;19(2):125–131

7. Calearo CV, Teatini G. Functional neck dissection. Anatomical grounds, surgical technique, clinical observations. Ann Otol Rhinol Laryngol 1983;92(3 Pt 1):215–222

8. Cabra J, Herranz J, Monux A, et al. Postoperative complications of functional neck dissection. Oper Tech Otolaryngol—Head Neck Surg 1993;4(8):318–321

9. Spiro JD, Spiro RH, Strong EW. The management of chyle fistula. Laryngoscope 1990;100(7):771–774

10. de Gier HHW, Balm AJM, Bruning PF, Gregor RT, Hilgers FJ. Systematic approach to the treatment of chylous leakage after neck dissection. Head Neck 1996;18(4):347–351

11. Scorza LB, Goldstein BJ, Mahraj RP. Modern management of chylous leak following head and neck surgery: a discussion of percutaneous lymphangiography-guided cannulation and embolization of the thoracic duct. Otolaryngol Clin North Am 2008;41(6):1231–1240, xi

12. Nussenbaum B, Liu JH, Sinard RJ. Systematic management of chyle fistula: the Southwestern experience and review of the literature. Otolaryngol Head Neck Surg 2000;122(1):31–38

13. Ilczyszyn A, Ridha H, Durrani AJ. Management of chyle leak post neck dissection: a case report and literature review. J Plast Reconstr Aesthet Surg 2011;64(9):e223–e230

14. Qureshi SS, Chaturvedi P. A novel technique of management of high output chyle leak after neck dissection. J Surg Oncol 2007;96(2):176–177

15. Martin IC, Marinho LH, Brown AE, McRobbie D. Medium chain triglycerides in the management of chylous fistulae following neck dissection. Br J Oral Maxillofac Surg 1993;31(4):236–238

16. Chantarasak DN, Green MF. Delayed lymphocoele following neck dissection. Br J Plast Surg 1989;42(3):339–340

17. Roh JL, Park CI. OK-432 sclerotherapy of cervical chylous lymphocele after neck dissection. Laryngoscope 2008;118(6):999–1002

18. Nouwen J, Hans S, Halimi P, Laccourreye O. Lymphocele after neck dissection. Ann Otol Rhinol Laryngol 2004;113(1):39–42

19. Müller HR, Hinn G, Buser MW. Internal jugular venous flow measurement by means of a duplex scanner. J Ultrasound Med 1990;9(5):261–265

20. Shankar L, Hawke M, Mehta MH. The radiologic diagnosis of internal jugular vein thrombosis. J Otolaryngol 1991;20(2):138–140

21. Prim MP, de Diego JI, Fernández-Zubillaga A, García-Raya P, Madero R, Gavilán J. Patency and flow of the internal

jugular vein after functional neck dissection. Laryngoscope 2000;110(1):47–50

22. Harada H, Omura K, Takeuchi Y. Patency and caliber of the internal jugular vein after neck dissection. Auris Nasus Larynx 2003;30(3):269–272

23. Docherty JG, Carter R, Sheldon CD, et al. Relative effect of surgery and radiotherapy on the internal jugular vein following functional neck dissection. Head Neck 1993;15(6):553–556

24. Cotter CS, Stringer SP, Landau S, Mancuso AA, Cassisi NJ. Patency of the internal jugular vein following modified radical neck dissection. Laryngoscope 1994;104(7):841–845

25. Lake GM III, DiNardo LJ, Demeo JH. Performance of the internal jugular vein after functional neck dissection. Otolaryngol Head Neck Surg 1994;111(3 Pt 1):201–204

26. Leontsinis TG, Currie AR, Mannell A. Internal jugular vein thrombosis following functional neck dissection. Laryngoscope 1995;105(2):169–174

27. Zohar Y, Strauss M, Sabo R, Sadov R, Sabo G, Lehman J. Internal jugular vein patency after functional neck dissection: venous duplex imaging. Ann Otol Rhinol Laryngol 1995;104(7):532–536

28. Quraishi HA, Wax MK, Granke K, Rodman SM. Internal jugular vein thrombosis after functional and selective neck dissection. Arch Otolaryngol Head Neck Surg 1997;123(9):969–973

29. Wax MK, Quraishi H, Rodman SM, Granke K. Internal jugular vein patency in patients undergoing microvascular reconstruction. Laryngoscope 1997;107(9):1245–1248

30. Cappiello J, Piazza C, Berlucchi M, et al. Internal jugular vein patency after lateral neck dissection: a prospective study. Eur Arch Otorhinolaryngol 2002;259(8):409–412

31. Weiss KL, Wax MK, Haydon RC III, Kaufman HH, Hurst MK. Intracranial pressure changes during bilateral radical neck dissections. Head Neck 1993;15(6):546–552

32. Dulguerov P, Soulier C, Maurice J, Faidutti B, Allal AS, Lehmann W. Bilateral radical neck dissection with unilateral internal jugular vein reconstruction. Laryngoscope 1998;108(11 Pt 1):1692–1696

33. Aydin O, Memisoglu I, Ozturk M, Altintas O. Anterior ischemic optic neuropathy after unilateral radical neck dissection: case report and review. Auris Nasus Larynx 2008;35(2):308–312

34. Suárez-Fernández MJ, Clariana-Martín A, Mencía-Gutiérrez E, Gutiérrez-Díaz E, Gracia-García-Miguel T. Bilateral anterior ischemic optic neuropathy after bilateral neck dissection. Clin Ophthalmol 2010;4:95–100

35. Balm AJM, Brown DH, De Vries WAEJ, Snow GB. Blindness: a potential complication of bilateral neck dissection. J Laryngol Otol 1990;104(2):154–156

36. Marks SC, Jaques DA, Hirata RM, Saunders JR Jr. Blindness following bilateral radical neck dissection. Head Neck 1990;12(4):342–345

37. de Vries WA, Balm AJ, Tiwari RM. Intracranial hypertension following neck dissection. J Laryngol Otol 1986;100(12):1427–1431

38. Lydiatt DD, Ogren FP, Lydiatt WM, Hahn FJ. Increased intracranial pressure as a complication of unilateral radical neck dissection in a patient with congenital absence of the transverse sinus. Head Neck 1991;13(4):359–362

39. Ferlito A, Rinaldo A, Devaney KO. Syndrome of inappropriate antidiuretic hormone secretion associated with head neck cancers: review of the literature. Ann Otol Rhinol Laryngol 1997;106(10 Pt 1):878–883

40. Freeman SB, Hamaker RC, Rate WR, et al. Management of advanced cervical metastasis using intraoperative radiotherapy. Laryngoscope 1995;105(6):575–578

41. Mathis JM, Barr JD, Jungreis CA, et al. Temporary balloon test occlusion of the internal carotid artery: experience in 500 cases. AJNR Am J Neuroradiol 1995;16(4):749–754

42. Standard SC, Ahuja A, Guterman LR, et al. Balloon test occlusion of the internal carotid artery with hypotensive challenge. AJNR Am J Neuroradiol 1995;16(7):1453–1458

43. Citardi MJ, Chaloupka JC, Son YH, Ariyan S, Sasaki CT. Management of carotid artery rupture by monitored endovascular therapeutic occlusion (1988-1994). Laryngoscope 1995;105(10):1086–1092

44. Morrissey DD, Andersen PE, Nesbit GM, Barnwell SL, Everts EC, Cohen JI. Endovascular management of hemorrhage in patients with head and neck cancer. Arch Otolaryngol Head Neck Surg 1997;123(1):15–19

45. Warren FM, Cohen JI, Nesbit GM, Barnwell SL, Wax MK, Andersen PE. Management of carotid 'blowout' with endovascular stent grafts. Laryngoscope 2002;112(3):428–433

46. Nason RW, Binahmed A, Torchia MG, Thliversis J. Clinical observations of the anatomy and function of the marginal mandibular nerve. Int J Oral Maxillofac Surg 2007;36(8):712–715

47. Nahum AM, Mullally W, Marmor L. A syndrome resulting from radical neck dissection. Arch Otolaryngol 1961;74:424–428

48. Piazza C, Cappiello J, Nicolai P. Sternoclavicular joint hypertrophy after neck dissection and upper trapezius myocutaneous flap transposition. Otolaryngol Head Neck Surg 2002;126(2):193–194

49. van Wilgen CP, Dijkstra PU, van der Laan BF, Plukker JT, Roodenburg JL. Shoulder and neck morbidity in quality of life after surgery for head and neck cancer. Head Neck 2004;26(10):839–844

50. Nori S, Soo KC, Green RF, Strong EW, Miodownik S. Utilization of intraoperative electroneurography to understand the innervation of the trapezius muscle. Muscle Nerve 1997;20(3):279–285

51. Miyata K, Kitamura H. Accessory nerve damages and impaired shoulder movements after neck dissections. Am J Otolaryngol 1997;18(3):197–201

52. Krause HR, Bremerich A, Herrmann M. The innervation of the trapezius muscle in connection with radical neck-dissection. An anatomical study. J Craniomaxillofac Surg 1991;19(2):87–89

53. Krause HR, Kornhuber A, Dempf R. A technique for diagnosing the individual patterns of innervation of the trapezius muscle prior to neck dissection. J Craniomaxillofac Surg 1993;21(3):102–106

54. Kierner AC, Zelenka I, Heller S, Burian M. Surgical anatomy of the spinal accessory nerve and the trapezius branches of the cervical plexus. Arch Surg 2000;135(12):1428–1431

55. Kierner AC, Zelenka I, Burian M. How do the cervical plexus and the spinal accessory nerve contribute to the innervation of the trapezius muscle? As seen from within using Sihler's stain. Arch Otolaryngol Head Neck Surg 2001;127(10):1230–1232

56. Kierner AC, Burian M, Bentzien S, Gstoettner W. Intraoperative electromyography for identification of the trapezius muscle innervation: clinical proof of a new anatomical concept. Laryngoscope 2002;112(10):1853–1856

57. Chepeha DB, Taylor RJ, Chepeha JC, et al. Functional assessment using Constant's Shoulder Scale after modified radical and selective neck dissection. Head Neck 2002;24(5):432–436

58. Bradley PJ, Ferlito A, Silver CE, et al. Neck treatment and shoulder morbidity: still a challenge. Head Neck 2011;33(7):1060–1067

59. Rafferty MA, Goldstein DP, Brown DH, Irish JC. The sternomastoid branch of the occipital artery: a surgical landmark for the spinal accessory nerve in selective neck dissections. Otolaryngol Head Neck Surg 2005;133(6):874–876

60. Prim MP, De Diego JI, Verdaguer JM, Sastre N, Rabanal I. Neurological complications following functional neck dissection. Eur Arch Otorhinolaryngol 2006;263(5):473–476

61. Weisberger EC, Kincaid J, Riteris J. Cable grafting of the spinal accessory nerve after radical neck dissection. Arch Otolaryngol Head Neck Surg 1998;124(4):377–380

62. Guo C-B, Zhang Y, Zou L-D, Mao C, Peng X, Yu GY. Reconstruction of accessory nerve defects with sternocleidomastoid muscle–great auricular nerve flap. Br J Plast Surg 2005;58(2):233–238

63. Wiater JM, Bigliani LU. Spinal accessory nerve injury. Clin Orthop Relat Res 1999;368(368):5–16

64. Salerno G, Cavaliere M, Foglia A, et al. The 11th nerve syndrome in functional neck dissection. Laryngoscope 2002;112(7 Pt 1):1299–1307

65. Gacek RR. Neck dissection injury of a brachial plexus anatomical variant. Arch Otolaryngol Head Neck Surg 1990;116(3):356–358

66. de Jong AA, Manni JJ. Phrenic nerve paralysis following neck dissection. Eur Arch Otorhinolaryngol 1991;248(3):132–134

67. Weber RS, Hankins P, Rosenbaum B, Raad I. Nonwound infections following head and neck oncologic surgery. Laryngoscope 1993;103(1 Pt 1):22–27

68. McCulloch TM, Jensen NF, Girod DA, Tsue TT, Weymuller EA Jr. Risk factors for pulmonary complications in the postoperative head and neck surgery patient. Head Neck 1997;19(5):372–377

69. Strickland RA, Stanton MS, Olsen KD. Prolonged QT syndrome: perioperative management. Mayo Clin Proc 1993;68(10):1016–1020

70. Rassekh CH, Dellsperger KC, Hokanson JA, et al. QT interval changes following neck dissection. A stratified prospective study. Ann Otol Rhinol Laryngol 1997;106(10 Pt 1):869–872

71. Nosan DK, Gomez CR, Maves MD. Perioperative stroke in patients undergoing head and neck surgery. Ann Otol Rhinol Laryngol 1993;102(9):717–723

72. Rechtweg J, Wax MK, Shah R, Granke K, Jarmuz T. Neck dissection with simultaneous carotid endarterectomy. Laryngoscope 1998;108(8 Pt 1):1150–1153

26 Complications in Surgery of the Parapharyngeal Space

M. O. Old, R. L. Carrau, B. A. Otto, D. M. Prevedello, A. B. Kassam

Preoperative Considerations

The most important factors in avoiding or managing complications from surgery of the parapharyngeal space are appropriate patient selection and informed consent. Thorough preoperative assessment of patients with parapharyngeal space pathology is critical. Parapharyngeal space surgery can result in significant morbidity, typically related to lower cranial nerve deficits. In experienced hands and with proper patient selection and counseling, morbidity can be significantly reduced. A multidisciplinary tumor board and team are critical to management of these patients. Depending upon the extent and nature of the lesion, team members include the head and neck surgeon, neuro-otologist, laryngologist, vascular surgeon, neurosurgeon, neuro-ophthalmologist, speech pathologist, audiologist, physical therapist, and a variety of other ancillary staff.

Preoperative lower cranial neuropathies (e.g., glossopharyngeal, vagus, accessory, and hypoglossal cranial nerves) are common in patients with tumors that originate at or invade the parapharyngeal space.[1–3] These patients present a wide spectrum of swallowing or speech problems including hypernasal or slurred speech, nasal regurgitation, dysphagia, aspiration, and dysphonia (because of deficits in CNs of glossopharyngeal, vagus, and hypoglossal cranial nerves). These and other preexistent neurologic and functional deficits need to be considered during the preoperative planning, because they significantly impact postoperative recovery and the functional rehabilitation of the patient. For example, pulmonary aspiration, caused by lower cranial neuropathies, has a significant morbidity and mortality. If the patient has long-standing deficits, then compensation may have occurred. However, even if a patient has adjusted well to deficits preoperatively, the effects of additional cranial nerve deficits should be considered and discussed with the patient.

Elderly and unhealthy patients require special consideration preoperatively. A majority of complications involving parapharyngeal space surgery involve lower cranial deficits (glossopharyngeal, vagus, accessory, and hypoglossal cranial nerves). If no deficits exist preoperatively, then proper counseling and discussion of alternative therapies should occur depending upon the pathology. If the cranial nerves are already affected by the tumor, patients have generally already compensated for the deficits and do better postoperatively. If little or no cranial nerve dysfunction is present preoperatively, acute denervation by the surgery can have a higher probability of causing significant morbidity in individuals, particularly the elderly population.[4] In nonaggressive pathologies, radiotherapy or observation should be strongly considered in elderly or infirm patients.

A thorough physical examination will reveal specific cranial nerve dysfunction, such as decreased elevation of the ipsilateral palate causing deviation of the uvula to the unaffected side (glossopharyngeal and vagus cranial nerves) (**Fig. 26.1**), decreased mobility/strength of the tongue with deviation to the involved side upon protrusion (hypoglossal cranial nerve) (**Fig. 26.2**), decreased supraglottic sensation, pooling of secretions in the hypopharynx with spillage into the laryngeal airway, ipsilateral vocal cord paralysis (vagus cranial nerve), and atrophy and paralysis of the sternocleidomastoid and trapezius muscles (accessory cranial nerve). These findings suggest the possible need for a tracheotomy for tracheopulmonary toilet and a gastrostomy tube for nutrition, hydration, and administration of medications.

Patients with a high vagal paralysis may benefit from a medialization laryngoplasty and an arytenoid adduction procedure.[5–8] These may be performed in a single stage with the tumor removal or during the early postoperative period. The authors prefer to delay the medialization and perform it in standard fashion under local anesthesia with sedation.[4,8] Laryngeal framework surgery improves

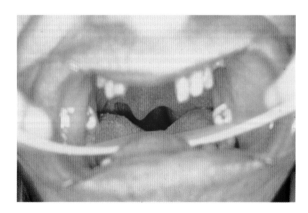

Fig. 26.1 Paralysis of the left palate causing deviation of the uvula to the patient's right and symptomatic velopharyngeal insufficiency.

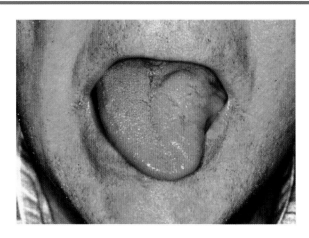

Fig. 26.2 Paralysis of the left hypoglossal nerve causing deviation of the tongue to the patient's left.

the glottic competency; therefore, decreasing the risk for aspiration and improving the effectiveness of the coughing mechanism. This may avoid the need for a tracheotomy for the sole purpose of tracheopulmonary toilet.

It should be noted, however, that laryngeal framework surgery improves the compensatory mechanisms related to motor dysfunction but does not improve the dysfunction related to afferent denervation; hence, patients remain at risk for aspiration and nutritional deficiencies.[5–8] An experienced speech and language pathologist can assist with the monitoring of the patient, recommend modifications in diet, and provide intensive swallowing therapy; therefore complementing the improvements produced by the laryngeal framework surgery.

Patients with severe deficits who do not respond to conservative treatment or those with severe cognitive problems that do not allow them to comply with the rehabilitation benefit from a tracheotomy for tracheopulmonary toilet and from a gastrostomy tube to facilitate postoperative nutrition and decrease the risk of prandial aspiration.

Velopharyngeal insufficiency may be treated with a palatal lift prosthesis although this may not be tolerated in some.[9] Patients who do not tolerate the prosthesis may undergo a pharyngeal flap or a palatopexy (palatal adhesion surgery).[4,9]

Eustachian tube dysfunction due to mechanical or functional obstruction caused by tumors of the infratemporal fossa, may lead to conductive hearing loss. Such tumors may destroy the temporal bone or posterior cranial fossa leading to sensorineural hearing loss. Persistent presbyacusis may also compound the hearing loss. A myringotomy or amplification facilitates communication with the patient.

Trigeminal sensory dysfunction is commonly overlooked. Preoperatively evaluation of the corneal sensation and reflex will reveal any significant deficit. This is especially relevant if the patient also presents incomplete

closure or a dry eye. Limitations of the extraocular movements usually present with diplopia and may occur as a result of direct tumor invasion of the orbit or extraocular muscles or through invasion or compression of the oculomotor, trochlear, and abducens cranial nerves. We recommend a neuro-ophthalmologic evaluation to elucidate these problems and to provide objective measures of the deficit. Similarly, patients with optic nerve problems or with tumor adjacent to the optic nerve, chiasm, or optic tract, are also referred for neuro-ophthalmologic evaluation.

Tumors that invade the facial nerve may cause facial paresis or paralysis, facial spasms, and epiphora (**Figs. 26.3 and 26.4**). A gold weight (implanted in the upper eyelid) or surgical tightening (lateral tarsal strip procedure) of the lower lid may be necessary to protect the cornea. Corneal anesthesia associated with lagophthalmos due to facial nerve palsy or other causes requires aggressive measures (e.g., tarsorrhaphy) to prevent corneal injury.

Lateral deviation of the mandible upon mouth opening may indicate paralysis or tumor invasion of the pterygoid muscles or dysfunction of the temporomandibular joint. Similarly, trismus may be due to mechanical effects of the bulk of the tumor, tethering of the mastication muscles due to scarring or tumor invasion, ankylosis of the temporomandibular joint, or pain. Severity and etiology of the trismus must be considered to ascertain management of the airway during the induction of anesthesia and during the postoperative period. Trismus due to pain

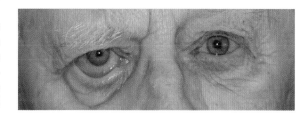

Fig. 26.3 Facial paralysis of the upper division of the facial nerve. The patient has significant ectropion with corneal exposure and lack of eye closure.

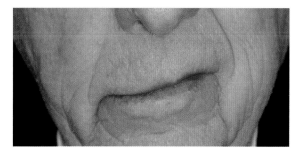

Fig. 26.4 Facial paralysis of the lower division of the facial nerve. The patient has significant facial asymmetry at rest and mild oral incompetence.

resolves with the induction of general anesthesia. If the extirpative surgery is expected to resolve the trismus, the patient may be managed with an awake nasotracheal intubation. Conversely, if the trismus is expected to persist even after tumor removal, the patient may require a tracheotomy performed under local anesthesia.

Preoperative Imaging

Owing to the relative inaccessibility of the infratemporal space to physical examination, radiologic imaging is a critical part of the evaluation. Computed tomography (CT) and magnetic resonance imaging scans provide valuable information. The CT scan is superior to demonstrate enlargement of neural foramina or erosion of bone. Magnetic resonance imaging provides better resolution of soft tissue planes and tumor invasion along neural and vascular structures (**Figs. 26.5 and 26.6**). CT and magnetic resonance imaging are often complementary for the evaluation of cranial base tumors.

A critical consideration is the relationship of the neoplasm to the internal carotid artery (ICA). Magnetic resonance angiography or CT angiography provides a noninvasive assessment of the ITF and intracranial vasculature. If preoperative embolization of the tumor is warranted, as is the case for some juvenile angiofibromas, paragangliomas, or other highly vascularized tumors, angiography is preferable to magnetic resonance angiography, because the tumor can be embolized during the initial angiogram. In addition to providing information about tumor vascularity and involvement of the ICA, the angiogram provides important information regarding intracranial circulation and collateral blood supply. Neither study is adequate, however, to reliably assess the adequacy of collateral intracranial circulation in the event that manipulation or sacrifice of the ICA is necessary. Whenever manipulation of the ICA is likely, evaluation of collateral cerebral blood flow with angiography balloon occlusion xenon CT (ABOX-CT) is recommended.[10]

During an ABOX-CT a nondetachable balloon is introduced into the ICA and it is inflated for 15 minutes, as the awake patient is monitored for sensory, motor, or higher cortical function deficits. The balloon is deflated, and the patient is transferred to a standard CT suite. The balloon is reinflated, and a mixture of 32% xenon and 68% oxygen is then administered to the patient via facial mask for 4 minutes. The CT scan will demonstrate the distribution of xenon within the cerebral tissue, which reflects the blood flow. This provides a quantitative assessment of millimeters of blood flow per minute per 100 g of brain tissue (mL/min/100 g tissue). This test accurately predicts those patients at risk for a cerebrovascular accident when blood flow through the ICA is compromised. This test, however, is fallible. Patients can still suffer ischemic brain injury despite negative ABOX-CT testing owing to embolic

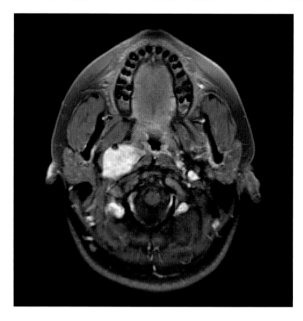

Fig. 26.5 Axial T1-weighted magnetic resonance imaging with contrast revealing a right parapharyngeal space sympathetic chain schwannoma pushing the internal carotid anteriorly. The patient has a preoperative Horner syndrome.

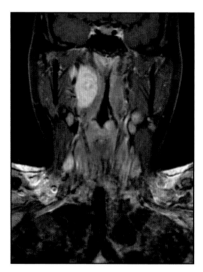

Fig. 26.6 Coronal T1-weighted magnetic resonance imaging with contrast of the same patient demonstrating the parapharyngeal space sympathetic chain schwannoma and medial deviation of the oropharynx. The internal carotid can be seen coursing the anterior surface of the tumor.

phenomena or the loss of collateral vessels, which are not assessed by balloon occlusion testing. For these reasons, every attempt is made to preserve or reconstruct the ICA when feasible. Other techniques that provide similar information regarding collateral cerebral blood flow include single photon emission CT (SPECT) with balloon occlusion and transcranial Doppler monitoring.

Need for blood replacement should also be considered; if deemed necessary, type and cross the patient for 2 to 6 units of packed red blood cells according to the extent and nature of the tumor and surgery. We advocate autologous blood banking when feasible, although it is frequently impractical. A cell-saver or autotransfusion device may be used during the resection of benign vascular tumors. Angiography and embolization in highly vascular tumors, such as glomus and angiofibromas, may curtail the need for blood replacement. Embolization of paragangliomas, however, is controversial. Vagal paragangliomas rarely have a single blood supply and their resection usually is not associated with excessive blood loss. Carotid body tumors do not have an obvious dominant vessel supply, but depend upon the adventitia of the carotid artery. Embolization of these lesions may result in an inflammatory response that obscures the subadventitial plane of the tumor; hence, adding to the difficulty of the dissection. We prefer not to embolize most carotid body tumors. In the rare cases when we choose embolization, it must be performed within 24 hours of the planned resection because of collateralization and the inflammatory response of embolization.

Complications

Although surgical intervention has improved greatly, the potential for complications and adverse effects is significant when operating in the parapharyngeal space. Complication rates vary from 25 to 40% with classic approaches.[1,11–13] Most are transient neurologic deficits and permanent sequelae are present in only 11%.[1] Rates of each particular complication vary significantly from study to study because of the rarity of the lesions and different pathology distributions. Complication rates are increased for malignant and neurogenic tumors compared with benign neoplasms such as pleomorphic adenomas. Patients should be adequately counseled regarding potential complications and expected course of recovery. Surgical complications are dependent on the etiology, nature and extent of the tumor; and, to some degree on the preferred surgical approach (different structures are exposed and manipulated). Much of the morbidity management related to the resection of tumors of the parapharyngeal space has been addressed in the previous section. We will complement this information by looking at the specific complications.

Cranial Neuropathies

> **Note**
> Deficits of the trigeminal nerve are common after surgery of the parapharyngeal space.

Loss of corneal sensation, especially in someone with facial nerve dysfunction, greatly increases the risk of a corneal abrasion or exposure keratitis. Facial anesthesia may predispose the patient to self-inflicted injuries, including neurotrophic ulcers. Loss of motor function of the mandibular nerve causes asymmetry of jaw opening and decreased force of mastication on the operated side, which may be further impaired by resection of the temporomandibular joint or mandibular ramus.

Temporary or permanent facial nerve dysfunction is a common occurrence, especially the marginal mandibular branch. During a transcervical approach to the parapharyngeal space with stylomandibular ligament or styloid bone resection, anterior displacement of the jaw should be performed with caution because this can cause traction injury to the facial nerve, specifically the lower division.

The risk increases with transparotid approaches, although avulsion of the nerve and cautery-induced electrical or thermal trauma are also possible. All these need to be considered during the surgery and avoided.

The removal of a vagal paraganglioma is associated with 100% incidence of permanent vocal cord paralysis and must be approached accordingly. Large paraganglioma involving the jugular foramen places the glossopharyngeal, vagus, accessory, and hypoglossal cranial nerves at risk and may require a combined skull base approach. During the surgical approach to a carotid body tumor, the vagus and hypoglossal nerves must be mobilized and preserved. These cranial nerves may occasionally lie on or be embedded within the tumor, but tumor invasion of cranial nerves is unusual.

Bilateral carotid body tumors are better addressed following a staged approach removing the larger tumor first. Subsequent treatment of the second lesion is dictated by postoperative assessment of cranial nerve function as the vagus nerve is at risk in each surgery. Bilateral vagal injury would be devastating and the patient will typically be tracheostomy and G-tube dependent. The patient should be counseled regarding baroreflex failure before contralateral resection (see section below) as the results can be debilitating.

Trismus

Postoperative trismus is also common because of postoperative pain and inflammation and subsequent scarring of the pterygoid muscles or temporomandibular joint. Trismus improves dramatically if patients perform active and passive stretching exercises for the jaw. Patients may also benefit from using devices such as the TheraBite Jaw Motion Rehabilitation System (Atos Medical Inc., West Allis, WI, USA) particularly if they will or have received radiotherapy. In severe cases, a dental appliance that gradually opens with a screw may be fabricated.

Sympathetic Chain Deficits: Horner Syndrome and First-Bite Syndrome

Damage or sacrifice of the cervical sympathetic chain can lead to two different problems—Horner syndrome and first-bite syndrome.[4] Horner syndrome consists of ptosis, miosis, and anhidrosis and is usually well tolerated (**Fig. 26.7**). This typically resolves if the sympathetic chain has been preserved. The Muller muscle may be resected or a levator-shortening procedure can be performed if the ptosis is troubling and does not resolve in cases where the sympathetic chain is preserved. First-bite syndrome results from unopposed parasympathetic stimulation of the myoepithelial cells after losing sympathetic input to the parotid gland, typically when the external carotid artery is ligated inferior to the parotid gland or the sympathetic chain is injured or sacrificed.[14]

Patients complain of mild to severe pain with the first bite of food that diminishes with time during the meal. Thinking of eating, spontaneous salivation, and strong sialogogs can increase the severity of symptoms, so patients will naturally gravitate to bland foods at the beginning of meals. The symptoms generally abate overtime but recovery is unpredictable. Thorough counseling should include dietary modifications. Eating bland foods at the start of a meal is the best treatment available at this time. Medications such as carbamazepine can be used but we have not encouraged this treatment because time and dietary modification work well for the majority of patients.

Infections

Infectious complications are rare. Predisposing factors include communication with the nasopharynx, seroma, or hematoma, and cerebrospinal fluid leaks. In general, we obliterate the dead space to prevent fluid collections, which subsequently can be colonized and infected. Separation of the cranial cavity from the upper aerodigestive tract is a requirement to avoid contamination with its flora. Vascularized tissue flaps are preferable, especially when dissection of the ICA or resection of the dura mater has been performed.

Wound Necrosis

This situation is rare. Poorly designed incisions and prolonged use of hemostatic clamps may result in areas of ischemia that can make the tissue susceptible to secondary infection. Patients who have undergone previous radiotherapy or chemoradiotherapy are at higher risk for this complication. Proper preoperative planning, minimizing retraction of tissue flaps during the procedure, viability assessment of the flaps at the end of cases, and the use of vascularized reconstruction can reduce this complication.

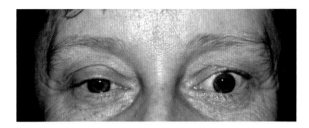

Fig. 26.7 Horner syndrome of the right side.

Neurovascular

Although not common, there is a risk of cerebrovascular injury during the removal of a carotid body paraganglioma. Similarly, proximal and distal vascular control of the internal carotid artery is necessary before tumor dissection. When dealing with a large carotid body tumor, distal control of the ICA at the skull base may be extremely difficult, as a minimum space of 1 cm is necessary to achieve vascular control of the ICA. Preoperative imaging may allow the surgeon to anticipate this scenario. When distal control of the ICA is not possible, preoperative angiography with balloon test occlusion and xenon-enhanced CT scan evaluation of contralateral circulation is necessary. The vessel can be sacrificed using endovascular techniques. Consultation with a vascular surgeon is prudent if a possibility of carotid resection or interposition grafting exists.

Postoperative cerebral ischemia may result from surgical occlusion of the ICA, temporary vasospasm, and thromboembolic phenomenon. Surgical dissection of the ICA can injure the vessel walls, resulting in immediate or delayed rupture and hemorrhage. In the event that a repair of the ICA is not possible, permanently occlude it by ligation or by the placement of a detachable balloon or vascular coil. Perform the occlusion as distally as possible (near the origin of the ophthalmic artery). The potential for thrombus formation decreases with a short column of stagnant blood above the level of occlusion.

Baroreflex Failure

Baroreflex failure occurs when bilateral carotid body-sinus complexes are denervated, leading to loss of the parasympathetic drive of this system. Complications occur when the unopposed sympathetic tone results in severe labile hypertension, hypotension, headache, diaphoresis, and emotional problems. Stress often induces a hypertensive crisis and antianxiety medications play a critical role in the prevention and treatment of these situations. Sodium nitroprusside can be used to control hypertension in the early postoperative period. Hypertension control postoperatively in these patients is critical, especially in those who underwent vascular repair or replacement.[15] Clonidine and phenoxybenzamine are helpful in these situations. Phenoxybenzamine is an α1 and α2 blocker and has a more rapid onset than clonidine, which is a selective α2-adrenergic agonist. Compensation does occur in these patients but the timing of this is unpredictable and variable.[4]

Cardiovascular Complications

It is also important to recognize that carotid body tumors may be associated with pheochromocytomas occasionally, and that they may produce catecholamines. A family history may elicit a familial form (paraganglioma type 1) of the disease or the possibility of multiple endocrine neoplasia syndromes. Tachycardia, hypertension, or intermittent flushing should prompt increased concern. Evaluation for elevated catecholamines and vanillylmandelic acid is mandatory under these circumstances (24-hour urine collection). Functional paragangliomas are more common in the hereditary syndromes. Presence of a pheochromocytoma in multiple endocrine neoplasia type 2B syndrome is a well-recognized association. When elevated catecholamines are present, the meta-iodinated benzylguanidine scan may localize the site of the secreting tumor. Failure to identify functional tumors may result in intraoperative cardiac arrhythmias and hypertensive crisis. Preoperative adrenergic blockage with phenoxybenzamine (α-adrenergic blocker) and propranolol (β-adrenergic blocker) can minimize these effects.

Conclusion

The complex neurovascular anatomy of the parapharyngeal space lends itself to increased morbidity during surgical procedures compared with other sites of the head and neck. Experience, preoperative assessment, informed consent, and a multidisciplinary approach are critical to the success of surgery in this region as well as the reduction and management of morbidities associated with these procedures.

Disclosure

ABK is a paid consultant for Karl Storz-Endoscopy and Stryker and holds an equity stake in NICO Corporation.

References

1. Carrau RL, Myers EN, Johnson JT. Management of tumors arising in the parapharyngeal space. Laryngoscope 1990;100(6):583–589
2. Myers E, Carrau R. Tumors arising in the parapharyngeal space. Revista Brasileira Cirugia Cabeca Pescoco. 1994;18:6–12
3. Cohen SM, Burkey BB, Netterville JL. Surgical management of parapharyngeal space masses. Head Neck 2005;27(8):669–675
4. Old M, Netterville JL. Head and Neck Paragangliomas. Head and Neck Cancer: Multimodality Management. Springer Science+Business Media. April 2011; 569–580
5. Carrau R, Eibling D, Myers E. Thyroplasty and arytenoid adduction for vocal cord medialization. Mexican Annals of Otolaryngology. 1994;39:23–28
6. Pou AM, Carrau RL, Eibling DE, Murry T. Laryngeal framework surgery for the management of aspiration in high vagal lesions. Am J Otolaryngol 1998;19(1):1–7
7. Carrau R, Pou A, Eibling DE, Murry T, Ferguson BJ. Laryngeal framework surgery for the treatment of aspiration. Oper Tech Otolaryngol–Head Neck Surg 1998;9:126–134
8. Jalisi S, Netterville JL. Rehabilitation after cranial base surgery. Otolaryngol Clin North Am 2009;42(1):49–56, viii
9. Netterville JL, Fortune S, Stanziale S, Billante CR. Palatal adhesion: the treatment of unilateral palatal paralysis after high vagus nerve injury. Head Neck 2002;24(8):721–730
10. Snyderman CH, Carrau RL, deVries EJ. Carotid artery resection: Update on preoperative evaluation. In: Johnson JT, Derkay CS, Mandell-Brown MK, Newman RK, eds. AAO-HNS Instructional Courses. Alexandria, VA: American Association of Otolayngologists-Head neck Surgery. 1993;341–346
11. Dimitrijevic MV, Jesic SD, Mikic AA, Arsovic NA, Tomanovic NR. Papapharyngeal space tumors: 61 case reviews. Int J Oral Maxillofac Surg 2010;39(10):983–989
12. Malone JP, Agrawal A, Schuller DE. Safety and efficacy of transcervical resection of parapharyngeal space neoplasms. Ann Otol Rhinol Laryngol 2001;110(12):1093–1098
13. Luna-Ortiz K, Navarrete-Alemán JE, Granados-García M, Herrera-Gómez A. Primary parapharyngeal space tumors in a Mexican cancer center. Otolaryngol Head Neck Surg 2005;132(4):587–591
14. Chiu AG, Cohen JI, Burningham AR, Andersen PE, Davidson BJ. First bite syndrome: a complication of surgery involving the parapharyngeal space. Head Neck 2002;24(11):996–999
15. Netterville JL, Reilly KM, Robertson D, Reiber ME, Armstrong WB, Childs P. Carotid body tumors: a review of 30 patients with 46 tumors. Laryngoscope 1995;105(2):115–126

27 Infectious Diseases (Lymphadenopathies, Abscesses, Necrotizing Fasciitis)

C. L. Oliver

Introduction

Infectious complications following head and neck surgery (HNS) can have devastating consequences for patients. Many major HNS breech the protective mucosa and expose "clean" anatomy to a bacterial inoculate, significantly increasing the risk of postoperative infection. Before the introduction of prophylactic antibiotic regimens, the postoperative infection rates for major HNS ranged from 36 to 87%.[1,2] Postoperative infections extend hospitalizations, increase patient-care costs, and limit immediate and long-term patient quality of life.[3–5] During a study period from 1977 to 1989, Blair et al[5] found postoperative infections resulted in an average increase in hospital stay of 15 days (at an estimated cost of $2,402 per day in 1992 US dollars). More recently, Penel et al[4] reported an increase of 16 hospitalization days and 17,000 Euros for surgical site infections (SSI) in HNS. Surgical site infections are a major healthcare cost. In a recent quantification of the costs of SSI, Broex et al[6] reported that SSI resulted in approximately double the costs, when compared with a patient without an SSI.

In an attempt to standardize the reporting of postoperative head and neck infections, Johnson et al[7] adapted a wound grading system from an American College of Surgeons Manual on control of infection in surgical patients. They defined a postoperative head and neck wound infection as a wound with purulent drainage by incision, spontaneous drainage, or development of a mucocutaneous fistula (**Fig. 27.1**). Most authors publishing in the head and neck literature subsequently have adopted Johnson's criteria. The Centers for Disease Control and the American College of Surgeons have adopted the terminology of SSI. This terminology was introduced in 1992 and was revised in 1999.[8] The basic schematic of SSI anatomy and appropriate classification is demonstrated in **Fig. 27.2** (see Horan et al[8] for full details and definitions). In keeping with Johnson's spirit of standardization, head and neck surgeons may want to adopt/modify the SSI terminology when reporting in the future.

In 1986, Becker stated, "Any method of wound infection control in patients undergoing HNS should address the following question: (1) who is likely to develop a wound infection; (2) what is the likely bacterial flora of the wound infection; (3) which antibiotic, or combination of antibiotics, should be used, and for how long; and (4) which adjunctive methods (other than the perioperative use of antibiotics) will decrease the rate of wound

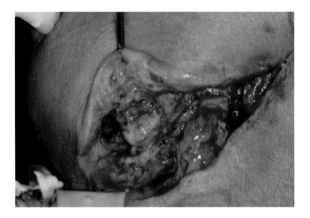

Fig. 27.1 Necrotizing fasciitis of the left neck. Note necrotic tissue within the reopened wound after neck dissection. (Image courtesy of F. Sabater, MD.)

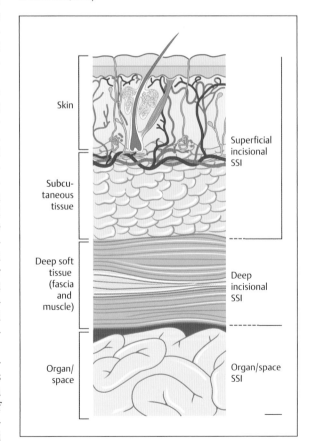

Fig. 27.2 Surgical site infection (SSI) anatomy and classification. (Adapted from Horan et al, 1992.[8])

Table 27.1 A summary of the risks of surgical site infections after head and neck surgery

	Reference number									
	10	11	12	13	14	15	16	17	18	19
Reported incidence of SSI (%)	22%	11%	25.4%	19.8%	45%	10%	18.4%	7%	38.8%	21%
Incidence of SSI in clean–contaminated cases	22%	NR	25.4%	20.6%	45%	18.6%	33.7%	7%	38.8%	21%
Total patients	159	119	59	400	260	209	697	245	258	66
Patient factors < 0.001										
Previous chemotherapy					0.009	< 0.001*	< 0.001			
Previous radiotherapy	0.05						0.001*			0.01
Extended perioperative hospitalization		Postop. 0.05			Preop. 0.013		Diabetes 0.002		0.018*	
Comorbidities			*							
Sex					Male 0.02		Male			
Smoking							< 0.001		0.044*	
Active alcohol use				< 0.05			0.02			
Nutrition/ Albumin/ Weight loss/ Anemia				0.001			Anemia 0.016/ Albumin 0.025			
Disease factors										
T3–4 versus T1–2			0.018*	0.001		0.028*	0.02	T4 < 0.01	0.025	0.05
Cervical metastasis			0.006*	< 0.05*			0.017		0.001*	
Tumor location[a]					HP 0.003		OC 0.028*			
Operative factors										
Tracheotomy				< 0.001		< 0.001*	< 0.001*			0.01
Length of surgery	0.005	0.015	< 0.001			< 0.001	< 0.001		0.009	
Clean–contaminated versus clean surgery				< 0.001*	NA	0.006*	< 0.001*	NA	NA	NA
Adequate antibiotic prophylaxis				0.003*					0.032*	
Flap reconstruction				0.003		Free flap < 0.001*	< 0.001	< 0.001	0.017*	Flap or STSG 0.005*
Transfusion				0.01		0.01	< 0.001			0.01

HP, hypopharynx; OC, oral cavity; SSI, surgical site infection; STSG, split-thickness skin graft.
*Indicates a statistically significant result.

III E Surgery of the Neck

infection?"[9] Multiple publications since Becker's statement have attempted to answer the basic question; what are the major risk factors for SSI after HNS. The results from several of these studies were analyzed and are summarized in **Table 27.1**.[10–19]

As underscored by Becker, substantial reductions in SSI following HNS were seen with the introduction of appropriate antibiotic prophylaxis. We will address the topic of prophylactic antibiotics initially and independently from other factors influencing SSI in HNS.

Prophylactic Antibiotics

The role of prophylactic antibiotics in clean (noncontaminated) surgery of the head and neck is limited, and should not be employed routinely.[20] The use of prophylactic antibiotics in uncontaminated neck dissections has been controversial. In a review of uncontaminated neck dissections, Carrau et al[21] reported a trend that did not reach statistical significance, favoring the efficacy of antibiotic prophylaxis. In 2004, Seven et al[22] reported on a prospective study (with historical controls) that reached statistical significance ($p = 0.02$) for the use of antibiotic prophylaxis in clean neck dissections. Most recently, Man et al[23] studied 273 uncontaminated neck dissections, comparing several antibiotic regimens. All wound infections occurred in patients receiving antibiotics. Infections were associated with extent of surgery (radical or extended neck dissections, $p = 0.006$), flap closure ($p < 0.001$), and extended length of surgery ($p < 0.001$). As demonstrated by Man et al,[23] it is my opinion that antibiotic prophylaxis for clean surgery of the head and neck should be be individualized based on the presence or absence of the risk factors outlined in **Table 27.1**.

In contrast to clean HNS, many studies have demonstrated the efficacy of prophylactic antibiotics in decreasing the incidence of SSI in the setting of clean–contaminated HNS. Burke[24] initially demonstrated that the timing of antibiotic delivery relative to bacterial inoculate was critical. Prophylactic antibiotics should be delivered intravenously before incision, and should be redosed according to half-life. Antibiotics delivered even 3 hours after the inoculate are ineffective at the prevention of infection. Rubin, Penel and others have described the polymicrobial nature of SSI after HNS, and prophylactic antibiotic regimens must include activity against gram-negative, aerobic, and anaerobic organisms.[14,20,25] Common single agents include cefazolin, cefotaxime, ampicillin, and clindamycin. Combinations with extended coverage are more effective than single agents and are recommended, including, clindamicin/metronidazole, amoxicillin/clavulanic acid, cefuroxime/metronidazole, clindamicin/gentamicin, and ampicillin/sulbactam.[20]

Multiple studies have attempted to define the optimal duration of perioperative antibiotics. In summary, the literature does not support the continuation of antibiotic coverage for > 24 hours following surgery, even in the setting of complex reconstruction.[26–29]

Preoperative Factors

> **Note**
>
> Preoperative consideration of patient risk factors for SSI may provide the opportunity to modify the likelihood of an SSI, or prepare both the patient and the surgical team for the possibility of an SSI.

Nutrition

One of the most commonly evaluated preoperative patient factors is nutrition. Reported in 1983, Hooley et al[30] successfully used the Prognostic Nutritional Index to predict major complications following HNS, whereas Daly et al[31] reported aggressive use of parenteral nutritional support to allow weight gain, and improved wound healing in patients with head and neck cancers. In spite of these findings, nutritional factors (serum albumin, anemia) have failed to reach statistical significance in many studies.[14,17,18] It is my feeling that severely malnourished head and neck cancer patients should undergo intense enteral nutrition regimens before definitive treatment, and that all other patients should have their nutritional needs addressed concurrently with treatment of disease.

Recurrence

Head and neck malignancies can recur or persist following treatment with chemotherapy and radiotherapy. Head and neck surgery in this salvage setting has been associated with increased rates of SSI (**Table 27.1**). In the setting of persistent disease, surgical timing may rely heavily on disease factors and the schedule for planned neck dissections following definitive treatment can be altered. Goguen et al[32] reported that eight out of nine SSI in posttreatment neck dissections occurred when neck dissections were performed less than 12 weeks after completion of chemoradiotherapy. In this study, patients undergoing neck dissection more than 12 weeks after completion of treatment had fewer postoperative complications without impact on disease-related outcomes. It should be noted that the increased risk of SSI is independently associated with previous chemotherapy or radiotherapy. In fact, Penel et al[33] reported previous chemotherapy as the only significant predictor of wound infections following clean HNS.

Alcohol and Tobacco Use

Both alcohol and tobacco use have been associated with an increased risk of perioperative complications following many types of surgery. In a review of the impact of smoking cessation, Wein[34] concludes that there are few data showing a significant change in perioperative morbidity from smoking cessation 1 to 4 weeks before surgery, as prevention of pulmonary complications requires 4 to 8 weeks of abstinence and wound healing benefits have been reported to require 4 or more weeks. In a population-based retrospective cohort study of postdischarge SSI, Daneman et al[35] found alcoholism to be a significant risk factor. Whereas the long-term benefits are clear, I have found that patients addicted to these drugs can be resistant to discontinuing their use before surgery.

Comorbidities

Comorbidities are common in patients with head and neck malignancies. Optimization of comorbidities such as diabetes mellitus, chronic obstructive pulmonary disease, and immunosuppression is recommended before HNS.

Methicillin-Resistant *S. aureus*

Methicillin-resistant *Staphylococcus aureus* (MRSA) is an aggressive nosocomial pathogen of increasing clinical importance worldwide. Watters et al[36] retrospectively investigated the effect of MRSA conversion in the postoperative period. They found a 45% postoperative conversion rate in 55 patients who underwent major HNS. Conversion was associated with an average hospital stay and average cost three times greater than for nonconverters. Of those that converted, 52% (13/25) required further surgery during acute management. More recently, Jeannon et al[37] reported on a retrospective uncontrolled case series of 31 patients regarding the role of MRSA on pharyngocutaneous fistula (PCF) formation following total laryngectomy. No patients were colonized before surgery. Ten patients (32%) acquired MRSA during the postoperative hospitalization. Ten patients (32%) developed PCF, eight of these were MRSA positive, whereas of the 21 patients that did not develop PCF, only two were MRSA positive ($p < 0.001$). Of the two MRSA-positive patients without PCF, both exhibited SSI, one, a wound cellulitis and the other, a carotid fistula (total number of SSI was not reported). These reports suggest the importance of (1) preoperative screening and treatment for MRSA in patients undergoing major HNS, (2) keeping a low index of suspicion for MRSA in postoperative SSI, and (3) hospital protocols to prevent/limit MRSA transmission and colonization. Further investigations are needed regarding the outcome of preoperative MRSA-positive patients to determine MRSA as a causative agent versus a consequence of postoperative wound healing issues in HNS.

Oral Health and Radiation Necrosis

The importance of dental disease/oral health and radiation necrosis has long been established, but the relationship to SSI after major HNS has been difficult to establish. Multiple studies have evaluated the effect of topical antibiotics on oral flora and postoperative SSI. A significant decrease in the absolute bacterial counts has been noted, and one study reported no postoperative infections in 10 patients undergoing laryngectomy with only topical clindamycin prophylaxis.[38–40] The majority of studies have found no significant benefit from the addition of topical antibiotics to established parenteral regimens, including in high-risk flap reconstruction.[41–43] In spite of these results there is some evidence that oral health care can impact postsurgical infections. Sato et al[19] prospectively studied risk factors for the development of SSI and the effect of systematic oral health care on 33 of 66 consecutive patients with oral cavity squamous cell carcinoma. The majority of their results are summarized in **Table 27.1**, but the finding that following multiple regression analysis only tissue transplantation (skin grafts and flap reconstruction) and oral health care emerged as independent risk factors was not included.

In a retrospective study investigating the optimal timing of dental extractions/edentulations with regards to major HNS, Doerr and Marunick[44] found a trend, not reaching statistical significance, of fewer postoperative wound complications in patients undergoing dental extraction at the time of ablative surgery rather than in a postoperative setting. Possible explanations of these findings could be a decreased bacterial load secondary to removal of grossly infected dentition, and a reduction in postoperative periodontal disease.

Postoperative Pneumonia

Postoperative pneumonia can be a significant non-SSI infectious cause of morbidity and mortality in HNS.[45] Most cases of postoperative pulmonary infections appear to be caused by aspiration of bacteria colonizing the upper aerodigestive tract. In a matched cohort study, Bágyi et al[46] compared the presence of periodontal disease in five patients who developed pneumonia following neurologic surgery with 18 matched controls. They reported significantly worse periodontal disease in the pneumonia group, with a high periodontal score resulting in a relative risk increase of 3.5 versus controls. In a prospective analysis of the effects of oral care in an institutionalized elderly population, Yoneyama et al[47] reported a relative risk increase of 1.67 for the development of pneumonia without versus with oral care. Given the frequency of pneumonia and SSIs in HNS, additional effort should be concentrated on delineating and potentially modifying the effect of dental disease.

Perioperative Factors

Many perioperative factors increasing the risk of postoperative SSI are difficult to modify, such as tumor stage, presence of cervical disease, tumor location, need for flap reconstruction and clean versus clean–contaminated wound. Other risk factors can be directly or indirectly modified, such as the timing of dental extractions and the choice for more time-consuming reconstruction. Following basic surgical principles in conjunction with sound surgical judgment is beyond the scope of this chapter but remains critical to optimal postoperative wound healing.

When additional tissue is needed for coverage/closure, it must have adequate vascularity or it will result in wound dehiscence and likely infection. Both adequacy of arterial inflow and adequacy of venous drainage are critical for free/pedicled flap viability. Common methods used to assess flap viability intraoperatively/postoperatively include implantable Doppler systems, color duplex sonography, near-infrared tissue oximetry (ViOptix; Fremont, CA, USA) and laser Doppler flowmetry.[48,49] I find the most practical and accurate combination to improve flap design and monitor for viability are preflap ultrasound to precisely localize vascular supply and intraoperative/postoperative ViOptix oximetry. For example, the fibular osteocutaneous free flap is a commonly employed method of mandibular reconstruction, the cutaneous portion of which relies on perforator vascularity and has historically been of questionable reliability.[50] In fact, Yu et al[51] recently published a study describing the location of 202 cutaneous perforators in 80 patients, and described the design of the cutaneous paddle for optimal vascularity. In my practice, all patients for whom a fibula osteocutaneous free flap reconstruction is contemplated undergo a brief surgeon-performed color-flow Doppler examination with localization of cutaneous perforators, confirmation of three-vessel outflow to the foot, and preliminary design of a cutaneous paddle (**Figs. 27.3 and 27.4**). Intraoperatively and postoperatively, I have found the ViOptix to be a sensitive method of flap monitoring, detecting even early venous outflow obstruction, and allowing flap salvage.

Many head and neck surgeons delay extubation following free-flaps and complex transoral resections when patients have not undergone tracheotomy. One must weigh the risk of postoperative hemorrhage, delayed airway edema, loss of a secured airway, and emergence-related agitation with the risks of delayed extubation or tracheotomy. Tracheotomy is a documented risk factor for the development of SSI after HNS (**Table 27.1**). A recent report comparing delayed versus immediate extubation following free-flap reconstruction found that delayed extubation resulted in longer intensive care unit stays, increased anxiolytic use, increased restraint use, and increased incidence of pneumonia; without difference in flap outcome.[52]

Postoperative Care

The postoperative period can often be a maze of medical/surgical issues that must be managed effectively for optimal patient outcomes. Of critical wound importance in the postoperative period are maintenance of drain suction/patency, early institution of enteral nutrition, and control of hyperglycemia. There is ample evidence that enteral nutrition should be instituted within 24 hours of admission to intensive care or surgery.[53] Early enteral nutrition has been found to decrease septic complications, abscess formation, the development of pneumonia, and mortality.[53,54] Preoperative gastric tube placement or a nasogastric feeding tube placed at the time of surgery should be used within the first 24 hours following surgery.

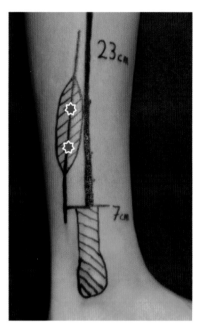

Fig. 27.3 Lateral leg with fibula free flap outlined. Note 8 × 2.5-cm skin paddle positioned over two septocutaneous perforators (red stars). Blue solid line delineates the posterior intermuscular septum.

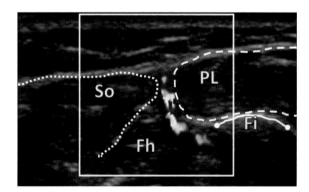

Fig. 27.4 Color duplex sonography. Transverse image at the level of septocutaneous perforator. PL, peroneus longus; So, soleus; Fh, flexor hallucis; Fi, lateral aspect of fibula.

In a retrospective study of 995 patients undergoing general or vascular surgery, bivariate and multivariate analysis demonstrated postoperative hyperglycemia as a risk factor for the development of postoperative infection. They reported that postoperative hyperglycemia increased the risk of postoperative infection by 30% with every 40-point increase above normoglycemia (< 110 mg/dL).[55] Insulin sliding scale protocols should be employed to control blood glucose because many HNS patients will become hyperglycemic in the early postoperative period due to the combination of stress, steroid administration, and tube feeding.

Postoperative SSI can be difficult to identify in the early postoperative period secondary to flap obstruction, edema, and erythema. Other clinical parameters of infection can be unreliable in this period such as mild white blood cell elevations and low-grade temperatures. Often wound dehiscence and overt drainage or purulent material in the drains is the first sign of an SSI. At the point of overt infection, efforts should be directed at control of the infection. If drains are functioning to decompress the area, every effort should be made to continue their effectiveness as a controlled fistula can often be managed by delayed drain removal and subsequent closure of the tract. If the drains are ineffective at evacuating the wound, it should be opened, drained, and managed with wound care until secondary reconstruction is appropriate if needed. Major considerations in this setting are the airway and the carotid artery. A significant number of wounds will heal with a variety of wound care techniques if given adequate time and nutrition.[56] I find an effective strategy is physician-performed dressing changes until the wound is clear of gross contamination, followed by less labor intensive methods such as vacuum-assisted dressings administered by support staff. Dhir et al[57] reported significant applicability and versatility of vacuum-assisted closure therapy in the management of head and neck wounds. The adhesion of the vacuum-assisted dressing can be effectively augmented by circumferential application of stoma paste adhesive. Exposure of the carotid artery should always be treated with extreme caution and usually warrants soft tissue coverage in an expedited fashion.

In summary, HNS patients are often at high risk for postoperative SSI because of the factors outlined in **Table 27.1**. Preoperative assessment may provide opportunities to institute clinical decisions that decrease overall risks, or at the very least, prepare the practitioner and patient for the likelihood of postoperative complications.

References

1. Becker GD, Parell GJ. Cefazolin prophylaxis in head and neck cancer surgery. Ann Otol Rhinol Laryngol 1979;88(2 Pt 1):183–186
2. Dor P, Klastersky J. Prophylactic antibiotics in oral, pharyngeal and laryngeal surgery for cancer: (a double-blind study). Laryngoscope 1973;83(12):1992–1998
3. Grandis JR, Snyderman CH, Johnson JT, Yu VL, D'Amico F. Postoperative wound infection. A poor prognostic sign for patients with head and neck cancer. Cancer 1992;70(8):2166–2170
4. Penel N, Lefebvre JL, Cazin JL, et al. Additional direct medical costs associated with nosocomial infections after head and neck cancer surgery: a hospital-perspective analysis. Int J Oral Maxillofac Surg 2008;37(2):135–139
5. Blair EA, Johnson JT, Wagner RL, Carrau RL, Bizakis JG. Cost analysis of antibiotic prophylaxis in clean head and neck surgery. Arch Otolaryngol Head Neck Surg 1995;121(3):269–271
6. Broex ECJ, van Asselt ADI, Bruggeman CA, van Tiel FH. Surgical site infections: how high are the costs? J Hosp Infect 2009;72(3):193–201
7. Johnson JT, Myers EN, Thearle PB, Sigler BA, Schramm VL Jr. Antimicrobial prophylaxis for contaminated head and neck surgery. Laryngoscope 1984;94(1):46–51
8. Horan TC, Gaynes RP, Martone WJ, Jarvis WR, Emori TG. CDC definitions of nosocomial surgical site infections, 1992: a modification of CDC definitions of surgical wound infections. Infect Control Hosp Epidemiol 1992;13(10):606–608
9. Becker GD. Identification and management of the patient at high risk for wound infection. Head Neck Surg 1986;8(3):205–210
10. Girod DA, McCulloch TM, Tsue TT, Weymuller EA Jr. Risk factors for complications in clean–contaminated head and neck surgical procedures. Head Neck 1995;17(1):7–13
11. Pelczar BT, Weed HG, Schuller DE, Young DC, Reilley TE. Identifying high-risk patients before head and neck oncologic surgery. Arch Otolaryngol Head Neck Surg 1993;119(8):861–864
12. Robbins KT, Favrot S, Hanna D, Cole R. Risk of wound infection in patients with head and neck cancer. Head Neck 1990;12(2):143–148
13. Cole RR, Robbins KT, Cohen JI, Wolf PF. A predictive model for wound sepsis in oncologic surgery of the head and neck. Otolaryngol Head Neck Surg 1987;96(2):165–171
14. Penel N, Fournier C, Lefebvre D, Lefebvre JL. Multivariate analysis of risk factors for wound infection in head and neck squamous cell carcinoma surgery with opening of mucosa. Study of 260 surgical procedures. Oral Oncol 2005;41(3):294–303
15. Ogihara H, Takeuchi K, Majima Y. Risk factors of postoperative infection in head and neck surgery. Auris Nasus Larynx 2009;36(4):457–460
16. Lee DH, Kim SY, Nam SY, Choi SH, Choi JW, Roh JL. Risk factors of surgical site infection in patients undergoing major oncological surgery for head and neck cancer. Oral Oncol 2011;47(6):528–531
17. Brown BM, Johnson JT, Wagner RL. Etiologic factors in head and neck wound infections. Laryngoscope 1987;97(5):587–590
18. Lotfi CJ, Cavalcanti RdeC, Costa e Silva AM, et al. Risk factors for surgical-site infections in head and neck cancer surgery. Otolaryngol Head Neck Surg 2008;138(1):74–80
19. Sato J, Goto J, Harahashi A, et al. Oral health care reduces the risk of postoperative surgical site infection in inpatients with oral squamous cell carcinoma. Support Care Cancer 2011;19(3):409–416
20. Simo R, French G. The use of prophylactic antibiotics in head and neck oncological surgery. Curr Opin Otolaryngol Head Neck Surg 2006;14(2):55–61
21. Carrau RL, Byzakis J, Wagner RL, Johnson JT. Role of prophylactic antibiotics in uncontaminated neck dissections. Arch Otolaryngol Head Neck Surg 1991;117(2):194–195

22. Seven H, Sayin I, Turgut S. Antibiotic prophylaxis in clean neck dissections. J Laryngol Otol 2004;118(3):213–216
23. Man LX, Beswick DM, Johnson JT. Antibiotic prophylaxis in uncontaminated neck dissection. Laryngoscope 2011;121(7):1473–1477
24. Burke JF. The effective period of preventive antibiotic action in experimental incisions and dermal lesions. Surgery 1961;50:161–168
25. Rubin J, Johnson JT, Wagner RL, Yu VL. Bacteriologic analysis of wound infection following major head and neck surgery. Arch Otolaryngol Head Neck Surg 1988;114(9):969–972
26. Righi M, Manfredi R, Farneti G, Pasquini E, Romei Bugliari D, Cenacchi V. Clindamycin/cefonicid in head and neck oncologic surgery: one-day prophylaxis is as effective as a three-day schedule. J Chemother 1995;7(3):216–220
27. Fee WE Jr, Glenn M, Handen C, Hopp ML. One day vs. two days of prophylactic antibiotics in patients undergoing major head and neck surgery. Laryngoscope 1984;94(5 Pt 1):612–614
28. Carroll WR, Rosenstiel D, Fix JR, et al. Three-dose vs extended-course clindamycin prophylaxis for free-flap reconstruction of the head and neck. Arch Otolaryngol Head Neck Surg 2003;129(7):771–774
29. Johnson JT, Schuller DE, Silver F, et al. Antibiotic prophylaxis in high-risk head and neck surgery: one-day vs. five-day therapy. Otolaryngol Head Neck Surg 1986;95(5):554–557
30. Hooley R, Levine H, Flores T, Wheeler T, Steiger E. Predicting postoperative head and neck complications using nutritional assessment: the prognostic nutritional index. Arch Otolaryngol Head Neck Surg 1983;109:83
31. Daly JM, Dudrick SJ, Copeland EM III. Parenteral nutrition in patients with head and neck cancer: techniques and results. Otolaryngol Head Neck Surg (1979) 1980;88(6):707–713
32. Goguen LA, Chapuy CI, Li Y, Zhao SD, Annino DJ. Neck dissection after chemoradiotherapy: timing and complications. Arch Otolaryngol Head Neck Surg 2010;136(11):1071–1077
33. Penel N, Fournier C, Lefebvre D, et al. Previous chemotherapy as a predictor of wound infections in nonmajor head and neck surgery: Results of a prospective study. Head Neck 2004;26(6):513–517
34. Wein RO. Preoperative smoking cessation: impact on perioperative and long-term complications. Arch Otolaryngol Head Neck Surg 2009;135(6):597–601
35. Daneman N, Lu H, Redelmeier DA. Discharge after discharge: predicting surgical site infections after patients leave hospital. J Hosp Infect 2010;75(3):188–194
36. Watters K, O'Dwyer TP, Rowley H. Cost and morbidity of MRSA in head and neck cancer patients: what are the consequences? J Laryngol Otol 2004;118(9):694–699
37. Jeannon JP, Orabi A, Manganaris A, Simo R. Methicillin resistant Staphylococcus aureus infection as a causative agent of fistula formation following total laryngectomy for advanced head & neck cancer. Head Neck Oncol 2010;2:14
38. Saito T, Hayashi Y, Inubushi J, Eguchi T, Ohmagari N. Oral microflora in reconstructive surgery for head and neck cancer. Paper presented at the IADR 86th General Session, July 4, 2008, Toronto
39. Grandis JR, Vickers RM, Rihs JD, et al. The efficacy of topical antibiotic prophylaxis for contaminated head and neck surgery. Laryngoscope 1994;104(6 Pt 1):719–724
40. Grandis JR, Vickers RM, Rihs JD, Yu VL, Johnson JT. Efficacy of topical amoxicillin plus clavulanate/ticarcillin plus clavulanate and clindamycin in contaminated head and neck surgery: effect of antibiotic spectra and duration of therapy. J Infect Dis 1994;170(3):729–732
41. Simons JP, Johnson JT, Yu VL, et al. The role of topical antibiotic prophylaxis in patients undergoing contaminated head and neck surgery with flap reconstruction. Laryngoscope 2001;111(2):329–335
42. Jones TR, Kaulbach H, Nichter L, Edlich RF, Cantrell RW. Efficacy of an antibiotic mouthwash in contaminated head and neck surgery. Am J Surg 1989;158(4):324–327
43. Kirchner JC, Edberg SC, Sasaki CT. The use of topical oral antibiotics in head and neck prophylaxis: is it justified? Laryngoscope 1988;98(1):26–29
44. Doerr TD, Marunick MT. Timing of edentulation and extraction in the management of oral cavity and oropharyngeal malignancies. Head Neck 1997;19(5):426–430
45. McCulloch TM, Jensen NF, Girod DA, Tsue TT, Weymuller EA Jr. Risk factors for pulmonary complications in the postoperative head and neck surgery patient. Head Neck 1997;19(5):372–377
46. Bágyi K, Haczku A, Márton I, et al. Role of pathogenic oral flora in postoperative pneumonia following brain surgery. BMC Infect Dis 2009;9:104
47. Yoneyama T, Yoshida M, Matsui T, Sasaki H; Oral Care Working Group. Oral care and pneumonia. Lancet 1999;354(9177):515
48. Keller A. Noninvasive tissue oximetry for flap monitoring: an initial study. J Reconstr Microsurg 2007;23(4):189–197
49. Smit JM, Zeebregts CJ, Acosta R, Werker PMN. Advancements in free flap monitoring in the last decade: a critical review. Plast Reconstr Surg 2010;125(1):177–185
50. Schusterman MA, Reece GP, Miller MJ, Harris S. The osteocutaneous free fibula flap: is the skin paddle reliable? Plast Reconstr Surg 1992;90(5):787–793, discussion 794–798
51. Yu P, Chang EI, Hanasono MM. Design of a reliable skin paddle for the fibula osteocutaneous flap: perforator anatomy revisited. Plast Reconstr Surg 2011;128(2):440–446
52. Allak A, Nguyen TN, Shonka DC Jr, Reibel JF, Levine PA, Jameson MJ. Immediate postoperative extubation in patients undergoing free tissue transfer. Laryngoscope 2011;121(4):763–768
53. Warren J, Bhalla V, Cresci G. Postoperative diet advancement: surgical dogma vs evidence-based medicine. Nutr Clin Pract 2011;26(2):115–125
54. Doig GS, Heighes PT, Simpson F, Sweetman EA, Davies AR. Early enteral nutrition, provided within 24 h of injury or intensive care unit admission, significantly reduces mortality in critically ill patients: a meta-analysis of randomised controlled trials. Intensive Care Med 2009;35(12):2018–2027
55. Ramos M, Khalpey Z, Lipsitz S, et al. Relationship of perioperative hyperglycemia and postoperative infections in patients who undergo general and vascular surgery. Ann Surg 2008;248(4):585–591
56. Hyman J, Disa JJ, Cordiero PG, Mehrara BJ. Management of salivary fistulas after microvascular head and neck reconstruction. Ann Plast Surg 2006;57(3):270–273, discussion 274
57. Dhir K, Reino AJ, Lipana J. Vacuum-assisted closure therapy in the management of head and neck wounds. Laryngoscope 2009;119(1):54–61

28 Complications of Myocutaneous and Local Flaps

T. Teknos, H. Arshad

Introduction

Every head and neck surgeon will encounter situations in which a primary closure will be inadequate. In these situations, local or pedicled myocutaneous flaps can be an excellent choice for coverage of these defects. When done properly, these types of flaps have an excellent success rate. This chapter will focus on the complications of local and pedicled flaps, how to avoid them, and what to do if they happen.

Complications of Pedicled Myocutaneous Flaps

Introduction

Despite the widespread use of microvascular reconstruction with free flaps, pedicled flaps are still important tools in head and neck reconstruction. These flaps are reliable and do not require the specialized postoperative care needed for free flaps. In general, these flaps can have complications with the donor and/or recipient site. Donor site complications include hematoma, seroma, and infection. Recipient site complications include partial or total flap loss, hematoma, seroma, infection, dehiscence, and fistula formation. Two pedicled flaps will be considered: the pectoralis major myocutaneous flap and the latissimus dorsi myocutaneous flap.

Pectoralis Major Myocutaneous Flap

> **Note**
> The best opportunity to avoid complications is when designing the flap.

Since Ariyan[1] described the use of the pectoralis major flap in the use of head and neck defects in 1979, it has remained an essential procedure in the head and neck surgeon's armamentarium. Four recent studies were reviewed for a total of 1,251 patients. The overall complication rate was 32.4%, including the donor and recipient sites. This seemingly high rate of complications is tempered by the fact that the incidence of total flap loss ranged from only 1% to 4%. Donor site complications ranged from 1 to 5.3% and included necrosis, hematoma, infection, and seroma. Recipient site complications

were reported in 9.5 to 29.7% of patients and involved dehiscence, fistula, partial or total flap loss, infection, or neck contracture. Radiation has been associated with an increased risk of complications.[2–5]

The best opportunity to avoid complications is when designing the flap. A simple skin pinch test can help to determine the maximum width of the skin paddle to avoid an overly tense closure at the donor site. Also, one should consider the amount of subcutaneous tissue between the skin paddle and muscle, as increased bulk in this area can compromise the health of the skin. This is especially an important consideration in women with large amounts of intervening breast tissue. If the flap is too bulky, then one should consider another flap. Keeping the skin paddle entirely over the pectoralis muscle, not extending the skin over the rectus abdominis, and beveling out from the skin to capture more muscle are all techniques to improve the number of perforator vessels to the skin paddle.[6]

Hematomas at the donor site can be avoided by meticulous attention to hemostasis before closing. Infection at the donor site is likely caused by cross-contamination from saliva at the primary tumor site. If there is any concern, the donor site should be copiously irrigated before closure. To avoid seromas, we routinely place two drains at the donor site: one at the lateral edge and one at the inferior edge. In this way, the gravity-dependent drainage will be captured both while sitting up and when in the recumbent position.

Fistula formation and dehiscence can be a result of a variety of factors such as poor nutrition, previous radiotherapy, and diabetes. Another factor is excessive tension or bulk. We avoid "tubing" a pectoralis flap because its excessive bulk is detrimental to the closure. Instead, if a total pharyngectomy defect is encountered and a free flap cannot be used, then the pectoralis flap will be sutured directly to the prevertebral fascia. Dehiscence can be avoided by designing a paddle with adequate length. It should be kept in mind that length will be lost during the rotation of the flap from the chest to the head/neck, and this must be accounted for.

Ischemia or venous congestion leading to total loss of the flap is rare but can be avoided by ensuring that there is no compression of the pedicle (**Fig. 28.1**). The flap should be brought through a subcutaneous tunnel, external to the clavicle, with at least four fingerbreadths of room. If there is too much tension still, as in previously irradiated patients, then the pedicle and surrounding muscle can be exteriorized and skin can be grafted. If ischemia is discovered in time (within 4 hours) it is best

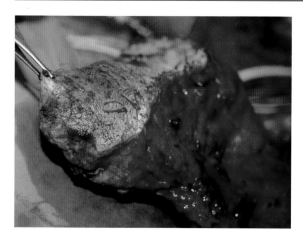

Fig. 28.1 Partial distal necrosis of a pectoralis major flap.

to re-explore. Venous congestion can be treated with medicinal leeches.[7] Another consideration is to remove some of the sutures at the recipient site.

A particularly difficult to treat but rare complication of pectoralis major flaps is costal osteomyelitis or necrosis. During the raising of the pectoral muscle off the ribs, one should take care to not apply cautery directly to the ribs. Conservative treatment involves appropriate antibiotic coverage.[8]

Latissimus Dorsi

> **Note**
>
> The latissimus dorsi pedicled myocutaneous flap offers a sizable skin paddle and bulk for large head and neck defects.

One of the main drawbacks of a latissimus dorsi pedicled myocutaneous flap is that it is difficult to raise concurrently with the primary tumor resection. The pedicle is also somewhat prone to kinking and so is not quite as reliable as a pectoralis flap, even in experienced hands.

In the recent literature, total flap loss ranges from 1 to 10%. The rate of any complication, major or minor, is 10 to 35%. Donor site complications include dehiscence, seroma, and hematoma. Recipient site complications include dehiscence, infection, hematoma, partial/total flap loss, and fistula.[9–13] Brachial plexus injuries were reported early in the experience of this flap and are likely to be the result of positioning and hyperadduction of the arm.[14]

Whereas earlier studies did not find significant shoulder weakness after flap transfer, more recent papers have detected some disability in a significant number of patients. Adams and Lassen[7] found that 39% of patients complained of at least moderate weakness. Another study identified six of 18 patients who were limited in their

ability to carry out housework.[15–17] Shoulder dysfunction can be minimized by not performing a concurrent pectoralis major myocutaneous flap on the ipsilateral side, or if that side already has spinal accessory nerve palsy.

As stated before, the vascular pedicle is prone to kinking at the site of tunneling. The pedicle can be tunneled between the pectoralis minor and pectoralis major or between the clavicle and skin. If there is excessive tension, an incision between the clavicle and recipient site can incorporate the proximal skin paddle. In one study, all 15 flaps recorded were successfully transferred via a subscapular tunnel (between the scapula and clavicle) and brought out into the posterior triangle.[18] Hayden et al[12] recommend preserving the circumflex scapular branches to "maintain a gentle curve of the vascular pedicle." They also advise preserving the humeral tendon until the pedicle dissection and tunnel are complete, to protect against excessive traction.

Complications of Local Flaps

Local cutaneous flaps are invaluable in reconstructing skin defects on the scalp, face and neck. Fortunately, with proper planning, complications are minimal. The types of complications that do occur can be divided into perioperative and cosmetic types. The complications considered below will apply to all types of local flaps, including rotational, advancement, transpositional, rhomboid, and bilobed flaps. The cervicofacial flap will be considered separately, as it has some unique complications bearing mention.

Peri-operative Complications

Ischemia/Necrosis

Ischemia and necrosis can be attributed to problems with flap design or systemic issues. Systemic issues include malnutrition, smoking, diabetes, and previous radiotherapy. Early studies showed an increased incidence of flap ischemia/necrosis with cigarette smoking, but a recent prospective trial comparing 439 smokers with 3,758 nonsmokers did not find any difference in ischemic complications.[19] The same group found no difference in ischemic complications when comparing patients with and without diabetes.[20] The overall low incidence of ischemia in local flaps of the face may be attributed to the excellent blood supply to facial soft tissues. We still advise, however, that patients stop smoking at least 48 hours before surgery. If there is concern for ischemia before surgery, then we advocate avoiding injection of subcutaneous epinephrine.

Flap design may have a greater role in preventing ischemic complications. One of the key concepts in designing any type of local skin flap is to have a resulting wound with the least possible tension. This can be accomplished with ample undermining, orienting vectors of maximal tension perpendicular to relaxed skin tension lines (especially for rhomboid flaps), and providing adequate donor skin. Rotational flaps should have a 4 : 1 to 5 : 1 ratio of flap circumference to wound diameter.[21] For bilobed flaps, the total axis of rotation should not exceed 100°. Careful attention to hemostasis can prevent a hematoma and resulting flap necrosis. However, one should not be overly aggressive in controlling bleeding areas because this can damage the blood supply to the flap.

Once ischemia has occurred, it is best to let the area of necrosis "declare itself" before debriding. If the problem is a result of excessive congestion or venous congestion, it may help to release some of the sutures. Medicinal leeches have also been used to salvage these flaps.[22] Patients receiving leech therapy should receive appropriate coverage for *Aeromonas*. Usually a fluoroquinolone, trimethoprim-sulfamethoxazole, or third-generation cephalosporin will suffice.

Hematoma

Wound hematoma usually occurs within the first 48 hours after surgery. Failure to treat the hematoma can lead to secondary complications such as ischemia, flap necrosis, or wound infection. Preoperative factors that predispose a patient to a hematoma can be identified with a thorough history. One should ask about any renal or hepatic disorders, history of blood coagulopathy, history of bleeding complications after previous surgery, malignancies, and medications. In addition to nonsteroidal anti-inflammatory drugs, clopidogrel, and warfarin use, patients should be questioned about herbal remedies and vitamins such as ginkgo biloba and vitamin E.[23] Unless medically contraindicated, patients should discontinue use of these medications 5 to 7 days before the surgery. One meta-analysis looking at patients undergoing cutaneous surgery showed only a significant difference in warfarin users versus patients on aspirin in causing moderate to severe bleeding complications.[24]

Bleeding can be minimized during surgery by subcutaneous infiltration of 1% epinephrine. However, the benefit of this should be weighed against the risk of ischemia in an at-risk patient. During the surgery, bleeding can be controlled with conservative measures such as pressure, topical epinephrine, or cautery. Bipolar cautery, rather than monopolar cautery, should be used to minimize thermal injury to the surrounding tissue. If a bleeding risk still remains at the end of the surgery, a passive drain can be placed. Although this will not decrease the incidence of bleeding complications, it may help to identify it earlier.

Signs of a hematoma include fluctuance under the flap, bruising on the overlying skin, or pain out of proportion to the normal postoperative course. When a hematoma has been identified, it can be evacuated with a needle and syringe or by opening a few sutures and pressing the blood out. If the hematoma is rapidly expanding or does not respond to conservative measures, then one should consider going back to the operating room and exploring the wound.[25]

Infection

Infectious complications have been reported to be less than 5%. Factors such as diabetes, hematoma, and site of surgery have been implicated as contributing factors.[20,26] Dixon et al[20] found a 4.2% infection rate in patients with diabetes undergoing cutaneous surgery versus 2% in those patients without diabetes. A 2008 advisory statement from the American Academy of Dermatology recommended antibiotic prophylaxis for high-risk cardiac patients, infected wounds, and wounds that breach the oral mucosa. Softer indications would include wounds involving the ear and nose.[27] The most important factor in preventing postoperative infection is probably adherence to sterile procedures.

Signs of postoperative infection include erythema and tenderness, with or without frank purulence. Usually, the infection is the result of *Staphylococcus* or *Streptococcus* spp. If the wound is perioral then oral anaerobes may also be involved. In addition, infections involving the ear may be caused by *Pseudomonas* spp. If the infection is superficial, an oral first-generation cephalosporin may be sufficient for treatment. A perioral infection may warrant clindamycin or amoxicillin-clavulanate. Ciprofloxacin can be given orally for infections involving the ear if the cartilage seems to be involved. More severe infections require partially or fully opening the wound with debridement. Once the infection has cleared and granulation has occurred, a revision procedure can be performed.

Cosmetic Complications

Trap-Door Deformity

This deformity can be seen with closures that are U-shaped or C-shaped. Various theories as to why this happens include scar contracture, redundant subcutaneous tissue, or lymphatic obstruction.[28] One way to help avoid this is to either plan the flap so the scar is not near-circumferential and to liberally undermine the surrounding skin.

Hypertrophic Scar

Hypertrophic scars can be seen anytime a skin incision is made. During the preoperative history and physical, a history of keloids should be elicited. At the time of surgery, care should be taken to evert the skin edges and reduce tension at the closure site. Various methods have been used to treat the scar hypertrophy. These include using silicone sheets, steroid injections, dermabrasion, cutaneous lasers, and injecting antimitotic agents.[29] Triamcinolone injections can be begun at 6 weeks postoperatively and reinjected every 6 weeks as needed. Finally, scar revision at a year after surgery can be used to camouflage the scar.

Cervicofacial Flap

The cervicofacial flap will be considered separately because it has the combined features of several types of local advancement flaps. This flap is used for extensive defects involving the cheek, midface, periorbita, and neck. Though it is technically a randomly blood supplied flap, it can have contributions from one or more of several named arteries such as the facial or transverse cervical. It can be extended onto the thorax and receive contributions from internal mammary perforators.

When assessing the complications of this flap, the literature varies because some studies included patients who had previously received radiation. However, in all studies reviewed for this chapter, none reported a total flap loss. Most complications were minor and mainly wound complications. These included partial wound-edge necrosis, epidermolysis, ectropion, facial nerve injury, decreased facial sensation, and hematoma. If there is a concern for flap ischemia, some authors have recommended a deep plane cervicofacial flap in which the dissection is sub-SMAS (superficial muscular aponeurotic system). This may, however, increase the incidence of ectropion. Most cases of ectropion are temporary, but if there is preoperative ectropion or concern for postoperative ectropion, a lower lid tightening procedure should be considered.[30-33]

In previously irradiated patients or those with large defects, excessive wound tension may be an issue. Not only can this cause wound edge necrosis or flap ischemia, it can result in seromas or hematomas because of the flap being "tented" up on the cervical portion. To help avoid this, one should not hesitate to extend the incision on to the anterior chest wall.

Conclusion

Local and pedicled flaps are important tools in the coverage of head and neck defects. The key to minimizing complications lies with appropriate preoperative planning. This includes proper patient selection, flap design, and choice of flap.

References

1. Ariyan S. The pectoralis major myocutaneous flap. A versatile flap for reconstruction in the head and neck. Plast Reconstr Surg 1979;63(1):73–81
2. McLean JN, Carlson GW, Losken A. The pectoralis major myocutaneous flap revisited: a reliable technique for head and neck reconstruction. Ann Plast Surg 2010;64(5):570–573
3. Liu R, Gullane P, Brown D, Irish J. Pectoralis major myocutaneous pedicled flap in head and neck reconstruction: retrospective review of indications and results in 244 consecutive cases at the Toronto General Hospital. J Otolaryngol 2001;30(1):34–40
4. Milenović A, Virag M, Uglešić V, Aljinović-Ratković N. The pectoralis major flap in head and neck reconstruction: first 500 patients. J Craniomaxillofac Surg 2006;34(6):340–343
5. Vartanian JG, Carvalho AL, Carvalho SM, Mizobe L, Magrin J, Kowalski LP. Pectoralis major and other myofascial/myocutaneous flaps in head and neck cancer reconstruction: experience with 437 cases at a single institution. Head Neck 2004;26(12):1018–1023
6. Ramakrishnan VR, Yao W, Campana JP. Improved skin paddle survival in pectoralis major myocutaneous flap reconstruction of head and neck defects. Arch Facial Plast Surg 2009;11(5):306–310
7. Adams JF, Lassen LF. Leech therapy for venous congestion following myocutaneous pectoralis flap reconstruction. ORL Head Neck Nurs 1995;13(1):12–14
8. Stack BC Jr, Klotch DW, Hubbell DS; C. SB. Costal osteomyelitis after pectoralis major myocutaneous flap use in head and neck reconstruction. Am J Otolaryngol 1995;16(1):78–80
9. Davis JP, Nield DV, Garth RJ, Breach NM. The latissimus dorsi flap in head and neck reconstructive surgery: a review of 121 procedures. Clin Otolaryngol Allied Sci 1992;17(6):487–490
10. Har-El G, Bhaya M, Sundaram K. Latissimus dorsi myocutaneous flap for secondary head and neck reconstruction. Am J Otolaryngol 1999;20(5):287–293
11. Haughey BH, Fredrickson JM. The latissimus dorsi donor site. Current use in head and neck reconstruction. Arch Otolaryngol Head Neck Surg 1991;117(10):1129–1134
12. Hayden RE, Kirby SD, Deschler DG. Technical modifications of the latissimus dorsi pedicled flap to increase versatility and viability. Laryngoscope 2000;110(3 Pt 1):352–357
13. Sabatier RE, Bakamjian VY, Carter WL. Craniofacial and head and neck applications of the transaxillary latissimus dorsi flap. Ear Nose Throat J 1992;71(4):173–182
14. Logan AM, Black MJ. Injury to the brachial plexus resulting from shoulder positioning during latissimus dorsi flap pedicle dissection. Br J Plast Surg 1985;38(3):380–382
15. Brumback RJ, McBride MS, Ortolani NC. Functional evaluation of the shoulder after transfer of the vascularized latissimus dorsi muscle. J Bone Joint Surg Am 1992;74(3):377–382
16. Koh CE, Morrison WA. Functional impairment after latissimus dorsi flap. ANZ J Surg 2009;79(1-2):42–47
17. Russell RC, Pribaz J, Zook EG, Leighton WD, Eriksson E, Smith CJ. Functional evaluation of latissimus dorsi donor site. Plast Reconstr Surg 1986;78(3):336–344
18. Prakash PJ, Gupta AK. The subscapular approach in head and neck reconstruction with the pedicled latissimus dorsi myocutaneous flap. Br J Plast Surg 2001;54(8):680–683
19. Dixon AJ, Dixon MP, Dixon JB, Del Mar CB. Prospective study of skin surgery in smokers vs. nonsmokers. Br J Dermatol 2009;160(2):365–367
20. Dixon AJ, Dixon MP, Dixon JB. Prospective study of skin surgery in patients with and without known diabetes. Dermatol Surg 2009;35(7):1035–1040
21. Lo CH, Kimble FW. The ideal rotation flap: an experimental study. J Plast Reconstr Aesthet Surg 2008;61(7):754–759
22. Zhao X, Higgins KM, Enepekides D, Farwell G. Medicinal leech therapy for venous congested flaps: case series and

review of the literature. J Otolarnygol Head Neck Surg 2009;38(2):E61–E64

23. Hurst EA, Yu SS, Grekin RC, Neuhaus IM. Bleeding complications in dermatologic surgery. Semin Cutan Med Surg 2007;26(1):40–46

24. Lewis KG, Dufresne RG Jr. A meta-analysis of complications attributed to anticoagulation among patients following cutaneous surgery. Dermatol Surg 2008;34(2):160–164, discussion 164–165

25. Vural E, Key JM. Complications, salvage, and enhancement of local flaps in facial reconstruction. Otolaryngol Clin North Am 2001;34(4):739–751, vi

26. Amici JM, Rogues AM, Lasheras A, et al. A prospective study of the incidence of complications associated with dermatological surgery. Br J Dermatol 2005;153(5):967–971

27. Wright TI, Baddour LM, Berbari EF, et al. Antibiotic prophylaxis in dermatologic surgery: advisory statement 2008. J Am Acad Dermatol 2008;59(3):464–473

28. Koranda FC, Webster RC. Trapdoor effect in nasolabial flaps. Causes and corrections. Arch Otolaryngol 1985;111(7):421–424

29. Jones N. Scar tissue. Curr Opin Otolaryngol Head Neck Surg 2010;18(4):261–265

30. Delay E, Lucas R, Jorquera F, Payement G, Foyatier JL. Composite cervicofacial flap for reconstruction of complex cheek defects. Ann Plast Surg 1999;43(4):347–353

31. Boyette JR, Vural E. Cervicofacial advancement-rotation flap in midface reconstruction: forward or reverse? Otolaryngol Head Neck Surg 2011;144(2):196–200

32. Moore BA, Wine T, Netterville JL. Cervicofacial and cervicothoracic rotation flaps in head and neck reconstruction. Head Neck 2005;27(12):1092–1101

33. Tan ST, MacKinnon CA. Deep plane cervicofacial flap: a useful and versatile technique in head and neck surgery. Head Neck 2006;28(1):46–55

29 Reconstructive Surgery: Free Fasciocutaneous Flaps and Bone-Containing Flaps

J. L. Llorente Pendas, C. Suárez

Introduction

Free flap reconstruction has become an integral part of the multidisciplinary care of head and neck cancers and the preferred reconstructive technique at many major medical oncology centers to repair complex defects of the head and neck. Current experience demonstrates that microvascular free tissue transfer frequently allows for reliable, single-stage, and immediate reconstruction in this patient population. The success rates for microsurgical procedures have greatly improved over the past few decades. Many centers have reported free flap success rates greater than 96%, and in some expert hands, close to 99%, making this operation one of the most reliable procedures in reconstructive surgery. However, because the use of these flaps permits advanced tumors to be more aggressively treated by surgery in a patient population with a high prevalence of coexisting diseases, complications are not uncommon and flap failures do occasionally occur.

Many aspects of resective surgery should be modified when a microsurgical transfer is anticipated, but once the resection is complete, attention focuses on analysis of the component parts of the defect. The complexities of the methods of reconstruction follow a "reconstructive ladder", beginning with simple split-thickness skin grafts at one end, proceeding to free tissue transfer at the other. Ascent of this ladder does not always imply a superior result because in the appropriate circumstances, for instance, a skin graft may provide the best functional and cosmetic result. When compared with pedicled locoregional flaps, these procedures prove more complex and demanding in terms of equipment, cost, and surgical experience.

The method of reconstruction with free flaps must be preselected depending upon the estimate size and shape of the defect and the structures involved and what donor site tissue is most appropriate. Thorough preoperative planning should also evaluate potential alternative methods of reconstruction.[1]

Controversy still exists about whether microvascular reconstruction is functionally superior to pedicled reconstruction of comparable defects. Intuition suggests that revascularized free-tissue transfer is functionally superior because it allows the reconstructive surgeon to customize reconstruction of defects of the head and neck. Free flaps can be designed to provide epithelium, subcutaneous tissue, muscle, and bone in proportions that closely resemble the missing tissue.[2]

Despite the best preoperative care, meticulous surgical technique, and attentive postoperative management, complications frequently arise in the patient with head and neck cancer. Many of these individuals are elderly with concomitant medical problems and pose a constant challenge for those involved in their care. About 20% of the patients will have perioperative medical complications, with pulmonary, cardiac, and infectious complications predominating,[3] and with multiple complications occurring in 10%.[4] Most of the medical literature suggests that comorbidity is likely to be the most important factor in determining the risk of perioperative complications. Early recognition of the symptoms and signs of complications can prevent amplification of existing problems. However, a perioperative mortality of 1 to 3% must be expected.

In some series, age remained a statistically significant predictor of medical complications,[3,4] but other investigators have concluded that age should not be considered when deciding whether a patient is an acceptable candidate to undergo a free flap reconstruction. Previous radiotherapy could increase the rate of complications for some authors but it is not a contraindication for free flaps.

The purpose of this chapter is to focus on the major surgical complications in free flap reconstructions and how they are best avoided or treated once they occur. It is beyond the scope of this chapter to review specific complications such as fistulas, dehiscences, or stenosis, because they do not only occur in free flaps and are usually multifactorial.

Fasciocutaneous flaps are tissue flaps that include skin, subcutaneous tissue, and the underlying fascia. Circulation to a fasciocutaneous flap is based on the prefascial and subfascial plexuses. They can be raised without skin and in some cases can include bone tissue.

Fasciocutaneous free flaps are gaining widespread popularity for the reconstruction of head and neck defects and in many units these flaps are used in preference to enteric free flaps (jejunum, omentum), especially in pharyngolaryngoesophageal reconstructions. This popularity is mainly because of the low donor site morbidity compared with the potential complications following opening the abdominal cavity.

Many different fasciocutaneous free flaps have been described for head and neck reconstruction. In this chapter we will focus mainly on the most widely used, such as the radial forearm, the anterolateral thigh, the scapular–parascapular, and the fibular osseocutaneous free flaps. Others free flaps that are much less used will not be reviewed, such as the ulnar forearm, lateral arm, lateral thigh, rectus abdominis, or osseocutaneous such as iliac crest.

The subject of this chapter is reviewing surgical complications in fasciocutaneous and osseocutaneous free flap reconstructions in head and neck as follows:
- Complications at donor site
- Complications at receiving site
  - Free flap failure
    - Causes for free flap necrosis
    - Microvascular technique and recipient vessels
    - Managing flap failure
    - Salvage reconstruction following flap loss.
  - Infection
  - Osteomyelitis.

Complications at Donor Site

The selection of donor tissues should first meet the needs of the defect. Beyond that, when the other choices are equal, the donor site morbidity should be kept to a minimum. Attention should be given to the donor site in terms of aesthetics and functional morbidity. Potential donor site sequelae and complications must be evaluated and taken into account in thorough preoperative planning.

Radial Forearm Flap

In the case of the radial forearm flap donor site morbidities are generally minor. The worst complication is the unrecognized lack of crossover circulation between the volar and palmar arches. This situation, seen in ~ 15% of the patients, must be identified preoperatively by the Allen test. If ulnar perfusion is inadequate, an alternative flap must be formed. In the rare event that this flap has to be chosen despite this anatomical variant, then reconstruction of the radial artery is mandatory.

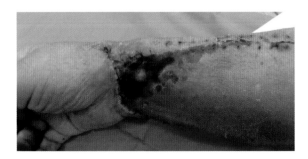

Fig. 29.1 Dehiscent area in a reconstruction radial forearm free flap defect.

When the distal radius is used as an osseous donor site, the complication of forearm fracture must be prevented with an adequate technique of osteotomy. When bony defects larger than ~ 10 cm are anticipated, reconstruction may require another free flap (i.e., fibula) or other reconstructive procedure.

Skin grafts are required to cover the donor site defect in the majority of patients so other potential complications are delayed healing of the skin graft, hypertrophic scar formation, sensory nerve damage, or minor functional deficits (**Fig. 29.1**). To prevent exposure, adhesions, or even rupture of the superficialis dissected tendons, peritenon should be preserved.

Another possibility is the closure of the radial forearm free flap donor site defect with an ulnar rotation-advancement flap that can avoid problems of delayed healing, tendon adhesion, and wrist stiffness (**Figs. 29.2 and 29.3**). However, the procedure required significant skin mobilization with the potential disadvantages of denervation of the volar forearm and temporary lymphedema.

Anterolateral Thigh Flap

The anterolateral thigh flap has become one of the preferred free flaps in the head and neck because of its minimal donor site morbidity. Scars on the thigh are well accepted, even if skin grafting is needed (rarely) (**Fig. 29.4**). Contraindications to harvesting the anterolateral thigh flap include previous surgery or injury to the upper thigh compromising the pedicle. Morbid obesity may make the flap too thick and compromise the vascularity. In hypopharynx reconstruction, our experience is that the anterolateral thigh flap seems to have a lower fistula rate even than the radial forearm flap.

Scapular/Parascapular Free Flap

The scapular/parascapular free flap even as osseocutaneous flap has proven to be excellent as a donor site.[1] The exception is when very large skin flaps are required, so that the skin graft closure needed leaves a poor donor site. The harvest of the scapular bone usually has no problems and decreased shoulder mobility can be avoided with a proper postoperative physical therapy. To prevent seromas, suction drains must be placed for several days.

Fibula Free Flap

Fibula free flap harvest is associated with a high rate of complications. Abnormalities of the lower leg vascular anatomy may preclude safe harvest of the fibula. Patients with peroneus magnus or impaired circulation to the leg should not undergo fibula transposition.

Caution is advised in patients who have had extensive leg trauma or surgery before planning fibular surgery. Patients who are diabetic and have significant venous

Section III   Complications of Head and Neck Surgery

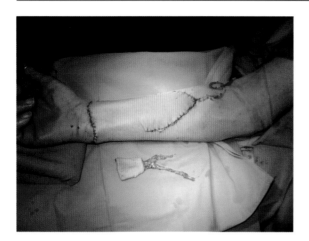

Fig. 29.2 Intraoperative view of a radial forearm free flap donor site wound closure with an ulnar advancement flap.

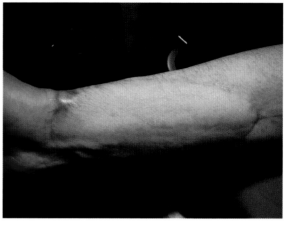

Fig. 29.3 Well-healed donor site following ulnar flap reconstruction.

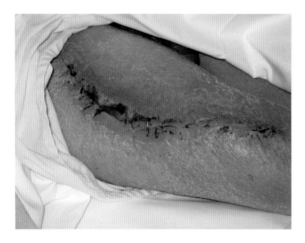

Fig. 29.4 Delayed healing anterolateral donor site in a patient with diabetes.

stasis or peripheral edema, poor circulation or healing, or cutaneous ulcers are poor candidates for this type of flap and an alternative reconstruction must be evaluated. The skin paddle may not be ideal for intraoral reconstruction because it is rather thick and orientation of the skin on the bone can make reconstruction difficult. Some authors have suggested that skin grafting may result in higher complication rates, because of poor graft take of the donor site wound bed. The peroneal nerve can be damaged during the dissection because it passes around the neck of the fibula. From a functional standpoint, most studies have shown that all or nearly all patients are able to successfully perform their activities of daily living without significant limitations. Reported long-term donor site morbidity has been variable, with some studies reporting no long-term morbidity and others suggesting that the majority of patients experience long-term problems with joint stiffness and instability, muscular weakness, or gait

abnormalities. However, complications requiring surgical intervention are rare, and the vast majority of patients have no long-term functional limitations.

Complications at the Receiving Site

Vascular occlusion or pedicle thrombosis remains the primary reason for free flap loss. The majority of flap failures occur within the first 48 hours with venous thrombosis being more common than arterial occlusion. Several authors have investigated the causes and timing of flap failure summarizing venous problems (35 to 80%) as the most common etiology of flap failure followed by arterial problems (30 to 45%), hematoma (20 to 30%), and recipient vessel problems (10%). Late flap failures (i.e., > 48 hours) were most often the result of infection or mechanical stress around the anastomosis. It can be estimated that 15% of patients require a return to the operating theater within 7 days for compromised flap or hematoma.

Free Flap Failure

Loss of vascular perfusion is the main complication associated with free flaps. The irreversible failure of reperfusion through a microvascular anastomosis is termed the "no reflow phenomenon" and has as its basis ischemia and endothelial cell swelling, luminal occlusion, and the release of toxic free radicals with ongoing distal soft tissue damage and necrosis. Free flap failure can lead to functional and cosmetic morbidity, as well as result in additional operative procedures, prolonged hospital stay, and increased health care costs. Moreover, free flap failure in some situations may increase the risk of lethal complications such as rupture of great vessels. All series report a certain incidence of flap failure ranging from 0 to 10%.[5] Early detection of flap compromise through careful monitoring and appropriate surgical revision can lead to significant improvements in overall success rates.

Even some authors in a retrospective study, with some bias, try to examine the predictive value of intraoperative physiologic variables in head and neck reconstructive surgeries. The results show that higher intraoperative maximum heart rates are associated with lower rates of mortality and major complications. There were no other independent predictors of morbidity and mortality in their patients.[6]

Causes for Free Flap Necrosis

There are many different causes for thrombosis or occlusion of the vascular pedicle. Technical errors with flap design and elevation, vessel suturing, tissue handling, or geometry of the pedicle may result in thrombosis. Extrinsic compression of the vascular pedicle by tight wound closure, tapes around the neck, or wound hematoma may also compromise the flap by obstruction of venous outflow (**Fig. 29.5**).

When the signs of vascular compromise occur some of the following measures should be immediately undertaken: reposition the patient to relieve possible vascular pedicle compression, remove compressive dressings, release tight sutures, or assess hydration of the patient. If these maneuvers at the bedside are not successful, immediate re-exploration in the operating room is critical.

Microvascular Technique and Recipient Vessels

Exploration and preparation of donor and recipient vessels must be adequate before flap transfer as reanastomosis has to be speedy to prevent flap loss due to ischemia. Fasciocutaneous free flaps seem to be more resistant to anoxia than visceral ones (for instance the free jejunal flap) and can tolerate warm ischemia for 4 to 6 hours and cold ischemia for up to 12 hours.

> **Note**
> Flap ischemia times should generally be minimized.

Recipient vessel selection is one of the most critical steps in ensuring a successful outcome in microvascular surgery of the head and neck. The optimum time for recipient site vessel selection is at the time of tumor resection or immediately after trauma. In case of "virgin neck" the opportunity to select and use different vessels is wide, but in secondary reconstructions of head and neck defects it is a much more difficult business. This is because of the scarring and fibrosis in the neck and surrounding vessels, especially if the neck has been previously irradiated. For

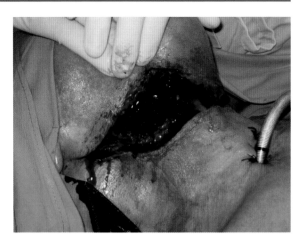

Fig. 29.5 Postoperative hematoma causes suffering of the forearm free flap.

these reasons careful preoperative planning for pedicle is required and studies by Doppler, computed tomography, magnetic resonance imaging, or arteriography could be mandatory. Control of infection and adequate debridement are necessary before flap transfer, if necessary.

A careful dissection of cervical vessels is very important, especially for patients who have had previous neck surgery and radiotherapy. When possible, we have to find multiple arteries and veins from which to choose, before flap harvest.

After that, the most important aspect for achieving patent anastomoses in the vessels is a perfect technique. The orientation and length of the vascular pedicle are important. The surgeon must measure the length of pedicle needed to reach the recipient vessels and compare that with the pedicle length available. The preparation of recipient vessels before flap harvest affords the surgeon the freedom and confidence to use the time during the ischemic period to inset the flap in a meticulous fashion.

In our practice, we usually complete the majority of final flap insetting before beginning the anastomoses. This is important because the definitive suturing of the flap is easier to perform if it is not limited by the pedicle or microsuture; we avoid the risk of vessel disruption and suture is facilitated by the ischemic flap. In spite of meticulous planning, it can be difficult to ascertain where the donor vessels and pedicle will lie after insetting.

Microsurgical anastomoses are performed using some of the following principles.

The diameter of the artery and vein, both for the flap and recipient site, should be 1 to 3 mm to permit adequate inflow and outflow. Either end-to-end or end-to-side anastomoses may be performed, depending on the recipient vessel, the orientation of the flap, and the match between the size of the vessels. These factors must be carefully assessed.

Some authors, including us,[1] recommended the use of a second venous anastomosis (external and internal jugular systems if possible) for the free flaps to guarantee the venous drainage. Moreover, like Ueda et al[7] and others, we support the theory that end-to-side anastomosis directly to the internal jugular vein, whenever possible, is the preferred procedure in vein anastomosis. The advantages are the potential for multiple anastomoses, potential beneficial respiratory venous pump effect, and ability to overcome size discrepancy.

Proper preparation of vessels is important; they must be free of all loose adventitia, with removal of intravascular clots and debris, and irrigation with heparinized saline (100 U/mL). The vascular approximation must be tension free and clamps should facilitate vascular exposure and manipulation. If the pedicle is short with excessive tension, or when other options are not available, vein graftings are used and if a vein graft is needed it should be prepared before dividing the vascular pedicle. Another recipient vein possibility is the use of mobilization of the ipsilateral cephalic vein.

Complete arterial and venous anastomosis is performed using either a vascular coupler or hand sewing. We prefer hand-sewn anastomoses, done with a microscope (or magnifying glass) and using 8–0, 9–0, or 10–0 nylon sutures placed in a simple, interrupted, and full-thickness fashion.

Once flow is established, the anastomotic sites are bathed with warm irrigation and papaverine/xilocaine to relieve vasospasm. Considerable bleeding may arise from the vessel side branches of the flap, which have to be examined and tied to prevent hematoma formation.

Vascular anastomoses are finally examined, and the vascular "patency test" is performed to check flow. The patency test is performed by occluding the vessel distal to the anastomosis with a microforceps and "stripping" the vessel with another microforceps proximally across the anastomosis. Brisk blood flow should then be observed to return across the anastomosis when the proximal microforceps are released. Finally, it is important to ensure that a closed suction drain is placed under the flap away from the anastomoses and then the flap is sutured in position.

Note

Avoidance of vessel tension, kinking, and twisting is important. Particular attention should be given to the position of the patient to avoid compression or pulling on the pedicle.

In the postoperative management, a reverse Trendelenburg position to ~ 30° is preferred. Maintenance of perfusion through normal blood pressure is essential. This can be ensured by euvolemic status and by not attempting to overly modulate blood pressure in patients with hypertension. Maintenance of normothermia also minimizes peripheral vasoconstriction.

Some authors found that significant medical comorbidities, such as diabetes, hypercoagulable disorders, atherosclerosis, and tobacco and alcohol abuse, may result in an increased risk of flap failure. However, others[8] found statistically nonsignificant negative outcome predictors for reoperation, including age, tobacco use, type of neck dissection, tumor staging, radiotherapy dosage, delay between radiotherapy and surgery, length of surgery, type of flap, flap indication, flap size, and postoperative radiotherapy.

Managing Flap Failure

Free flap monitoring depends on the operation and surgeon/team preference. Free flap loss is usually, but not always, an all-or-none phenomenon with the majority of failures occurring within the first 72 hours of revascularization.[5]

The first step in managing free-flap failure is early recognition of a compromised flap. The critical period of thrombus formation in the anastomosis is the first 3 to 5 days of healing. Currently, there is no consensus on which method is most effective for monitoring of free flaps, but physical examination and hand-held Doppler remain the standard of care in most institutions. Clinical observation remains the simplest method of identifying vascular compromise. Color, temperature, bleeding to pinprick, and capillary refill are inexpensive, simple, and reliable methods of flap monitoring (**Figs. 29.6 and 29.7**).

Vascular compromise includes congestion or ischemia of the flap, and it may develop very quickly or more slowly (**Fig. 29.8**). Arterial insufficiency is recognized clinically by a flap that is cool to touch, white, and non-blanching. Venous insufficiency gives the flap a bluish appearance, and causes swelling and dark bleeding on pin-prick testing. Other objective methods include temperature measurement, pH, intraflap blood pressure, light absorbancy,

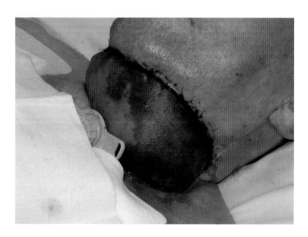

Fig. 29.6 Necrosis of a parascapular flap.

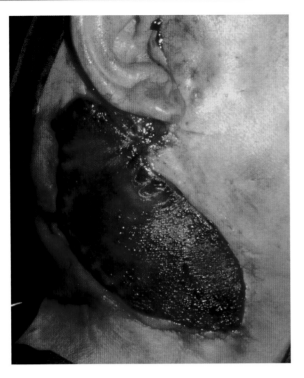

Fig. 29.7 Necrosis of an anterolateral thigh free flap.

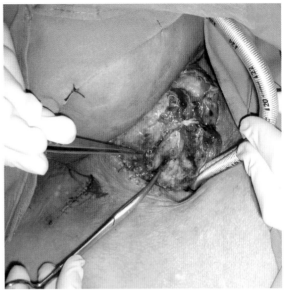

Fig. 29.8 Venous thrombosis in a free flap for hypopharynx reconstruction.

CO_2/O_2 content, and fluorescein dye inspection with a Wood light.

Buried flaps are more difficult or even impossible to monitor clinically. An external skin monitor paddle may be used, otherwise monitoring relies on Doppler signal, the loss of which should be a cause for immediate concern. An implantable Doppler has also been demonstrated as an effective tool for monitoring flaps and potentially improving salvage rates, especially if it is a buried flap. Kind et al[9] suggested that a miniature Doppler ultrasonic probe attached directly to the outflow vein of the flap may lead to a significant improvement in the salvage rates of free flaps (**Figs. 29.9 and 29.10**).

Upon suspicion of vascular compromise, the patient needs to be taken immediately to the operating room for exploration of the anastomotic site. The surgical method must be the first choice because it offers significantly higher salvage rates and nonsurgical procedures should only be used if surgical revision is not feasible or fails.

With re-exploration, initial attention should be directed at the vascular pedicle. Causes of extrinsic compression such as hematoma, pedicle kinking or misconfiguration are easily identifiable and potentially correctable.

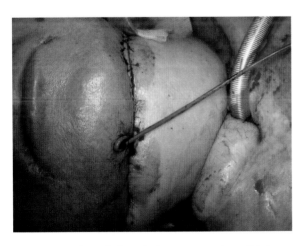

Fig. 29.9 Doppler probe buried adjacent to vascular pedicle in a cervical free flap reconstruction.

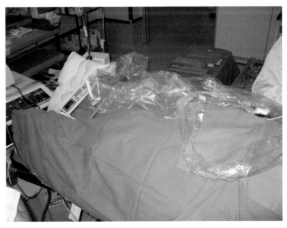

Fig. 29.10 Doppler system.

The internal jugular vein should also be examined for possible thrombosis. The arterial system should be examined under magnification for vascular spasm, for which topical papaverine or xilocaine may be used. Arterial flow can be assessed by looking for pulsation of the distal pedicle or use of an intraoperative Doppler ultrasound. A patency test of the venous system using microsurgical instruments may be used to assess venous outflow. Identification of thrombus should prompt opening the anastomosis and evacuation of the clot, flushing the arterial or venous ends with heparinized saline or using a Fogarty catheter.

Thrombolytic agents, such as streptokinase, urokinase, or tissue plasminogen activator, can be used if a thrombus is identified, particularly in the venous system. Their use has been well documented as a means to salvage vascular insufficiency and theoretically prevent irreversible ischemic reperfusion injury or no-reflow phenomena.

Thrombosed vessels require resection on either side of the anastomosis. Once normal vessel wall is reached and good blood flow is re-established a reanastomosis can be performed.

> **Note**
> Vasodilators and low-molecular-weight dextrans have been used with little evidence of success in a case of impending flap compromise.

The venous anastomosis should be taken down before flushing the flap with any of these thrombolytic agents to avoid systemic effects. Systemic antithrombotic therapy with intravenous heparin may be considered in selected salvage cases of arterial or venous thrombosis, where flow is re-established, particularly if thrombus formation rapidly occurs at the time of reanastomosis. The drawback to intravenous heparin use is the potential for bleeding and hematoma formation. If thrombosis occurs at the time of reanastomosis the initial recipient vein or artery may not be appropriate, in which case another should be chosen.

> **Note**
> Late thromboses are mainly the result of fistula and local infection or mechanical stress around the anastamotic site, rather than technical failure.

Venous congestion can be "non-surgically managed" with the application of leeches. Several successful cases of venous congested flaps salvaged by leeches have been described, suggesting that relief of congestion for 4 to 10 days may allow enough time for neovascularization. However, surgical re-exploration should be the first line of management of a compromised flap. Salvage rates with late exploration are generally poor and the chance of surgical salvage is low after the first 48 hours and even

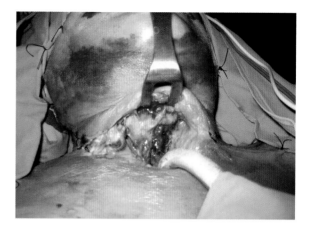

Fig. 29.11 Necrosis of a forearm free flap in hypopharynx reconstruction.

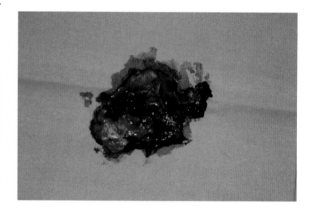

Fig. 29.12 Specimen of necrotic free flap from **Fig. 29.11**.

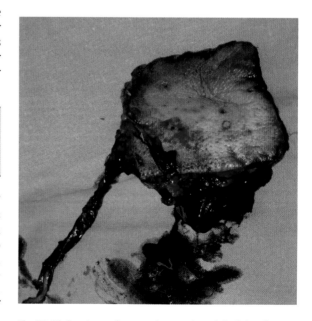

Fig. 29.13 Specimen of a necrotic anterolateral thigh free flap.

impossible if thrombosis occurred more than 3 days after surgery[10] (**Figs. 29.11, 29.12, 29.13**). This might be the reason why flap loss was much higher in buried flaps (7%) compared with nonburied flaps (2%) with a longer time to re-exploration in the buried group because of unreliable flap monitoring. Mean re-exploration time for salvage cases was 1.3 days compared with 3.9 days for those not salvaged.[10]

As we have mentioned, free flap loss is usually an all-or-nothing phenomenon. However, occasionally, partial free flap loss occurs and in these cases it could be managed with conservative treatment such as debridement and secondary healing (**Figs. 29.14, 29.15, 29.16, 29.17**). However, one must take into consideration the risk of conservative management, such as infection, or exposure of vital structures, as well as the type of flap, location, and indication for the flap when deciding on conservative management.

Prompt re-exploration and revision is crucial because most flaps fail to recover after 10 to 12 hours of ischemia. The success of salvage with re-exploration alone is related to the etiology and timing of flap failure and return to the operating room. The greatest chance of success will be in patients with a technical failure that is identified early with an immediate return to the operating room.

The attempted salvage of compromised flaps significantly increases flap survival rates and an aggressive approach to early exploration is recommended. With early recognition and intervention, flap revision has a quoted success rate of 60 to 80%, although a more realistic figure is ~ 50%. Most of these were within 24 hours of initial operation and salvage rates were significantly higher for unique flaps than for composite flaps. It seems that salvage rates are higher when venous thrombosis is identified as the problem and this may be related to the fact that venous compromise is easier to detect via traditional methods of monitoring.

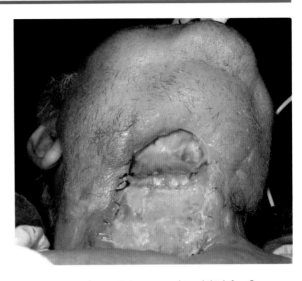

Fig. 29.15 Partial necrosis in an anterolateral thigh free flap conservatively managed.

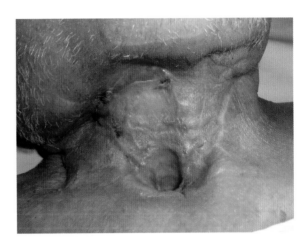

Fig. 29.16 Definitive aspect of flap from **Fig. 29.15** after complete healing.

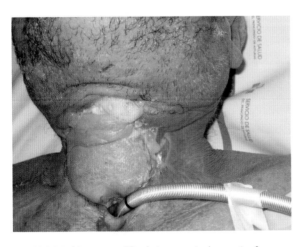

Fig. 29.14 Dehiscence and fistula in a marginal necrosis of an anterolateral thigh free flap.

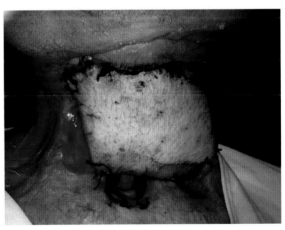

Fig. 29.17 Right small necrosis from cervical skin in an anterolateral thigh free flap reconstruction.

Salvage Reconstruction Following Flap Loss

When salvage is not possible despite re-exploration and conservative management, a second flap usually needs to be performed. The timing and choice of flap used for salvage depends upon several factors including the original surgical defect, risk of wound infection, number of available flap options, and patient comorbidities.

> **Note**
>
> Salvage with a second flap may be performed in an immediate or delayed fashion, and may be either a second free flap or a regional flap.

Once the free flap used in the original reconstruction is deemed to be unsalvageable, salvage reconstruction should be performed as early as possible to avoid a severely compromised wound bed.

Salvage reconstruction is technically very challenging because it occurs in a previously operated and often contaminated surgical bed and the ideal flap has already been used in the initial setting. It is particularly difficult in the head and neck, because critical structures, such as the great vessels or brain, require coverage; infection, saliva, and previous radiotherapy or chemoradiotherapy create a compromised wound bed, and patients are frequently malnourished with medical comorbidities.

Moreover, salvage surgery is more complicated due to factors such as depleted vessels for anastomosis. Pedicled flaps are particularly useful in the vessel-depleted neck. The reasons for free tissue transfer should be carefully considered at salvage surgery in order to correct any predisposing factors. Flap failure can be 4.6 times more likely in a salvage setting with a success rate of only 53%;[11] however, other complication rates were similar to those reported in other series and to those seen in primary flap operations.[12]

In cases where a severely compromised wound bed has developed, initial conservative management with a delay in salvage reconstruction is recommended to increase the chance of success. The goals of salvage reconstruction are to select the simplest reconstructive option that will have the highest chance of survival but also able to restore form, function, and cosmesis. These goals are usually best achieved with a second free flap or a regional flap (i.e., pectoralis pedicled major flap or a pedicled latissimus dorsi). However, in cases of infected wound beds conservative management may be required initially, followed by secondary reconstruction once an ideal wound bed is achieved

Availability of adequate vessels may be a significant problem in second free tissue transfer. Any patient with a suspected paucity of recipient vessels should undergo preoperative angiography (i.e., patients with multiple neck operations or infected wounds) to better identify potential sites for vascular anastomosis.

When recipient veins are scarce for end-to-end anastomosis, the internal jugular vein may be used if available. This method of venous drainage is preferred due to size, constant anatomy, high patency rates, and ready availability in most necks. In addition, it is thought that the configuration problems associated with kinking will be less likely, even when the neck is turned.

Thoracoacromial trunk vessels are a feasible option when carotid vessels are not available. Unfortunately, sometimes these may be of a variable size or may have been damaged by previous surgery. A useful extra option for vascular supply in patients with vessel depletion on both sides of the neck is transposition of the internal mammary artery and vein.[12,13] These authors[12,13] prefer these techniques to vein interposition grafting, which has been associated with higher failure rates.

Infection

One of the major challenges in studying wound and soft tissue infection in a clinical setting is the lack of a precise definition of infection, especially in irradiated patients.

Infection is of particular interest in the study of free flaps in an irradiated bed for three reasons: it is common in irradiated tissues even without further surgical intervention, it has been associated with flap failure, and it is preventable to some extent.[8] Partial flap failure along with bone and hardware exposure are identified as the complications most significantly associated with infection and flap size. Infection can delayed healing or discharge and the median length of hospital admission is greater for patients that acquired infection.

> **Note**
>
> Because the presence of infection predicts other complications and is often associated with reoperation, it should be treated aggressively in patients who have been irradiated in an attempt to decrease other complications.

Osteomyelitis

Mandible reconstructions with osseocutaneous free flaps have revolutionized mandibular reconstruction. Even when these bone flaps are transferred from distant sites into areas of irradiation, compromised blood flow, and salivary contamination, the union of bone segments is the usual result. Osseointegrated implants can also be successfully placed within vascularized bone free flaps, contributing to rehabilitation and a stable dental arch. Complex, composite defects such as these can only be restored effectively with osseocutaneous free tissue transfers that include the fibula, iliac crest, and scapula.

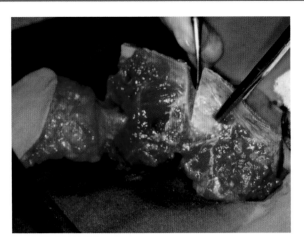

Fig. 29.18 Osteotomy after harvest, a scapular osseocutaneous free flap that retains medial periosteal attachments that allows anatomical skeletal reconstruction and centripetal perfusion.

However, the development of the fibula free flap for mandibular reconstruction has overcome many of the disadvantages of the other donor sites and has been demonstrated to be an ideal replacement for the mandible. This is particularly true for anterior defects for which the unique bone and soft tissue attributes of this flap ideally satisfy the reconstructive requirements. Massive defects requiring large amounts of mucosa, bone, and external skin replacement are often not ideally reconstructed with a fibula free flap. Adequate soft tissue replacement is the highest priority in these cases. Reconstruction with a single flap can be accomplished with the osseocutaneous scapula flap, which provides maximum soft tissue as well as up to 14 cm of bone or iliac crest free flap. In the massive defect there is a rare but justifiable indication for the use of two simultaneous free flaps: fibula for bone and forearm for soft tissue replacement.[14]

In the majority of patients the bone contouring and stabilization of the bone should be carried out before microvascular anastomosis of the flap. If possible, some of this work can even be done before removing the flap from the donor site. However, most is usually done after harvest on a back table (**Fig. 29.18**). If a reconstruction plate is used, the plate is usually fixated on top of the flap periosteum. When miniplates are used, the fixation should be under the periosteum, and the periosteum is draped back over the plates. In composite flaps and complex reconstructions, it is occasionally easier to suture in the more posterior soft tissues before plating the bone into position.

Complications are free flap failure, unstable situation of the flap, unfavorable soft tissue situation, or trismus (**Figs. 29.19 and 29.20**). Bone resorption is surprisingly minimal, even when patients undergo postoperative radiotherapy and the viability of the bone can be confirmed by scintigraphy.

The majority of patients are able to tolerate a regular diet and to either wear dentures or acquire osseointegrated implants. Acceptable speech and appearance are restored and continue to be a source of patient satisfaction at least a decade after surgery.

Bourget et al[8] found that the risk of reoperation was 1.5 times greater in patients with a segmental mandibulectomy reconstructed with a bony flap compared with patients without segmental mandibulectomy. However, the odds ratio increased to 20 times when the segmental mandibulectomy was reconstructed only with plates and soft tissues compared with patients without segmental mandibulectomy.

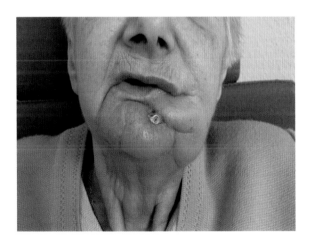

Fig. 29.19 Skin dehiscence and plate reconstruction exposure.

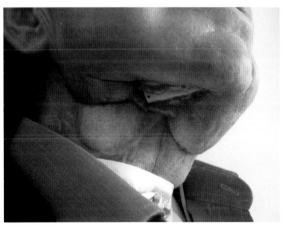

Fig. 29.20 Mandible exposure and tumor recurrence.

There is consensus that free-flap mandibular reconstruction and implant placement are worthwhile, but only a small percentage of patients will benefit from complete dental rehabilitation (~ 25%).[15]

The main reason in this series was the poor survival rate of the patient population with malignant disease. Moreover, it seems that the beneficial effects of dental rehabilitation with an implant-retained denture or fixed appliances, mainly favored cosmetic aspects, rather than oral function.[15]

References

1. Llorente Pendás JL, Suárez Nieto C. Colgajos Libres en las reconstrucciones de cabeza y cuello. Madrid: Editorial Garsi; 1997
2. Swartz WM, Banis JC. Head and neck Microsurgery. Baltimore, MD: Williams & Wilkins; 1992
3. Suh JD, Sercarz JA, Abemayor E, et al. Analysis of outcome and complications in 400 cases of microvascular head and neck reconstruction. Arch Otolaryngol Head Neck Surg 2004;130(8):962–966
4. Singh B, Cordeiro PG, Santamaria E, Shaha AR, Pfister DG, Shah JP. Factors associated with complications in microvascular reconstruction of head and neck defects. Plast Reconstr Surg 1999;103(2):403–411
5. Novakovic D, Patel RS, Goldstein DP, Gullane PJ. Salvage of failed free flaps used in head and neck reconstruction. Head Neck Oncol 2009;1:33
6. Jaggi R, Taylor SM, Trites J, Anderson D, MacDougall P, Hart RD. Review of thromboprophylaxis in otolaryngology-head and neck surgery. J Otolaryngol Head Neck Surg 2011; 40(3):261–265
7. Ueda K, Harii K, Nakatsuka T, Asato H, Yamada A. Comparison of end-to-end and end-to-side venous anastomosis in free-tissue transfer following resection of head and neck tumors. Microsurgery 1996;17(3):146–149
8. Bourget AT, Chang JT, Wu DB-S, Chang CJ, Wei FC. Free flap reconstruction in the head and neck region following radiotherapy: a cohort study identifying negative outcome predictors. Plast Reconstr Surg 2011;127(5):1901–1908
9. Kind GM, Buntic RF, Buncke GM, Cooper TM, Siko PP, Buncke HJ Jr. The effect of an implantable Doppler probe on the salvage of microvascular tissue transplants. Plast Reconstr Surg 1998;101(5):1268–1273, discussion 1274–1275
10. Hyodo I, Nakayama B, Kato H, et al. Analysis of salvage operation in head and neck microsurgical reconstruction. Laryngoscope 2007;117(2):357–360
11. Bozikov K, Arnez ZM. Factors predicting free flap complications in head and neck reconstruction. J Plast Reconstr Aesthet Surg 2006;59(7):737–742
12. Alam DS, Khariwala SS. Technical considerations in patients requiring a second microvascular free flap in the head and neck. Arch Otolaryngol Head Neck Surg 2009;135(3):268–273
13. Urken ML, Higgins KM, Lee B, Vickery C. Internal mammary artery and vein: recipient vessels for free tissue transfer to the head and neck in the vessel-depleted neck. Head Neck 2006;28(9):797–801
14. Hidalgo DA, Disa JJ, Cordeiro PG, Hu Q-Y. A review of 716 consecutive free flaps for oncologic surgical defects: refinement in donor-site selection and technique. Plast Reconstr Surg 1998;102(3):722–732, discussion 733–734
15. Hundepool AC, Dumans AG, Hofer SOP, et al. Rehabilitation after mandibular reconstruction with fibula free-flap: clinical outcome and quality of life assessment. Int J Oral Maxillofac Surg 2008;37(11):1009–1013

30 Reconstructive Surgery: Pedicled and Free Visceral Flaps

C. Suárez, J. L. Llorente Pendas

Indications

Pedicled or free visceral flaps are used in the reconstruction of pharyngolaryngeal and esophageal defects. They are an alternative to reconstruct defects limited to the pharynx or the cervical esophagus microvascular fasciocutaneous free flaps; however, their use is mandatory in extensive defects including those of the thoracic esophagus.

Reconstruction of circumferential defects limited to pharyngolaryngeal and cervical esophagus is accomplished by means of jejunum free flaps (**Figs. 30.1 and 30.2**). The gastric pull-up is indicated when a thoracic esophagectomy is necessary (**Figs. 30.3 and 30.4**). For patients in whom a gastric pull-up is not an option because of previous gastric surgery, or in very extensive tumors invading up to the oropharynx, a free colon transfer or pedicled colon interposition, with or without vascular supercharge, is the second best option. If neither the stomach nor the colon flaps are feasible options, then a long jejunal segment with two vascular pedicles is the next alternative.

Salvage reconstruction of the esophagus after failure of a gastric pull-up is still considered a challenging procedure because of its associated risks of postoperative infection and delayed wound healing, as well as the unavailability of recipient vessels for free tissue transfer. In these patients a free jejunal transfer including two long segment transfers

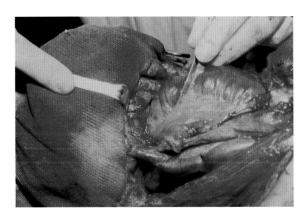

Fig. 30.1 Microvascular transfer of jejunum after total laryngopharyngectomy.

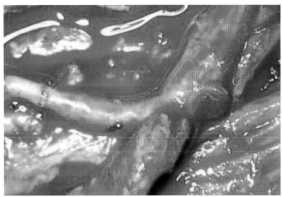

Fig. 30.2 Detail of the arterial anastomosis.

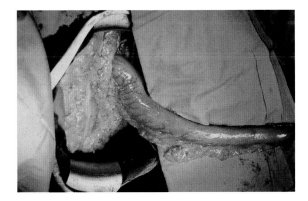

Fig. 30.3 Gastric tube after transhiatal nonthoracic esophagectomy.

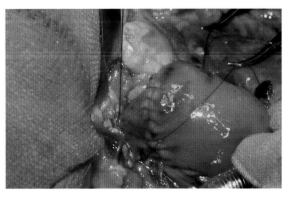

Fig. 30.4 Proximal suture of stomach to the oropharyngeal mucosa.

with double vascular pedicle or colon interposition with vascular supercharge can be performed. Total esophageal reconstruction with supercharged pedicled jejunum has also been proposed as an alternative in patients receiving a total resection of the esophagus.

In general terms, the surgeon must possess a reconstructive algorithm that progresses according to the defect, the available donor sites, and surgical experience.

Jejunal Free Flaps

Complications

Postoperative complications, including those considered minor or not related to the graft, are frequently encountered, and occur in up to 80% of patients (**Table 30.1**). In a series of 79 free jejunal transfers, medical complications and complications at the recipient and donor sites occurred in 67%, 56%, and 11%, respectively.[1] Rates of major complications ranged between 7 and 20%, including death and total flap failure. Minor complication rates ranged between 25 and 45%. To achieve a more objective and accurate evaluation of postoperative morbidity, it has been recommended to stratify postoperative complications according to a standard classification (i.e., Clavien–Dindo[2]).

In general terms, mortality after a jejunal free flap is rare, and occurs in less than 5% of patients; however, in some series it has been reported to be as high as 17%. Overall failure rate of jejunal free flaps is also low; a successful flap is attained in 90 to 100% of patients and most series show flap survival rates higher than 95%.

Oral Bleeding

Oral bleeding is the most prominent sign of a failed flap; and, most flap failures occur within 2 weeks of surgery.

Most failures are due to venous thrombosis, and in ~ 80% of cases thrombosis develops within 3 days after surgery (**Figs. 30.5 and 30.6**). Sometimes this circulatory crisis can be restored with emergency exploration; however, most of these flaps do not survive because of the poor ischemic tolerance of the jejunum (mainly in cases of arterial thrombosis).

Flap Failure

Flap failure is significantly more frequent in patients with a history of previous surgery and postoperative infection, but it also occurs as the result of inadequate microsurgical technique. After a complete loss of the jejunal flap, the risk of postoperative infection and delayed wound healing is high because of thick scar formation and persistent inflammation, and; furthermore, recipient vessels for free tissue transfer are not always available. Nevertheless, in most cases of flap failure the cervical esophagus is usually reconstructed with a second free jejunal transfer or with a fasciocutaneous free flap. Surgical options depend on time of detection of flap necrosis, control of wound bacterial count, vascular status, and the patient's general conditions. A pectoralis major myocutaneous flap should be considered to cover the reconstructed esophagus, because it is a reliable technique and primary wound closure is often difficult during a secondary reconstruction of the cervical esophagus (**Fig. 30.7**). When regional or general conditions do not permit further free flap transfer or when defects are comparatively small, reconstruction with a pedicled flap is a preferable option.

Pharyngocutaneous Fistula

Postoperative pharyngocutaneous fistula is a common complication, that is observed in 5 to 30% of patients. Chang et al[3] identified 13.7% of patients with fistulas in a series of 168 patients who underwent free jejunal

Table 30.1 Comparative studies of visceral flap complications (%)

Reference	Jejunum flap						Gastric pull-up						Colon interposition					
	Nec.	Fis.	Ste.	C-P	Abd.	Dea.	Nec.	Fis.	Ste.	C-P	Abd.	Dea.	Nec.	Fis.	Ste.	C-P	Abd.	Dea.
Ferahkose[15]	7	0	7	28	–	7	5	3	0	40	–	5						
Keereweer[16]	8	35	10	8	14	4	11	53	31	32	11	16						
Kolh[17]							2	7	1	26	2	11	0	0	0	18	3	3
Bardini[18]	–	6	50	–	–	0	11	23	–	–	–	15	18	18	–	–	–	18
Carlson[19]	4	19	15	12	12	0	0	26	13	22	22	9	5	11	21	16	5	11
Daiko[20]	6	4	–	0	–	0	11	11	–	11	–	11						
Triboulet[21]	6	32	12	7	–	5	2	16	7	22	–	5						

Nec., necrosis of the flap; Fis., fistula; Ste., stenosis; C-P, cardiopulmonary complications; Abd, abdominal complications; Dea., death.

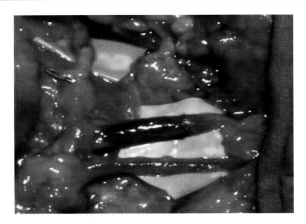

Fig. 30.5 Immediate intraoperative venous thrombosis.

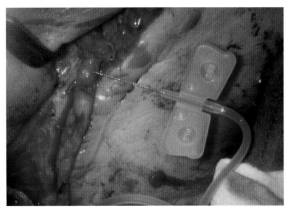

Fig. 30.6 Intraoperative injection of a thrombolytic agent (streptokinase) into a recipient facial artery in a jejunum free flap to improve flap perfusion.

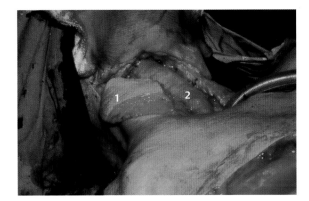

Fig. 30.7 Pectoralis major flap (1) covering a reconstructed esophagus with a jejunum free flap (2).

transfers following total laryngopharyngectomy. In this series the mean onset of fistula formation was 16 days, with a similar frequency of fistulas occurring at the proximal and distal anastomoses. The incidence of fistula formation was highest in patients with a single-layer repair and in patients who received preoperative radiotherapy. Postradiotherapy fistulas, however, were mainly located at the distal anastomosis. Most of the fistulas closed spontaneously (65%), particularly at the proximal anastomosis in patients who had not been irradiated. Distal fistulas in patients who have been irradiated usually need surgical repair; therefore, the use of a "prophylactic" pedicled pectoralis major myofascial flap to prevent fistula formation in previously irradiated patients has been advocated.

Wound Infection

Wound infection at the recipient site is also a frequent complication, mainly occurring in patients with a history of previous local cervical surgery and after fistula formation. Late anastomotic strictures have been reported in

2 to 30% of patients, preventing them from resuming a solid diet (**Fig. 30.8**). Early fistula formation significantly increases the risk of subsequent anastomotic stricture. Significant strictures require repeated dilatations or even open surgery. Some authors recommend the use of mitomycin-C after dilatation of the stenotic segment.

Pulmonary Diseases

Pulmonary diseases are the most frequent general complications, followed by thyroid and parathyroid dysfunction, cardiovascular, neurologic, renal, and multiple organ failure. Donor site morbidity of the jejunal flap (i.e., abdominal), however, is low and is related to prolonged ileus, abdominal pain, wound infection or dehiscence and intra-abdominal hemorrhage.

Factors Influencing Complications

Early venous or arterial thrombosis is the culprit for the failure of free jejunal flaps. During the first 2 weeks, re-establishment of axial blood flow is essential to flap survival, whereas after 2 to 3 weeks, vascularization from the recipient bed is adequate to maintain viability.[4] In the case of venous occlusion, venous neovascularization of a free jejunal flap is complete within 5 weeks after the operation. Using a large animal model, Cordeiro et al[5] showed that a free jejunal transfer can develop collateral circulation that is adequate to maintain viability after division of the pedicle. Jejunal flap survival rate after dividing the flap was 60% at 2 weeks, 83% at 3 weeks, and 100% at 4 weeks. Nevertheless, when a jejunal flap is transferred to an irradiated and scarred recipient bed, revascularization may never occur. If pedicle division is required under such circumstances, reanastomosis of the pedicle would be ideal regardless of the time after the transfer.

Critical factors that determine the level of function of the flap include the duration of ischemia and the

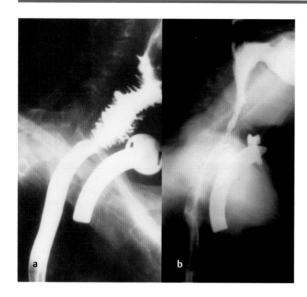

Fig. 30.8a, b Jejunal flap.

a Normal postoperative barium swallow in a jejunum free flap.
b Stricture of a jejunum flap that suffered postoperative ischemia with damage of the mucosa.

degree of venous congestion. When smaller veins are used as recipient vessels, the chance of venous congestion is higher than when larger recipient veins are used. Method of anastomosis (end-to-end versus end-to-side) and previous radiotherapy are significant determinants of venous congestion. End-to-side anastomosis to large vessels is a more reliable method that has a significant influence on minimizing venous congestion. According to Tsao et al[6] venous problems accounted for 87.5% of all re-explorations, and in 75% of the re-explored patients, a pharyngocutaneous fistula was noted. Perisanidis et al[1] reported that site of the tumor, alcohol consumption, neck dissection, and duration of surgery were significantly associated with the development of complications.

Free tissue transfer in the previously treated neck (surgery and radiotherapy) is not as risky as was generally believed. A pectoralis major musculocutaneous flap is advocated to cover the reconstructed esophagus, as skin flaps may be damaged by neck dissection and/or irradiation.

Prevention of Complications

Ultimate free flap success is enhanced by the rapid identification and salvage of failing flaps. Conventional free flap monitoring techniques effectively monitor free flaps with an external component; however, internal or buried free flaps lack an external component. In consequence, the overall salvage rate of external flaps is significantly higher than that of buried flaps. To enhance earlier identification of flap compromise in buried free flaps, alternative monitoring techniques such as implantable Doppler

probes, the use of the lactate : glucose ratio, or exteriorization of flap segments are recommended. Nevertheless, when a jejunum "watch window" is designed for postoperative monitoring, false-positive thrombosis can occur due to torsion or tension of the pedicle of the monitoring flap.

Fistula formation after free jejunal transfer is a serious complication with potentially critical consequences. Use of a circular mechanical stapler does not reduce the fistula and stricture rates compared with grafts that are hand sewn.[7] Barium swallow has been used postoperatively to check for anastomotic competence before feeding; however, it is unreliable as a predictor of leak.

Previous radiotherapy often leads to vascular damage of the usual recipient arteries for free jejunal transfer. Under these conditions, Müller et al[8] reported that 17% of patients with microvascular anastomoses to the smaller vessels needed surgical intervention for ischemia. Nevertheless, in patients with anastomosis to the external carotid artery no significant failure of perfusion occurred. End-to-side anastomosis of the flap artery to the external carotid artery is also recommended in the case of marked size discrepancy between the jejunal artery and potential recipient arteries, or the lack of an available branch artery because of poor regional conditions. When the cervical recipient vessels are buried in extensively scarred fibrous tissues, and they are thought to be less reliable, a secondary vascular anastomosis to the healthy chest vessels (i.e., thoracoacromial artery) is recommended.

An end-to-side anastomosis to the internal jugular vein also has the advantage of overcoming the problems of vessel size discrepancy. In addition, the internal jugular vein has a wide capacity to be the recipient of two or more end-to-side anastomoses, and the respiratory venous pump effect may act directly on the venous drainage of the transferred flap through the internal jugular vein.

Finally, complications associated with conventional harvesting of the jejunal segment through a midline open laparotomy can be reduced using a completely endoscopic jejunum harvest, bowel reanastomosis, and placement of a feeding jejunostomy tube.

Gastric Pull-up

Gastric pull-up has been widely used for reconstruction of the esophagus after esophagectomy for cervical and thoracic esophageal cancer. In a series of 208 patients, Shuangba et al[9] reported that 42% of them developed complications, including pneumonia (11%), anastomotic leak (9%), pleural effusion (7%), wound infection (4%), anastomosis stricture (3%), heart failure (2%), chylous fistula (2%), hemothorax (1%), hemoperitoneum (1%), and evisceration (1%), but there was no gastric necrosis. Segmental proximal necrosis of the gastric pedicled flap has been reported in 0 to 12% of patients. Postoperative mortality was only 2%. In general terms, surgical and medical morbidity rates hover around 27% and 32%, respectively with a total complication rate of 40%.[10]

Postoperative mortality is higher than that of the jejunal free flaps, and in most of the series ranges between 7 and 20%. Fatal complications mainly result from local sepsis and medical problems (pneumonia, heart failure). No difference between mortality rate associated with pharyngogastric anastomosis and that with cervical esophagogastric anastomosis has been reported.

Complications

Dehiscence of the Anastomosis

Dehiscence of the anastomosis, or smaller fistulas, usually leads to an infection in the neck and mediastinum that is potentially lethal (**Fig. 30.9**). They occur in 4 to 15% of patients, independent of whether they received a hand-sewn or mechanically stapled anastomosis. Thoracic anastomotic leaks can be closed through endoscopic insertion of a self-expanding covered metal stent at the site of the anastomotic leak, whereas cervical leaks often require an open repair. Main complications, such as dehiscence or stenosis, result from insufficient blood flow at the distal end. To overcome this problem, it has been proposed (with satisfactory results) to perform an

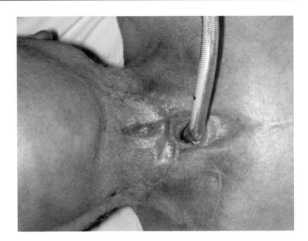

Fig. 30.9 Gastrocutaneous fistula.

additional microvascular anastomosis using the short gastric vessels of the gastric tube.

Stricture

Persistent stricture at the cervical esophagogastric anastomosis is a troublesome complication of gastric pull-ups that occurs in 3 to 25% of the patients. Suturing technique does not appear to influence the incidence of stricture (**Fig. 30.10**). When the stricture is the result of ischemia of the stomach, the strictures are long, often not responsive

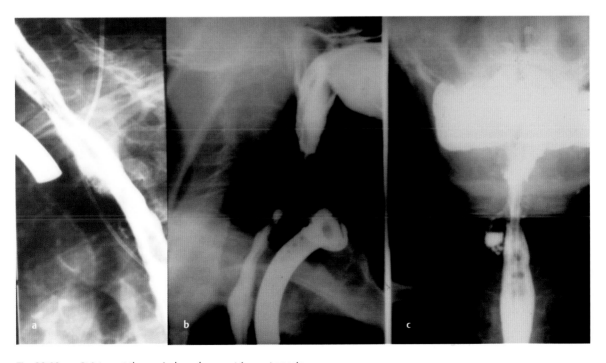

Fig. 30.10a–c Stricture at the cervical esophagogastric anastomosis.
a Normal postoperative barium swallow in a gastric pull-up.   **b, c** Stricture at gastropharyngeal junction.

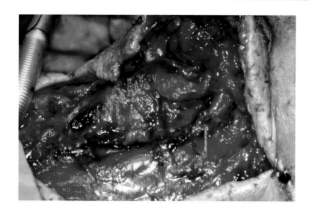

Fig. 30.11 Neck hematoma in a gastric pull-up.

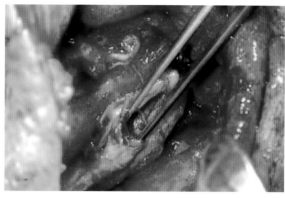

Fig. 30.12 Carotid artery rupture caused by fistula formation and neck infection.

to dilatation, and may require reoperations with jejunal interposition or replacement with colonic pull-up. In these cases the radial forearm flap is an excellent option for handling persistent stricture because it obviates a laparotomy to harvest jejunum and fits easily into the neck.

Other Surgical Complications

Other surgical complications include neck, thoracic, or abdominal hemorrhage (**Figs. 30.11 and 30.12**), laceration of the posterior tracheal wall, neoesophagotracheal fistula, and pyloric stenosis. Laparoscopic dissection and mobilization of the stomach, extended cranially until connecting with cervical dissection, is a useful technique for reduction of abdominal and thoracic complications.

As reported before, medical complications are more frequent than surgical, particularly pulmonary complications (pneumonia, pleural effusion, pulmonary embolus) that account for more than 20%. Aspiration of gastric contents in patients who retained the larynx is a common phenomenon, particularly during the first 24 hours after transthoracic esophagectomy. Gastric pull-up through the posterior mediastinum appears to correlate with the development of postoperative pneumonia. Heart complications (heart failure, myocardial infarction) occur at a much lower rate. Pharyngolaryngoesophagectomies often involve a total thyroidectomy, so hypocalcemia is of special concern.[11]

Long-term complications or sequelae of the gastric pull-up include severe reflux esophagitis in more than 50% of patients, particularly in those who underwent intrathoracic anastomosis. Postprandial discomfort and bilious eructation related to intragastric bile acid concentration are commonly observed symptoms, as well as vomiting, anemia, and anorexia.

Colon Interposition

Colon can be used as a pedicled or free microvascular flap for the reconstruction of the entire esophagus or pharyngoesophageal defects. Pedicled flaps with the ileocolon, the entire ascending colon, or the descending colon have been employed to restore the continuity of the digestive tract. Free transverse colon transfers based on the middle colic vessels and ileocolic free grafts have been used also. Most authors prefer to perform the interposition using descending colon. Anatomical variations of the veins and the tiny venous network of the right colon lead to a lower success rate when using ascending colon compared with the left colon segment. Nevertheless, colon interposition and colon free flaps are associated with a higher rate of functional failure (inability to maintain adequate nutrition without tube feedings); therefore, they should be considered only if a gastric pull-up or a jejunum free flap are not available.

Generally, colonic grafts are not associated with increased postoperative mortality or complications compared with other procedures. Fürst el al[12] reported major complications in 23% of the patients, whereas minor complications occurred in 20% of them. Postoperative mortality has been observed in 2.5 to 23% of patients.

In pharyngoesophageal reconstruction with colon interposition, the oral segment of the colon graft suffers from a high incidence of ischemia necrosis because of the insufficient blood supply of the distal colon. This leads to increased rates of fistula formation and hence, increased mortality. This implies meticulous assessment and care of colic vessels, and the addition of microvascular reinforcement of colonic circulation when the colon is taken to the neck. Supercharging the flaps with ileocolic vessels reduces the rate of distal necrosis and fistula formation. Partial necrosis occurs in 5 to 18% of the colon interpositions, but the incidence is less if the colon is used as a free flap.

Complications

A comparison of the potential complications of using visceral flaps is shown in **Table 30.1**.

Anastomotic Leakage

Anastomotic leakage is the most frequent complication and has been reported in 10 to 26% of colon interpositions. According to Briel et al[13] risk factors for leak are ischemia, neoadjuvant therapy, and comorbid conditions. Pharyngocutaneous fistula, in turn, leads to neck infections and dehiscences.

Strictures

Strictures at the anastomotic point are also very frequent, and occur in up to 22% of patients. Risk factors for development of a stenosis are ischemia, anastomotic leak, and increasing preoperative weight.[14] In most of the patients these strictures are solved with repeated dilatations, but some of them require further surgery.

Donor Site Morbidity

Donor site morbidity of free ileocolon flap has been studied.[13] Fifty-six percent of patients experienced temporary diarrhea, and 18% suffered from upper gastrointestinal tract problems (gastroduodenal ulcer, erosive gastritis, and minor bleeding), probably because of insufficient gastric protection. Therefore, donor site morbidity is comparable to that of the other intestinal flaps.

References

1. Perisanidis C, Herberger B, Papadogeorgakis N, et al. Complications after free flap surgery: do we need a standardized classification of surgical complications? Br J Oral Maxillofac Surg 2012;50(2):113–118
2. Clavien PA, Barkun J, de Oliveira ML, et al. The Clavien–Dindo classification of surgical complications: five-year experience. Ann Surg 2009;250:187–196
3. Chang DW, Hussussian C, Lewin JS, Youssef AA, Robb GL, Reece GP. Analysis of pharyngocutaneous fistula following free jejunal transfer for total laryngopharyngectomy. Plast Reconstr Surg 2002;109(5):1522–1527
4. Chen HC, Tan BK, Cheng MH, Chang CH, Tang YB. Behavior of free jejunal flaps after early disruption of blood supply. Ann Thorac Surg 2002;73(3):987–989
5. Cordeiro PG, Santamaria E, Hu QY, DiResta GR, Reuter VE. The timing and nature of neovascularization of jejunal free flaps: an experimental study in a large animal model. Plast Reconstr Surg 1999;103(7):1893–1901
6. Tsao CK, Chen HC, Chuang CC, Chen HT, Mardini S, Coskunfirat K. Adequate venous drainage: the most critical factor for a successful free jejunal transfer. Ann Plast Surg 2004;53(3):229–234
7. Schneider DS, Gross ND, Sheppard BC, Wax MK. Reconstruction of the jejunoesophageal anastomosis with a circular mechanical stapler in total laryngopharyngectomy defects. Head Neck 2012;34(5):721–726
8. Müller DF, Lohmeyer JA, Zimmermann A, et al. The carotid artery as recipient vessel: troubleshooting for free jejunal transfer after esophagectomy in preradiated patients. [Article in German] Chirurg 2011;82(8):670–674
9. Shuangba H, Jingwu S, Yinfeng W, et al. Complication following gastric pull-up reconstruction for advanced hypopharyngeal or cervical esophageal carcinoma: a 20-year review in a Chinese institute. Am J Otolaryngol 2011;32(4):275–278
10. Cahow CE, Sasaki CT. Gastric pull-up reconstruction for pharyngo-laryngo-esophagectomy. Arch Surg 1994;129(4):425–429, discussion 429–430
11. Clark JR, Gilbert R, Irish J, Brown D, Neligan P, Gullane PJ. Morbidity after flap reconstruction of hypopharyngeal defects. Laryngoscope 2006;116(2):173–181
12. Fürst H, Löhe F, Hüttl T, Schildberg FW. Esophageal replacement by interposition of pedicled ascending colon flap supplied by the inferior mesenteric artery. [Article in German] Chirurg 1999;70(12):1434–1439
13. Briel JW, Tamhankar AP, Hagen JA, et al. Prevalence and risk factors for ischemia, leak, and stricture of esophageal anastomosis: gastric pull-up versus colon interposition. J Am Coll Surg 2004;198(4):536–541, discussion 541–542
14. Rampazzo A, Salgado CJ, Gharb BB, Mardini S, Spanio di Spilimbergo S, Chen HC. Donor-site morbidity after free ileocolon flap transfer for esophageal and voice reconstruction. Plast Reconstr Surg 2008;122(6):186e–194e
15. Ferahkose Z, Bedirli A, Kerem M, Azili C, Sozuer EM, Akin M. Comparison of free jejunal graft with gastric pull-up reconstruction after resection of hypopharyngeal and cervical esophageal carcinoma. Dis Esophagus 2008;21(4):340–345
16. Keereweer S, de Wilt JH, Sewnaik A, Meeuwis CA, Tilanus HW, Kerrebijn JD. Early and long-term morbidity after total laryngopharyngectomy. Eur Arch Otorhinolaryngol 2010;267(9):1437–1444
17. Kolh P, Honore P, Degauque C, Gielen J, Gerard P, Jacquet N. Early stage results after oesophageal resection for malignancy—colon interposition vs. gastric pull-up. Eur J Cardiothorac Surg 2000;18(3):293–300
18. Bardini R, Ruol A, Peracchia A. Therapeutic options for cancer of the hypopharynx and cervical oesophagus. Ann Chir Gynaecol 1995;84(2):202–207
19. Carlson GW, Schusterman MA, Guillamondegui OM. Total reconstruction of the hypopharynx and cervical esophagus: a 20-year experience. Ann Plast Surg 1992;29(5):408–412
20. Daiko H, Hayashi R, Saikawa M, et al. Surgical management of carcinoma of the cervical esophagus. J Surg Oncol 2007;96(2):166–172
21. Triboulet JP, Mariette C, Chevalier D, Amrouni H. Surgical management of carcinoma of the hypopharynx and cervical esophagus: analysis of 209 cases. Arch Surg 2001;136(10):1164–1170

Index

Note: Illustrations and tables are comprehensively referred to in the text. Therefore, significant material in illustrations or tables has usually only been given a page reference in the absence of its concomitant mention in the text referring to that figure or illustration.